Client-Centered Care
for Clinical
Medical Assisting

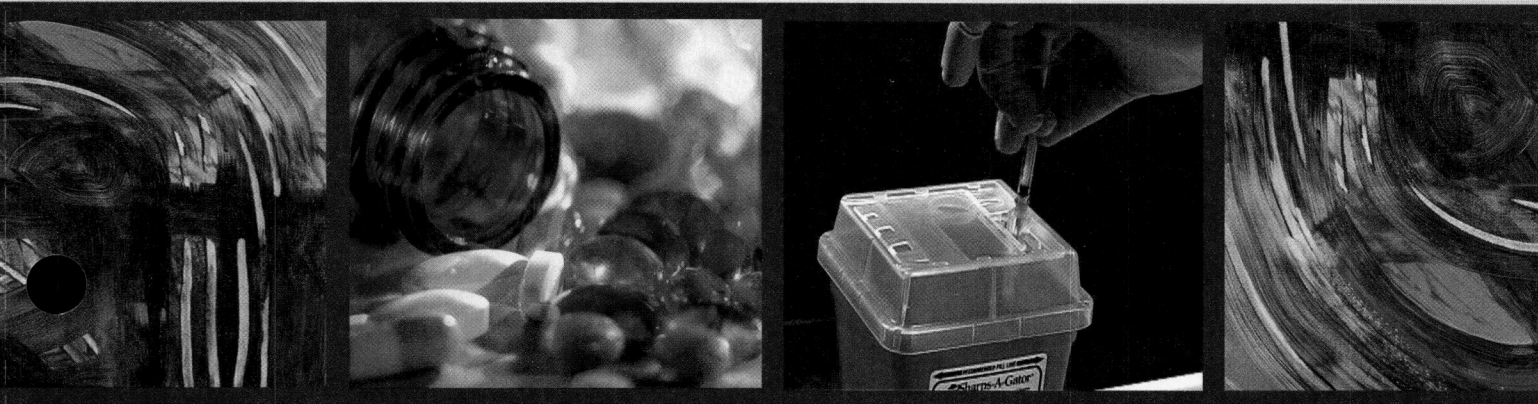

Victoria Roehmholdt Koprucki
Ed.D, M.S. (Nursing), M.S.Ed, CRRN, CMA

THOMSON

DELMAR LEARNING — Australia   Canada   Mexico   Singapore   Spain   United Kingdom   United States

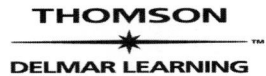

THOMSON

DELMAR LEARNING

Client-Centered Care for Clinical Medical Assisting

by Victoria Roehmholdt Koprucki

Vice President,
Health Care Business Unit:
William Brottmiller
Director of Learning Solutions:
Matthew Kane
Acquisitions Editor:
Rhonda Dearborn
Product Manager:
Sarah Duncan

Editorial Assistant:
Debra S. Gorgos
Marketing Director:
Jennifer McAvey
Marketing Coordinator:
Andrea Eobstel
Technology Director:
Laurie K. Davis

Technology Project Manager:
Carolyn Fox
Production Director:
Carolyn Miller
Production Manager:
Barbara A. Bullock
Content Project Manager:
Kenneth McGrath

Library of Congress Cataloging-in-Publication Data
Koprucki, Victoria Roehmholdt.
   Client-centered care for medical assisting / Victoria Roehmholdt Koprucki.
          p. ; cm.
   ISBN 1-4018-6178-4
   1. Medical assistants—Handbooks, manuals, etc. I. Title.
   [DNLM: 1. Patient Care—methods—Handbooks. 2. Allied Health Personnel—Handbooks. 3. Patient-Centered Care—methods—Handbooks. W 49 K83c 2006]
      R728.8.K67 2006
      610.73'7069—dc22

2006010718
ISBN 1-4018-6178-4

NOTICE TO THE READER

DEDICATION

This book is dedicated to my supportive husband, Richard Henry Koprucki; to our children, Michael, Victoria, Elizabeth, and Therese; and to my parents, Robert and Mary Roehmholdt, who led by love and example.

Contents

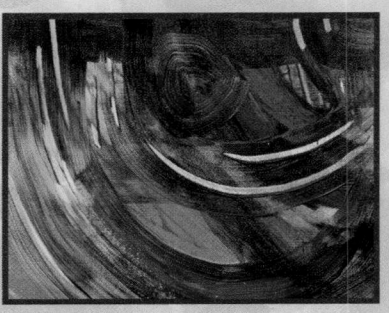

UNIT ONE

The Nature of Medical Assisting

UNIT TWO

Introduction to Clinical Medical Assisting

CHAPTER 4   Vital Signs ■ 44

CHAPTER 5   Client Examination ■ 78

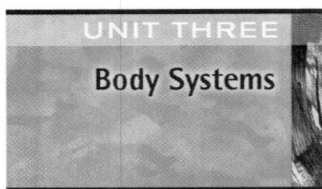

UNIT THREE
Body Systems

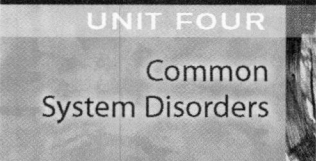

UNIT FOUR

Common
System Disorders

UNIT FIVE

Specialty Topics
in Clinical
Medical Assisting

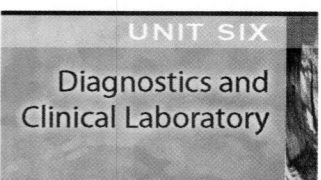

UNIT SIX

Diagnostics and
Clinical Laboratory

Preface

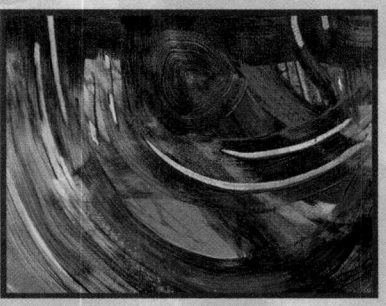

"Help people!" When asked why they had decided to enter medical assisting, the recurring theme expressed by students was the desire to help people. Students want to help sick people get better and help healthy people stay that way.

Client-Centered Care for Clinical Medical Assisting is designed to keep the focus on the client and the medical assistant's role in working with each client. It introduces the medical assisting student to the world of health care and the role that the medical assistant will play in that world.

This textbook of clinical medical assisting highlights the rapidly changing nature of health care and the evolving role of the clinical medical assistant within the new structure. The textbook material is geared toward students who desire to work as clinical medical assistants in a physician's office, an ambulatory care setting, or a hospital setting. The text is appropriate for a one-semester course, but it can easily be divided into a two-semester course by separating units into physician office skills and diagnostic and clinical laboratory skills. In addition, this textbook can become a reference source in medical practice settings for clinical medical assistants.

The essential features are the text's client-centered focus and its emphasis on communication between the client and the medical assistant. This approach is unique among medical assisting textbooks. The course of treatment, the client's response, and client satisfaction are all greatly affected by the way the client is approached in the medical setting. In addition to skill competency, the professional interaction between the medical assistant and the client directly affects the outcome of care.

As a direct care provider, the medical assistant needs to understand how to communicate effectively. What are the client's needs? How does one best establish rapport and trust? How does one share information and assist the client while performing clinical skills? These are all challenges facing the medical assistant every day. Medical assisting is a people-oriented profession. In all clinical skill areas, *Client-Centered Care for Clinical Medical Assisting* facilitates students' mastery of entry-level clinical procedures and their ability to adapt these procedures to the needs of a particular client group.

■ KEY IDEAS

Several key ideas provide the foundation for the organization and focus of this book:

- Caring about people and having a desire to assist them are fundamental to the medical assisting profession.
- Being connected to others promotes health and well-being. In light of this, this textbook encourages medical assistants to communicate caring to all clients in an open and supportive manner.
- The way in which a health care provider speaks with a client can have a huge effect on the client's response to health care. In this text, the language is simple and concise. Whenever possible, medical terms are put into everyday language. Because the medical assistant works with the doctor and other health care professionals and providers, the medical assistant must understand technical medical terms and be able to communicate on a professional level. However, another major role of the medical assistant is to work with clients, establishing rapport and trust while providing competent care. The language of this book makes it easier to translate complex medical concepts into language that clients can easily understand.

■ ORGANIZATION OF THIS TEXTBOOK

Client-Centered Care for Clinical Medical Assisting is organized to introduce the medical assistant student to the clinical role of medical assisting. The book is divided into six units:

- **Unit One**
  Material on the medical assisting profession introduces students to the profession upon which they are embarking. It attempts to answer two questions: "What does it mean to be a medical assistant?" and "How does a person become a medical assistant?" This is followed by a description of the ever-changing health care environment in which medical assistants are employed.
- **Unit Two**
  Students are introduced to the world of clinical medical assisting. An entire chapter is devoted to explaining the cycle of infection and the medical assistant's role in breaking that cycle, to create a healthy environment for clients. Measuring vital signs and assisting with client examinations are large parts of the everyday world of the clinical medical assistant. Because accurate measurement and recording of vital signs are so critical to the assessment, diagnosis, and treatment of clients, a full chapter is devoted to vital signs. This unit also acquaints students with the basic preparation, positioning, and testing associated with client examinations.
- **Unit Three**
  This unit reviews the structure and working of the various body systems. In many medical assisting curricula, students cover this material in anatomy and physiology courses. Unit Three is meant as a refresher. When learning clinical skills, students must correlate each skill with normal body functioning. Combining the skill with the body system in the clinical part of this

textbook allows easy access to information. Each of the major body systems is explained in terms of the parts or structures that make up that system. The function and working of these body system parts are then discussed. Each chapter is organized in the same way, for ease in learning and location of information. This unit on the makeup and working of the body corresponds to the following unit, which discusses common disorders of each body system.

- **Unit Four**

Common disorders often seen in the primary care clinical setting are presented in the fourth unit. The disorders are presented in the same body-system order as in Unit Three. Each chapter includes a client teaching plan for the student to use as a blueprint for client teaching and instruction.

- **Unit Five**

Clients whose needs present challenges for the medical assistant are discussed in this unit. Many clients have special needs, from physical impairments such as hearing, sight, mobility, or speech impairments to cognitive impairments such as those seen with some developmental disabilities, Alzheimer's, and other brain disorders. In caring for these clients, the medical assistant must adapt the clinical skills learned to the individual situation. All clients are to be treated with dignity, and individual clients help the medical assistant to grow in respecting the uniqueness of every client.

Children also need different and special care. Care of children involves understanding growth and development over the life span. Students are introduced to care of the infant and child during well-child visits. Clinical competencies that are routinely done on infants and children are outlined for skilled practice.

For medical assistants working in primary care, the majority of client care is provided to older clients. This unit presents information to help medical assisting students meet the needs of the elderly. Sensory and physical changes that come with aging affect medication use, medication effectiveness, and client compliance. Special considerations for this client population are highlighted.

This unit also introduces the basics of pharmacology and medication administration, while stressing promotion of healthy lifestyle and prevention of chronic health care disorders—a major goal of health care providers. The medical assistant's helping role in this effort includes discussion and teaching regarding lifestyle choices. The text is organized so that students can compare and correlate lifestyle choices and their effects with the body systems, system functions, and disorders presented in Units Three and Four.

Minor surgery is a specialized clinical skill area. Students will gain competencies in surgical asepsis, sterile technique, setup for procedures, and assisting the doctor within the scope of their practice and education.

Medical assistants working in an ambulatory medical setting will most likely have to respond to emergencies. Common emergencies that may be encountered in such a setting are explained in the context of the medical assistant's role in resolving those emergencies.

- **Unit Six**

  Medical assistants are multiskilled professionals who perform various tasks in accordance with their scope of practice, law and regulations, and education. In keeping with that, Unit Six introduces the student to the clinical and diagnostic laboratory. This text acquaints the student with basic competencies and stresses the importance of understanding the rationale—the why of a test—and applying critical thinking skills to laboratory procedures. Students learn to collect specimens, perform some specific tests, and prepare clients for more complex laboratory procedures. With this knowledge, medical assistants will quickly be able to master any new technology as different pieces of equipment are added to their places of employment.

■ KEY FEATURES

The following features are incorporated into the chapters to aid students in mastering the information, content, and competencies covered in the chapters:

- *Anticipatory Statements.* Students' own life experiences help them form opinions on health care issues. Students from various backgrounds and with varying experiences will have different knowledge levels. Sometimes what may seem to be common knowledge either is not common knowledge or is myth. Students read and respond to the Anticipatory Statements appearing at the beginning of each chapter based on their current understanding. As they read the chapters, students become active participants in the learning process, finding out for themselves if their opinions can be supported by newly encountered, correct information.

- *Learning Objectives.* The objectives at the beginning of each chapter focus on what students will gain in content knowledge or skill competency. By reading these before beginning the chapter, students can easily follow the direction of the chapter.

- *Key Terms.* Words and phrases that describe or are used to explain ideas in the chapter are listed and defined at the beginning of each chapter. Key Terms are not limited to medical terms. Familiarity with other words and phrases that students will encounter in the health care setting is helpful in building the conceptual understanding needed by the medical assistant.

- *Note to Student.* At strategic points within the chapters, additional brief statements are inserted. These statements alert students to an exceptional or critical point to keep in mind about the concept just discussed.

- *Legal/Ethical Thoughts.* Medical assisting is a service to people, so medical assistants interact with clients during the performance of both administrative and clinical tasks. All the activities within medical assisting involve ethics, in addition to being governed by laws and regulations. Clients must always be treated with dignity and respect. Many chapters present a legal/ethical thought or reminder, which students can apply to the world of medical assisting. These reminders also help students identify other situations that involve legal/ethical issues.

- *Points of Highlight.* A bulleted list at the end of each chapter helps students refocus on important ideas presented in the chapter. Students can also compare their choices of key ideas to this listing.

- *Critical Thinking Questions.* These questions help students go beyond mere learning of facts, to solving fact-based problems. Every work day, medical assistants must problem-solve. Often these questions ask students to explain the "why" to a client. The questions also stimulate students to think about how they would respond to clients' questions. To answer Critical Thinking Questions well, students must understand medical terminology and then put their responses into everyday language that is easy for clients to comprehend.

- *Student Portfolio Activity.* These activities are designed to help students become more marketable in a health care setting. By doing these suggested activities, students perform specific tasks that improve their professional skills for entry-level medical assisting. Upon completion of each activity, students have written documentation to place in their individual portfolios for future employers to view. These portfolio activities also help students to monitor and guide their future interests in medical assisting.

- *Applying Your Skills.* From the chapters, students learn the health and medical content and competencies involved in medical assisting. However, when students graduate, they need to apply the information learned to their work situations. Therefore, at the end of each chapter, a situation or scenario is given. Students must think critically to decide what skills learned in the classroom apply in this professional role.

- *Client Teaching Plans.* This is a new area for medical assisting textbooks. *Client-Centered Care for Clinical Medical Assisting* highlights interactions between medical assistant and client. Teaching is increasingly becoming part of the provider-client relationship, as medical assistants help clients to become active participants in their own health care. The Client Teaching Plans in this book act as samples to help students in working with clients. The Client Teaching Plans are especially useful for students who are just beginning and have no formal coursework in client teaching theory. For more advanced students, these plans will refresh and reinforce knowledge. The teaching plans can also be used as blueprints for developing other teaching plans. Medical assisting students can adapt these plans to the specific client populations they serve and the health care setting in which they work.

■ LEARNING PACKAGE

Instructor's Manual

An Instructor's Manual is available to help instructors plan the course and implement activities, quizzes, and more. The manual includes the following tools:

- Learning Objectives, Classroom Methodology and activities
- Evaluation Criteria for Competency Checklists

- Comprehensive Final Exam
- Answer Keys

Electronic Classroom Manager

An Electronic Classroom Manager is available on CD-ROM to provide instructors with complete support in the classroom, in preparing for class, delivering effective presentations, and monitoring student progress throughout the course. This comprehensive CD-ROM contains the following tools:

- A Computerized Test Bank in ExamView, organized by chapter
- PowerPoint presentations by chapter, covering key concepts presented in the text
- Complete, customizable Instructor's Manual files
- An Image Library with the photos and illustrations from this book.

List of Procedures

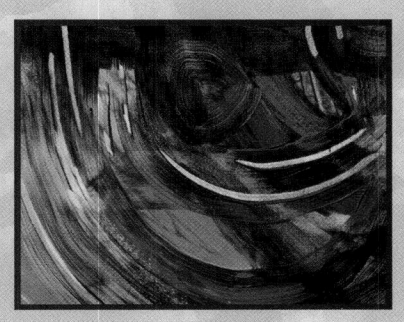

List of Client Teaching Plans

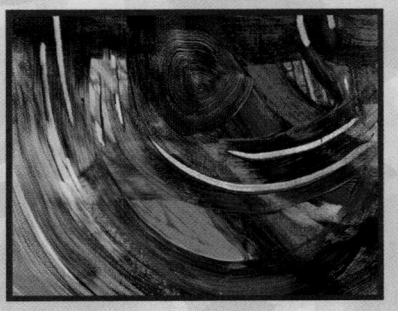

Reviewers

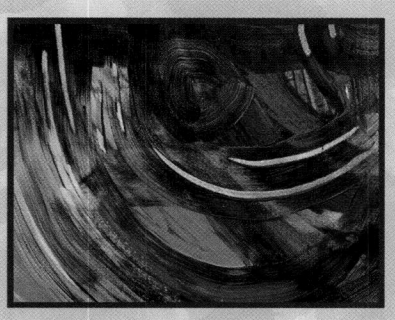

David Drumm, PCMA, ASB, AE
Medical Director
Computer Learning Network
Mechanicsburg, PA

James W. Ferraro, DDS, MD

Frank Harbison, BS Ed
Manager of Education
Vatterott College
St. Louis, MO

Kris A. Hardy, CMA, CDF, RHE
Program Director
Brevard Community College
Cocoa, FL

Sharon Harris-Pelliccia, RPAC
Division Chair
Mildred Elley
Latham, NY

Jean L. Kooda, RN, RMT
Clinic Nurse
Richland College
Dallas, TX

Brigitte Niedzwiecki, RN, MSN
Medical Assistant Program Director
Chippewa Valley Technical College
Eau Claire, WI

Fred Valdes, MD
Medical Department Chair
City College
Ft. Lauderdale, FL

How to Use This Book

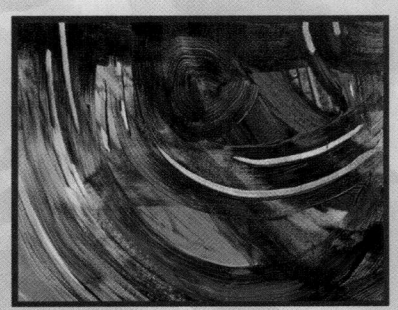

The following features are integrated throughout the text to assist you in learning the clinical concepts and terms.

ANTICIPATORY STATEMENTS

Special Feature! At the beginning of each chapter, statements about the chapter content are presented. Some are true; some are not. Read and respond to each of these based on your knowledge and understanding before you read the chapter. After reading the chapter, you will be asked to go back and review these, to discover whether you were correct, and review why your answers may not have been correct.

LEARNING OBJECTIVES

The objectives at the beginning of each chapter focus on what learners will gain in content knowledge or skill competency. If you read these before beginning the chapter, you should be able to easily follow the direction of the chapter.

KEY TERMS

Words or phrases that describe or are used to explain ideas in the chapter are listed and defined at the beginning of each chapter.

CHAPTER **6** Organization of the Human Body

Anticipatory Statements

People have different ideas of how the body is organized and how it works. Read and think about the following statements based upon what you believe now. Decide whether you agree or disagree. Write the word **agree** after the statement if you think the statement is true. Write the word **disagree** after the statement if you think the statement is false. Read the chapter to find out if your current beliefs can be supported.

1. Systems of the body depend upon each other to work smoothly. _____

2. Only doctors need to know the organization of the body and how it functions. _____

3. Using medical terms helps the medical assistant to communicate with other health care professionals. _____

4. Organs in the body function on their own. _____

5. Knowing anatomical positions and directions helps in describing where a point is on the body. _____

Learning Objectives

Upon completion of this chapter, the medical assistant student should be able to:

■ List the four basic units in the body
■ State the four types of tissue
■ Define each major body system
■ Demonstrate the anatomical position
■ Identify the main body cavities and the major organs in each
■ Point out body directions on an anatomical chart

Key Terms

anatomical Position of the body when standing straight, facing forward, arms down at side with the palms of the hands forward.
cell The basic unit of all living organisms.
cranial cavity Space in the head that contains the brain.
epithelial tissue Tissue that covers structures inside and on the surface of the body, thereby protecting these structures.
organs Groups of tissue(s) that have the same function.
pelvic cavity The space in the body that contains the reproductive organs, urinary

bladder, rectum, part of the large intestine, and the appendix.
system A group of organs that work together to perform the same function.
thoracic cavity The space in the body that contains the lungs, heart, trachea, esophagus, thymus gland, and large blood vessels.
tissue A group of cells the function of which is similar.
visceral cavity The space in the body that contains abdominal organs; also called the *abdominal cavity*.

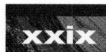

NOTE TO THE STUDENT

Each note makes clear or alerts you to an exceptional or critical point to keep in mind about the concept being discussed.

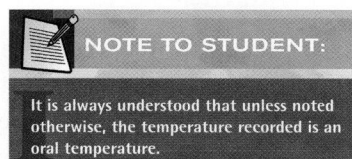

NOTE TO STUDENT:
It is always understood that unless noted otherwise, the temperature recorded is an oral temperature.

LEGAL/ETHICAL THOUGHTS

All activities within medical assisting involve ethics. Clients must always be treated with dignity and in a respectful way. In addition to ethical issues, legal issues and the law are involved in all client interactions. These boxes point out concepts that you should be familiar with, to help you perform your job to the highest standards.

LEGAL/ETHICAL THOUGHTS
Family members may ask questions such as "What is her blood pressure?" Remember that it is up to the client to decide what information can be given out and to whom.

POINTS OF HIGHLIGHT

Bulleted lists at the end of each chapter summarize the chapter material and help you refocus on the most important ideas contained in the chapter.

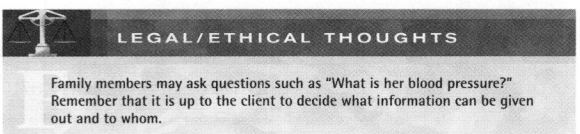

POINTS OF HIGHLIGHT
- The internal organs of the female reproductive system are found in the pelvic cavity.
- The uterus is a pear-shaped, hollow organ that expands to hold and nourish the growth and development of a baby.
- Menarche is the beginning of the first menstrual cycle in a woman at puberty.
- Puberty is the beginning of the reproductive years.
- Menopause is the end of a woman's reproductive years; it is a gradual process that is considered complete when the woman has not had a menstrual period for one full year.

PROCEDURES

Step-by-step procedures give instruction on all entry-level clinical competencies as defined by CAAHEP and ABHES. Each procedure contains a competency objective, instructions, and charting examples, where applicable. Use the Competency Skill checklists, found at the back of the book, to track your mastery of these procedures.

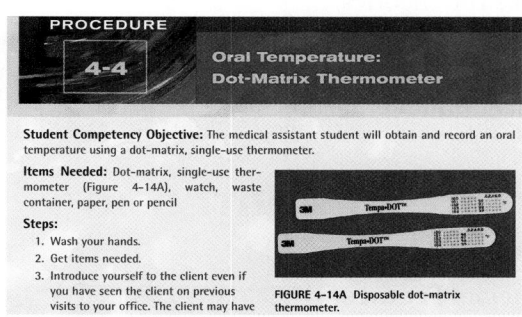

PROCEDURE

4-4 Oral Temperature: Dot-Matrix Thermometer

Student Competency Objective: The medical assistant student will obtain and record an oral temperature using a dot-matrix, single-use thermometer.

Items Needed: Dot-matrix, single-use thermometer (Figure 4-14A), watch, waste container, paper, pen or pencil

Steps:
1. Wash your hands.
2. Get items needed.
3. Introduce yourself to the client even if you have seen the client on previous visits to your office. The client may have

FIGURE 4-14A Disposable dot-matrix thermometer.

CRITICAL THINKING

Every day on the job, medical assistants must solve problems. These critical thinking questions often ask you to explain the "why" of something; that is, you will be asked to explain a concept to the client in a medical office. Other times, you will be asked to think about how you would respond to questions clients may have. These questions allow you to apply the concepts learned in the chapter and encourage further discussion and thought about the concepts.

CRITICAL THINKING QUESTIONS
1. A client has been diagnosed with otitis media. The doctor has ordered antibiotics for the client and has asked you (the medical assistant) to teach the client about the medication. What are some key points that you would include on the teaching plan?

2. A client with early-stage dementia comes to the office with a family member. What are some changes that you expect to see as the dementia progresses?

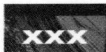

APPLYING YOUR SKILLS

At the end of each chapter, a situation or scenario is given relating to the chapter content. These scenarios take the theories

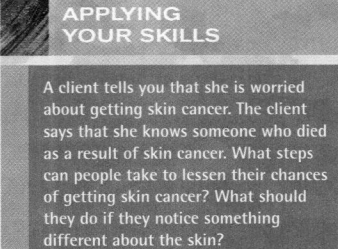

you have learned in the chapter and ask you to apply them to a situation that you may encounter on the job.

STUDENT PORTFOLIO ACTIVITY

Special Feature! During the course of study, you can perform these suggested activities, all of which are useful for

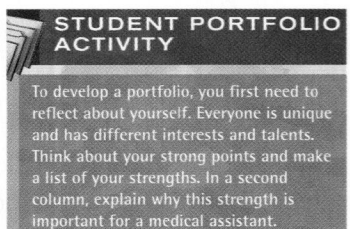

improving professional skills for entry-level medical assisting. Upon completion of the activity, you will have written documentation to place in your individual portfolios for future employers to view.

CLIENT TEACHING PLANS

Special Feature! Sample teaching plans are provided in many chapters, on many subjects. Medical assisting students can adapt these plans to client situations specific to the client populations you serve and the health care situations in which you will work.

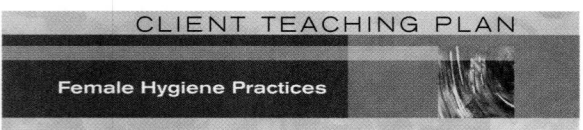

SOFTWARE CD-ROM THE CRITICAL THINKING CHALLENGE

Interactive Software! The Critical Thinking Challenge is a game simulation on the Student Software CD-ROM accompanying this book. You are on a three-month externship in a medical office. You will be confronted with a series of situations in which you must use your critical thinking skills to choose the most appropriate action in response to the situation.

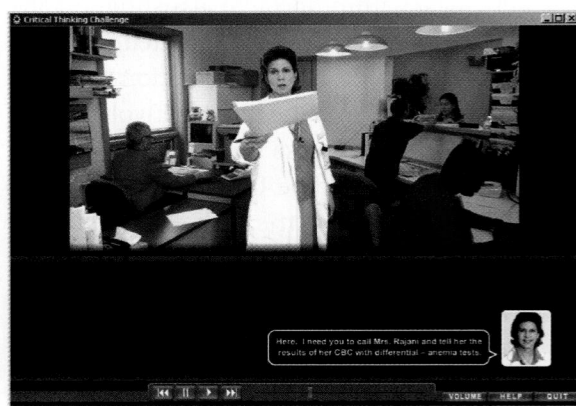

MEDICAL TERMINOLOGY AUDIO LIBRARY

Practice your pronunciation and recognition of medical terms using the Audio Library, included on the Student Software CD-ROM accompanying this book. You may search for terms by word or body system. Once you select a word, it is pronounced correctly and defined on the screen.

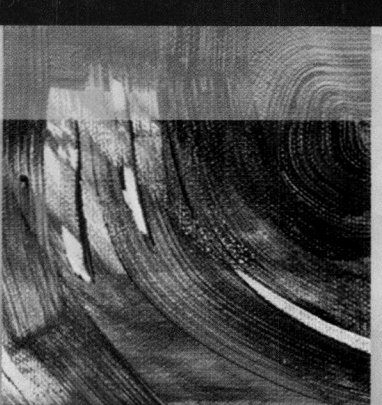

CHAPTER 1
The Medical
Assisting Profession

CHAPTER 2
The Health Care
Environment

The first unit of *Client Centered Care for Clinical Medical Assisting* introduces you, the student, to the profession of medical assisting and to the health care environment. First, we define the role of the multiskilled medical assistant professional. Making a difference in a client's life can be a major part of a medical assistant's professional life. You will also explore the characteristics and qualities necessary to become a medical assistant. The steps that you will take in education, clinical experience, laboratory situations, and testing on your journey to becoming a medical assistant are all mapped out for you in this unit. You can see where your decision to become a medical assistant can lead you and what to expect along the way.

Change, with its challenges and opportunities for improving the health of clients, is inevitable. The settings where clients seek health care, and the method of payment for that care, reflect these changes. This unit describes the many places where the medical assistant is a vital health care team member, and explores the medical assistant's work with clients in these settings.

At the end of each chapter in the unit, you will be given a professional situation, or problem, to solve by using what you have learned in the chapter and applying your critical thinking skills. Now let's begin!

Anticipatory Statements

People have different ideas about what medical assisting is and what a medical assistant does. Read and think about the following statements based upon what you believe now. Decide whether you agree or disagree. Write the word **agree** after the statement if you think the statement is true. Write the word **disagree** after the statement if you think the statement is false. Read the chapter to find out if your current beliefs can be supported.

1. Caring about people is an important quality in a medical assistant.   _____

2. A medical assistant is the same as a nurse.   _____

3. Medical assisting involves only clinical skills.   _____

4. A person can become a medical assistant without attending any formal education program.   _____

5. There are many benefits for the medical assistant who belongs to a national professional association representing medical assistants.   _____

Learning Objectives

Upon completion of this chapter, the medical assistant student should be able to:

- Define the medical assisting profession
- Explain how a person becomes a medical assistant
- Explain what is meant by the initials CMA
- List at least five clinical competencies of a medical assistant
- List at least five administrative competencies of a medical assistant

The Medical Assisting Profession

- Describe the personal characteristics of a medical assistant
- Explain the role of the AAMA
- Explain what is meant by the initials RMA
- Describe the relationship between American Medical Technologists (AMTs) and medical assisting

Key Terms

accredited Standing awarded to a school program that meets the standards of an accrediting organization.

Accrediting Bureau of Health Education Schools (ABHES) A national organization that grants accreditation to medical assisting programs.

administrative Skills and tasks regarding the business aspects of the office setting.

American Association of Medical Assistants (AAMA) A national professional organization of medical assistants. The AAMA is a three-level group with local, state, and national divisions. It certifies medical assistants and maintains professional standards.

American Medical Technologists (AMT) A national professional organization that certifies medical assistants and other health professionals.

certificate Diploma or document given to an individual who has successfully completed a program of study.

certified medical assistant (CMA) Medical assistant who has met the criteria for certification, including passing a national certification examination of the American Association of Medical Assistants.

client The person seeking help from a health care provider; also called *patient* or *health care consumer.*

clinical Medical skills and tasks regarding direct care in a health care setting.

Commission on Accreditation of Allied Health Education Programs (CAAHEP) National organization that sets standards and accredits allied health programs such as medical assisting programs.

medical assistant Multiskilled professional who performs both clinical and administrative tasks in a variety of health care settings.

registered medical assistant (RMA) Medical assistant who has met the professional examination requirements set by the American Medical Technologists.

■ INTRODUCTION

Have you ever walked into a medical office and observed an employee greeting **clients,** asking questions and guiding clients back to the examination rooms? Later on, that same employee could be seen working on the computer and then talking with clients and scheduling additional clinic or laboratory appointments. This individual was most likely a **medical assistant,** a valuable member of the health care team. Medical assistants are multiskilled professionals, who have both an administrative and a clinical role in health care.

■ MEDICAL ASSISTING EDUCATION

Medical assistant programs vary in length. Some schools offer a **certificate** program that may take only one year. Other medical assistant programs, especially those offered by two-year or community colleges, take two years to complete. The student earns an associate's degree with a major in medical assisting.

The courses offered will reflect the variety of skills needed to work as a medical assistant. Schools of higher education will organize or present required courses in slightly different ways. What the accredited schools have in common are the type of skills or competencies taught; these requirements are defined by the accrediting bodies or organizations. The content, although grouped under different course titles, will cover the areas defined by either the **American Association of Medical Assistants (AAMA)** and the **Commission on Accreditation of Allied Health Education Programs (CAAHEP),** or the **Accrediting Bureau of Health Education Schools (ABHES).**

Administrative or Business

Administrative or business courses provide the student with the knowledge and skills needed to perform the many administrative tasks of an entry-level medical assistant. Students may hear this job referred to as "front desk" or "front office," because the individual performing these tasks is often found at the front of the office where clients first enter the health care setting. In the business courses, the student will gain the knowledge and skills necessary for a medical assistant who works in the business aspects of a health care setting. The administrative procedures are critical to the functioning of the entire health care setting, so they must be competently performed in a manner friendly to and considerate of clients.

Computer literacy and competency are now a must for every health care setting. The student will be introduced to the use of computers in the medical office (Figure 1-1). Computer software programs commonly used in health care settings will be discussed. The student will practice to gain speed and accuracy in applying electronic technology to the medical setting.

The doctor examines and treats clients. Afterward, the doctor must record his or her findings in the client's chart. If the client was referred by one doctor (the *referring* doctor) to another doctor (who is called a *consulting doctor*), the consulting doctor will document the findings and send a letter to the referring doctor. The medical assistant listens to the doctor's recorded voice on a dictation machine, or "Dictaphone," and inputs the verbal information

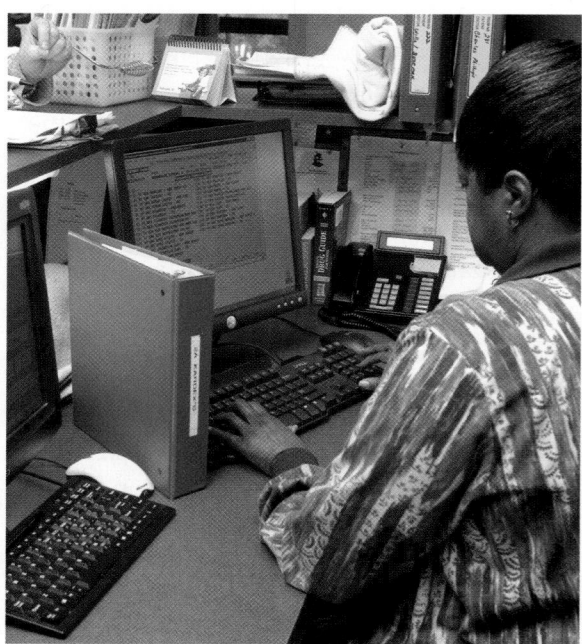

FIGURE 1–1 Computers are an important component of the medical office.

into the computer in the proper format. This process of listening to and typing information into the computer is called *transcription*. Transcription skills are in high demand.

Later in this book, we will explore communication courses focusing on types of written communication in the medical office. The medical assistant will be introduced to written communication first; then other courses will focus on oral communication among professionals, as well as therapeutic communication with clients.

Basic medical office functions are taught in administrative courses. The client is the center of all medical office functions. The **client** is the person who is seeking help or care for health concerns. The purpose of the office functions is to provide quality health care to each client. The student will learn to make appointments for clients with doctors and schedule appointments for laboratory and diagnostic work. This will involve coordinating appointments among health care providers and monitoring those appointments. Arranging admission to a hospital and scheduling surgery are also part of a medical assistant's administrative responsibilities. Monitoring includes reminders and follow-up calls.

Accounting basics and bookkeeping are taught within the program. Visits to the doctor for treatments and services cost money. Employees in the office are paid through the process of payroll. Submitting fees, accepting payment, giving receipts, and keeping records are part of basic accounting and bookkeeping. The student will be introduced to accounts receivable and accounts payable, banking, and records. These areas may be covered in medical office courses or in separate accounting or bookkeeping courses.

Bills for treatments and services are often sent to a client's insurance company for payment. The medical assisting student will learn about health insurance and other third-party payers. Claims may have to be sent to insurance companies electronically, using the company guidelines, to obtain payment or reimbursement. All conditions and treatments given must be coded before the health care provider can apply for payment. Each condition or disorder and treatment is assigned a specific, individual code number.

Without that correct number, payment will be denied. Because insurance coding is a major part of all health care practices, and because medical assistants often perform these tasks, separate courses devoted to insurance and coding may be offered in medical assisting programs.

The ordering of office supplies and tracking of equipment services are part of the administrative responsibilities called *operational functions*. These tasks are grouped under facility management topics.

Clinical

The second major focus of a medical assistant program is the clinical responsibilities of a medical assistant. **Clinical** refers to activities done during direct, hands-on client care. The clinical courses explain fundamental or basic principles upon which client care procedures are based.

Asepsis and infection control are the first and most fundamental principles of medical assisting, and are the basis for the clinical procedures. The student will learn many clinical procedures through these courses (Figure 1-2). Each program may group the clinical knowledge and tasks in a slightly different way. All

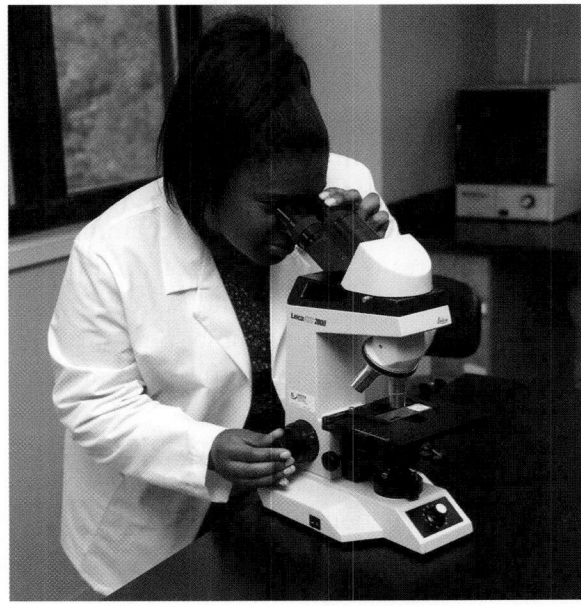

FIGURE 1-2 Medical assisting students learn fundamental clinical skills to help them succeed on the job.

accredited programs will contain information on the content as outlined by the AAMA and CAAHEP or ABHES core areas.

Laboratory tests are an integral part of a complete physical examination. The results are used to help the doctor to diagnose, treat, and monitor the client. Diagnostic and laboratory testing and the collection and processing of specimens are important components of clinical courses in medical assisting programs.

Medications are often part of the client's treatment plan. Medications and medication interactions can have a dramatic effect on a client's health. Clients may be prescribed medication by the doctor. They may also be taking over-the-counter (OTC) drugs. Vitamins or herbal supplements are also considered drugs. The study of medications—including groups, actions, and side effects—is called *pharmacology.* Basic pharmacology for medical assistants focuses on medication and the client.

During the course of daily operations in a health care setting, medical emergencies may occur. Common emergencies and the response of the medical assistant are explained in either a clinical course or a CPR and First Aid course.

Clients can be sent to a radiology office or department for X-ray pictures or films of designated body areas. X-ray studies can help the doctor determine a clinical diagnosis. X-rays can also be used to treat disorders. An understanding of the principles of radiology is essential, as the medical assistant will instruct clients on how to prepare for having X-rays taken.

Assisting the doctor with examinations and procedures is a major part of the medical assistant's clinical responsibilities. Courses will provide information on examinations and treatments that are common in the medical office setting.

Additional treatments that the medical assistant student will learn throughout the program of instruction are: taking vital signs; positioning the client; caring for the treatment area; and performing selected tests, such as EKGs, pulmonary or lung function tests, and client height and weight measurements. These are just

samples of what will be taught in clinical courses. As part of the courses, students will learn to take a client history, find out about the client's past medical history, and how to record all of this in the medical record (a legal document).

Medical assisting is a people-oriented, caring profession. Therefore, the ability to communicate effectively is critical. Communication skills are needed in all areas of competence as defined by the AAMA.

Externship

An *externship* is the practical application of theory and skills learned in the classroom and laboratory. This practical application takes place in health care settings. At this point in the curriculum, students have been evaluated as competent in clinical and administrative skills within a laboratory setting. The externship is a valuable and exciting part of the learning experience. Students have the opportunity to work with professional medical assistants as they interact with and provide care to clients. This is also an opportunity for students to develop in their professional role as part of a health care team (Figure 1-3). Working with administrative personnel and other health care professionals in different fields provides students with experiences to help them in the real work world.

When students successfully complete the course of study and graduate from an **accredited** medical assisting program, they may apply to and take the national certification examina-

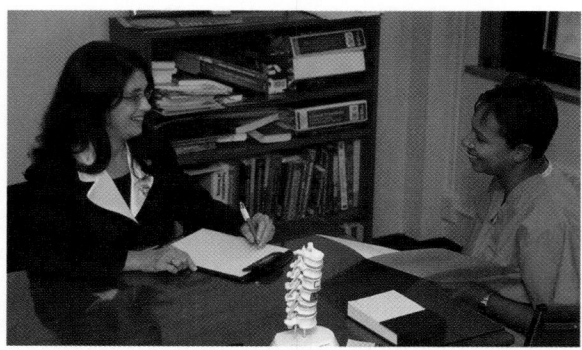

FIGURE 1-3 Medical assisting student speaking with office manager at externship site.

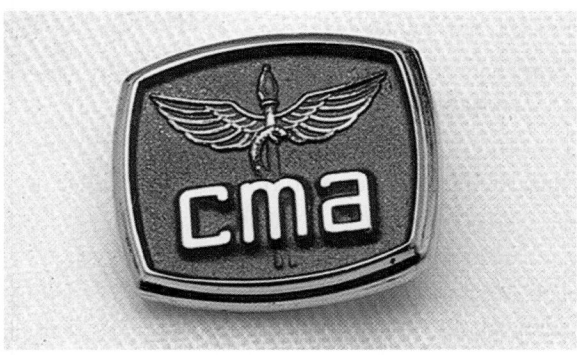

FIGURE 1-4 CMA pin awarded by the American Association of Medical Assistants.

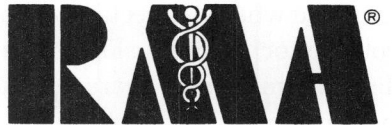

FIGURE 1-5 Logo of the registered medical assistant credential. (Courtesy of the American Medical Technologists)

tion to become certified medical assistants. The accrediting body is the Commission on Accreditation of Allied Health Education Programs. The national certification examination tests competencies that are required of an entry-level medical assistant. It includes all three major areas (administrative, clinical, and general competencies). This examination is offered at a specific time during the year at various sites throughout the country. Those who pass the exam become **certified medical assistants (CMA)** (Figure 1-4). These individuals may use the initials CMA after their name.

Education and learning do not end with initial certification. To continue as a CMA, a person must recertify every five years. This can be done in one of two ways. First, the CMA can earn educational credits in a variety of ways, such as attending meetings or conferences, sponsored by the medical assistant chapter or state organization, that award continuing education credits. The CMA can also retake the examination instead of earning the required number of continuing education credits. Learning is a lifelong process, and these continuing education requirements help to keep the standards high and ultimately help provide the most competent client-centered care.

Medical assistants who have met the requirements established by the **American Medical Technologists (AMT)** can take a national examination to become **registered medical assistants (RMA)** (Figure 1-5). To take this

exam, the individual must be a graduate of an approved program accredited by the Accrediting Bureau of Health Education Schools. There are other approved educational and professional employment ways for an individual to earn the title of registered medical assistant. The medical assistant must also successfully complete the registered medical assistant examination given by the AMT organization.

■ QUALITIES OF A MEDICAL ASSISTANT

Certain qualities are important in medical assistants. Ask yourself if the following qualities describe you as a person:

- Voice is calm and easy to listen
- Likes people
- Friendly personality
- Easy smile
- Intelligent
- Neat, clean appearance
- Dependable
- Reliable
- On time
- Able to adapt to change
- Honest
- Enthusiastic
- Tactful
- Accurate
- Understanding of others' feelings
- Careful with information received

Medical assisting is a very people-oriented service profession. Medical assistants meet new clients every day. Some of these people are sick or injured. They may be afraid, angry, hesitant, or worried. Some are comfortable about coming to a health care provider; others may be nervous or unsure about what to expect. All clients bring their problems or worries, along with all the physical and emotional characteristics that make them unique. The procedural skills of a medical assistant affect the health and lives of clients, so the medical assistant must be accurate, responsible and professional in all interactions. The medical assistant who possesses and uses the qualities listed here will greatly influence client outcomes. Medical assistants make a difference in a client's life!

■ PORTFOLIOS

A *portfolio* is an organization or collection of items that illustrate parts of an individual's professional growth and development (Figure 1-6). Portfolios benefit both the student and the employer and ultimately the clients.

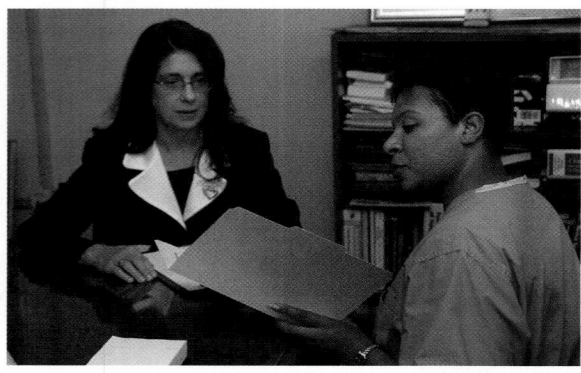

FIGURE 1-6 Portfolios display items that reflect your professional skills.

How to Organize Your Portfolio

Think about yourself and how you want others to see you. What expresses who you are as a professional medical assistant? What sets you apart from the rest? When you have decided these factors, you will want to gather items that reflect your professional skills. When you have gathered the items, you need to organize and display them so that your future employer can recognize your special skills (Table 1-1).

Consider the following when gathering and putting together your portfolio:

- Do you want to organize by year?
- Do you want to organize by area of medical assisting, such as clinical skills, administrative skills, and transdisciplinary skills?
- Are there other categories or ways to organize?
- Do you want to divide according to the type of item (such as letters, certificates, term papers, etc.) without regard to whether the item is clinical, administrative, or transdisciplinary?
- Should the dividers that separate items be one solid color, or color-coded? (It will depend on the image you are trying to present.)

Benefits to Students

- A portfolio is an organized way to document your growth and development as an entry-level medical assistant.

TABLE 1-1 Advantages and disadvantages of different ways of displaying your positive characteristics.

TYPE OF ORGANIZER	ADVANTAGES	DISADVANTAGES
Binder	Easy to put in and take out materials; stays updated.	Not very professional-looking (unfinished look).
Expandable folder	Holds many items that are easy to put in and take out.	Need to take items out of each section to look at them.
Photo album	Easy to add to or subtract from and for employers to flip through pages.	Only single sheets of paper can fit in each page.
Plastic sleeves	Protect items from wear and tear.	Bulky items will not fit in the sleeves.

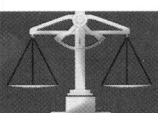

LEGAL/ETHICAL THOUGHTS

All the personal characteristics that help you become an excellent professional medical assistant will affect the clients you care for. All your actions while performing your job have legal and ethical consequences.

- Portfolios give a clear picture of where your strengths are and what areas still have to be developed, while you are still in the educational process.
- Putting together a portfolio helps you to prepare for job interviews.
- Portfolios demonstrate the extent to which the medical assisting program is guiding students from simple to complex competencies.
- The process helps you decide how to present yourself professionally.
- Through portfolio development, you can examine interest areas that you might like to develop in more depth after graduation.
- The process builds your confidence as you prepare to enter the professional world of an employed medical assistant.

Benefits to Employers

- Employers see the qualities of possible future employees.
- Portfolios provide documentation of medical assisting competencies.
- Employers can view letters that describe a medical assisting student's abilities.
- Portfolios can give additional support to substantiate traditional reference letters.
- Potential employers can see if the attributes or qualities of an individual medical assisting graduate match the needs of their health care setting.
- Employers can plan for inservices to strengthen employee competencies.
- Using portfolios for guidance, employers can become partners with new employees to professionally develop to advanced-level skills.

POINTS OF HIGHLIGHT

- Medical assisting is a valued allied health care profession.
- Medical assistants are multiskilled professionals who perform both administrative and clinical roles in health care.
- An externship provides an opportunity for students to apply competencies learned in theory and practiced in the lab to real-life work experiences.
- The initials CMA stand for certified medical assistant.
- To become a CMA, an individual must graduate from an accredited program and successfully pass the national certification examination.
- The American Association of Medical Assistants is a national organization representing the medical assisting profession.
- The initials RMA stand for registered medical assistant.
- To become a RMA, an individual must meet the requirements set by the American Medical Technologists.
- Portfolios are an excellent way for medical assistants to document and display their special qualities as medical assistant professionals.

BRIDGE TO CAAHEP

This chapter, which discusses the medical assisting profession, provides information or content related to CAAHEP standards for Anatomy and Physiology, Medical Terminology, Law and Ethics, Communication, Psychology, Administrative Medical Assisting Procedures, and Medical Assisting Clinical Procedures.

 ## ABHES LINKS

This chapter, which discusses the medical assisting profession, links to ABHES course content for medical assisting for Orientation, Medical Law and Ethics, Psychology of Human Relations, Medical Office Business Procedures/ Management, Medical Office Clinical Procedures, and Externship.

 ## AAMA AREAS OF COMPETENCE

This chapter, which discusses the medical assisting profession, provides information or content within several areas listed in the Medical Assistant Role Delineation Study. These areas include: clinical, fundamental principles, diagnostic orders, patient (client) care, general transdisciplinary, professionalism, professional conmmunication skills, communication skills, legal concepts, and instruction.

 ## AMT PATHS

Medical assisting provides a path to AMT competencies for general medical assisting knowledge, medical law, medical ethics, human relations, and patient (client) education.

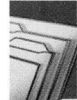
STUDENT PORTFOLIO ACTIVITY

To develop a portfolio, you first need to reflect about yourself. Everyone is unique and has different interests and talents. Think about your strong points and make a list of your strengths. In a second column, explain why this strength is important for a medical assistant.

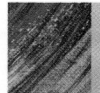
APPLYING YOUR SKILLS

You tell a friend that you are a medical assistant student and excited about the career choice. Your friend then asks you, "What is a medical assistant? Is it the same as a nurse?" What do you say? How do you explain the profession? (Note: Those who are unfamiliar with your work will often ask this question.)

CRITICAL THINKING QUESTIONS

1. A person is wondering if becoming a medical assistant is right for him. What are some ways to help the person make this decision?

2. How does an externship help the medical assistant student?

3. What steps must a person take to earn the CMA credentials?

4. What is the role of the medical assistant? What are some clinical tasks of a medical assistant in a health care setting?

5. A friend is not planning on joining the AAMA because she is just interested in working at a local health care facility. What would you say to your friend? What are some of the benefits of joining the AAMA?

6. If a student wants to work as a clinical medical assistant after graduation, why must the externship still include administrative areas?

7. "Enjoys being with people" is an important quality in a medical assistant. Why is this personal characteristic critical in a person who wishes to become a medical assistant?

8. While working at your externship site, a client refers to you as the "student nurse." How do you respond?

9. Your instructor has told the class about attending continuing education classes after completion of the program. Why do you think this is important for health care professionals?

10. Another student in the medical assistant program announced that she is not going to waste her time working on a portfolio, as this is just the first semester. What could you say to your classmate to influence her not to wait until the end of the program to think about a personal portfolio?

11. Go back to the beginning of this chapter and review the Anticipatory Statements. Reread each statement and then indicate whether it is true or false. If the statement is false, rewrite it to make it a true statement.

CHAPTER

2

Anticipatory Statements

People hold various beliefs regarding the health care environment in the United States. Read and think about the following statements based upon what you believe now. Decide whether you agree or disagree. Write the word **agree** after the statement if you think the statement is true. Write the word **disagree** after the statement if you think the statement is false. Read the chapter to find out if your current beliefs can be supported.

1. A medical assistant may work in a variety of settings. _____

2. Ambulatory care centers perform only general physicals and checkups. _____

3. The medical assistant is an important part of the health care team. _____

4. Subacute units are the same as long-term care units. _____

5. The medical assistant works with other health care professionals to care for clients. _____

The Health Care Environment

Learning Objectives

Upon completion of this chapter, the medical assistant student should be able to:

- Identify the causes of the rapid change in the health care environment
- Describe the two areas that have undergone major changes in the health care environment
- List the major health care professions
- Explain the health care services that are grouped under the title of long-term care
- Discuss the meaning of ambulatory care

Key Terms

activities of daily living (ADLs) Tasks that a person performs in everyday life, such as walking, eating, and toileting.

ambulatory Describes health care settings where a client who is not hospitalized receives care; the client ambulates (walks) into these settings.

health care team Individuals from different professions who work together to give quality health care to a client.

Health Insurance Portability and Accountability Act (HIPAA) Law passed by Congress in 1996 dealing with privacy of client information, among other matters.

Medicaid Joint venture between the states and the federal government to help finance health care for those who are in financial need or disabled.

Medicare Federal program to help finance health care for people who are over the age of 65 or disabled.

occupational therapist Rehabilitation specialist who helps clients with ADLs.

physical therapist Rehabilitation specialist who helps clients with use of their muscles and movement.

preventive Steps taken to maintain health and avoid medical problems or disorders.

protected health information (PHI) Health information that identifies an individual.

rehabilitation Process to help a client attain the highest possible level of functioning after an injury or illness.

subacute A level of care that is less intense than the acute level, but where the client is still not independent and needs skilled health care.

■ INTRODUCTION

Change is the key word in describing the health care environment. Traditional ways, methods of care, those who give care, and the places where care is given are all changing. As science advances, new and better ways are discovered to diagnose and treat disorders. Technology has saved lives and added quality of life for many. Babies who are born too early can now be helped to survive and live healthy lives because of new technology. What was not possible 15 years ago is now everyday practice. Clients with respiratory problems who once had to stay at home, attached to an oxygen tank, now can be more independent with the aid of portable machines. New technology has made it possible for frail clients with walking difficulties to move more independently with the use of motorized wheelchairs. Special machines, such as magnetic resonance imaging (MRI) and computerized tomography (CT) units, allow doctors to see structures inside the body in new and different ways, and thus more accurately diagnose disorders. The science of medical knowledge has expanded so rapidly that many disorders can be found earlier, thereby permitting earlier treatment and yielding better client outcomes. New medications have been discovered to treat conditions that a few years ago could not have been treated successfully. The quality of life, and not just the quantity or amount of time in a life, has been expanded with new medications.

With the discovery of new and better ways to help people has come a problem: The costs of medical care have increased dramatically. The places where care is given and the way that care is given have also dramatically changed.

In response to the changing health care environment, many new health care professions have been developed and blended with the traditional health care roles. The medical assistant needs to recognize these different professions and the skills that workers in these fields possess. Members of each profession contribute to health care. The individual members of the health professions, working together,

become an effective **health care team**. The focus of all health care teamwork is the client; the client is the center of the team.

NOTE TO STUDENT:

Your attitude as a medical assistant will help determine whether you are happy in your chosen work. Do you look upon the changing environment as challenging, with exciting new possibilities, or do you see it only in negative terms, with changes meaning confusion or more work?

■ PLACES AND COSTS OF CLIENT CARE

As health care providers and clients struggle to keep costs reasonable and yet still have quality care, many new ideas are being tested. Two areas that have received much attention are: (1) places where health care is delivered, and how that health care is delivered; and (2) finances or payment for health care.

■ PLACES WHERE CLIENT CARE IS GIVEN

The places where care is given have undergone many changes. The organization of health care facilities and the care that is delivered at each specific setting are much different from before. The medical assistant needs to be aware of these differences, as the medical assistant's role varies with the specific place or clinical site.

Health care services are provided at many different places or settings. The client can receive **preventive** medicine or health care, which is aimed at keeping the client as healthy as possible and avoiding the development of any disorders. When a client is sick or injured, services to diagnose and treat the problem can be given in many different settings.

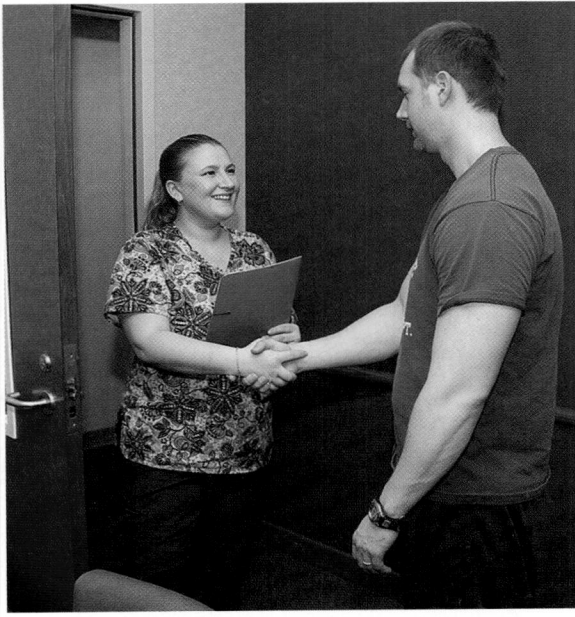

FIGURE 2-1 The medical assistant greets a client in a medical office.

Medical Offices

The medical assistant works most frequently in a medical office (Figure 2-1). Medical offices are organized in various ways. Some treat only adults; others, only children. Some provide care to the entire family. Medical offices may see clients who have disorders in a specific system. For example, some offices, called *cardiology* practices, see clients who have disorders of the cardiovascular system. Still other offices are grouped according to who owns and who works in the practice. Years ago, most doctors worked by themselves in *solo practice.* This is much less common now. Today, it is more common for doctors to work in a group. There are several ways to organize a group practice. Sometimes the doctors see their own clients and just "cover" one another for weekends and holidays. *Coverage* means that one doctor assumes responsibility for another doctor's clients for a short, specified amount of time. This means that the doctor is *on call.* In other situations, clients see all the doctors in a group. The medical assistant will need to find out before being employed how the office is organized.

Ambulatory Centers

Ambulatory centers are clinical sites where clients receive care on an outpatient basis. Clients do not stay overnight, as in hospitals. The organizational structure of an ambulatory center can vary greatly. In some centers, every client must have an appointment; in others, walk-in clients are welcomed. A *walk-in* is a client who feels that he or she needs to see a health care provider but does not have an appointment. Usually, the problem just arose and the client does not want to wait until there is a scheduled opening. Sometimes ambulatory centers have clinics as part of the structure. Clinics can also stand alone, or they may be attached to a hospital. Sometimes the terms *clinic* and *ambulatory center* are used interchangeably, but they are not exactly the same. Clinics usually are open on set days at specific times. Clinics may be grouped according to the specialty; for example, allergy clinic on Monday, orthopedic clinic on Tuesday, and so on. This is especially true if the clinic is attached to a hospital.

Hospitals

For the past 100 years or so, hospitals were commonly the places where most health care services were provided. In recent years, though, hospitals have undergone drastic changes. In the past, clients would stay overnight in the hospital while undergoing diagnostic testing. Now overnight hospital stays are reserved for the acutely sick, and the length of stay for all patients has been shortened considerably.

Hospitals may be privately or publicly operated. Public hospitals are usually owned and operated by a local government. State hospitals are often facilities for the mentally ill. The federal government operates hospitals to serve the needs of veterans. Religious groups or other individuals may operate private facilities.

Medical centers are usually large hospitals located in cities. In addition, they frequently offer specialized, highly technical services unavailable in smaller hospitals. Research laboratories are often located at these centers.

Long-Term Care Facilities

Many clinical settings can be grouped under the heading *long-term care facility*. **Rehabilitation,** skilled nursing, and **subacute** are some of the divisions in this category. With shorter hospital stays, clients may not be ready to go home to live independently. After a cerebrovascular accident or stroke, for example, a client may need intensive therapy to regain lost skills (Figure 2-2). After hip replacement surgery, the client needs time to heal before trying to walk with full weight bearing. These clients benefit from staying in a rehabilitation facility. Rehabilitation sites may be freestanding or located on a specific floor of a hospital. Subacute units provide services for the client who is not acutely sick any more but is still not well enough to care for herself independently. Subacute units may also provide rehabilitation services. These units are often special, separate units in a long-term care facility or nursing home.

Skilled nursing facilities (SNFs) are similar to the traditional long-term care facility. The difference is that only clients who have medical conditions requiring the skills of a registered nurse are admitted to the SNF. These facilities provide around-the-clock nursing care. Long-term care nursing homes do not provide this intensive care.

Laboratories

A *laboratory* is a place where specimens or samples from clients are obtained and tested. A *client sample* or *specimen* is something that is removed from the body and tested. The sample can be urine, blood, or tissue. The test results can help identify health problems, or check if the treatment is helping the client. The medical assistant may be employed in a physician's office laboratory. Wherever he is employed, the medical assistant will work with the laboratory personnel (Figure 2-3). The role of the medical assistant in the laboratory is more fully discussed in Chapter 40.

■ PAYING FOR HEALTH CARE

Financing of, or payment for, health care is the subject of much discussion. Who is to receive care? How much care will that patient receive? Who will pay for the care? Is it up to the individual, the family, the employer, the state or government? What if a person cannot pay? Who pays then? Who decides if someone can pay? Who is responsible? These are serious questions with no easy answers. The medical assistant student will explore these questions in more detail in administrative and medical ethics courses.

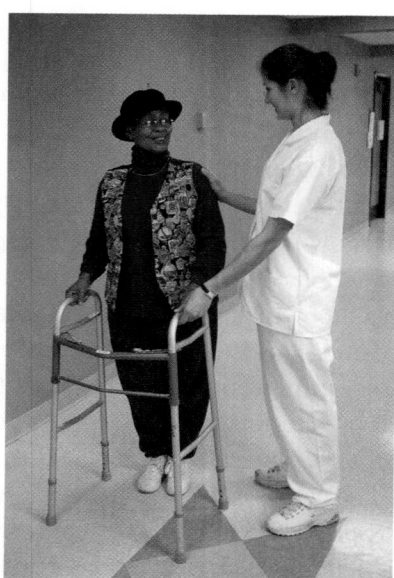

FIGURE 2-2 The medical assistant helps a client learn to walk with a walker to gain independence.

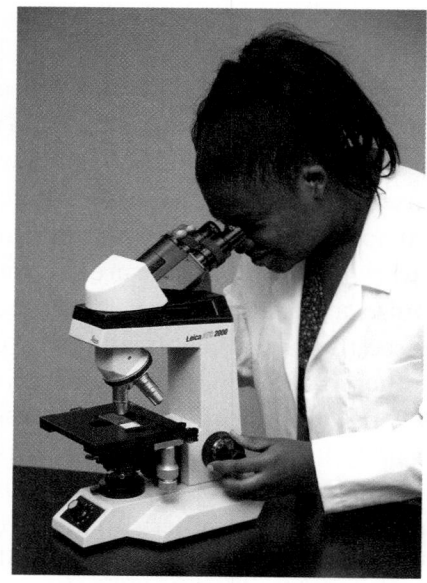

FIGURE 2-3 Medical assistant using a microscope in a laboratory setting.

Chapter 2 THE HEALTH CARE ENVIRONMENT   **19**

The medical assistant will be part of this debate as both a provider and a consumer of care.

Health care costs are the main determinant of what health care is provided and how it is financed. Health care costs are paid either through public government funding or through the private sector. Many individuals have health insurance through their employers. Health insurance pays for much health care service, but many people in the United States do not have health insurance coverage.

Medicare and **Medicaid** are the two major government sources of health care funding. Medicare is federally funded health insurance for those over the age of 65. Medicaid is a joint effort between the federal government and the states. There are federal guidelines for service reimbursement, but benefits vary from state to state. Financial need is the major qualification for obtaining Medicaid benefits, though there are other criteria as well. Medical assistants need to become knowledgeable about these two programs, as many clients of health care practices are participants in these programs. Eligibility criteria and procedures for payment to the provider for services rendered to clients are detailed in administrative or business courses.

Many insurance companies offer insurance to individuals and groups. Employers frequently offer their workers health insurance through a group plan. Paperwork required to receive payment for services, as well as deductibles and co-pays, vary with the company. Medical assistants need to become comfortable with this process, as it is important to both the client and the health care provider.

Many interrelated factors affect the high costs of health care. Advanced technology has made it possible to save lives and improve the quality of those lives through early diagnosis and treatment with technology. Life expectancy is longer, but with advancing age health problems increase. Medications needed to treat these illnesses are expensive. Research to find cures and develop technology to help people is costly. Health care and the providers who give health care are highly regulated by government agencies, insurance companies, and other groups.

Compliance with regulations also contributes to the high cost of health care.

■ HEALTH CARE WORKERS

Many professions focus on only one aspect of client care. Working together, professionals from these various fields can provide quality, client-centered care. The medical assistant will work with many of these people while giving care to clients. The medical assistant may work directly in the same office with different professionals, or may act as a liaison or advocate for the client (Figure 2-4). It is important to know the professions and the skills their practitioners use.

Some of the professionals are:

- Physician—The physician or doctor is a highly trained individual who has a medical degree. After medical school, the doctor completed years of additional training. This additional training is called *residency,* and the number of years for which a person is a resident varies depending on his or her medical specialty. After completion of a residency and receipt of a license to practice medicine, the doctor may enter private practice. A doctor may take further training and years of work to become board certified. Board certification indicates additional training and demonstration of specialized knowledge. Continuing education throughout the doctor's lifetime is necessary to keep that board certification. A physician who is board certified will have additional letters

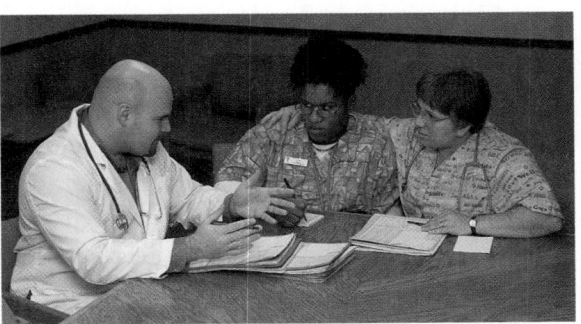

FIGURE 2-4 Medical assistants participate in a team conference about a client's treatment plan.

after his or her name and the M.D. designation. The medical assistant should be familiar with this, as many clients ask if a doctor is board certified. The doctor is responsible for making the medical diagnosis (what is the health concern) and deciding on the course of treatment and follow-up. The medical assistant works under the direction of the physician.

- Physician's assistant—The physician's assistant works directly with the physician. This individual has a bachelor's or master's degree. The physician's assistant often performs physical examinations of clients and provides routine follow-up care. The assistant may care for clients before and after surgery in the hospital, depending on the physician's specialty.
- Nurse practitioner—The nurse practitioner has a master's degree in nursing. This person has duties similar to those of the physician's assistant.
- Nurse—The nurse may be a registered nurse or a licensed practical nurse. The roles and responsibilities vary depending on whether the person is an RN or an LPN, and according to office policy. The education level and scope of practice are not the same. The medical assistant and the nurse often have very similar clinical duties.
- Nursing assistant—The nursing assistant helps the nurse give basic client care. This person usually works in a hospital or long-term care facility.
- **Physical therapist**—The physical therapist works with clients who have movement problems. The therapist helps the client to use bones, muscles, and joints to move or ambulate. The therapist has a master's degree or doctoral academic preparation.
- **Occupational therapist**—An occupational therapist, like a physical therapist, has a master's or doctoral degree. The occupational therapist helps the client keep or regain the ability to perform **activities of daily living (ADLs)**. For example, the physical therapist helps the client regain movement in the hand, and the occupa-

tional therapist helps that client use the hand in eating, dressing, and writing.
- Social worker—The social worker helps individuals with problems in everyday life. For example, clients may be referred to a social worker if they need help with living arrangements or in getting to and from medical appointments. The social worker often has a master's degree.

The medical assistant will work with many other professions while providing client-focused care. The profession and the amount of time spent with the professional or practitioner will depend on the medical setting in which the medical assistant works.

Changes in the Health Care Environment

The health care environment is constantly changing as it strives to meet the needs of clients in a changing society. Knowledge of the structure of the health care environment is important. The medical assistant needs to keep current with new scientific developments and changes in health care delivery. As technology advances, many clients are able to become more independent and are not restricted to remaining in health care facilities. Many treatments and even some surgeries are now performed on an outpatient or **ambulatory** basis. This can be an exciting time to be part of the health care team in providing client-centered care. Knowledge and attitude are key for the medical assistant. A positive attitude toward changes in the health care environment will help determine professional job satisfaction. Ultimately, it is up to the medical assistant.

■ HEALTH INSURANCE PORTABILITY AND ACCOUNTABILITY ACT

Clients need to know that information about them is confidential. The **Health Insurance Portability and Accountability Act (HIPAA)**, passed by Congress in 1996, established privacy regulations among other things. A "Notice of

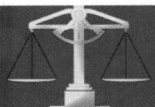

LEGAL/ETHICAL THOUGHTS

Check where regulated information is kept in the office. Rules apply not only to the client's health care providers, but also to the people who provide accounting, bookkeeping, and statistical services (among others). You will need to keep updated as to the current regulations.

Privacy Practices" tells clients how the medical office keeps client information safe and secure. There are many parts of the HIPAA law. The following discusses the parts of HIPAA that the medical assistant will be most concerned with.

The key idea underlying all the HIPAA provisions and regulations is the privacy of the client's health information. The privacy rules center around sending, receiving, and using protected health information. Most often, this is called **protected health information (PHI).** Protected health information is health information that can identify individuals. The rules specify how that information may be sent, received, and stored.

The medical assistant constantly obtains client information, through the performance of administrative tasks such as gathering information to put together a client's medical chart. The administrative medical assistant also sends and receives PHI via telephone calls, faxes, and the Internet. The medical assistant discusses client care issues with other members of the health care team. During the performance of clinical tests, medical assistants obtain and have access to much protected health information.

■ PRIVACY GUIDELINES

Four criteria should be observed in regard to protected health information:

1. Workers may not use or give out PHI unless regulations permit it.

2. An individual must give authorization before PHI may be used or given out. Client authorization or permission is very specific. It is granted within a limited time frame, and permission can be taken back at any time.

3. When using, asking for, or receiving information, every effort must be made to keep the information shared to a minimum to meet the need.

4. Individual clients have the right to access their medical information and to restrict the sharing of their private health information.

Privacy Standards

Health information that is shared verbally or sent or stored in paper form must be processed according to the HIPAA privacy standards.

Security Rule

The security rule of HIPAA became effective in April of 2005. The security rule applies to health information that is sent, transmitted, or stored electronically. If the health information can identify an individual person, the security rule covers this information. *Security* means safety. These rules are meant to keep those who have no legitimate reason or need to know from finding or using clients' confidential, personal information.

Outside and Inside Risks

Security breaches can occur outside the medical office or within the health care setting.

Outside Factors

- E-mail viruses
- Firewall breakthrough (firewalls are meant to keep unauthorized people from accessing computer information)
- Easy passwords

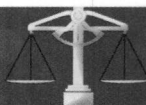

LEGAL/ETHICAL THOUGHTS

You must check that the client has signed a PHI notice (and possibly an authorizaton to release PHI) as you prepare the client for the office visit.

Inside Factors

- Staff who are not trained to recognize and protect health information unknowingly become a threat to security within the medical setting
- Staff who receive training but do not incorporate the security measures into their everyday handling of protected information
- Staff who choose to ignore the rules and become careless and sloppy while handling PHI

Precautions

Precautions must be taken to comply with all security rules. The entire health care team can help to develop, put in place, and evaluate steps specific to their work setting. The steps can be grouped into workplace or worker precautions.

Workplace Precautions

- Limit access to information
- Enforce rules as to who may and may not use computers
- Keep work areas secure
- Restrict who can enter the health care setting
- Keep information confidentially stored
- Guard confidential information
- Use alarms triggered by any attempt to enter without proper authorization

Worker Precautions

- Multiskilled medical assistants, especially those who perform administrative tasks, must implement worker precautions.

- Medical assistants can review and update policies and procedures specific to the health care setting on how to work with personal health care information.
- All employees must attend inservices on security awareness (attendance and participation should be documented with date, time, and type of training).
- Workers must familiarize themselves with recovery plans.
- Workers must know the steps to follow for any possible incident involving personal health information.
- Employees must have individual identifiers.
- Employees must never share their passwords.
- Workers who can see data must be authorized.
- Everyone is responsible for maintaining the integrity of the system. Specific individuals or teams should review and then report on the integrity of the system.

HIPAA Security Incidents

Even if all the security measures are put into effect for an office, a HIPAA security incident may happen. The medical assistant must know what to do if such an event occurs. Any breach, no matter how small or insignificant, it may seem, must be reported to the risk management department. If the health care setting is small, a specific individual may be identified as the officer for risk management. The medical assistant must use the appropriate reporting form, which should be found in the office policy manual. As members of the health care team, medical assistants are responsible to report any security incidents. This applies to verbal or paper transmission as well as electronic incidents.

BRIDGE TO CAAHEP

This chapter, which describes the health care environment, provides information or content related to CAAHEP standards for Medical Terminology, Medical Law and Ethics, Communication, Medical Assisting Administrative Procedures, Medical Assisting Clinical Procedures, and Professional Components.

ABHES LINKS

This chapter, which describes the health care environment, links to ABHES course content for medical assisting for Orientation, Medical Terminology, Medical Law and Ethics, Medical Office Business Procedures/Management, Medical Office Clinical Procedures, and Career Development.

AAMA AREAS OF COMPETENCE

This chapter, which describes the health care environment, provides information or content within several areas as listed in the Medical Assistant Role Delineation Study. The areas included are: administrative, administrative pro-

NOTE TO STUDENT:

In any health care setting, the medical assistant needs to be aware of the type of client information that is used in that setting. The information that comes in, the uses made of it, and the way it is shared must comply with the HIPAA provisions and regulations.

cedures, clinical, patient (client) care, general transdisciplinary, professionalism, professional communication skills, communication skills, legal concepts, instruction, and operational functions.

AMT PATHS

Health care environment provides a path to AMT competencies in general medical assisting knowledge, medical terminology, medical law, medical ethics, human relations, and patient (client) education. It also includes administrative medical assisting, insurance, and medical-secretarial-receptionist information.

POINTS OF HIGHLIGHT

- Health care environments have experienced much change as the result of new technology.
- Keeping costs down while maintaining quality care is a major discussion topic in the United States.
- Medical assistants work in a variety of settings, the most common being the medical office.
- Clients receive the majority of health care services in ambulatory care settings. Ambulatory care settings or outpatient sites are organized in a variety of ways.
- Rehabilitation, skilled nursing, and subacute care are often grouped under the title of long-term care.
- Medical assistants work together with a variety of health care professionals.
- Knowledge of and a positive attitude toward changes in the health care environment contribute to professional job satisfaction.

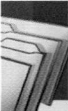

STUDENT PORTFOLIO ACTIVITY

You have learned about health care settings and the health professionals who work there. Select a health facility in your community and arrange to interview a health care provider employed there. Afterward, take time to describe in writing your impression of your visit. Would you want to work there as a medical assistant? Why or why not? If not, explain why it is still important for you as a medical assistant to be familiar with the health care setting. (Why is this important for your future employer to know? Remember critical thinking.)

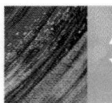

APPLYING YOUR SKILLS

You work in a doctor's office and today you are answering phone calls at the front desk. A female caller identifies herself and asks questions about her mother's health. You know that the mother is a client and once in a while you have seen them together at the office. What do you do? What issues are involved? How does HIPAA affect your actions?

CRITICAL THINKING QUESTIONS

1. Describe ways in which the health care environment has changed in recent years. Give examples of some of those changes.

2. What effect have the changes in the health care environment had on the places where client care is provided?

3. How does the medical assistant's attitude toward change affect work performance and job satisfaction?

4. What are some health care professions that the medical assistant will be working with to give client-centered care? Select one profession and explain how the medical assistant would work with a practitioner of this profession.

5. What are some steps the medical assistant could take to help clients adjust to a changing health care environment?

6. Select a recent advance in technology. In what ways has this changed treatment for clients who need this technology?

7. Medical assistants work in a variety of settings. Choose a health care environment and think about a typical day for a medical assistant in this setting. What are some tasks the medical assistant might perform during the day?

8. What is the role of the medical assistant on the health care team in a primary care office? Who are some of the other professionals that the medical assistant will be working with in the office?

9. What are some ways that rising costs of medical care affect a medical assistant as a health care provider?

10. A client complains to you about the bill she received from your office. She appears upset. How should you respond? What are some steps you could take to help this client?

11. Go back to the beginning of this chapter and review the Anticipatory Statements. Reread each statement and then indicate whether it is true or false. If the statement is false, rewrite it to make it a true statement.

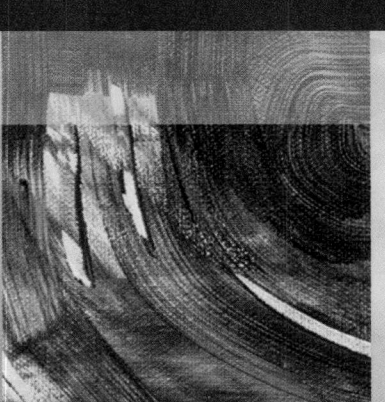

This second unit moves learners from the foundation of the medical assistant profession to the clinical skills part of the medical assistant profession.

The fundamental responsibility of a health care provider in a clinical setting is to provide clients with a safe and healthy environment that is free from harmful organisms. This unit discusses the infection cycle and the role of the medical assistant in breaking that cycle, the measurement of vital signs, and the physical examination and procedures commonly performed in the medical office. Procedures are first explained and then shown step by step. You can practice these competencies in the clinical laboratory by following the procedural steps, using the competency skill checklist found in each chapter. Your instructor can then use these checklists to guide and observe you in the laboratory setting.

At the end of each chapter, you are presented with a client-centered care situation. You are asked to solve the problem by using what you have learned in the chapter and applying your critical thinking skills.

Much of the role of the medical assistant involves client teaching. A sample client teaching plan is included at the end of each chapter, and these plans can be used when working with clients. They can also be used as a starting point and modified to meet the needs of a client in your specific job setting.

Anticipatory Statements

Read and think about the following statements based upon what you believe now. Decide whether you agree or disagree. Write the word **agree** after the statement if you think the statement is true. Write the word **disagree** after the statement if you think the statement is false. Read the chapter to find out if your current beliefs can be supported.

1. If health care workers wear gloves, they need not wash their hands after taking off the gloves. _____

2. All microorganisms cause diseases. _____

3. A person can become infected if he comes into contact with blood from an infected person. _____

4. Some people are more prone to catching colds or the flu than others. _____

5. An individual who has a virus should wash his hands and limit contact with others until well. _____

Infection Control

Learning Objectives

Upon completion of this chapter, the medical assistant student should be able to:

- Define the term *microorganism*
- Explain the difference between pathogenic and nonpathogenic microorganisms
- Describe the importance of handwashing in activities of daily living
- State the difference between resident and transient flora
- Explain the infection cycle (chain of infection)
- State the difference between medical asepsis and surgical asepsis
- List six ways for a medical assistant to break the infection cycle

Key Terms

asepsis A state of being free from pathogenic microorganisms.

microorganism A tiny living plant or animal that is too small to be seen with the eye unless aided by an instrument.

nonpathogenic Describes microorganisms that do not normally cause disease.

pathogenic Disease-causing.

resident flora Microorganisms found in the deeper layers of the skin; most are usually harmless, but they are not removed by routine handwashing.

transient flora Microorganisms found in and on the upper layers of skin; picked up during the course of everyday activities. These can cause disease, but can easily be removed through use of correct handwashing technique.

■ INTRODUCTION

We are constantly being told that we must fight germs in our homes and in our bodies. Manufacturers advertise a myriad of products on television and radio, in newspapers and magazines, that supposedly fight those "nasty germs" and make our homes clean and fresh smelling. Others promote products to keep our bodies clean, fresh smelling, and free from odors caused by "germs." People's ideas about cleanliness and infection control often are based on such advertisements, but the medical assistant must understand the scientific principles and basis of infection control. This chapter introduces students to microorganisms and the medical assistant's role in breaking the infection cycle.

■ MICROORGANISMS

Microorganisms are around us at all times and all places. These tiny plants and animals, which are invisible without the aid of a special instrument such as a microscope, surround us where we work, where we live, and where we play. Not all microorganisms are harmful. Some are even beneficial to humans, helping to keep other harmful organisms under control. **Pathogenic** microorganisms can cause disease. Microorganisms that normally are not harmful and generally do not cause disease are **nonpathogenic.**

Growth Factors

Microorganisms are living plants or animals, and therefore need certain conditions in which to survive and reproduce. In this they are just like humans and other animals and plants, which need certain conditions in order to live.

All microorganisms need a food source and certain gases. The temperature, the amount of light and moisture, and the pH of the environment all affect microorganisms' ability to survive. Food sources for microorganisms include both inanimate materials and other living organisms. Some organisms, called *aerobes*, need oxygen. Others, called *anaerobes*, do not need oxygen; in fact, oxygen may be poisonous to these microbes.

Normal human body temperature often encourages the growth of microorganisms. A dark, moist environment that is neither too acidic nor too basic (neutral pH) fosters the multiplication of many microorganisms.

Medical assistants need to understand common factors that influence the growth of pathogenic organisms, especially conditions that favor reproduction. The medical assistant can use this knowledge to help maintain a safe, healthful environment for the health care setting by breaking the chain of infection and thus preventing sickness.

■ MAINTAINING A SAFE, HEALTHFUL ENVIRONMENT

A medical assistant can help to limit the growth and spread of harmful microorganisms in several ways.

Handwashing

Frequent medical **asepsis** handwashing by the medical assistant is the single most important action to prevent the spread of pathogens and infection. People's hands are a major source of bacterial transmission. Hands are used for most activities of daily living, such as preparing and eating food, dressing, and personal hygiene. People communicate with each other through handshakes and touching (Figure 3-1), and as a result pathogenic organisms can easily be passed from one person to another through direct contact.

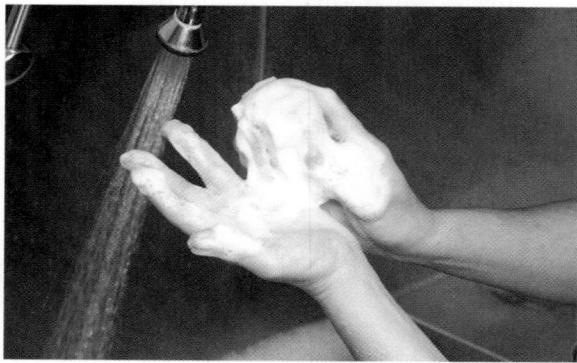

FIGURE 3-1 A major source of transmission of microorganisms is through the hands.

Microorganisms are always present on the hands. Normal flora found on the hands are called **resident flora** because these microbes normally lives there, firmly attached to the skin. It can be difficult to remove resident flora. Also, as people go through activities of daily living and come into contact with the environment, they pick up **transient flora.** Transient flora can be either pathogenic or nonpathogenic. Even if the transient flora that a person picks up are pathogenic, these microorganisms are easily removed by proper handwashing.

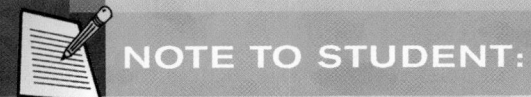

NOTE TO STUDENT:

Remember to use friction when washing your hands with soap. The friction helps to loosen and remove dirt and transient flora. Handwashing is primarily a mechanical action.

Health

Eating a well-balanced diet, in combination with exercise and an adequate amount of sleep, will help you maintain health. A healthy person is less susceptible to infection by harmful organisms. A healthy person can defend against and fight off infections.

Personal Hygiene

Bathe often and keep your skin healthy. Practice good oral hygiene. In the course of daily work activities, do not hold items against your uniform. For example, when changing the paper cover on an exam table, do not allow the dirty paper to brush against your uniform. This also applies to client gowns and other items. Follow all office procedures to limit the amount of exposure to potentially infectious materials.

Cleanliness

Maintain a clean environment. Consider the floor contaminated; anything that falls on the floor is also considered contaminated. Keep all surfaces clean and dry. Wipe up any spills or moisture immediately (Figure 3-2). Keep the office free from dust. If your place of employment uses a cleaning service, make sure that cleaning is done properly. Rooms should be kept well lit and well ventilated.

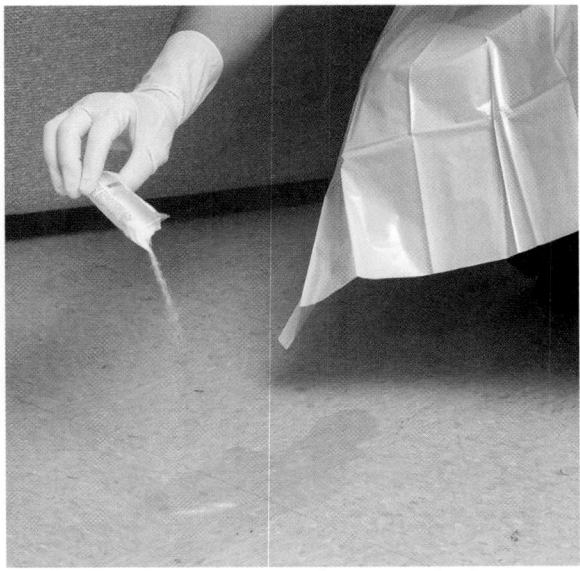

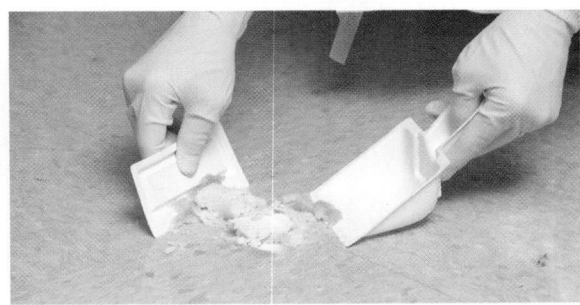

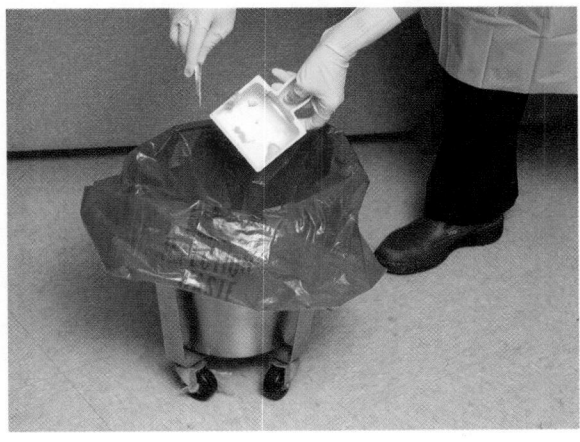

FIGURE 3-2 Medical assistants should wipe up any spills on the floor immediately.

Contact with Others

Health care workers are generally cautious when working with contagious individuals. However, the medical assistant should treat bodily fluids from all clients as potentially contagious.

■ THE INFECTION CYCLE

The process of infection is like a circular chain with five links (Figure 3-3). If any one of these links is broken, the cycle will be disrupted and the process of infection cannot continue.

The infection process begins with a source of pathogens. The source or *reservoir host* is usually an animal or person that has become infected; the pathogen survives and reproduces in this host. The reservoir host can then transfer the infecting pathogen to others.

The second link is the way out or the *means of exit* from the reservoir host. Any opening on the infected person or animal can become the means of exit. Some diseases are spread through specific openings. The mouth, nose, throat, urinary opening, reproductive tract, and any open areas on or breaks in the skin are common means of exit.

The third link, the *means of transmission,* is how the pathogen comes into contact with another person. The means of transmission can be direct or indirect. *Direct contact* means that another person actually comes into contact with an infected host and picks up the pathogen through that contact. *Indirect contact* occurs by touching contaminated items, such as objects that an infected person has handled. Food and water can also be a means of transmission. Water vapor, such as that produced by coughing or sneezing, is yet another means of transmission.

To cause infection, a pathogenic organism must find a way into another host, that is, a *means of entry.* The means of entry are the same as the means of exit. In other words, bodily openings (including breaks in the skin) can be both a way for pathogens to get in and a way for pathogens to get out of the host.

The fifth link is the *susceptible host,* someone or something that can become infected. Not everyone who comes into contact with patho-

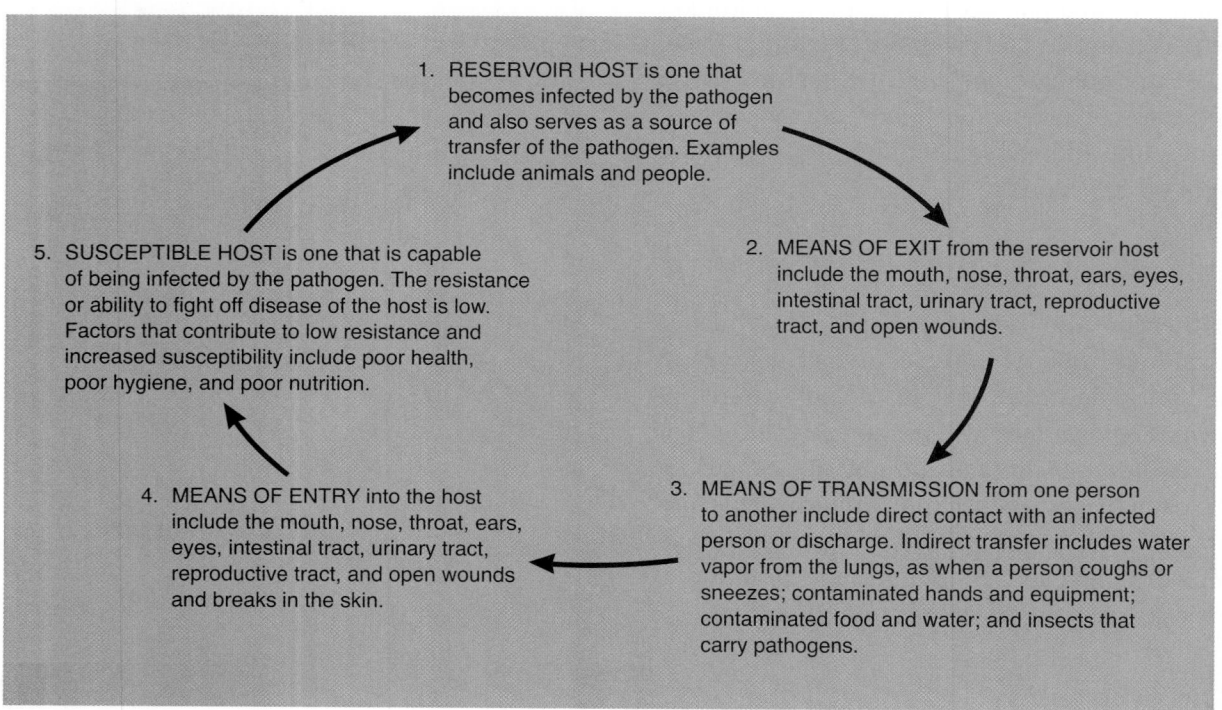

FIGURE 3–3 The chain of infection (infection cycle).

genic organisms will become sick. Some people are more likely to develop an infection (that is, they are more susceptible to getting sick), whereas other individuals are more resistant. Good health, good nutritional status, and low levels of stress help to protect a person because these factors support the body's immune system, which defends against infection (see Chapter 14 and Chapter 27).

■ HOW THE BODY PROTECTS ITSELF

Unbroken skin is the best defense for keeping out harmful organisms from the environment. Because of frequent handwashing, medical assistants are prone to have dry, cracked, and chafed skin. Broken skin means easy access for bacteria and other pathogens! After handwashing, gently pat the skin dry, and apply moisturizing lotion frequently.

The body also defends itself against the invasion of harmful organisms through its secretions: tears wash away foreign objects in the eyes, mucus in the nose and respiratory tract helps trap and expel foreign objects; hair in the nose and cilia in the respiratory tract help to trap foreign organisms and remove them to the outside of the body. Perspiration helps to wash bacteria off the skin. Chemicals in the stomach help to render harmless or destroy any ingested pathogens. Harmful organisms may also be excreted in urine and feces, through the urinary and digestive systems.

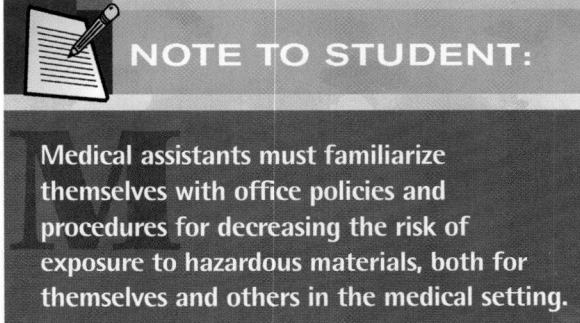

NOTE TO STUDENT:

Medical assistants must familiarize themselves with office policies and procedures for decreasing the risk of exposure to hazardous materials, both for themselves and others in the medical setting.

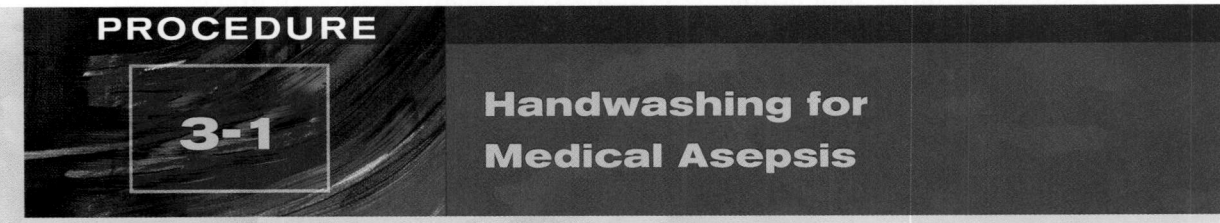

PROCEDURE 3-1

Handwashing for Medical Asepsis

Student Competency Objective: The medical assistant student will wash hands to maintain medical asepsis.

Items Needed: Liquid soap in dispenser, paper towels, orange stick or nail brush, sink with warm water, wastebasket

Steps:
1. Take off your watch and any rings (they harbor bacteria).
2. Make sure your sleeves are above your elbows.
3. Stand close to the sink without touching it (a wet uniform encourages the growth and transmission of bacteria).
4. Turn on the faucet with a paper towel, unless the faucet is operated with a foot or knee control or is motion-activated.

(Continues)

PROCEDURE 3-1 (Continued)

5. Adjust the water temperature.

6. Rinse hands under warm running water (Figure 3-4A). Very hot or cold water is damaging to the skin.

7. Keep hands lower than forearms.

8. Let soap from the soap dispenser squirt into the palm of your hand.

9. Rub your hands together, working the soap into a lather.

10. Rub soap over palms, back of hands, and between fingers, using a circular motion. Friction helps to loosen dirt and mechanically remove pathogens (Figure 3-4B).

11. Put fingertips of your right hand into the palm of your left hand and scrub. This also helps to get soap under the fingernails.

12. Put fingertips of the left hand into the palm of the right hand and scrub. This also helps to get soap under the fingernails.

13. Take an orange stick and clean under fingernails of both hands. If using a nail brush, brush under each nail and around the cuticle.

14. Rinse well, making sure to get off all soap. Do not touch the inside of the sink with your hands.

15. If your hands have come into contact with blood, drainage, pus, or body fluids, repeat the handwashing.

16. Dry hands gently and thoroughly with paper towels.

17. Discard used paper towels and the orange stick or nail brush.

18. Using a paper towel, turn off the faucet (unless automatic or knee-controlled).

19. Discard the paper towel.

20. Put on your watch and rings (if worn).

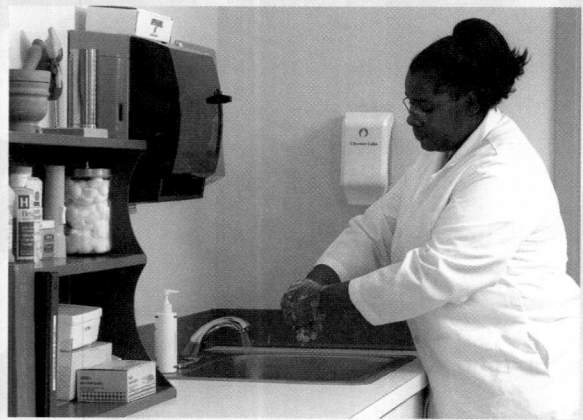

FIGURE 3-4A Rinse your hands under warm running water, keeping hands lower than forearms.

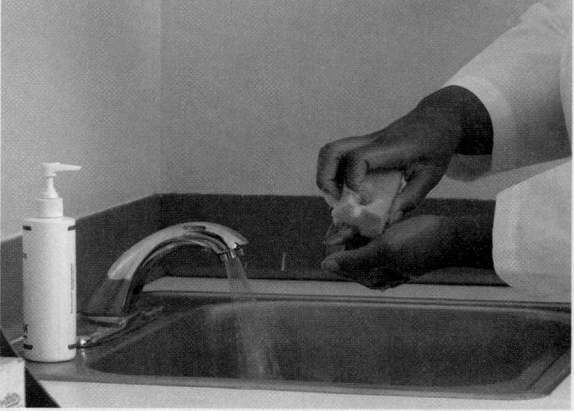

FIGURE 3-4B Rub your hands together, working soap over palms, the backs of the hands, and between fingers, using a circular motion.

NOTE TO STUDENT:

Handwashing for medical asepsis should last from one to two minutes, and should include both the hands and the wrists.

PROCEDURE

3-2 Handwashing for Surgical Asepsis

Student Competency Objective: The medical assistant student will wash hands as a part of surgical asepsis.

Items Needed: Liquid antibacterial soap in dispenser, sterile towels, paper towels, orange stick or nail brush, sink with warm water, wastebasket

Steps:

1. Take off your watch and any rings (they harbor bacteria).
2. Make sure your sleeves are above your elbows.
3. Stand close to the sink without touching it (a wet uniform encourages the growth and transmission of bacteria).
4. Turn on the faucet with a paper towel, unless the faucet is operated with a foot or knee control or is motion-activated (Figure 3-5A).

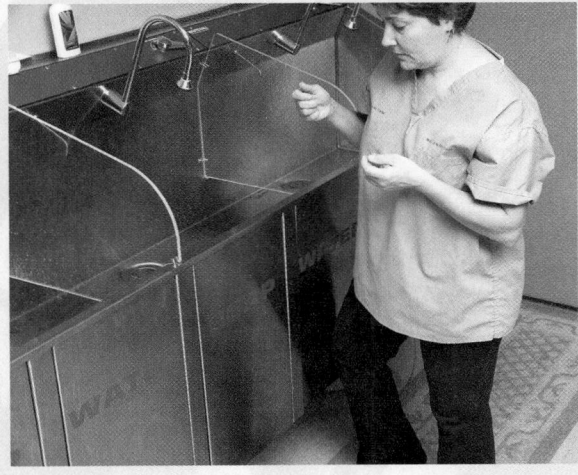

FIGURE 3-5A With hands free of watches and jewelry and sleeves above elbow level, turn on the faucet, using a paper towel or knee or foot control.

(Continues)

PROCEDURE 3-2 (Continued)

5. Adjust the water temperature.

6. Hold hands under the faucet above waist level.

7. Rinse hands under warm running water. Very hot or cold water is damaging to the skin.

8. Keep hands lower than forearms.

9. Let soap from the soap dispenser squirt into the palm of your hand.

10. Rub your hands together, working soap into a lather.

11. Rub soap over palms, back of hands, and between fingers, using a circular motion. Friction helps to loosen dirt and mechanically remove pathogens (Figure 3–5B).

12. Put fingertips of the right hand into the palm of the left hand and scrub. This also helps to get soap under the fingernails.

13. Put fingertips of the left hand into the palm of the right hand and scrub. This also helps to get soap under the fingernails.

14. Take an orange stick and clean under fingernails of both hands (Figure 3–5C).

15. Pick up a nail brush and scrub palms and backs of hands, nails, wrists, and forearms (Figure 3–5D).

16. Start rinsing from the tips of the fingers to the forearms.

17. Rinse well, making sure to get off all soap. Do not touch the inside of the sink with your hands.

18. Continue to keep your hands higher than your elbows. This prevents water from running down to the clean fingers (Figure 3–5E).

19. Pick up a sterile towel.

20. Dry hands gently and thoroughly with the sterile towel, starting with the fingers and hands and working your way up the forearms.

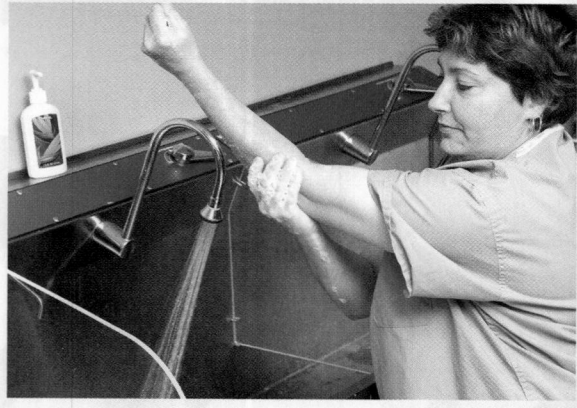

FIGURE 3–5B Work soap into a lather, rubbing the palms, backs of the hands, and between fingers, being sure to keep hands above waist level.

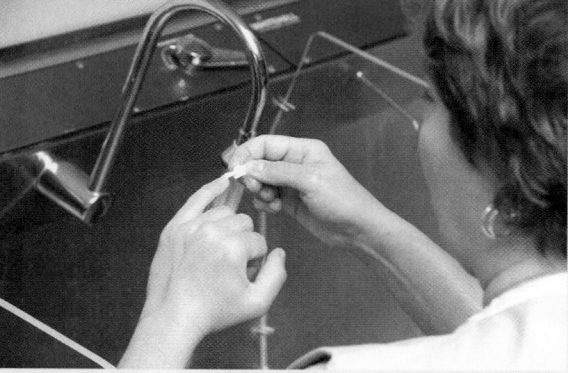

FIGURE 3–5C Use a stick to clean underneath the fingernails.

(Continues)

PROCEDURE 3-2 (Continued)

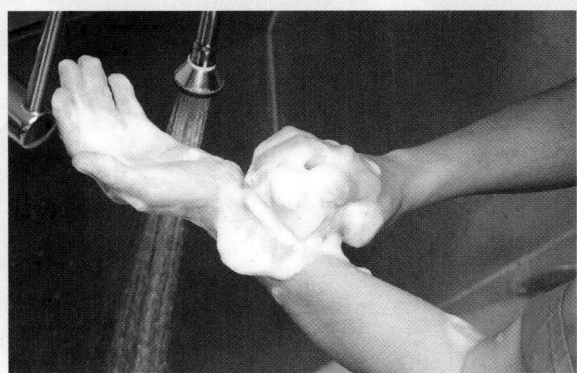

FIGURE 3–5D Scrub the palms, backs of the hands, fingernails, wrists, and forearms.

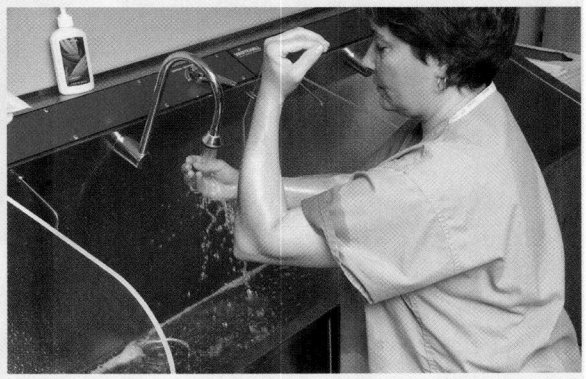

FIGURE 3–5E Rinse off the soap, keeping hands above waist level and higher than elbows.

21. Discard the used sterile towel, orange stick, and nail brush.
22. Take a dry sterile towel and turn off the faucet, or turn it off with an elbow (unless the faucet is automatic or knee–controlled).
23. Discard the used sterile towel.

 NOTE TO STUDENT:

A surgical scrub should last from five to ten minutes, depending on the policy and procedure established for the particular health care setting.

PROCEDURE

3-3

Application of Sterile Gloves

Student Competency Objective: The medical assistant student will open and put on a pair of sterile gloves.

Items Needed: One pair of sterile gloves, soap and water

Steps:

1. Remove rings from hands.
2. Wash hands.
3. Select the correct glove size. Gloves that are too big will make finger actions clumsy. Gloves that are too tight will tear easily.
4. Read the package label. Some packages contain two gloves; others include only a single glove.
5. Place the glove package on a clean surface with the left glove in front of your left hand and the right glove in front of your right hand.
6. Break the seal on the package for the left glove.
7. Open the flap and fold it away from you.
8. Make sure that the cuff of the glove is closest to you.
9. Break the seal on the package for the right glove.
10. Open the flap and fold it away from you.
11. Make sure that the cuff of the glove is closest to you.
12. Using the thumb and forefinger of your nondominant hand (if you are right-handed, your nondominant hand is your left hand; if you are left-handed, your nondominant hand is your right hand), grab the cuff of the glove for the dominant hand (Figure 3–6A).
13. Fit your dominant hand into the glove, being careful not to let your ungloved nondominant hand touch any other area of the glove (Figure 3–6B).

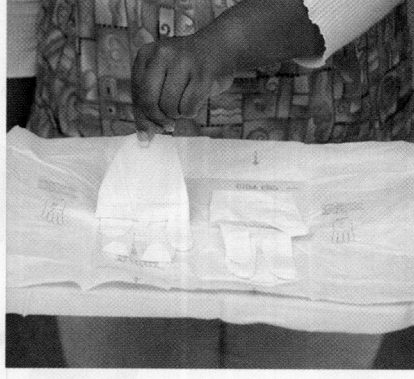

FIGURE 3-6A Use the thumb and forefinger of your nondominant hand to grab the cuff of the glove.

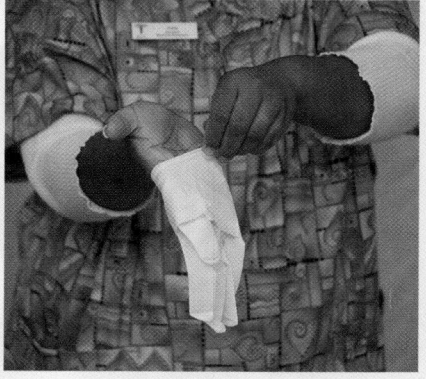

FIGURE 3-6B With palm up, slide your hand into the glove.

(Continues)

PROCEDURE 3-3 (Continued)

14. Using your sterile-gloved dominant hand, slip your four fingers under the cuff of the other sterile glove. Be careful not to let your thumb touch the other glove (Figure 3-6C).

15. Fit your nondominant hand into the glove (Figure 3-6D).

16. Do not touch anything that is not sterile.

17. While waiting to assist the doctor or undertake a procedure, interlace your fingers.

18. Keep sterile gloved hands above your waist.

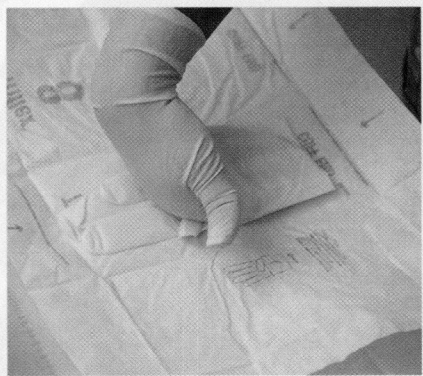

FIGURE 3-6C Using the sterile-gloved dominant hand, slip four fingers under the cuff of the other sterile glove, being careful not to let your thumb touch the other glove.

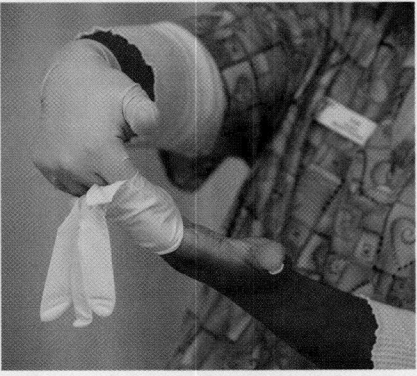

FIGURE 3-6D Fit your nondominant hand into the glove. Keep sterile-gloved hands above your waist and interlace your fingers while waiting to assist the doctor.

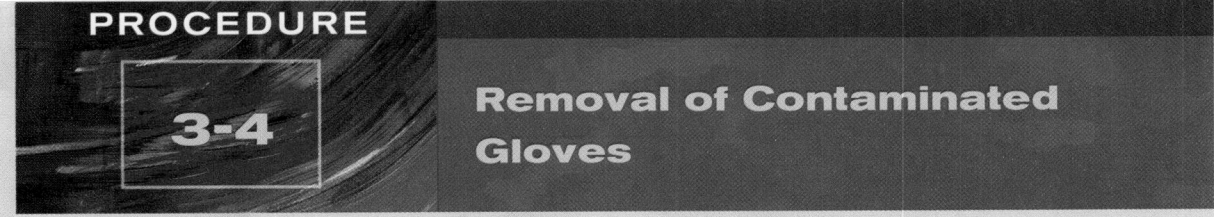

PROCEDURE 3-4

Removal of Contaminated Gloves

Student Competency Objective: The medical assistant student will remove contaminated (used) gloves.

Items Needed: Gloves, biohazard bag

Steps:

1. With your nondominant hand, grab the outside of the sterile glove on the dominant hand at the palm (Figure 3-7A).

2. Pull that glove off and hold it in the sterile-gloved nondominant hand (Figure 3-7B).

3. Slip the fingers of your dominant hand (ungloved) under the cuff of the sterile glove on your nondominant hand (Figure 3-7C).

(Continues)

PROCEDURE 3-4 (Continued)

4. Pull the glove off the nondominant hand inside out, inverting it over the first glove. The gloves will be in a ball with the insides out (Figures 3-7D and E).
5. Dispose of the contaminated gloves in a biohazard bag (Figure 3-7F).
6. Wash your hands.

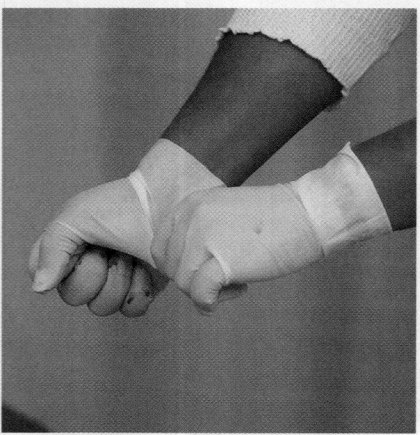

FIGURE 3-7A Using the thumb and forefinger of your nondominant hand, grab the outside of your sterile-gloved dominant hand at the palm to begin removing contaminated gloves.

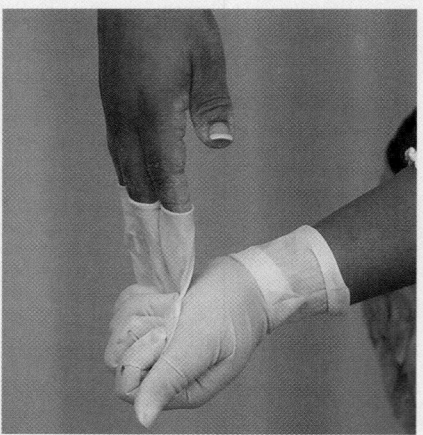

FIGURE 3-7B Pull the glove off your dominant hand and hold it in your sterile-gloved nondominant hand.

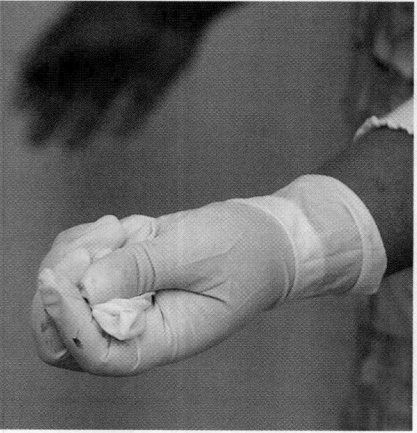

FIGURE 3-7C Slip the fingers of your ungloved dominant hand underneath the cuff of the sterile glove on your nondominant hand.

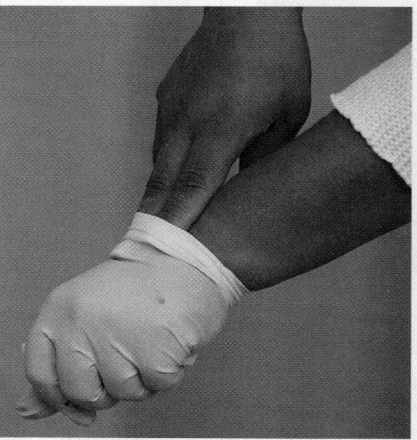

FIGURE 3-7D Pull the glove off inside out. The contaminated gloves are now in a ball in your hand.

(Continues)

PROCEDURE 3-4 (Continued)

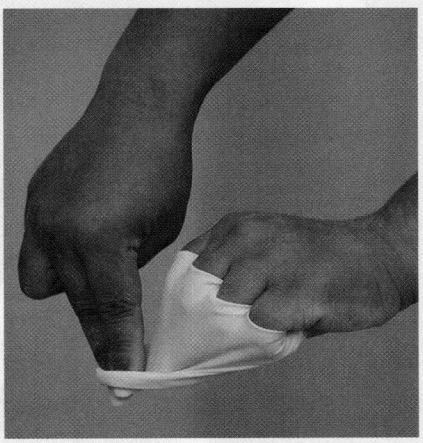

FIGURE 3–7E Invert the second glove over the first.

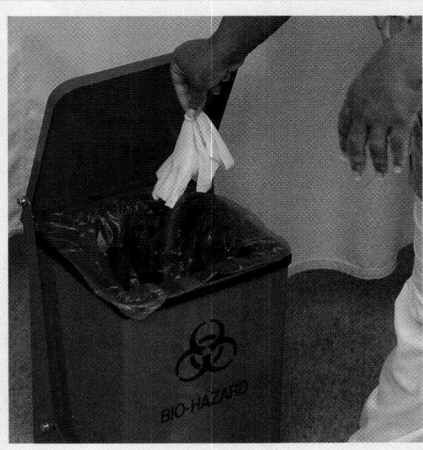

FIGURE 3–7F Dispose of gloves in a biohazard container.

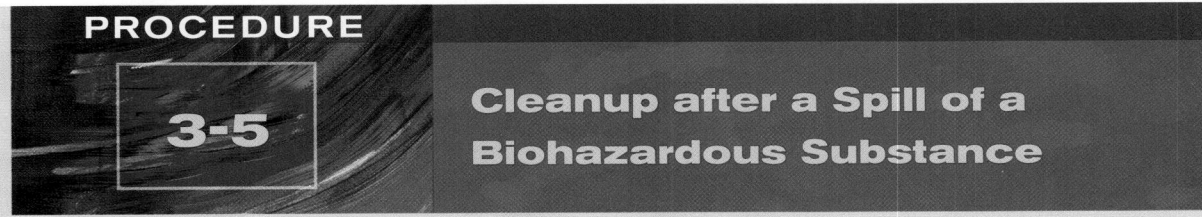

PROCEDURE
3-5   Cleanup after a Spill of a Biohazardous Substance

Student Competency Objective: The medical assistant student will clean up a biohazard spill (contaminated surface).

Items Needed: 1:10 bleach solution or other prepared germicide, disposable towels, biohazard containers, gloves and other personal protective equipment (goggles, gown, face mask)

Steps:

1. Gather the items needed for cleanup.
2. Put on gloves.
3. Put on other personal protective equipment (as needed, in case of splashing).
4. Wipe with disposable towels any spill that can be seen.
5. Dispose of used towels in the biohazard container.
6. Spray or pour germicide solution or bleach onto the surface to decontaminate it, being careful not to splash outside of the contaminated area.
7. Wipe the surface with disposable towels.
8. Dispose of used towels in the biohazard container.
9. Put away unused supplies.
10. Take off personal protective equipment.
11. Take off your gloves.
12. Wash your hands.

BRIDGE TO CAAHEP

This chapter, which discusses infection control, provides information and content related to CAAHEP standards for Anatomy and Physiology, Medical Terminology, Communication, Medical Assisting Clinical Procedures, and Professional Components.

 ## ABHES LINKS

This chapter, which discusses infection control, links to ABHES course content for medical terminology, medical law and ethics, psychology of human relations, and medical office clinical procedures.

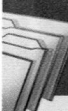 ## STUDENT PORTFOLIO ACTIVITY

Becoming a knowledgeable consumer about products that claim to produce a healthful, germ-free environment can help you work with clients. Prepare a list of common products and note their claims and cost. Compare the products, noting exactly what germs are rendered harmless and at what cost. Look at the ingredients. Are common household products just as beneficial? What about the cost to the client? Your findings can help you guide your clients. This demonstrates awareness of the environment in which your clients live and your desire to help clients protect themselves in a cost-conscious, healthful way.

 ## AAMA AREAS OF COMPETENCE

This chapter, which discusses infection control, provides information or content within several areas listed in the Medical Assistant Role Delineation Study. These areas include: clinical, fundamental principles, patient (client) care, general transdisciplinary, professionalism, communication skills, legal concepts, and instruction.

 ## AMT PATHS

Infection control provides a path to AMT competency in general medical assisting knowledge, medical terminology, medical ethics, human relations and patient(client) education, clinical medical assisting, and asepsis.

 ## APPLYING YOUR SKILLS

Another medical assistant complains to you about his painfully chapped hands, caused by handwashing many times a day. What suggestions can you give him to prevent this in the future? Why is it so important to prevent dry, cracked skin?

POINTS OF HIGHLIGHT

- Microorganisms are tiny, living plants or animals that are invisible to the naked eye.
- Pathogenic organisms can cause disease; nonpathogenic organisms do not.
- During the course of daily activity, individuals pick up transient flora that might be harmful.
- Handwashing is the single most important activity for preventing the spread of disease.
- The five links in the chain of infection (the infection cycle) are: (1) reservoir host; (2) means of exit (from reservoir host); (3) means of transmission; (4) means of entry; (5) susceptible host.
- Medical assistants can help break the chain of infection by practicing medical asepsis.

CRITICAL THINKING QUESTIONS

1. The doctor tells a client that the client is a susceptible host for a type of infection. The client asks you to explain what the doctor meant. What do you tell him?

2. Why is it important to use friction, as well as soap, when washing your hands?

3. During your externship at a clinical site, you observe a health care worker drawing blood. He has gloves on, but you notice that one fingertip is torn off. He tells you that he cannot feel the client's vein through gloves. What is wrong with this situation, and why?

4. How do you decide if medical asepsis or surgical asepsis should be used for a procedure?

5. At what points in the day should a medical assistant wash his hands? What factors help the medical assistant to decide if handwashing is needed?

6. Think about the cycle of infection. Select one point in this cycle. How can you as a medical assistant prevent the spread of infection at this point? Give an example.

7. Explain ways in which you as a medical assistant can promote a clean and healthful environment for yourself and your co-workers.

8. You hear the claim, "This will kill all microorganisms." Are all microorganisms harmful? Can you think of some reasons why you might not want to kill all microorganisms in the everyday environment?

9. Identify ways in which you as a medical assistant can protect clients from infection and disease.

10. Go back to the beginning of this chapter and review the Anticipatory Statements. Reread each statement and then indicate whether it is true or false. If the statement is false, rewrite it to make it a true statement.

Anticipatory Statements

People have different ideas about body temperature, pulse, respiration, blood pressure, and pain and what these measurements and numbers mean to a person's health. Read and think about the following statements based upon what you believe now. Decide whether you agree or disagree. Write the word **agree** after the statement if you think the statement is true. Write the word **disagree** after the statement if you think the statement is false. Read the chapter to find out if your current beliefs can be supported.

1. When a person holds a cold object, heat will be transferred from the person to the object. _____

2. Only people who are sick have a temperature. _____

3. An adult has a faster pulse rate than a child. _____

4. It is very important to tell a client when you are counting her breaths. _____

5. A person who is confused or cognitively (mentally) impaired does not experience pain. _____

Learning Objectives

Upon completion of this chapter, the medical assistant student should be able to:

- Define temperature, pulse, respiration, and blood pressure
- Explain the process of heat production/heat loss in the human body
- Measure temperature, pulse, respiration, and blood pressure
- Record temperature, pulse, respiration, and blood pressure
- Recognize variations in temperature, pulse, respiration, and blood pressure
- Define pain
- Identify ways to assess pain

Vital Signs

- Describe ways of measuring and assessing pain
- List ways to treat pain
- Recognize a client's verbal and nonverbal behaviors when obtaining vital signs
- Prepare a teaching plan for obtaining and recording a radial pulse
- Teach another person how to obtain and record a radial pulse

Key Terms

acupressure Use of fingers and hands to press on certain body points to ease pain and decrease harmful stress.

acupuncture Therapy that uses needles, inserted at specific body points, for relief of pain.

aromatherapy Use of scents or odors from herbs or flowers to promote wellness or relief from stress and pain.

blood pressure Force of the blood against the walls of the blood vessels.

diastole Phase in the cardiac cycle when the heart relaxes.

hypothalamus Part of the brain that regulates body temperature.

medulla Area in the brain that controls respirations.

pain Unpleasant bodily feeling caused by a stimulus that alerts the body to damage or a problem. May be described as sharp, dull, aching, or throbbing.

pulse Beating of the heart. May be felt or heard as a tapping sound over artery near a bony prominence.

respirations Taking in and letting out of air, during which oxygen and carbon dioxide are exchanged in the alveoli of the lungs. One inhalation (breathing in) and one exhalation (breathing out) is counted as one respiration.

sphygmomanometer Instrument used to measure blood pressure.

stethoscope Instrument used to hear sounds from inside the body; often used to listen to heart and lung sounds.

systole Phase in the cardiac cycle when the heart contracts.

temperature A measurement of the hotness or coldness of the body.

therapeutic touch Use of the practitioner's hands and the energy from the client to promote a sense of well-being. The practitioner's hands, held a few inches off the skin, are passed over the client's body.

thermometer Instrument used to measure temperature.

45

■ INTRODUCTION

Vital signs are signs of life. They are sometimes called *cardinal signs* because they are basic indicators of life itself. These include:

1. **Temperature**
2. **Pulse** or heart rate
3. **Respirations** or breathing rate
4. **Blood pressure**
5. **Pain**

The vital signs are a measurement of the working of body processes that sustain life. These processes are dependent upon each other. As one function or process is affected, the other functions are also affected. The vital signs will then be different from the usual, showing that change. For example, if a person's temperature increases because of a fever, that person's pulse (heart rate) and respiratory rate (breathing rate) will also increase as part of the body's overall response to the problem.

Obtaining and recording vital signs are entry-level competencies for a medical assistant, and are a basic part of office visits. The vital signs are important to client outcomes for several reasons. First, obtaining and recording a person's vital signs gives a baseline of what is normal or regular for that specific client. When the vital signs are obtained on future office visits, the new numbers can be compared with the previous ones. After a while, a client's normal range can be determined by looking at the records for a period of time. Second, vital-sign measurements that are outside the normal range for a specific client may mean a problem. The difference from normal may indicate sickness, or may be due to medication or treatments.

The doctor prescribes treatment based on vital signs, along with information from other examinations and tests. Thus, it is crucial to client care outcomes that medical assistants be knowledgeable about and competent in obtaining, recording, and reporting vital signs.

As a medical assistant, you will need to know what the vital signs are and understand what body functions they measure. You must be competent in obtaining these measurements.

After you obtain the vital signs, you must write the numbers correctly in the client's chart or medical record. In addition, the medical assistant must recognize and report to the doctor any findings that are outside the normal range.

You want to be professional, competent, and caring in your work with clients. In addition to competency, relating in a therapeutic way with clients will put them at ease. This will ensure that the numbers you obtain are an accurate reflection of that client's vital signs.

Finally, the medical assistant may need to teach the client, and sometimes the client's family, how to obtain some vital signs. Preparation to teach others and a sample teaching plan are included at the end of this chapter. This will guide you as you work with clients.

■ BODY TEMPERATURE

The term *temperature* refers to how hot or cold a substance, item, or body is. To sustain life, body temperature must be maintained within a specific range. (This range varies slightly depending on the way the temperature is measured.) To understand body temperature and temperature changes, it is first necessary to understand heat production and heat loss.

Heat Production

The human body constantly tries to maintain its normal temperature. To do this, it must perform a balancing act between heat production and heat loss. Within the **hypothalamus** of the brain, there are thermoregulatory centers that balance heat production and heat loss as the environment around us and conditions within us change. For example, the body must adjust when we walk into an air-conditioned room after spending time outdoors on a hot, humid day.

Heat Loss

The majority of heat loss (85%) occurs through the skin. The skin, which is the largest organ of the body, accomplishes this in several ways. First, heat is transferred to a colder object when the two objects are in contact. This is called *con-*

duction. If a person is very warm and holds onto a cold glass filled with ice, heat will be transferred from the warm hands to the glass. Second, in *radiation,* energy such as heat is transferred in the form of waves into the surrounding air. Heat radiates from the body to the cooler air around the person. Third, air currents moving over a person or substance cause heat loss by *convection.* The air currents remove the heated air closest to the person's body. For example, when a person fans herself on a hot day, the heated air closest to the skin is removed by the air currents caused by the movement of the fan. Fourth, during *evaporation,* liquid becomes a gas. When a person perspires, perspiration or sweat on the skin changes from a liquid to a gas. This process of evaporation cools the person's skin.

Measuring Body Temperature

There are several ways to obtain or take a person's temperature. A common method of measuring body temperature is to place a **thermometer** in the mouth under the tongue (Figure 4-1). This is called taking an *oral temperature.* The normal range for oral temperature is 97.5 to 99.5 degrees Fahrenheit (97.5°F to 99.5°F).

A rectal thermometer may be placed into a person's rectum; this method of measurement will yield a temperature that is 0.5°F to 1.0°F (0.28 to 0.56 degrees Celsius, or 0.28°C to 0.56°C) higher than a temperature taken orally (Figure 4-2). This is called taking a *rectal temperature.* The normal body temperature, taken rectally, ranges from 98°F to 100.6°F.

An *axillary temperature* is obtained by placing a thermometer under the arm, in the armpit (Figure 4-3). This temperature is approximately 0.5°F (0.28°C) lower than an oral temperature. The normal body temperature, taken in the axilla, ranges from 97°F to 99°F.

A person's temperature can also be measured by placing a tympanic thermometer into the external auditory canal of the ear (Figure 4-4). This is called taking an *aural temperature* or a *tympanic temperature.* (Be sure not to confuse the word *aural* with *oral,* which means "by mouth" and would indicate a temperature taken orally.)

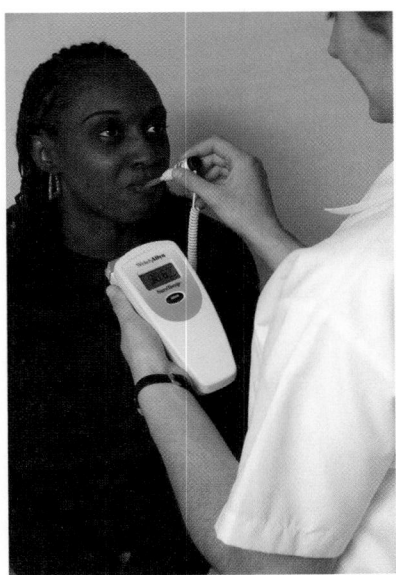

FIGURE 4-1 A medical assistant taking a client's oral temperature.

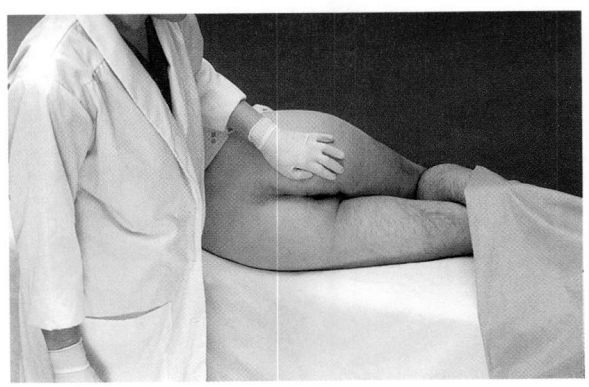

FIGURE 4-2 The medical assistant positions a client before taking a rectal temperature.

The tympanic thermometer usually has two settings, oral and rectal. If the thermometer is placed on the oral setting, the normal range would be 97.5°F to 99.5°F. If it is placed on the rectal setting, the normal range would be 98°F to 100.6°F.

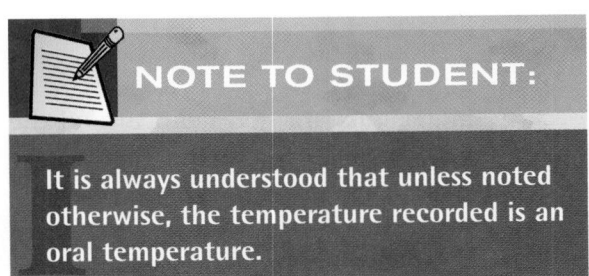

NOTE TO STUDENT:

It is always understood that unless noted otherwise, the temperature recorded is an oral temperature.

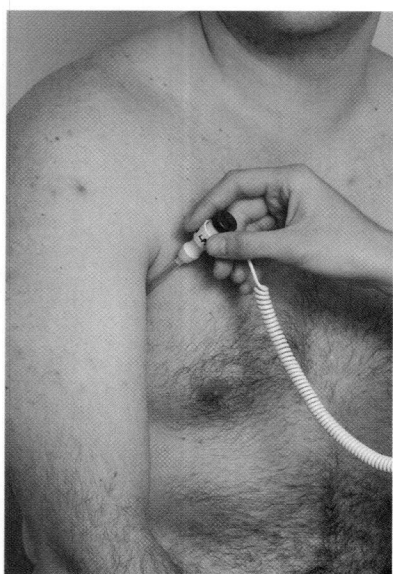

FIGURE 4-3 A medical assistant obtaining a client's axillary temperature.

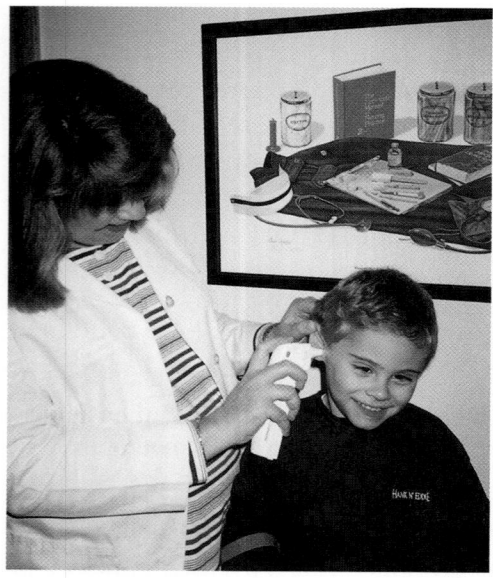

FIGURE 4-4 A medical assistant obtaining a client's temperature with a tympanic, or aural, thermometer.

Variations in Body Temperature

Because individuals are not identical and the body is constantly adjusting to the internal and external environments (stimuli), clients may show minor variations in temperature that are not caused by disease or pathological condi-

tions. Steps may be taken to prevent these variations or adjust to the cause when obtaining a temperature. Knowing the causes of these variations and their effect on body temperature will help the medical assistant. Some causes of temperature variations include:

- **Exercise.** Physical aerobic exercise will increase the body temperature as the muscles work and heat production increases.
- **Time of day.** The temperature will be the lowest in the early morning just after arising. The highest temperature within the normal variation will be observed during the late afternoon.
- **Gender.** Before menopause, women may have a slightly higher temperature at certain times of the month. At the middle of the ovulation cycle, the temperature rises and remains that way until menses (flow of menstrual blood).
- **Age.** A wider range of temperature is seen in infants and children (see Chapter 35). Elderly individuals often have temperatures lower than the usual adult range (see Chapter 34).

■ PULSE

During the cardiac cycle, the heart contracts and relaxes in a rhythmical pattern. It contracts and then relaxes, contracts and then relaxes, and so on continuously. As the ventricles contract to send blood through the body, the arteries expand and recoil. This expansion and recoiling sends a wave throughout the body. This wave is felt as a pulsation called a *pulse.* The pulse correlates to the number of heartbeats. The medical assistant needs to understand the significance of the pulse, which is an important indicator of heart function (Figure 4-5). Measuring the pulse includes noting the *aspects* of rate, rhythm, and volume or force.

Measuring Pulses

Several easily accessible sites on the body are used to determine the rate, rhythm, and volume

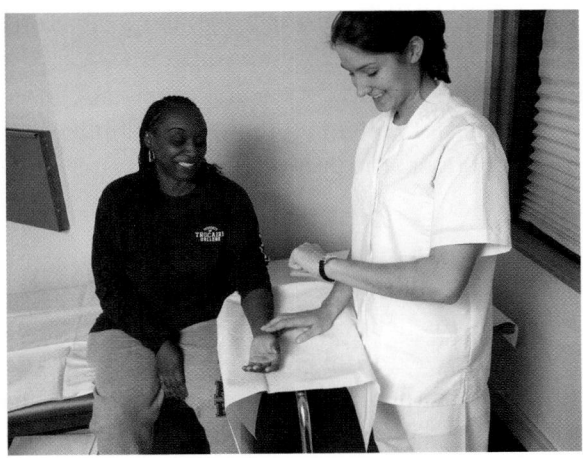

FIGURE 4–5 A medical assistant obtaining a client's radial pulse.

of a pulse (Table 4-1 and Figure 4-6). The medical assistant uses the pads of the first two fingers of either hand to feel the pulse; at some body points, a **stethoscope** is used to listen for the pulse (Figure 4-7).

Rate, Rhythm, and Volume

The medical assistant can check all three aspects of the pulse, which include the rate, rhythm, and volume. The *pulse rate* or number is determined by counting the number of beats or taps felt or heard in one minute.

The rhythm of the pulse is also an important part of pulse measurement. *Rhythm* refers to the interval or space between each beat. A healthy heart will have equal intervals or spaces between beats; these are referred to as *regular*. If the time between beats is unequal or erratic, the pulse is referred to as *irregular.*

The *volume* is the force of the pulse. The force of the pulse will be felt as strong if the heart is pumping effectively. If the heart is not beating effectively, the pulse may feel weak or thready. A very forceful pulse is called *bounding.*

Variations in Pulse

The normal pulse range for an adult is 60 to 100 beats per minute. Several factors can influence the pulse rate:

- **Age.** Infants and young children have a faster pulse than adults.
- **Fitness or athletic condition.** An athlete will have a slower pulse as a result of having a well-conditioned, effective heart muscle.
- **Sleep.** During periods of sleep or deep relaxation, the pulse will be slower.

Certain conditions and/or substances can also have an effect on the pulse (heart) rate:

- The nicotine in cigarette smoke will increase the heart rate.
- Cocaine and other drugs increase the heart rate.

TABLE 4–1 Pulse sites.

Apical	Pulse heard over the apex of the heart. A stethoscope is placed at the fifth intercostal space at the junction (connecting point) of the left midclavicular line.
Brachial	Pulse felt over the brachial artery, in the bend of the elbow in either arm.
Carotid	Pulse felt over the carotid artery on each side of (lateral to) the midline of the neck.
Dorsalis pedis	Pulse felt over the dorsalis pedis artery between the first and second metatarsal bones, midway up from the great toe of either foot.
Femoral	Pulse felt over the femoral artery, in the middle of the groin of either leg.
Popliteal	Pulse felt over the popliteal artery, behind the knee of either leg.
Radial	Pulse felt over the radial artery, on the inside of either wrist near the bony prominence by the thumb.
Temporal	Pulse felt over the temporal area of the head, above and in front of either ear.

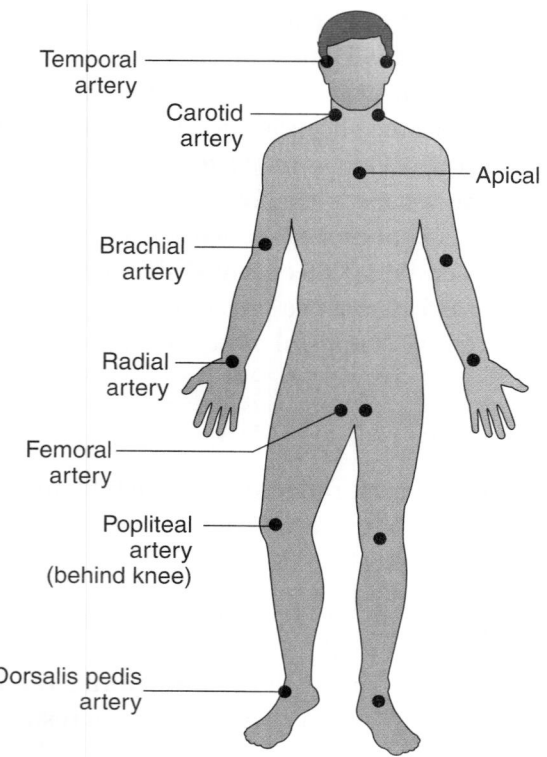

FIGURE 4–6 Pulse sites on the body.

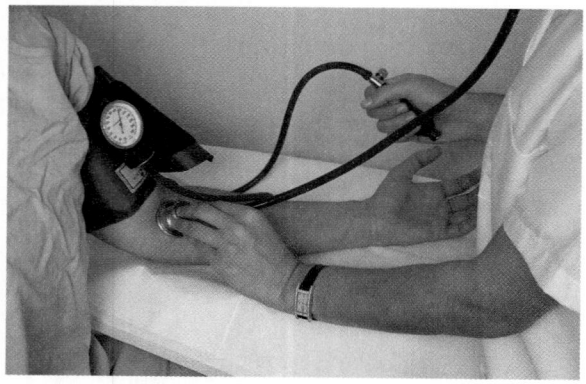

FIGURE 4–7 The medical assistant listens with a stethoscope at the brachial pulse.

- The caffeine found in many products, such as coffee and cola drinks, will speed up the heart rate.
- Medications may increase the heart rate. For example, theophylline (a bronchodilator used in the treatment of respiratory conditions) and other sympathomimetic drugs will stimulate the heart and thus increase the pulse rate. Other medications may also have the same effect.
- During illness accompanied by fever (febrile), anemia (low hemoglobin levels), or shock, the pulse rate will be faster.

■ RESPIRATION

Respiration is defined as the exchange of gases between the external environment (outside the person) and the internal environment (cells in the body). This process is controlled by the **medulla** area of the brain and the buildup of carbon dioxide (CO_2) in the blood. The medulla is also called the respiratory center of the brain.

Ventilation is the act of breathing. When a person takes in air (inhalation), the diaphragm (a large, disc-shaped muscle between the thoracic chest cavity and the abdominal cavity) contracts and flattens. This creates more space for the chest cavity to expand. When a person lets out the air (exhalation), the diaphragm relaxes and the chest cavity decreases in size (see Chapter 15).

Measuring Respiration

The rate of respiration is measured by counting the number of breaths per minute (Figure 4-8). Breathing in (one inhalation) and then breathing out (one exhalation) are counted as one respiration or one full breath. The normal range of respiration for an adult is 12 to 20 breaths per minute.

NOTE TO STUDENT:

Avoid staring at a client's chest when counting respirations. The person may become uncomfortable and, without realizing it, alter or change the breathing pattern. As a result, the number of breaths counted may not be an accurate reflection of the client's breathing pattern.

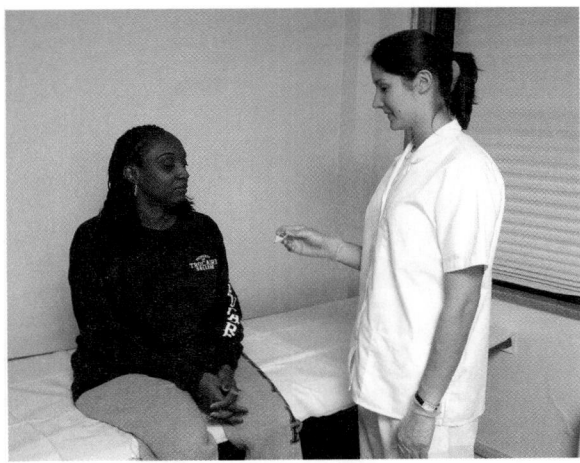

FIGURE 4-8 A medical assistant counting a client's respirations.

Variations in Respiration

The medical assistant needs to recognize causes of variations in the rate of respiration. Some common causes that are not related to disease conditions are:

- **Exercise.** Aerobic exercise, or any strenuous work or activity for which a person is not conditioned, can increase the respiratory rate.
- **Emotion.** Fear, anger, and excitement can increase the respiratory rate.
- **High altitude.** Individuals who are unaccustomed to high altitudes may experience an increase in respirations when in high-altitude areas.

■ BLOOD PRESSURE

Blood pressure is the force exerted by the blood against the arterial walls. When the ventricles of the heart contract (during the **systole** phase of the cardiac cycle), the pressure created is termed *systolic.* The normal systolic range is 90 to 139 millimeters of mercury (mm Hg). When the ventricles of the heart relax while refilling with blood (during the **diastole** phase of the cardiac cycle), the pressure measured is called *diastolic.* The normal diastolic range is 60 to 89 mm Hg.

The normal range for a blood pressure reading is 90 to 139 mm Hg systolic and 60 to 89 mm

Hg diastolic. This is expressed as 90–139/60–89. Healthy individuals may exhibit lower blood pressure. It is essential that a client's blood pressure be taken at all visits (Figure 4-9). This helps to establish the individual's baseline and aids in understanding any variations in readings obtained for future visits.

Measuring Blood Pressure

The medical assistant will measure a client's blood pressure using a stethoscope and a **sphygmomanometer** (Figure 4-10). A common site for measuring blood pressure is the brachial artery on either arm. (For complete step-by-step measurement of blood pressure, see Procedure 4-9.)

Variations in Blood Pressure

Several factors can cause the blood pressure to vary from the normal range:

- **Talking.** The client should remain silent while the medical assistant obtains the blood pressure. Talking during the procedure can increase the blood pressure.
- **Smoking.** Smoking can increase blood pressure.
- **Caffeine.** The caffeine found in coffee, tea, and many cola drinks can elevate the blood pressure.
- **Emotion.** Clients are often anxious or worried when they come to a health care provider, whether or not they have a serious

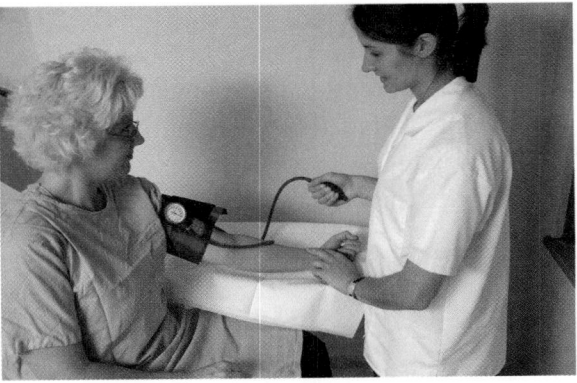

FIGURE 4-9 The medical assistant obtains a client's blood pressure as part of taking the vital signs.

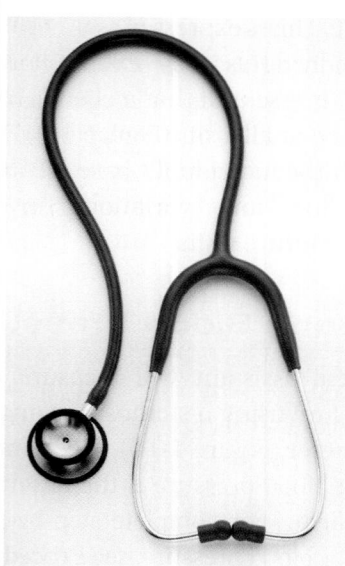

FIGURE 4-10A Stethoscope. *(Courtesy of Welch Allyn)*

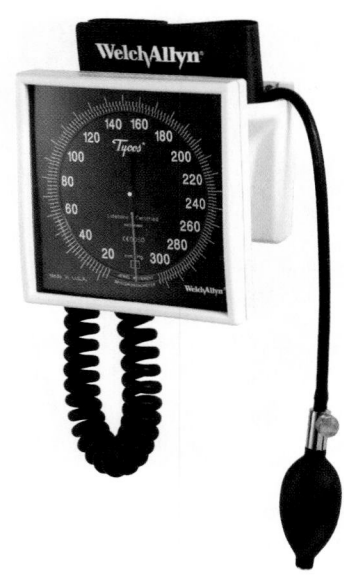

FIGURE 4-10B Aneroid sphygmomanometer. *(Courtesy of Welch Allyn)*

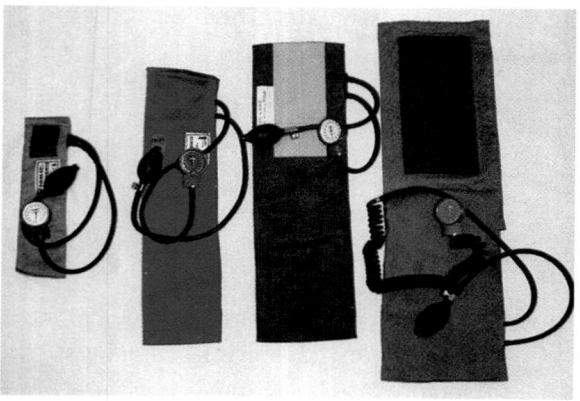

FIGURE 4-10C Different sizes of blood pressure cuffs, ranging from cuffs small enough to fit a child's arm to large enough to fit an adult's thigh.

condition or are in **pain.** Even when scheduled for a routine visit, some people worry about what might be done or what the doctor might say. These clients may or may not express their feelings of nervousness.

NOTE TO STUDENT:

The medical assistant must be aware of client behaviors that might indicate nervousness. Nervousness or agitation can cause a common condition called "white coat hypertension," which is temporary. To verify this temporary rise in blood pressure and not miss true hypertension, the medical assistant should take the blood pressure in a more relaxing setting. If the medical assistant suspects that a client has white coat hypertension, she should wait until the examination or procedures are complete, thereby allowing the client to relax, and then repeat the blood pressure measurement.

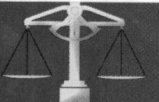

LEGAL/ETHICAL THOUGHTS

Family members may ask questions such as "What is her blood pressure?" Remember that it is up to the client to decide what information can be given out and to whom.

◼ PAIN

According to the International Association for the Study of Pain (IASP), "Pain is an unpleasant sensory and emotional experience associated with actual or potential tissue damage, or described in terms of such damage." Pain is both a physical and an emotional experience. The Joint Commission on Accreditation of Healthcare Organizations (JCAHO) has set standards or rules about pain assessment and management that accredited health care organizations must follow and most other health care providers follow voluntarily. As a medical assistant, you want to be aware of a client's pain and her perception of that pain (Figure 4-11). How you communicate with the client and your response to the client's concerns will greatly affect the client's course of care.

Pain can prevent a person from performing everyday activities. This is especially true of acute, sudden-onset pain. Pain is the body's warning sign that something is wrong. Acute pain is not a sensation that a person can ignore or pretend that it does not exist. It interferes with normal activities. The purpose of pain is to alert the individual to remove or relieve the cause of the pain. Therefore, acute pain does not stop until it is responded to or the cause of the pain no longer exists.

Chronic pain (also called *persistent pain)* is defined as pain that lasts over a period of time.

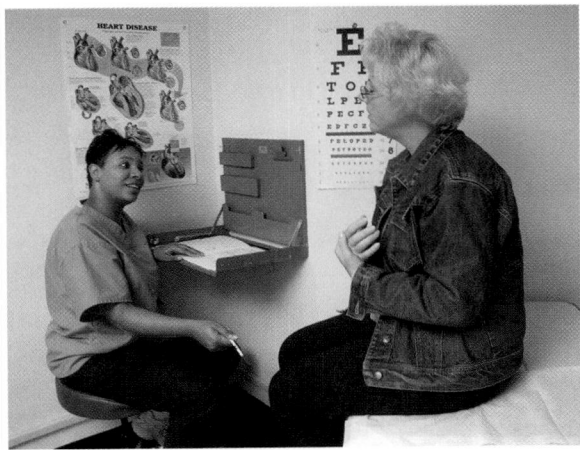

FIGURE 4–11 The medical assistant listens attentively to a client talking about her painful arm.

Chronic pain that is not controlled is exhausting, because the client's mental and physical energy are focused on the pain or working around the pain. Thus, the client may complain of fatigue or feeling extremely tired. People cope with pain in different ways. Some ways are helpful, but other coping mechanisms are harmful. Ineffective coping mechanisms or strategies can even raise a person's risk of depression. Also, the client's ability to carry out ADLs (activities of daily living) may be hindered. This loss of independence can further complicate a person's health outcomes.

Measuring Pain

Instruments to standardize the measurement of pain are available, and new ones are currently being developed. The medical assistant will need to gather data regarding clients' pain. This data can come from both verbal and nonverbal cues.

The medical assistant needs to ask the client if she is experiencing pain. Not every person who has pain will raise the issue first; the client may be waiting for the health care provider to ask about it. Some clients may not want to bother the busy health care provider with this problem. Especially if the client is older, she may also feel that pain is something a person just has to live with.

Variations in Pain

The medical assistant will gather as much information as possible regarding the client's pain, including:

- **Location.** Ask the client to locate the pain. Where does it hurt? The client may be able to point to the area. (Remember anatomical position and points when charting the location.)
- **Description.** Ask the client to use her own words and terminology to explain what the pain is like. When charting, use the client's words to describe the pain.
- **Intensity.** How strong or uncomfortable is the pain? Can the client perform everyday activities? Does the pain affect going out of the home? Does the client cancel plans because of the pain?

TABLE 4-2 Treatments for pain.

NAME	DESCRIPTION	CAUTION
Herbal supplements	Substances taken by mouth or applied directly to a body part.	May have harmful effects or interactions with client's other medications.
Acupuncture	Needles inserted at specific points in the body; stimulate electrical/energy pathways to help the body heal itself.	Need to know the qualifications of the acupuncture provider who inserts the needles.
Acupressure	Similar to acupuncture, but uses finger pressure at specific body sites instead of needles.	Need to know the qualifications of the acupressure provider.
Massage	Uses provider's hands to rub or knead the body's muscles; may be helpful for mild to moderate pain.	If pain increases, need to inform therapist and seek assistance for other pain relief measures.
Therapeutic touch	Palms of hands held about two inches from client's body to sense problems and increase/rebalance energy flow.	Because there is no direct contact with the client's body, there is little chance of any problem with this method.
Aromatherapy	Essential oils are applied to the skin or sprayed into the air. The client inhales the aroma.	Make sure client is not allergic to the substance and does not dislike the aroma before using it as a treatment.
Imagery	Uses thought or imagination of different scenes and situations to calm and reduce pain. Another person may talk a client through this process, or the client may follow a CD or tape.	Works best when led by a skilled person who can guide the client until the client can do the imagery process independently.
Music therapy	Uses various types of music to help decrease pain.	Client should select type of music; a poor choice may cause agitation or an increase in pain.

- **Duration.** When does the pain occur, and how long does it last? Does activity make the pain worse? Is it worse in the morning or at night?
- **Precipitating factors.** What seems to cause the pain? If the client does not know, ask what is going on right before the pain begins.
- **Alleviation.** Does anything make the pain better? If so, what?

Treatment for Pain

In addition to medication, several other treatments are available to ease pain. Although the doctor will decide which treatments are best suited to the particular client, medical assistants need to be aware of these treatments. This will help the medical assistant to answer questions while observing for pain relief in the client. Table 4-2 lists some of the more common treatments used for pain relief.

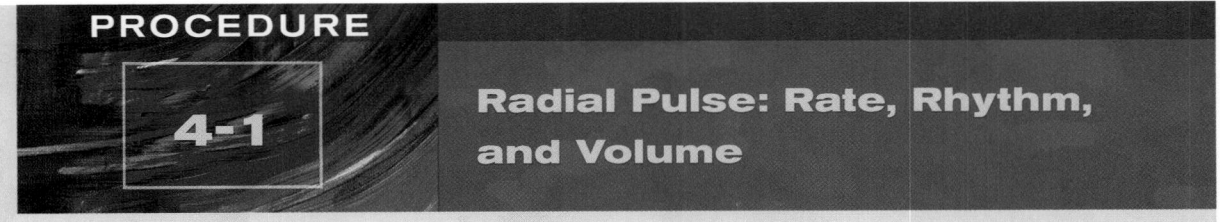

PROCEDURE

4-1

Radial Pulse: Rate, Rhythm, and Volume

Student Competency Objective: The medical assistant student will find, obtain, and record the radial pulse rate, rhythm, and volume.

Items Needed: Watch with sweep second hand, paper, pen or pencil

Steps:

1. Wash your hands.
2. Get items needed.
3. Introduce yourself to the client even if you have seen the client on previous visits to your office. The client may have forgotten your name. This also helps to establish a provider-client relationship, because it shows the client that you want her to know who you are.
4. Identify the client. Ask the client to state her name to establish that this is the right client, and then compare the name given to the name on the chart. Never enter a room and call out a client's name to determine if this person is the correct client. The client may not have heard you clearly and may just nod, smile, or answer yes. Clients almost never question if the medical assistant professional has the right client. It is up to the medical assistant to identify the right client before performing any procedure.
5. Tell the client, in everyday language, what you are going to do.
6. Ask if the client has any questions. If she does, give short and simple answers. Sometimes clients will start (and continue) talking because they are nervous about the procedure.
7. If the client is sitting, ask her to rest her arm comfortably on a table or other supportive surface that will keep the wrist at heart level (Figure 4–12).
8. If the client is lying down, place her arm across her chest.
9. Place the pads of your first two fingers on the radial site, which is located near the wrist on the thumb side.
10. Apply steady, gentle pressure. Too much pressure will obliterate or cause the pulsation to disappear. Never use your thumb, because the thumb has its own pulse and you may mistakenly count your own heart rate.
11. Count each tap or pulsation felt for 30 seconds and multiply by 2.

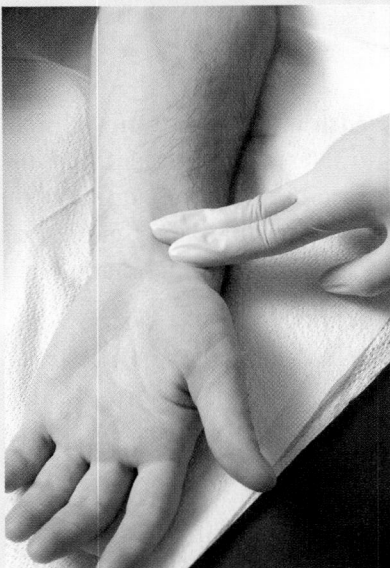

FIGURE 4–12 Instruct the client to rest the arm comfortably on a table (or other supportive surface) that will keep the wrist at heart level. The medical assistant places the pads of the first two fingers on the client's radial site.

(Continues)

PROCEDURE 4-1 (Continued)

12. While counting the pulse beats, note if the beats are regular and equally spaced (that is, whether the time between each beat is the same).

13. Note the volume or force while counting. Does the pulse feel strong, bounding (too forceful), or thready (weak)?

Charting Example:

You counted 40 beats in 30 seconds, equally spaced, and the pulse felt strong as you counted. You would record the following:

P80 regular and strong

Mary Smith, S. M. A.

Mary Smith, S.M.A. (printed name)

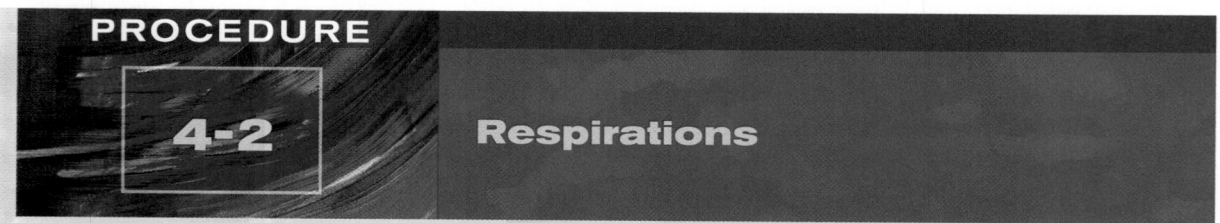

PROCEDURE 4-2 Respirations

Student Competency Objective: The medical assistant student will find, obtain, and record respiration rate, rhythm, and depth, while noting any sounds heard while the client is breathing in and out.

Items Needed: Watch with sweep second hand, paper, pen or pencil

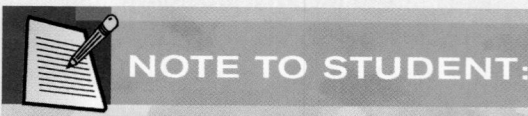

NOTE TO STUDENT:

One inhalation (breathing in) and one exhalation (breathing out) counts as one respiration.

Steps:

1. Wash your hands.

2. Get items needed.

3. Introduce yourself to the client even if you have seen the client on previous visits to your office. The client may have forgotten your name. This also helps to establish a provider-client relationship, because it shows the client that you want her to know who you are.

4. Identify the client. Ask the client to state her name to establish that this is the right client, and then compare the name given to the name on the chart. Never enter a room and call out a client's name to determine if this person is the correct client. The client may not have heard you clearly and may just nod, smile, or answer yes. Clients almost never question if the medical assistant professional has the right client. It is up to the medical assistant to identify the right client before performing any procedure.

5. Tell the client, in everyday language, what you are going to do.

(Continues)

PROCEDURE 4-2 (Continued)

6. Ask if the client has any questions. If she does, give short and simple answers. Sometimes clients will start (and continue) talking because they are nervous about the procedure.

7. If the client is sitting, ask her to rest her arm on a surface (table, chair arm, etc.) that will comfortably support the arm.

8. If the client is lying down, rest the client's arm across her chest.

9. Place the pads of the first two fingers of your hand on the radial site (the same as the radial pulse position).

10. Watch the rise and fall of the client's chest and count the number of respirations for 30 seconds (breathing in and out counts as one respiration). Do not stare at the client's chest, as this may make the client uncomfortable. Without being aware of it, the client who knows that her respirations are being counted may alter her breathing pattern. As a result, the respiration measurement may not accurately reflect the client's true breathing pattern.

11. Multiply the number of respirations counted by 2 and record that number.

12. Record the rhythm. Is the time (space) between each breath equal or the same? (If spacing is equal, the pattern is recorded as regular; if the time between breaths is not equal, the pattern is recorded as irregular.)

13. Record the depth. Is the rise and fall of the chest minimal, small (shallow), moderate (easy to see but not exaggerated), or deep (very noticeable rise and fall)?

Charting Example:

If you counted a respiration rate of 16, with equal spacing and small movement of the chest. You would record the following:

R16 regular and shallow

Mary Smith, S.M.A.

Mary Smith, S.M.A. (printed name)

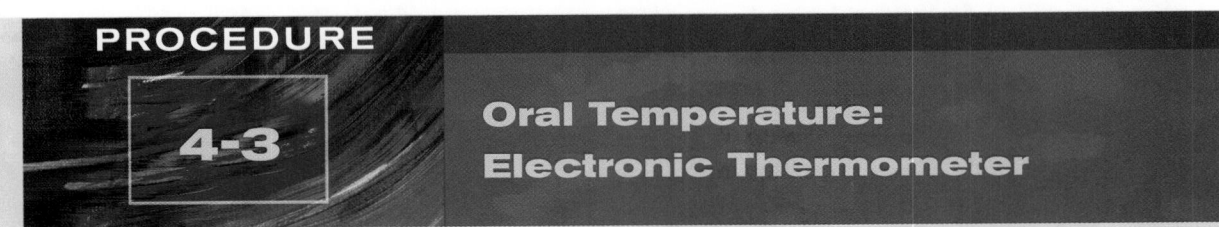

PROCEDURE 4-3

Oral Temperature: Electronic Thermometer

Student Competency Objective: The medical assistant student will obtain and record an oral temperature using an electronic thermometer.

Items Needed: Electronic thermometer, probe cover, biohazardous waste container, paper, pen or pencil

Steps:

1. Wash your hands.
2. Get items needed.

(Continues)

PROCEDURE 4-3 (Continued)

3. Introduce yourself to the client even if you have seen the client on previous visits to your office. The client may have forgotten your name. This also helps to establish a provider–client relationship, because it shows the client that you want her to know who you are.

4. Identify the client. Ask the client to state her name to establish that this is the right client, and then compare the name given to the name on the chart. Never enter a room and call out a client's name to determine if this person is the correct client. The client may not have heard you clearly and may just nod, smile, or answer yes. Clients almost never question if the medical assistant professional has the right client. It is up to the medical assistant to identify the right client before performing any procedure.

5. Tell the client, in everyday language, what you are going to do.

6. Ask if the client has any questions. If she does, give short and simple answers. Sometimes clients will start (and continue) talking because they are nervous about the procedure.

7. If there is a probe connector for the electronic thermometer, put it in the unit base holder (Figure 4–13A).

8. Holding the probe by the collar (the thick piece between the probe and the connecting coiled cord), take the probe from its holder.

9. Push the probe into a probe cover. You must do this with a firm movement to make sure the probe cover does not fall off (Figure 4–13B).

10. Ask the client to open her mouth; then place the probe in her mouth (Figure 4–13C).

11. Tell the client to keep the lips closed.

12. Hold the thermometer probe cover to keep it steady while in the probe is in the client's mouth. The probe and coiled cord are heavy.

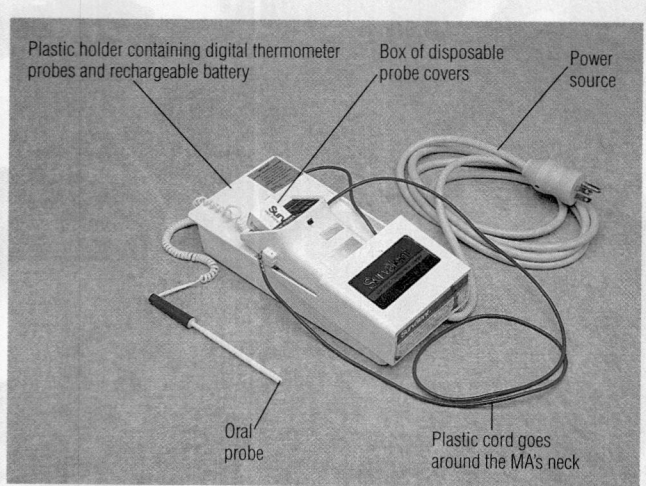

FIGURE 4–13A An electronic thermometer.

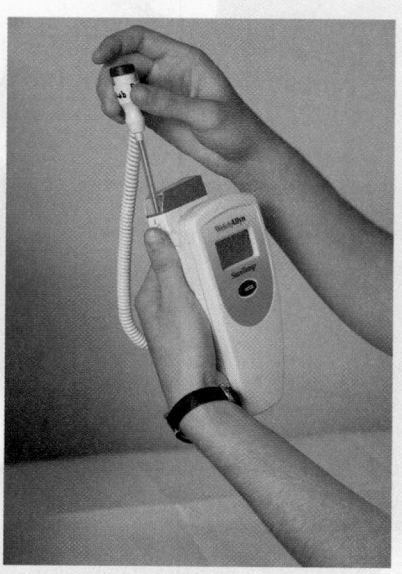

FIGURE 4–13B When using an electronic thermometer, take the probe by the collar, remove it from its holder, and push the probe into the probe cover.

(Continues)

PROCEDURE 4-3 (Continued)

13. Hold the probe steady for approximately 10 seconds until the unit makes a noise meaning that the measurement is complete.

14. Remove the probe from the client's mouth without touching the probe cover (Figure 4-13D).

15. Read the temperature number that is showing on the thermometer's screen.

16. Push the button to eject the probe cover directly into the biohazardous waste container (Figure 4-13E).

17. Put the probe back into its unit. The thermometer will shut off.

18. Wash your hands.

19. Make sure to record the temperature reading immediately.

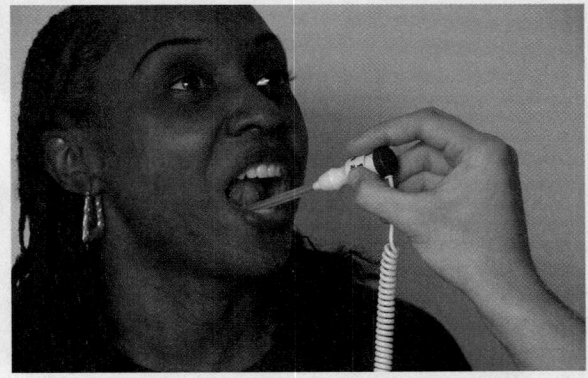

FIGURE 4–13C Place the thermometer under the client's tongue.

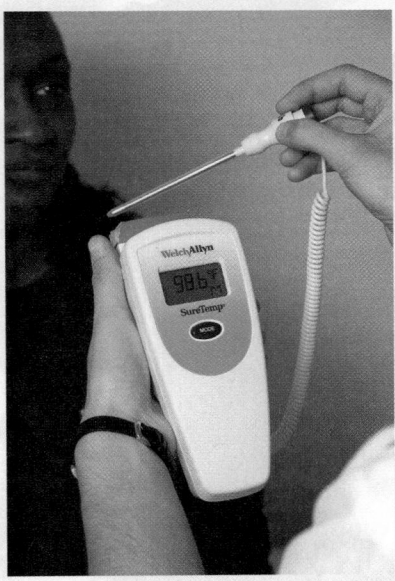

FIGURE 4–13D Remove the thermometer from the client's mouth without touching the probe cover, and read the number on the display.

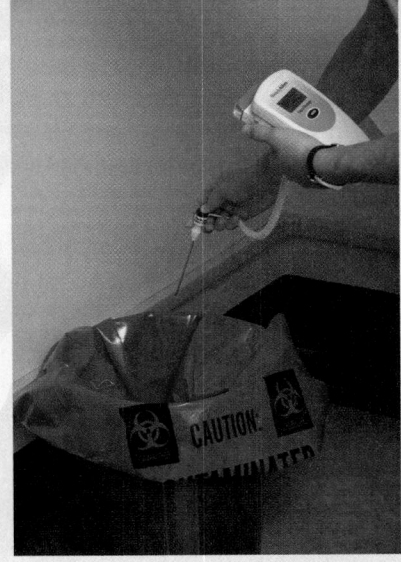

FIGURE 4–13E Push the ejection button to discard the probe cover; dispose of the cover directly into a biohazardous waste container.

Charting Example:

The thermometer screen reads 98.2. You would record the following:

      10/12/20xx   T 98.2

      Thomas Jones, S.M.A

      Thomas Jones, S.M.A. (printed name)

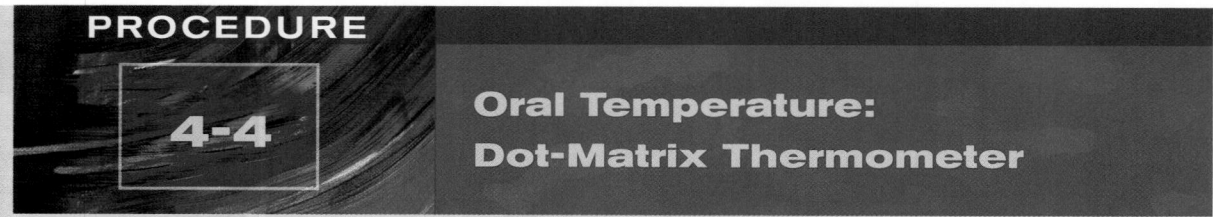

PROCEDURE

4-4

Oral Temperature: Dot-Matrix Thermometer

Student Competency Objective: The medical assistant student will obtain and record an oral temperature using a dot-matrix, single-use thermometer.

Items Needed: Dot-matrix, single-use thermometer (Figure 4-14A), watch, waste container, paper, pen or pencil

Steps:

1. Wash your hands.
2. Get items needed.
3. Introduce yourself to the client even if you have seen the client on previous visits to your office. The client may have forgotten your name. This also helps to establish a provider-client relationship, because it shows the client that you want her to know who you are.
4. Identify the client. Ask the client to state her name to establish that this is the right client, and then compare the name given to the name on the chart. Never enter a room and call out a client's name to determine if this person is the correct client. The client may not have heard you clearly and may just nod, smile, or answer yes. Clients almost never question if the medical assistant professional has the right client. It is up to the medical assistant to identify the right client before performing any procedure.
5. Tell the client, in everyday language, what you are going to do.
6. Ask if the client has any questions. If she does, give short and simple answers. Sometimes clients will start (and continue) talking because they are nervous about the procedure.
7. Ask the client to open her mouth. Put the thermometer under her tongue toward the back. The dots on the thermometer may be facing up or down.
8. Ask the client to keep her tongue down on the thermometer and keep the thermometer in her mouth for 60 seconds.
9. After 60 seconds, remove the thermometer. Wait a few seconds as the color on the dots locks in.
10. Read and write down the number at the last colored dot. Ignore any skipped dots (Figure 4-14B).

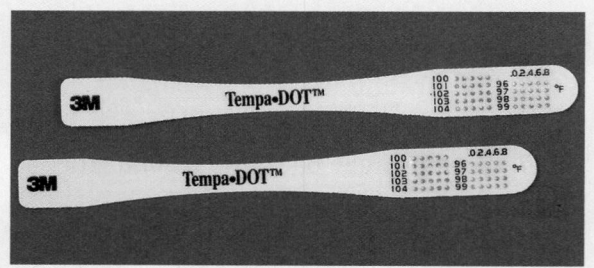

FIGURE 4-14A Disposable dot-matrix thermometer.

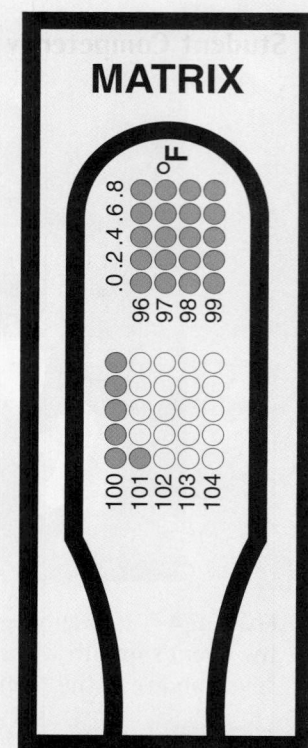

FIGURE 4-14B Read the temperature by looking at the last changed colored dot.

(Continues)

PROCEDURE 4-4 (Continued)

11. Dispose of the used thermometer in a waste container.
12. Wash your hands.

Charting Example:
The colored dots on the thermometer read 101.0. You would record the following:

10/16/20xx   T = 101.0

Jim Smith, S.M.A.

Jim Smith, S.M.A. (printed name)

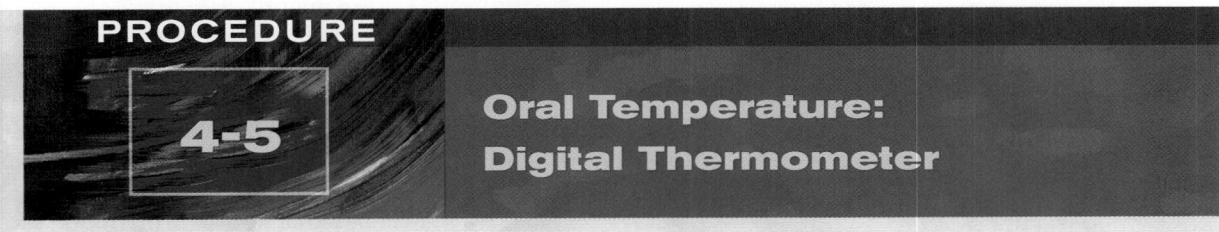

PROCEDURE

4-5 Oral Temperature: Digital Thermometer

Student Competency Objective: The medical assistant student will obtain and record an oral temperature using a digital thermometer.

Items Needed: Digital thermometer, probe cover, biohazardous waste container, paper, pen or pencil

Steps:
1. Wash your hands.
2. Get items needed.
3. Familiarize yourself with the parts of a digital thermometer: the probe or sensor, the display window, and the on-off or multifunction button.
4. Introduce yourself to the client even if you have seen the client on previous visits to your office. The client may have forgotten your name. This also helps to establish a provider-client relationship, because it shows the client that you want her to know who you are.
5. Identify the client. Ask the client to state her name to establish that this is the right client, and then compare the name given to the name on the chart. Never enter a room and call out a client's name to determine if this person is the correct client. The client may not have heard you clearly and may just nod, smile, or answer yes. Clients almost never question if the medical assistant professional has the right client. It is up to the medical assistant to identify the right client before performing any procedure.
6. Tell the client, in everyday language, what you are going to do.
7. Ask if the client has any questions. If she does, give short and simple answers. Sometimes clients will start (and continue) talking because they are nervous about the procedure.
8. Push the on-off button on the thermometer.
9. The display window will read 188.8 F ~ M. (This shows that the unit is functioning properly.) If a different symbol is flashing, the battery may be low.

(Continues)

PROCEDURE 4-5 (Continued)

10. The display window will flash F or C (Fahrenheit or Celsius) to show that the unit is ready. Digital thermometers can be switched between Fahrenheit and Celsius scales. To switch to the other measurement scale, hold down the multifunction button (follow the manufacturer's directions for the specific unit you are using).

11. Ask the client to open her mouth. Put the thermometer under the client's tongue, toward the back.

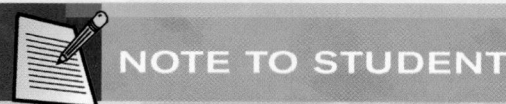

NOTE TO STUDENT:

The temperature recorded is stored in a digital thermometer's memory until the next temperature measurement is made. If you need to recheck, push the on-off button. The figure "188.8" will light up and then the stored temperature reading will display for 2 seconds.

12. Ask the client to keep her tongue down on the thermometer and keep it in her mouth.

13. After the number has stopped flashing, remove the thermometer from the client's mouth. The display window will continue to flash until the temperature reading is complete.

14. Read and write down the number from the display window.

15. Discard the probe cover directly into the biohazardous waste container.

16. Push the on-off button.

17. Clean the thermometer tip with an alcohol wipe.

18. Store the thermometer in its protective case.

19. Wash your hands.

20. Record your findings in the client's chart.

Charting Example:
The display window on the digital thermometer reads 98.8. You would record the following:

      08/17/20xx   T = 98.8

      Jennifer Bench, S.M.A.

      Jennifer Bench, S.M.A. (printed name)

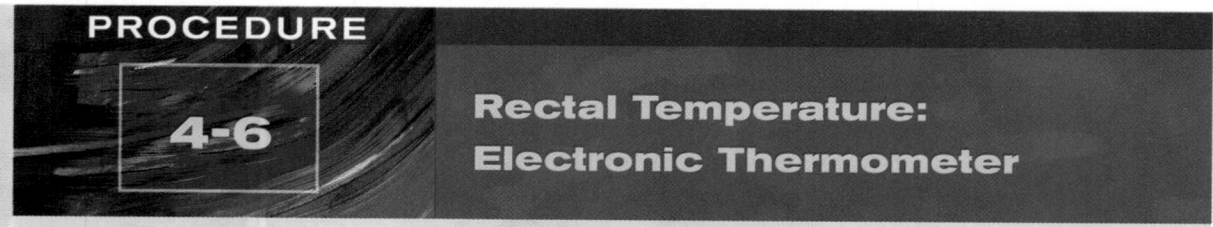

PROCEDURE

4-6

Rectal Temperature: Electronic Thermometer

Student Competency Objective: The medical assistant student will obtain and record a rectal temperature using an electronic thermometer.

Items Needed: Electronic thermometer, rectal probe cover, gloves, biohazardous waste container, paper, pen or pencil

(Continues)

PROCEDURE 4-6 (Continued)

Steps:

1. Wash your hands.
2. Get items needed.
3. Introduce yourself to the client even if you have seen the client on previous visits to your office. The client may have forgotten your name. This also helps to establish a provider-client relationship, because it shows the client that you want her to know who you are.
4. Identify the client. Ask the client to state her name to establish that this is the right client, and then compare the name given to the name on the chart. Never enter a room and call out a client's name to determine if this person is the correct client. The client may not have heard you clearly and may just nod, smile, or answer yes. Clients almost never question if the medical assistant professional has the right client. It is up to the medical assistant to identify the right client before performing any procedure.
5. Tell the client, in everyday language, what you are going to do (Figure 4-15).
6. Ask if the client has any questions. If she does, give short and simple answers. Sometimes clients will start (and continue) talking because they are nervous about the procedure.
7. Put on gloves.
8. If there is a probe connector for the electronic thermometer, put it in the unit base holder.
9. Holding the probe by the collar (the thick piece between the probe and the connecting coil cord), take the probe from its holder.
10. Push the probe into a probe cover. You must push with a firm movement to make sure the probe cover does not fall off.

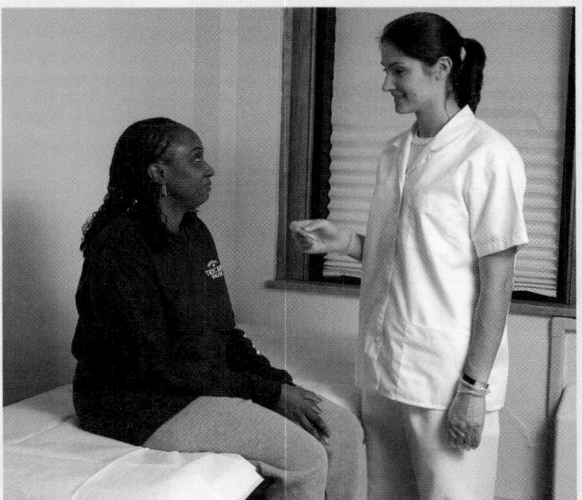

FIGURE 4-15 Explain the procedure and allow the client to ask any questions she may have about the procedure.

11. Assist the client to lie on her side. If the client is on the left side, her left leg should be slightly flexed (bent) at the knee and the right leg sharply flexed at the knee.
12. Drape the client to ensure privacy.
13. Make sure the probe is lubricated (with a water-soluble lubricant).
14. With one gloved hand, lift the client's buttock to expose the anus (rectal opening).
15. With the other gloved hand, gently insert the probe into the client's anus.
16. Hold the probe in place until the thermometer makes a noise meaning that the temperature measurement is complete.
17. Remove the probe from the client without touching the probe cover.
18. Cover the client's buttock with the drape.

(Continues)

PROCEDURE 4-6 (Continued)

19. Read the temperature number shown on the thermometer's screen.
20. Push the button to eject the probe cover directly into the biohazardous waste container.
21. Remove your gloves and dispose of them in a waste container.
22. Put the probe back into the unit. The thermometer will shut off.
23. Assist the client as needed to adjust clothing and sit up.
24. Wash your hands.

Charting Example:

The thermometer screen reads 100.2. You would record the following:

      11/2/20xx   T100.2 R.

      Jean Martin, S.M.A.

      Jean Martin, S.M.A. (printed name)

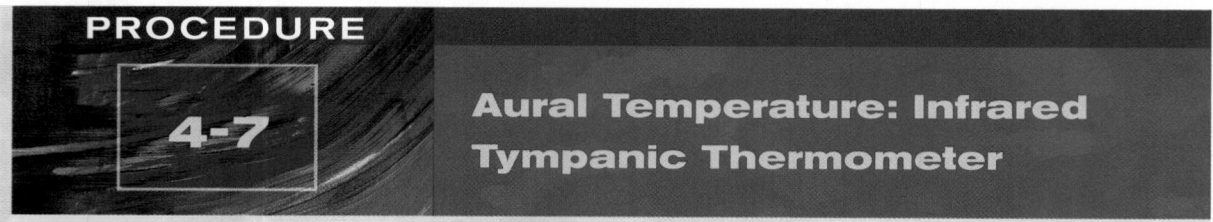

PROCEDURE 4-7

Aural Temperature: Infrared Tympanic Thermometer

Student Competency Objective: The medical assistant student will obtain and record a body temperature using an infrared tympanic (aural, ear) thermometer.

Items Needed: Tympanic thermometer, probe cover, waste container, paper, pen or pencil

Steps:

1. Wash your hands.
2. Get items needed.
3. Introduce yourself to the client even if you have seen the client on previous visits to your office. The client may have forgotten your name. This also helps to establish a provider–client relationship, because it shows the client that you want her to know who you are.
4. Identify the client. Ask the client to state her name to establish that this is the right client, and then compare the name given to the name on the chart. Never enter a room and call out a client's name to determine if this person is the correct client. The client may not have heard you clearly and may just nod, smile, or answer yes. Clients almost never question if the medical assistant professional has the right client. It is up to the medical assistant to identify the right client before performing any procedure.
5. Tell the client, in everyday language, what you are going to do.
6. Ask if the client has any questions. If she does, give short and simple answers. Sometimes clients will start (and continue) talking because they are nervous about the procedure.

(Continues)

PROCEDURE 4-7 (Continued)

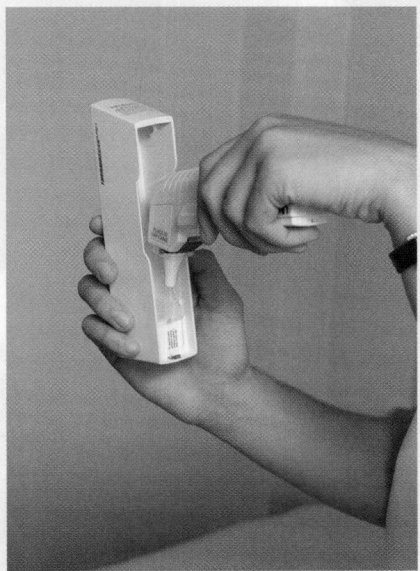

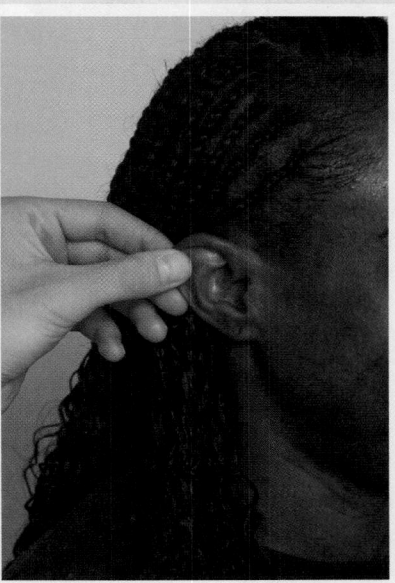

FIGURE 4–16A Put the disposable cover over the thermometer probe.

FIGURE 4–16B Gently pull the client's ear back and up to straighten the ear canal.

7. Put the probe cover on the ear–probe part of the thermometer (Figure 4–16A). The screen should flash "READY."

8. Pull gently on the client's ear to straighten the ear canal (Figure 4–16B).

9. Put the covered probe into the client's ear canal. The probe must fit securely and make a good seal, but be gentle when inserting it (Figure 4–16C).

10. Press the scan button; this will start the thermometer.

11. The thermometer will sound (beep) in about five seconds.

12. Take the probe out of the client's ear.

13. Read the temperature number shown on the screen (Figure 4–16D). Write down the number followed by T (for Fahrenheit measurements) or Tc (for Celsius measurements).

14. Press the release button to dispose of the probe cover directly into a waste container (Figure 4–16E).

15. Place the thermometer unit back on its base.

16. Wash your hands.

Charting Example:

The thermometer screen shows 99.2. You would record the following:

        11/1/20xx   99.2 T

        Andrew Harmon, S.M.A.

        Andrew Harmon, S.M.A. (printed name)

(Continues)

PROCEDURE 4-7 (Continued)

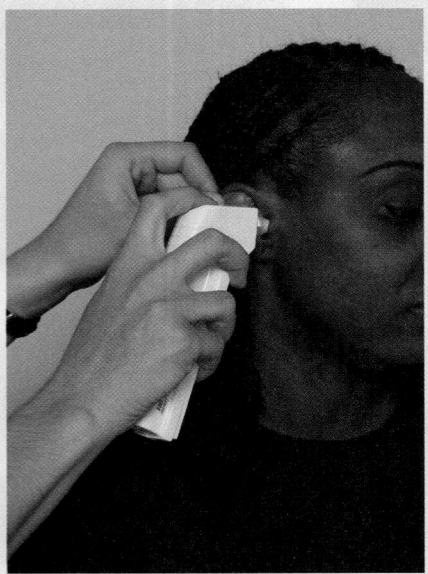

FIGURE 4–16C Place the probe in the client's ear so that it fits securely.

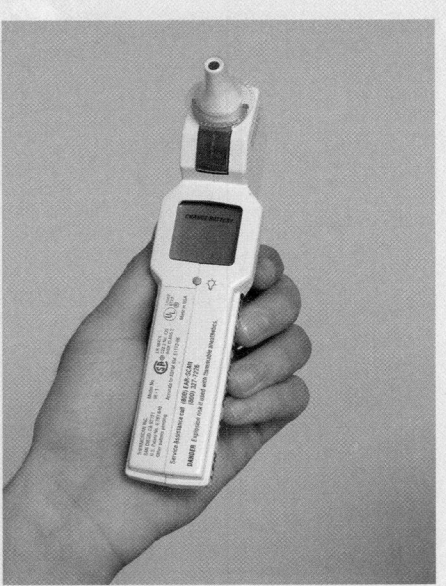

FIGURE 4–16D Remove the probe after the signal, and read the number displayed.

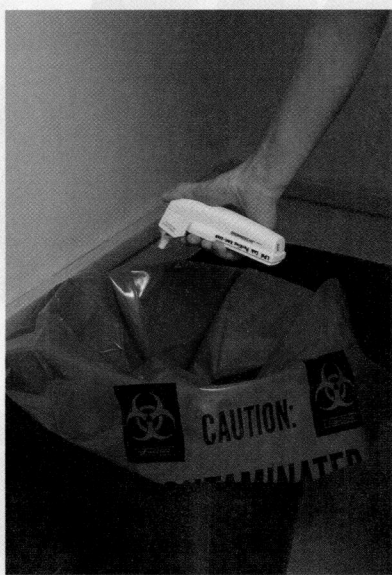

FIGURE 4–16E Eject the disposable probe cover directly into an appropriate waste container.

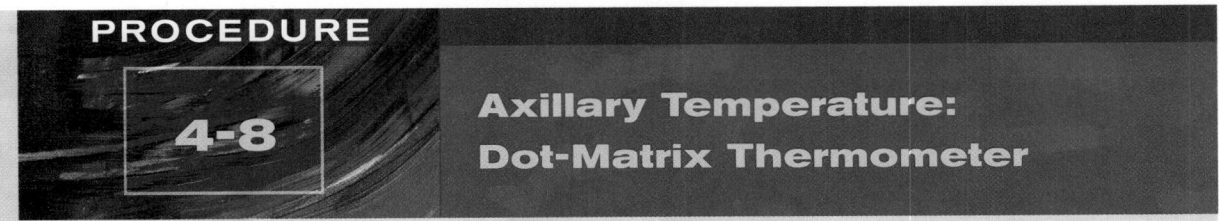

PROCEDURE

4-8

Axillary Temperature: Dot-Matrix Thermometer

Student Competency Objective: The medical assistant student will obtain and record an axillary (armpit) temperature using a dot-matrix, single-use plastic thermometer.

Items Needed: Dot-matrix, single-use thermometer, watch, waste container, paper, pen or pencil

Steps:

1. Wash your hands.
2. Get items needed.
3. Introduce yourself to the client even if you have seen the client on previous visits to your office. The client may have forgotten your name. This also helps to establish a provider-client relationship, because it shows the client that you want her to know who you are.
4. Identify the client. Ask the client to state her name to establish that this is the right client, and then compare the name given to the name on the chart. Never enter a room and call out a client's name to determine if this person is the correct client. The client may not have heard you clearly and may just nod, smile, or answer yes. Clients almost never question if the medical assistant professional has the right client. It is up to the medical assistant to identify the right client before performing any procedure.
5. Tell the client, in everyday language, what you are going to do.
6. Ask if the client has any questions. If she does, give short and simple answers. Sometimes clients will start (and continue) talking because they are nervous about the procedure.
7. Ask the client to lift her arm.
8. Place the thermometer high up in the armpit, vertically (straight up and down, the long way).
9. Place the dots on the thermometer against the client's torso (body).
10. Move the client's arm down to hold the thermometer in place.
11. Check your watch to note the time. The thermometer must be held in place for 3 minutes.
12. After 3 minutes, ask the client to lift her arm; remove the thermometer.
13. Read and write down the number at the last colored dot on the thermometer.
14. Dispose of the used thermometer in a waste container.
15. Wash your hands.

Charting Example:

The thermometer reads 99.2. You would record the following:

      10/17/20xx   T=99.2 Ax

      James Oliver, S.M.A.

      James Oliver, S.M.A. (printed name)

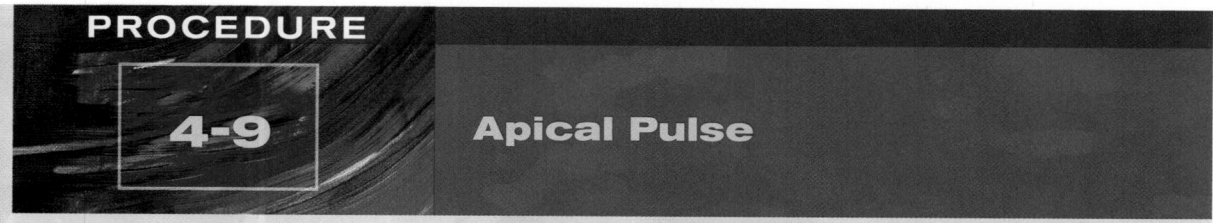

PROCEDURE 4-9   Apical Pulse

Student Competency Objective: The medical assistant student will find, obtain, and record the apical pulse rate, rhythm, and volume.

Items Needed: Stethoscope, watch with sweep second hand, alcohol wipes, paper, pen or pencil

Steps:

1. Wash your hands.
2. Get the items needed.
3. Introduce yourself to the client even if you have seen the client on previous visits to your office. The client may have forgotten your name. This also helps to establish a provider–client relationship, because it shows the client that you want her to know who you are.
4. Identify the client. Ask the client to state his name to establish that this is the right client, and then compare the name given to the name on the chart. Never enter a room and call out a client's name to determine if this person is the correct client. The client may not have heard you clearly and may just nod, smile, or answer yes. Clients almost never question if the medical assistant professional has the right client. It is up to the medical assistant to identify the right client before performing any procedure.
5. Tell the client, in everyday language, what you are going to do.
6. Ask if the client has any questions. If she does, give short and simple answers. Sometimes clients will start (and continue) talking because they are nervous about the procedure.
7. Remove clothing from the left side of the client's chest; provide a gown, if needed.
8. The client may either sit or lie down.
9. Put the stethoscope earpiece in your ear (Figure 4–17A).
10. Find the apical pulse site by starting at the midclavicular line and counting the intercostal spaces on the left side of chest. Stop at the fifth intercostal space (Figure 4–17B).
11. Put the chestpiece of the stethoscope directly on the client's skin at this spot, which is over the apex of the heart.
12. Listen for the heartbeat. Using your watch, begin counting when the second hand is at 12.
13. Count the number of beats for one full minute.
14. While counting, pay attention to the pulse rhythm. Is the time between each beat equal (regular) or unequal (irregular)?
15. Note also the volume or quality of the apical pulse.
16. Remove the stethoscope earpieces from your ears.
17. Record your findings. Be sure to write that this measurement is an apical pulse.
18. Ask the client if he needs help to dress; assist as needed.
19. Clean stethoscope earpieces and chestpiece with disinfectant wipes.
20. Wash your hands.

(Continues)

PROCEDURE 4-9 (Continued)

Charting Example:
You counted 76 beats for 1 full minute, and noted that the time between beats was unequal—first rapid, then slow. You would record the following:

    6/9/20xx   Apical pulse 76 irregular

Sally O'Brien, S.M.A.

    Sally O'Brien, S.M.A. (printed name)

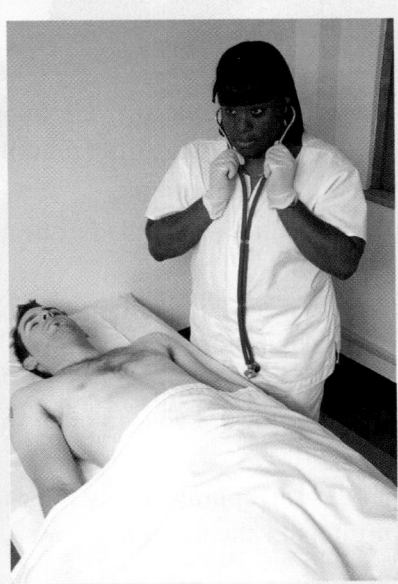

FIGURE 4-17A The medical assistant positions a client on the exam table. She then puts the stethoscope earpieces into her ears.

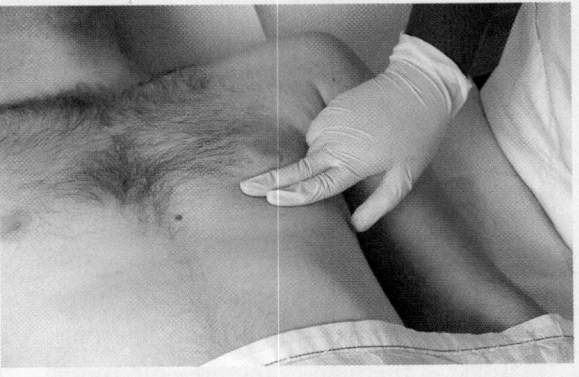

FIGURE 4-17B Find the apical pulse site by starting at the midclavicular line and counting the intercostal spaces on the left side of the chest. The apical pulse site is found at the fifth intercostal space. Count the number of beats for one full minute.

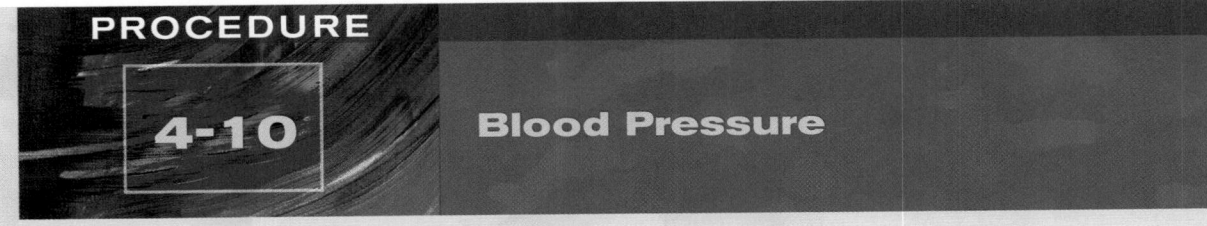

PROCEDURE

4-10   Blood Pressure

Student Competency Objective: The medical assistant student will obtain and record a client's palpatory and auscultatory blood pressure.

Items Needed: Stethoscope, sphygmomanometer, alcohol wipe, paper, pen or pencil

Steps:

1. Wash your hands.
2. Get items needed.

(Continues)

PROCEDURE 4-10 (Continued)

3. Introduce yourself to the client even if you have seen the client on previous visits to your office. The client may have forgotten your name. This also helps to establish a provider–client relationship, because it shows the client that you want her to know who you are.

4. Identify the client. Ask the client to state her name to establish that this is the right client, and then compare the name given to the name on the chart. Never enter a room and call out a client's name to determine if this person is the correct client. The client may not have heard you clearly and may just nod, smile, or answer yes. Clients almost never question if the medical assistant professional has the right client. It is up to the medical assistant to identify the right client before performing any procedure.

5. Tell the client, in everyday language, what you are going to do.

6. Ask if the client has any questions. If she does, give short and simple answers. Sometimes clients will start (and continue) talking because they are nervous about the procedure.

7. Wipe the earpieces and chestpiece of the stethoscope with alcohol wipes.

8. The client may either sit or lie down. If sitting, her arm should be extended at heart level with the palm of the hand facing up.

9. Remove any clothing from the client's arm. Although it is possible to obtain a blood pressure reading over light clothing, the clothing can make it more difficult for the medical assistant to hear the sounds.

10. Turn the valve on the bulb of the cuff counterclockwise (or toward you) to open the valve and completely empty the air from the blood pressure cuff.

11. Wrap the blood pressure cuff snugly around the client's arm, approximately 2 inches above the elbow (Figure 4–18A). Most cuffs have arrows printed on them; these arrows should be

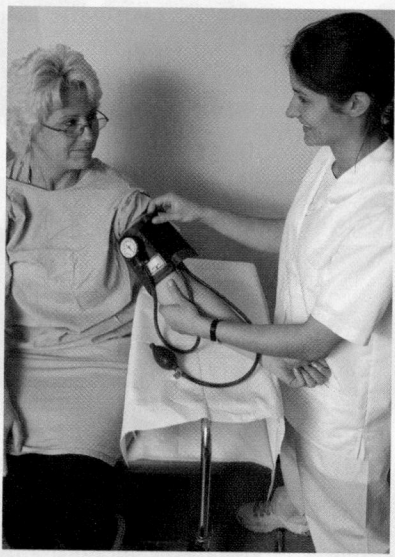

FIGURE 4–18A The client may sit or lie down on the exam table. Wrap the blood pressure cuff snugly around the arm, approximately 2 inches above the elbow.

(Continues)

PROCEDURE 4-10 (Continued)

placed pointing downward toward the brachial artery. You may also fold the cuff in half to find the center point and then place that point toward the brachial artery.

12. The cuff should be loose enough for you to fit two fingers under the cuff, but not so loose that the cuff can slide down.

13. If using an aneroid sphygmomanometer, make sure the dial is placed so that you can clearly see the numbers. Make sure the ends of the cuff are tucked in and do not block your view of the numbers. If using a mercury sphygmomanometer, make sure it is placed on a flat surface where the numbers are easily visible.

14. With the pads of your first two fingers, find the client's radial pulse (the radial artery is at the thumb side of the wrist, near a bony prominence).

15. With the other hand, turn the valve on the bulb clockwise (or away from yourself) to close it. Do not tighten it too much.

16. Pump the bulb to inflate the cuff to 30 mm Hg above where you no longer feel the radial pulse (Figure 4–18B).

17. Turn the valve counterclockwise (or toward you) to deflate the cuff, until you feel the radial pulse.

18. Make note of the number where you felt the radial pulse. This is called the palpatory systolic pressure. (For example, if you felt the radial pulse at 110, the BP = 110 palpatory.)

19. Quickly finish turning the valve to release the rest of the air.

20. Place the earpieces of the stethoscope in your ears.

21. Find the brachial artery at the client's inner forearm, near the bend of the elbow (medial antecubital space).

22. Put the stethoscope chestpiece at this site. Do not let the chestpiece touch the cuff, or what you hear may sound scratchy (Figure 4–18C).

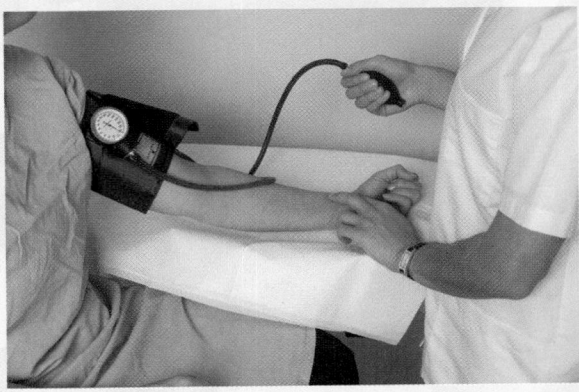

FIGURE 4–18B Find the client's radial pulse; then pump the bulb to inflate the cuff to 30 mm Hg above where you no longer feel the radial pulse. Then, turn the valve counterclockwise to deflate the cuff, until you feel the radial pulse again. This is the palpatory systolic pressure.

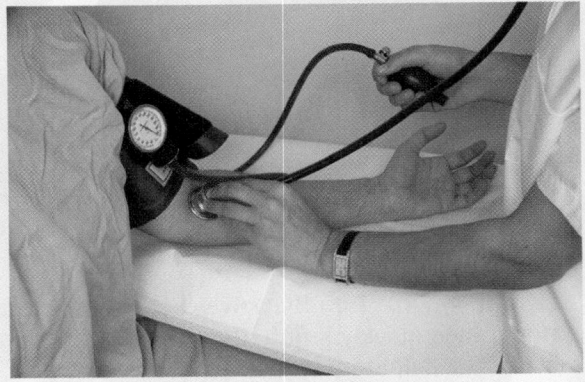

FIGURE 4–18C Find the brachial artery at the medial antecubital space, near the bend of the elbow. Place the stethoscope chestpiece over this site.

(Continues)

PROCEDURE 4-10 (Continued)

23. Turn the valve clockwise (away from you) to close it. Quickly inflate the cuff 30 mm Hg above the palpatory systolic pressure.

24. Turn the valve counterclockwise (toward you) to open the valve and slowly keep turning to release 2 to 3 mm Hg per second (Figure 4–18D). If the air is released too quickly, you will be unable to note the number when you heard the sound or thought the sound changed. If it is released too slowly, the needle on the aneroid dial will bounce and the client will complain of pain. Either action can cause inaccurate/false blood pressure readings.

25. The number at which you first heard the sound is called the systolic pressure.

26. Keep turning the valve until you hear the sound change to a softer, less clear sound. This is called the diastolic pressure (if directed). Keep turning the valve slowly and steadily (evenly) until you no longer hear any sound. The number at the last sound heard is the diastolic pressure.

27. Quickly release the rest of the air.

28. Take the cuff off the client.

29. Write down the blood pressure measurement as systolic over diastolic (when diastolic is requested): systolic/diastolic.

30. Using alcohol wipes, clean the stethoscope chestpiece and earpieces (Figure 4–18E).

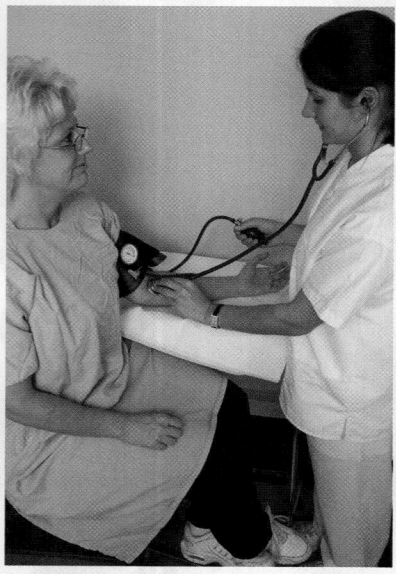

FIGURE 4–18D Turn the valve clockwise to close it and then quickly inflate the cuff to 30 mm Hg above the palpatory systolic pressure. Turn the valve counterclockwise to open the valve and slowly keep turning it so that the pressure goes down about 2 to 3 mm Hg per second. Note the number at which you first hear a sound. This is the systolic pressure.

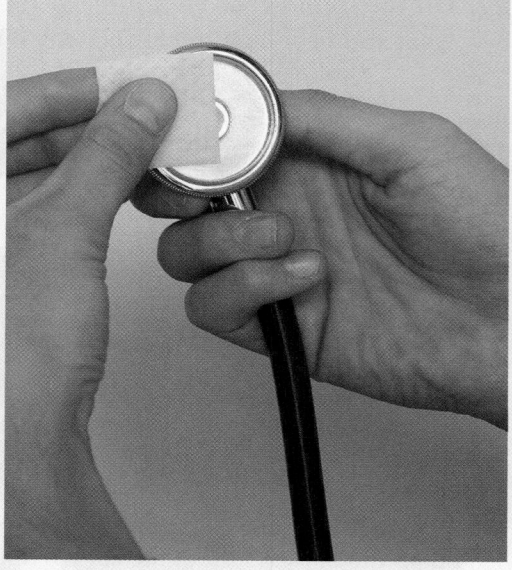

FIGURE 4–18E After you find the systolic pressure (and diastolic, if so directed), document your findings and clean the stethoscope chestpiece and earpieces with alcohol wipes.

(Continues)

PROCEDURE 4-10 (Continued)

31. Fold the cuff and put it away with the sphygmomanometer and stethoscope.
32. Wash your hands.

Charting Example:

You used the client's right arm and you heard the first sign at 130; the sound became softer at 80 and 60 was the last sound you heard. You would record the following:

8/8/20xx   Right arm BP = 130/80/60

James Fox, S.M.A.

James Fox, S.M.A. (printed name)

POINTS OF HIGHLIGHT

- Vital signs are indicators of life and client status.
- Temperature, pulse, respiration, and blood pressure are routinely taken and recorded by the medical assistant.
- The body tries to maintain a balance between heat production and heat loss.
- The majority of heat loss occurs through the skin.
- A client's temperature may be obtained orally, rectally, in the axilla (axillary), or in the ear (aurally, using a tympanic thermometer).
- Exercise, time of day, gender, and age can affect a person's temperature.
- Pulse corresponds to the number of heartbeats.
- The eight areas on the body at which one can easily obtain a pulse are temporal, carotid, apical, brachial, radial, femoral, popliteal, and dorsalis pedis.
- The rate, rhythm, and volume of the pulse give clues to the working of the heart.
- The medulla area in the brain controls respirations.
- Breathing in (inhalation) and then breathing out (exhalation) is counted as one respiration.
- The ratio of the pulse to respirations is normally 4:1.
- Blood pressure is the force of the blood against the walls of the arteries.
- A blood pressure reading consists of two numbers: the systolic measurement and the diastolic measurement.
- A stethoscope and a sphygmomanometer are used to measure blood pressure; BP is often taken at the brachial artery.
- Pain alerts the body that something is wrong.
- Pain can either be acute (sudden-onset) or chronic (long-term).
- Uncontrolled pain can prevent a person from doing everyday activities.

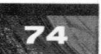

 ## BRIDGE TO CAAHEP

This chapter, which discusses vital signs, provides information and content related to CAAHEP standards for Anatomy and Physiology, Medical Terminology, Communication, Medical Assisting Clinical Procedures, and Professional Components.

 ## ABHES LINKS

This chapter, which discusses vital signs, links to ABHES course content for medical terminology, medical law and ethics, psychology of human relations, and medical office clinical procedures.

 ## AAMA AREAS OF COMPETENCE

This chapter, which discusses vital signs, provides information or content within several areas listed in the Medical Assistant Role Delineation Study. These areas include: clinical, fundamental principles, patient (client) care, general transdisciplinary, professionalism, professional communication skills, legal concepts, and instruction.

 ## AMT PATHS

This chapter provides a path to AMT competency in general medical assisting knowledge, medical terminology, medical ethics, human relations and patient (client) education, clinical medical assisting, asepsis, and vital signs.

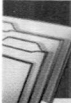 ### STUDENT PORTFOLIO ACTIVITY

Obtaining and recording vital signs are critical procedures that are performed at almost every office visit on almost every client. The evaluation or competency checklist form is an important documentation of your skill competency. Obtain a copy showing that you have achieved competency in obtaining and recording vital signs. Place this in your portfolio.

 ### APPLYING YOUR SKILLS

Part of the clinical responsibilities of a medical assistant is to obtain and record vital signs at each office visit. A client appears very anxious when you take her into an examination room. How will this affect her vital signs? What steps would you take to make sure that the numbers you record are an accurate reflection of the client's vital signs and functioning?

CRITICAL THINKING QUESTIONS

1. You are having problems obtaining a radial pulse. What other area on the client might you use to obtain a pulse? Explain why you chose that site.

2. In addition to counting the number of beats in a minute, what else should the medical assistant note about the pulse?

3. Why should the medical assistant avoid staring at a client's chest while counting respirations?

4. You have to obtain a client's blood pressure. What items do you need to carry out this clinical skill?

5. How is acute pain different from chronic pain?

6. A client with chronic pain complains of being unable to do everyday work activities. Explain how chronic pain is related to this complaint.

7. What are some questions the medical assistant can ask the client who complains of pain?

8. How does vigorous physical activity affect body temperature?

9. How does perspiration help to cool a person?

10. What are some advantages to obtaining a client's temperature with a tympanic thermometer?

11. Go back to the beginning of this chapter and review the Anticipatory Statements. Reread each statement and then indicate whether it is true or false. If the statement is false, rewrite it to make it a true statement.

CLIENT TEACHING PLAN

Taking a Radial Pulse

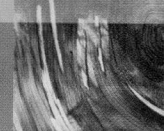

What Is to Be Taught:

- How to take a radial pulse and report the findings.

Objectives:

- Client will be able to find and count own radial pulse.
- Client will be able to report pulse number to doctor's office.

Preparation Before Teaching:

- Review the cardiovascular system and pulse rate, rhythm, and volume.
- Remember to put technical medical terms into simple, everyday language that clients will be able to understand.
- Look over the step-by-step procedure for finding and counting the pulse (even though the medical assistant does this clinical procedure frequently in the medical office).
- Get together teaching materials, such as a watch with a second hand, paper, pen, and diagrams and pictures to explain the pulse and counting the pulse.
- Make sure that the area is free from distractions while you are teaching.

Steps for the Medical Assistant:

1. Wash your hands.
2. Introduce yourself to the client.
3. Explain what you are going to teach and why.
4. Tell the client, in simple words, what a pulse is and its importance to health.
5. Show the client a diagram of the many pulse sites and point out the radial site.
6. Inform the client that she will learn how to find and count the radial pulse.
7. Take the client's arm and hand and rest them on a solid surface.
8. Find the radial pulse.

9. Ask the client to put the pads of the first two fingers of her other hand on that spot.
10. Instruct the client never to use the thumb (because the thumb has its own pulse).
11. Tell the client to use steady pressure but not to press too hard; the pulse will disappear with too much pressure and will not be felt.
12. Tell the client to look at her watch and begin counting when the second hand gets to the 12. Each beat counts as one.
13. Count for one full minute.
14. Write the number on a piece of paper, along with the date and time.
15. Tell the client to count and record her pulse every day.
16. Instruct the client to call the doctor if the pulse goes below 60 beats per minute.
17. Tell the client to bring the paper with the pulse rates written to the doctor's office at the next visit.
18. Ask the client if she has any questions.
19. Ask the client to find her radial pulse on the other wrist. Provide prompts and cues as needed.
20. Give written, step-by-step directions for the client to use at home as a reference.

Special Needs of the Client:

- Look at the client's chart to see if anything might interfere with the client's ability to find, count, and record the radial pulse.
- Ask the client, both before and after the teaching, if there is anything you should know that might affect her performance of this procedure.

Evaluation:

- Client will be able to explain what is meant by a pulse.
- Client will be able to find, count, and record the radial pulse.

(Continues)

CLIENT TEACHING PLAN (Continued)

- Client is able to state what to do if the radial pulse count is below 60 beats per minute.

■ Further Plans/Teaching:

- Provide written instructions and information about the pulse.
- In writing, give the client the name and telephone number of the doctor to call if the pulse is less than 60 beats per minute.

■ Follow-up:

Medical Assistant

Name: _____

Signature: _____

Date: _____

Client

Date: _____

Follow-up Date: _____

5

Anticipatory Statements

People may or may not be familiar with the physical examinations that are performed in a medical setting. Read and think about the following statements based upon what you believe now. Decide whether you agree or disagree. Write the word **agree** after the statement if you think the statement is true. Write the word **disagree** after the statement if you think the statement is false. Read the chapter to find out if your current beliefs can be supported.

1. By the time a person becomes an adult, he is familiar with and comfortable at the doctor's office. _____

2. All adults should be able to get on the examination table and position themselves correctly without any help from the medical assistant. _____

3. Testing how well a client can see using a vision chart is a procedure done by a medical assistant. _____

4. It is not necessary to measure a person's height once he has reached adulthood. _____

5. A person who is overweight (obese) is at increased risk for certain diseases. _____

Learning Objectives

Upon completion of this chapter, the medical assistant student should be able to:

■ Discuss the importance of communication between the medical assistant and the client
■ Measure the client's height and weight
■ Record the client's height and weight
■ Describe a client's mobility

Client
Examination

- Measure a client's vision with a Snellen chart
- Measure a client's hearing with an audiometer
- Be sensitive to clients' fears and concerns about medical procedures
- Define and explain the standard client position for examinations

Key Terms

audiometer Instrument used to measure sharpness (acuity) of hearing.

auscultation Listening to sounds in the body.

bruit Abnormal noise or sound, usually heard with a stethoscope.

chief complaint (CC) The main reason or problem that made the client seek help from the health care provider.

dorsal recumbent position Examination position in which the client lies on the back with the knees bent and feet flat on the exam table surface.

Fowler's position Examination position in which the client's back is supported at a 90-degree angle.

inspection Looking closely; a careful examination.

interview Meeting during which one person seeks information from another in order to reach a decision (job interview, client interview).

lithotomy position Examination position in which the client is on the back with the legs bent and the feet supported in stirrups.

mobility Ability to move or change position.

palpation Process of examining by touch, using the fingers.

percussion Process of examining by tapping a surface to listen to internal sounds.

prone position Examination position in which the client lies flat with the face downward.

review of systems (ROS) Organized, step-by-step review of major body systems.

semi-Fowler's position Examination position in which the client's back is supported at a 45-degree angle.

Sims' position A side-lying position in which the upper leg is sharply flexed.

Snellen chart A chart with letters or symbols used to measure visual acuity.

stirrups Metal supports attached to an exam table in which the client places the feet (or heels) to assume the lithotomy position; so named because the attachments look like the stirrups on a saddle.

supine position Lying on the back with the face up.

■ INTRODUCTION

The medical assistant is often the first member of the health care team to interact with a client. A good provider-client relationship depends, to a large extent, on the atmosphere of trust established by the medical assistant. The course of treatment, the client's response, and client satisfaction are all greatly influenced by the way the client is approached in a medical setting. The client's first impression of the health care setting and practice is based on the first encounter or appointment.

The medical assistant professional has many responsibilities. The medical assistant must be technically competent, and be able to communicate in a professional, therapeutic, caring way with clients. A major responsibility for any medical assistant is to assist the doctor during the examinations. The type and amount of assistance are determined by office policy and the medical assistant's scope of practice.

Medical assistants perform clinical skills as part of client examinations. Among other things, medical assistants prepare clients for examinations and procedures. This preparation includes positioning; common positions used for specific examinations include supine, prone, Fowler's, semi-Fowler's, dorsal recumbent, Sims', and lithotomy. Medical assistants must know these positions and when and how to place the client in these positions.

Client examination includes both the gathering of information and the physical examination of the client. Initial information about the chief complaint, past medical history, family history, and social history is obtained by the medical assistant. The information is reviewed and supplemented by the doctor. The doctor then performs a **review of systems (ROS)**, which involves asking specific questions about each of the major body systems. This helps to ensure that key signs and symptoms found in the other parts of the examination are reinforced.

Inspection (looking), palpation (feeling), percussion (tapping), and auscultation (listening with a stethoscope) are methods used by doctors to aid in the examination of clients. The medical assistant's role is to understand these examination methods and assist the doctor and client as the doctor uses them during an examination.

Medical assistants also perform clinical procedures during office visits. Client height and weight are measured and recorded. Administration of some types of vision and hearing tests is often part of the clinical tasks.

A major responsibility for the medical assistant is to assist the doctor during the examination. The type and amount of assistance is determined by office policy and the medical assistant's scope of practice.

■ WELCOMING THE CLIENT

The welcoming process begins as the medical assistant greets each client with a smile and a friendly "hello." The manner in which the medical assistant communicates with the client while asking questions and performing clinical tasks has a direct effect on client outcomes. All clients must be treated respectfully and with dignity. This is a basic, fundamental goal. If the medical assistant fails to do this, the negative effects can be enormous. These effects range from the patient receiving suboptimal care to the patient changing to another doctor or abandoning the health care system altogether. Ultimately, it is the client who suffers if providers fail in this part of care.

NOTE TO STUDENT:

Especially if this is the client's first visit, your interaction can greatly affect client satisfaction and client outcome. The medical assistant is often the first professional to work with the client. Your interaction sets the tone for the client-doctor relationship.

■ COURSE OF TREATMENT

Clients are looking for help when they make appointments to see the doctor. During their appointments, clients often must undergo procedures that are uncomfortable and invasive, such as the drawing of blood. Unfamiliar health care providers ask many personal questions, often the same ones the clients have answered before.

Based on all the information gathered, the doctor prescribes a course of treatment. The information comes from laboratory and diagnostic procedures, the doctor's review of body systems and the physical examination of the client, the medical assistant's procedures (such as taking vital signs), and verbal communication with the client. This important decision as to the course of treatment is based on input from all members of the health care team, including the medical assistant.

Client's Response

The course of treatment prescribed does not guarantee or ensure that the client's outcomes will be positive. Nevertheless, the client's response to the course of treatment is often influenced by how the client feels he was treated by the provider. Did the medical assistant or other provider act in a way that communicated respect, interest, and friendliness? The medical assistant can affect the client's response in a very positive way.

Client Satisfaction

Is your client happy about his experience or encounter with the health care system? The client may agree to follow the course of treatment, and in fact get better, but this does not guarantee that the client is satisfied with or happy about the quality of care received. The medical assistant contributes much by understanding the client and his feelings and responding in a professional way.

■ INTERVIEWING

Getting to know the client is a cornerstone of quality medical care. The administrative med-ical assistant creates an impression beginning with the initial phone call or the client's first conversation when he arrives at the front desk. The clinical medical assistant's first encounter often takes place when the client is brought back to the examination room.

The client looks to the medical assistant as a helper and an expert in health care. At the first **interview** or meeting, be aware of verbal and nonverbal communication:

- State the client's name. Ask the client how he wants to be addressed or called. Never assume that the client wants you to use only his first name. Depending upon age and culture, or for personal reasons, a client may feel disrespected if you call him by only his given name.
- Smile at the client (Figure 5-1). A smile sends the message that you are friendly and glad to see the other person.
- Make eye contact. This expresses your interest and desire to focus on the other person. A genuine smile will also show in your eyes. If the medical assistant avoids eye contact, the client may assume that he is not interested; this can hinder a client's sharing of feelings or concerns.

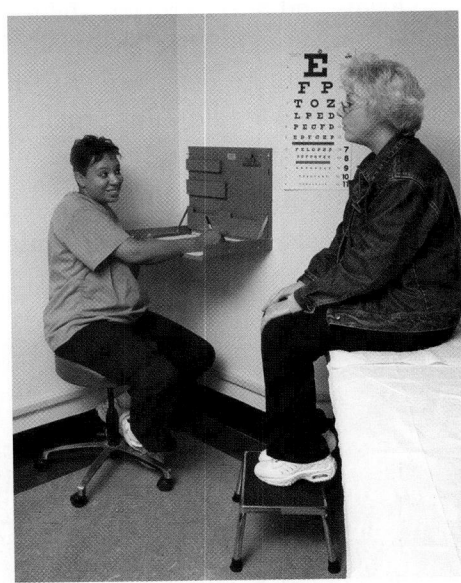

FIGURE 5-1 The medical assistant smiles encouragingly during the first interview with the client.

However, prolonged eye contact or staring can be intimidating or frightening to a client.

- Introduce yourself in a clear voice while making eye contact. Tell the client your name and title. For example, "I am Cecelia Jones, the medical assistant student . . . ."

- Shake hands. In addition to an introduction, the medical assistant can learn much about a person just from a handshake. Is the skin dry, sweaty, rough? Does the person have a strong grip? Is there evidence of arthritis or other swelling of the hand? Does the person's hand shake or tremble? Does the person have difficulty extending his arm and grasping another person's hand? All of these observations are important pieces of information that may indicate certain disease conditions or problems.

- Tell the client what you need to do. The medical assistant interviews or asks the client health-related questions. On an initial visit, there are many questions to ask and forms to complete. Frequently the office sends forms to the client in advance of the first visit. The medical assistant should offer to help the client complete the forms and also to review them if the client has already filled them out. This gives the client an opportunity to clarify any questionable points and provide additional information.

When the initial forms have been completed, the medical assistant must find out why the client came to the office for this particular visit. This problem is called the **chief complaint (CC)**. There are several ways to ask this: for example, "Why did you come to the office today?," "How can we help you today?," or "What seems to be your biggest concern or problem today?" The chief complaint must be noted in a clear, concise way. The problem, the part(s) of the body affected, and how long the problem has existed should be included. For example, the client states, "I have had chills all over and a high temperature for three days." The medical assistant would write down that exact statement. If the client does not offer information about how long the problem has persisted, the medical assistant should ask that specific question.

The client may come for a general physical and not have a specific health concern. In the charting space for chief complaint, the medical assistant would write: "Client came to office today for a general physical examination and expresses no specific complaint or problem."

Past Medical History

The client will always have to answer questions about his past personal medical history (Figure 5-2). If this individual has an established client-doctor relationship at the office, most likely he has already completed a form with this information. Nevertheless, past history should still be reviewed with the client.

NOTE TO STUDENT:

Be aware of your nonverbal behavior and what it communicates to clients. Do not act as if you are in a hurry. You are collecting important information that can affect a client's health outcome.

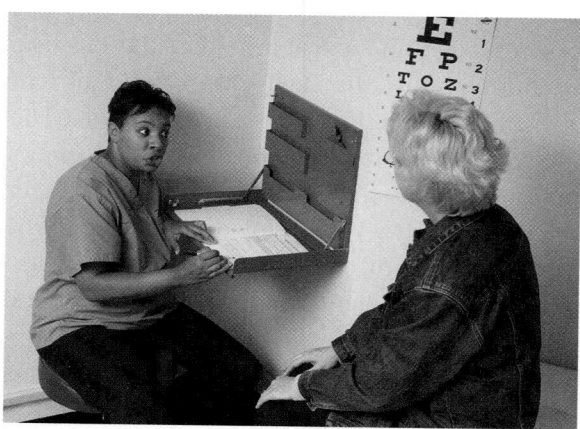

FIGURE 5-2 The medical assistant enters the client's medical history into a file.

Questions about past history include childhood illnesses, surgeries, and immunizations. For example, as an adult, has the client had any surgeries, injuries, immunizations, or serious illnesses (physical or emotional)? Allergies and any medication are included. If the client answers yes to an allergy, the file must be flagged in some way to alert providers to the allergy, in addition to the allergy information being recorded in the file. Allergies can cause life-threatening situations.

Medications taken, both past and present, must be recorded. The client should bring a list of current medications with him, including name of drug, dosage, and when and how often the dose is taken. Alternatively, he may bring the prescription bottle with him to the health care provider. When asking about medication, be sure to ask directly if the client takes any over-the-counter (OTC) medications, vitamins, hormones, or herbs. These can be very potent and can interfere with other prescribed medications and treatments. Many laypeople do not think of vitamins or herbs as drugs and will not mention them. It is up to the medical assistant to ask.

Family History. Questions are asked regarding the health history of family members. For example, if a family member is deceased, at what age did that person die, and what was the cause of death? Currently, the term *family* is often defined as whomever the individual is close with and considers to be family. For medical purposes, though, *family* includes only the client's biological father, mother, and siblings. In-laws, however close to the client they are emotionally, are not included, nor is the client's spouse, partner, or significant other.

Social History. Questions regarding lifestyle, sleeping patterns, smoking, risk-taking behavior (such as seat-belt use and driving habits), work, recreation, and living arrangements are included in the client interview. Some individuals may see this as an invasion of privacy. If the medical assistant has established a rapport with the client, it will be easier to proceed with questions of this nature. Explain that this information is important to the physician for understanding the person's health issues and prescribing a course of treatment.

Review of Systems

A medical assistant can begin a review of systems (ROS) during the client interview. This is done by asking the client questions about specific signs and symptoms, going through the body system by system. In most cases, the doctor does the **Review of Systems (ROS)** with the client to uncover any problem that may not have been raised in other parts of the examination. The medical assistant's role is to make sure to ask questions and complete all parts of the forms pertaining to the client's history and chief complaint. This will help to ensure that all necessary information is obtained.

Other Documentation

Other documentation required will vary according to the individual practice setting. More and more frequently, offices are switching from paper charts to computerized charting. (Through other courses in medical assisting programs, the student will become familiar with computer use.) Most offices conduct their own inservices (teaching and orientation) for new employees. During these orientation classes, employees are taught the computer programs used in that office and policies regarding charting. Privacy, client confidentiality, and HIPAA regulations play an important part in office policies regarding computer use.

■ STANDARD (COMMON) PROCEDURES

Certain standard or routine procedures are a basic part of any physical examination. These procedures are carried out in most primary care or family health offices by the medical assistant. Height is always measured on an initial or first visit, and periodically thereafter. Height is measured frequently for children. For adults, height measurements are taken periodically, which may point to possible problems with the vertebrae or bone structure. Weight should be measured at each visit. Although not considered a vital sign, baseline weight (as well as any increase or decrease from that weight) will be needed for comparison at later visits. Obesity (excessive weight) can put a person at risk of certain diseases. Unusual weight loss or gain can also be a sign of some disorders.

Vision (sight) changes and hearing loss usually happen gradually, so the medical assistant should test regularly for possible changes.

Mobility, or the degree to which a person can move part or all the body freely or without help, is an important function. In health care, *mobility* is commonly defined as the ability to walk and change positions without help. The person's ability to perform activities of daily living (ADLs) is greatly affected by his amount of mobility. Medical assistants can observe the client as they walk with the client from the waiting room to the examination room. Does the client have difficulty walking? Are his movements slow and unsteady? Does the client need help getting on and off the examination table or changing positions during procedures?

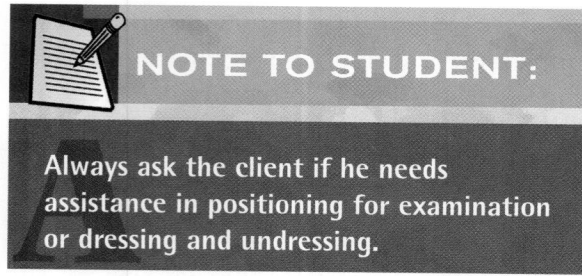

NOTE TO STUDENT:

Always ask the client if he needs assistance in positioning for examination or dressing and undressing.

Height

Measuring and recording a client's height is a common procedure performed by the medical assistant. Height is most frequently measured at the same time as a client's weight, as the balance-beam scale is used for both (Figure 5-3). Adults do not grow taller after reaching skeletal maturity, but certain disorders can cause a person to

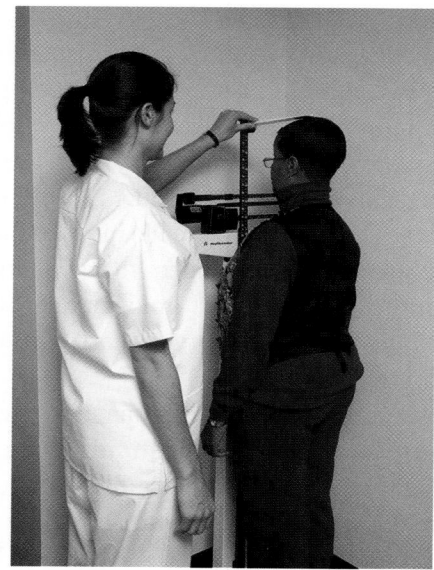

FIGURE 5–3 The medical assistant measures the client's height using a balance-beam scale.

lose height. For example, osteoporosis can cause skeletal changes by compression fractures of the vertebrae. Other degenerative conditions can also cause these changes.

Recent advances in the study of aging highlight the need to record the client's height periodically. Clients may question why height is being measured and are often worried if the measured height is less than before. They may fear that they are "shrinking" as they grow older. Explain to the client that height is periodically measured so that comparisons can be made. Note any discrepancy (change in height) from a previous visit or the client's stated height. Remind the client to talk about this worry with the doctor if the client is concerned.

Weight

A client's weight should be measured and recorded at every office visit. Obesity indicates an unhealthy addition of body fat and is a serious concern. In the United States, more than 50% of adults are overweight. Studies have shown that obesity decreases a person's life span (on the average, an obese person lives fewer years than a person within a healthy weight range). Overweight can also decrease the quality of the client's life, both physically and socially. Being obese puts a person at risk for many serious diseases and conditions, such as hypertension, heart disease, stroke, and diabetes mellitus.

It is important to obtain the baseline weight at the initial visit, and to weigh the client at each following visit to note any weight gain or loss (Figure 5-4). These changes can be positive or negative. An underweight person's gaining weight may be a positive finding and part of the treatment plan, just as with an obese individual who loses weight. However, weight loss may be due not to healthy eating and exercise, but to a disease process. A weight gain may be due not to overeating, but to the effects of a disorder such as cardiovascular disease.

Keep in mind that the medical assistant is not to judge the client on the basis of weight. Weight is the balance between what is taken in (eating calories) and what is burned (exercise, metabolism). This can become unbalanced for many reasons, many of which are not that simple. There are complex causes and explanations for overweight (and underweight). Researchers are studying why some people can apparently eat as much as they like and not gain weight, whereas others eat far fewer calories and are overweight.

Vision

Visual acuity (the ability to see clearly) is important to a person's ability to independently perform ADLs. Eye changes can occur slowly, without pain or discomfort to the person. It is important for the medical assistant to measure visual acuity; this is one part of caring for an individual's eye health. A common vision test done in the physician's office uses the **Snellen chart** (Figure 5-5). A Snellen chart has horizontal rows of black letters on a white background. The letters are biggest at the top and get smaller with each following line. Other charts are also available, such as a chart with objects or the letter "E" pointing in different directions. These charts can be used with young children or individuals who are not familiar with the English letter names or alphabet.

The right and left eyes should be tested separately, as well as both eyes together. Ask the client if he wears glasses or contact lenses. If the client wears glasses, vision should be tested first with the glasses and then without the glasses. Policy regarding testing without contacts differs according to the medical office. For example, some doctors require that contacts not be worn for a few days before vision testing. Ask the client if he has noticed any changes in his vision. Visual changes have many causes (see Chapter 10).

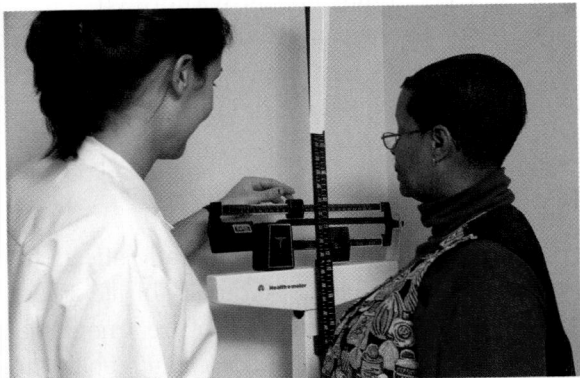

FIGURE 5-4 The medical assistant measures the client's weight using a balance-beam scale.

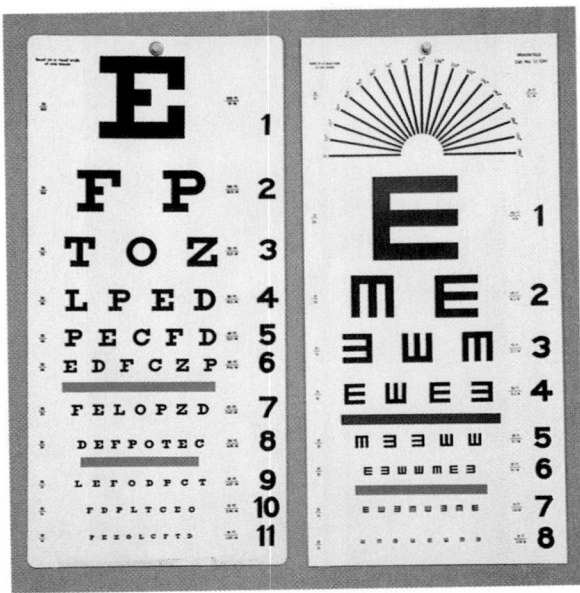

FIGURE 5-5 Snellen charts for screening visual acuity.

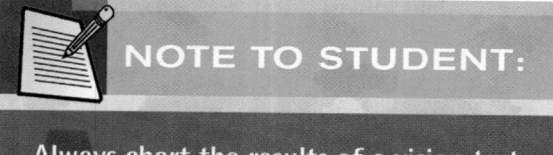

NOTE TO STUDENT:

Always chart the results of a vision test indicating if the client wore glasses or contact lenses during the testing. The results are stated using the phrase "with correction."

Hearing

The ability to hear and distinguish sounds is an important sensory function. Hearing changes can be acute or sudden, but most often they are subtle and occur slowly over time. The medical assistant will test hearing using an **audiometer,** an instrument that is used to measure hearing. The doctor may use a tuning fork to do a Rinne test and a Weber test (Figure 5-6).

The Rinne test compares air and bone conduction. Sound will be heard longer by air conduction than by bone conduction. A vibrating tuning fork is first held on the mastoid area of the skull (area behind the ear). When the client can no longer hear the vibrating sound, the fork is moved from the area behind the ear

and placed close to the external auditory canal. If the client can still hear the vibrating sound, his hearing is considered normal, because air conduction is better than bone conduction.

In the Weber test, the doctor places a vibrating tuning fork on the midline of the top of the client's head. A person who hears equally well with both ears will hear the sound equally in each ear. With certain diseases, the sound will be louder on the diseased side; with other conditions, the sound will seem louder in the unaffected ear.

Before any tests are done, ask the client if he has experienced any changes in hearing. Are certain sounds more muffled? Is it difficult to hear when there are other noises in the environment, such as in a restaurant or with a group of people (Figure 5-7)? Many clients are hesitant to complain about difficulty in hearing. Some clients are not even aware of their hearing losses. The client may also view poor hearing as a sign of old age, and thus not want to admit to hearing loss. During interaction with the client, the medical assistant should be alert to signs of hearing difficulty and record and report these findings to the doctor. Some signs of hearing problems are:

- The client may frequently ask to have a question repeated
- The client may seem to watch the speaker's lips
- The client may answer a question incorrectly (for example, saying "uh-huh" or nodding in response to an open-ended question)
- The client may appear withdrawn
- If the client comes with another person, the client may look to that person to repeat the question or for prompts or cues

Mobility

A person's degree of mobility greatly affects his activities of daily living and quality of life. Client mobility also affects the course of treatment prescribed by the doctor and the client's ability to participate in that course of treatment. For example, the doctor prescribes increased physical

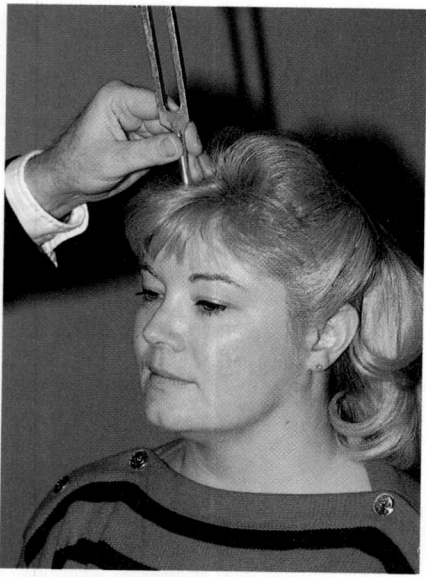

FIGURE 5-6 A tuning fork is placed against the client's head to perform the Weber test.

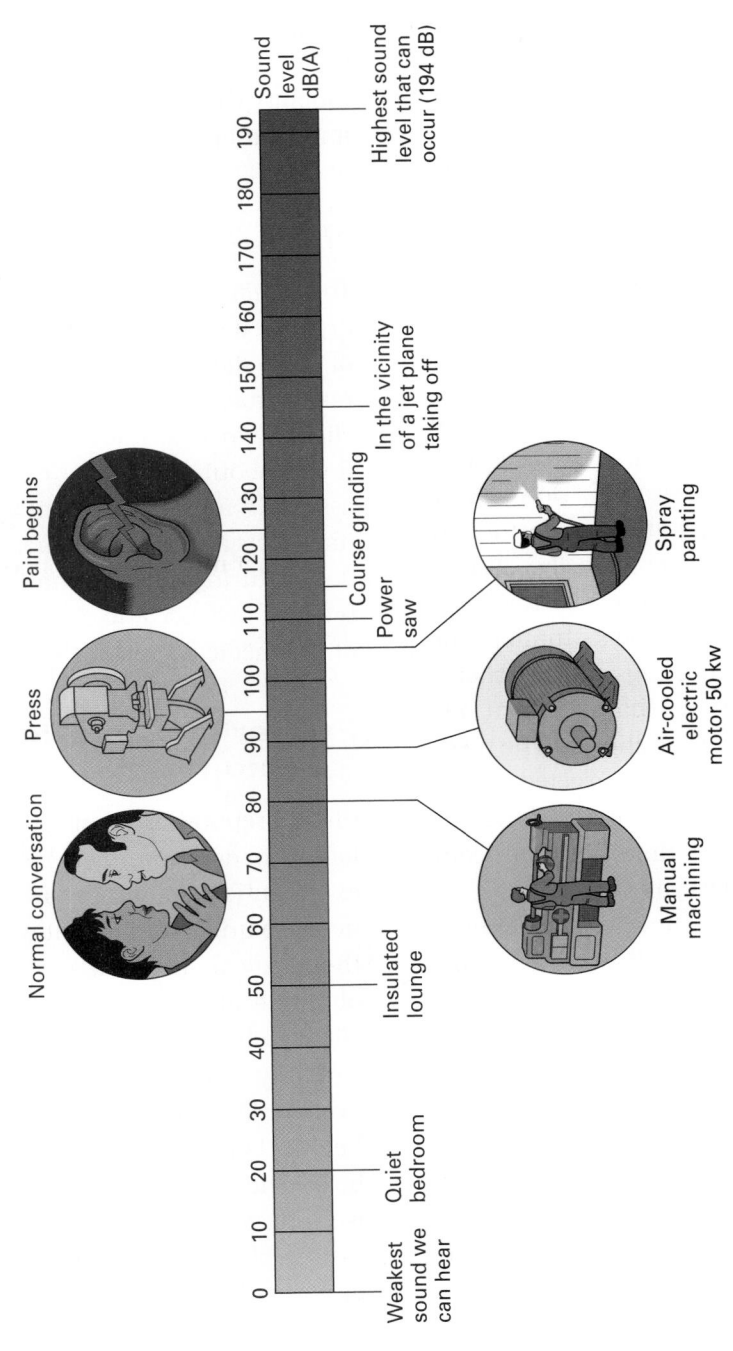

FIGURE 5-7 Noise levels of various operations.

activity as part of the treatment plan, but the client experiences knee pain when walking; this client probably will not follow the prescribed course of treatment. As a result of impaired mobility, client outcome can be negatively affected.

The skilled medical assistant can help clients in these situations. Difficulty with ambulation or walking is sometimes easy to observe. The person may use an assistive device, such as a wheelchair, walker, or cane. At other times, ambulation problems are harder to detect.

The medical assistant should incorporate assessment of mobility into every office visit by a client. During the assessment, the medical assistant should ask questions, observe, and document. Ask the client direct questions: "Are you able to walk, climb stairs, and get around freely?" "Have there been any changes recently?" "Can you go shopping or visiting?" "Do you stay home and turn down invitations because you don't think you can move about easily?" When the medical assistant knows the client, the questions can be specific to the person's situation. For example, from previous meetings with the client, the medical assistant knows that the client has been an active member of his church. The medical assistant can ask a question targeted to that client: "Does walking, getting up and down, or sitting for long periods of time stop you from going to church as often as you would like?"

Clients may say that they get around fine, but your observations may tell you differently. Clients may not want to complain, or may feel that a person just has to put up with decreased mobility. The medical assistant's observation skills can prove very valuable in this situation. Watch the client as you walk together to the examination room. Is the person unsteady? Is he limping, reaching for a handrail, or walking very slowly and hesitantly? In the examination room, does the client grimace, make a face, or groan when getting on the examination table? Watch facial expressions for signs of pain or discomfort when the client gets in and out of a chair.

The next step in assessment of mobility is to share your findings. Make sure the doctor is aware of what you observed and the client's response before the doctor does an examination or test. Information gathered from questions and observations should also be documented in the client's chart. This helps in continuity of care and maintenance of the quality of care. The findings gathered at the next visit can be compared with previous findings. Is there improvement, worsening, or is the client's mobility the same? Assessment of mobility is an important part of any office visit.

■ EXAMINATION

To *examine* means to look closely, in a detailed, organized way. An examination is a critical part of the client's visit. The medical assistant's major role is to prepare the client, ease the client's worries, and answer the client's questions about what to expect. The medical assistant must competently perform preliminary tests and ask vital questions. Assisting the doctor during the examination, according to the scope of practice and office policy, is a large part of the medical assistant's role.

Preparing the Client for Examination

Client preparation is one of the most important factors in determining a positive outcome of an examination or procedure. First, the client needs to understand what will happen. Second, the medical assistant can help the client to obtain and follow pre-exam instructions. A client who follows the pre-exam directions carefully helps ensure that the results of the exam or lab tests truly reflect the client's state of health. For example, if a client eats breakfast before having blood drawn for fasting chemistry tests, the results would not reflect true fasting blood levels. If the health care provider discovers that a client did not follow instructions, the tests will probably have to be repeated, causing more client discomfort and increasing the cost of care. If the doctor does not learn that the results were inaccurate, because of poor client compliance, the doctor could prescribe treatment or medication that will harm rather than help the client.

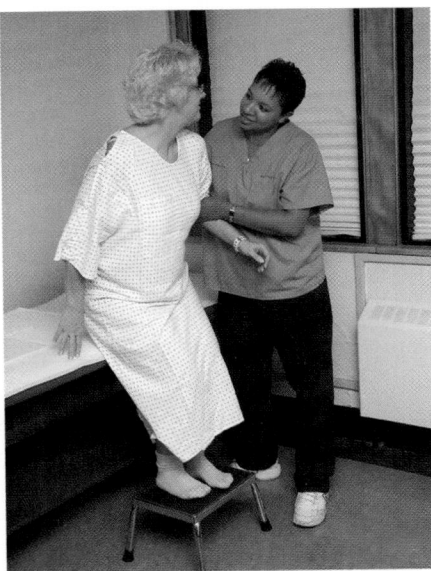

FIGURE 5-8 The medical assistant helps the client onto the exam table, using a friendly and professional manner.

Part of the preparation for examinations or procedures is done on the day of the exam. Before the client arrives, make sure that the examination room is clean and that all items needed for the examination are available in the room and ready for use.

When the client arrives, introduce yourself to the client. Put the client at ease with your friendly, professional, competent manner (Figure 5-8). The procedure about to be done may be common and routine to the health care provider, but remember that much of what health care providers do may seem unfamiliar and strange to clients. Never assume that a person knows what is going to happen or what to expect.

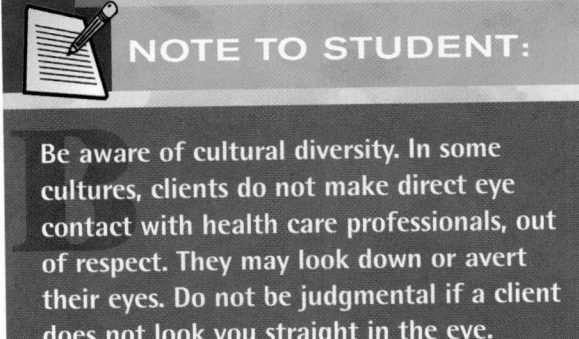

NOTE TO STUDENT:

Be aware of cultural diversity. In some cultures, clients do not make direct eye contact with health care professionals, out of respect. They may look down or avert their eyes. Do not be judgmental if a client does not look you straight in the eye.

If any special preparation was needed for the exam, review the preparation with the client. Ask the client if he experienced any problems in following the instructions. If the client answers yes, ask for specific details and inform the doctor of those findings.

Check to see if a urine sample is needed. Even if not needed, ask the client if he needs to use the bathroom to urinate, or void. A full bladder may cause client discomfort during an examination. The client who has a full bladder may also have to interrupt the procedure to void.

Client gowning varies according to office policy and for various procedures. Explain gowning by showing the client how the gown should go on. Does the gown open in front or back? Does the procedure require that the client remove all clothing, including underwear? Give clear instructions and offer to help the client change into the gown (Figure 5-9). Some people may need help with zippers or buttons but are hesitant to ask for assistance.

Explain to the client what will happen at this visit and during this examination. An explanation helps to gain the client's cooperation, ease any fears, and correct any misconceptions about what to expect. Many procedures are somewhat uncomfortable but not actually painful. Nevertheless, do not say, "It won't hurt a bit," or "You

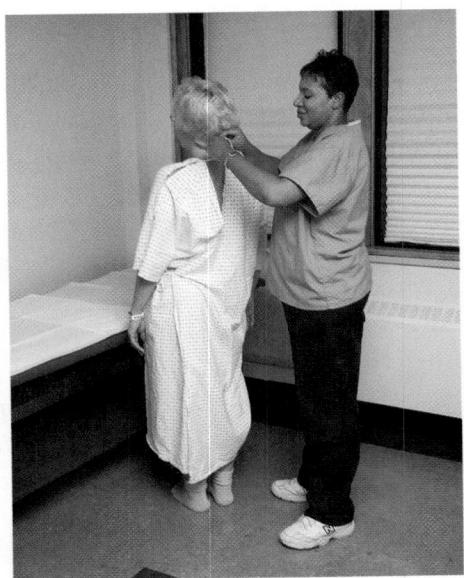

FIGURE 5-9 The medical assistant helps the client into a gown for the examination.

won't feel any pain." Instead, tell the client that if he does feel pain during the examination or procedure, he should tell the doctor immediately.

Depending on office policy, the medical assistant often remains with the client during the procedure. The medical assistant assists the doctor and comforts the client. When the client feels that a health care provider really cares, client comfort, cooperation, and satisfaction are all increased. Trust between the heath care provider and the client is critical to positive client outcome.

Methods of Examination

During client examinations, the doctor uses different methods to obtain data. The information gathered from the different methods is added together. This assists the doctor in arriving at a diagnosis and prescribed course of treatment.

Inspection. **Inspection** involves examining the client by looking at the body, movement, and form. The medical assistant uses inspection and observation to gather information about the client. The physician uses an in-depth knowledge of anatomy, physiology, and pathophysiology to choose a method of inspection. This first method of examination enables the physician to determine what the next step in the examination should be.

Palpation. **Palpation** involves applying the fingers or hands to a body surface for examination (Figure 5-10). The physician uses palpation to feel for any abnormalities that might indicate a disease or disorder. For example, the physician uses bimanual (two-handed) palpation during a pelvic exam to determine size and location of the client's uterus and ovaries. Internal organs located within the abdominal cavity can also be palpated by feeling the abdomen. The medical assistant can help by reminding the client to take slow, deep, easy breaths; this will help to relax tense muscles that make palpation of internal organs difficult. The medical assistant also uses palpation when locating pulses to count the heart rate or obtain a blood pressure reading.

Percussion. **Percussion** involves using the fingers to strike or hit a body surface. This is done to assess the size, location, or thickness of structures under the surface. The physician rests one hand at a point on the client's body (Figure 5-11). With the fingers of the other hand, he taps the fingers that are resting on the body. This should not be painful for the client.

Auscultation. The process of listening for sounds that come from within the body is called **auscultation.** This listening for internal sounds is normally done with a stethoscope (Figure 5-12). The bell or chestpiece of the

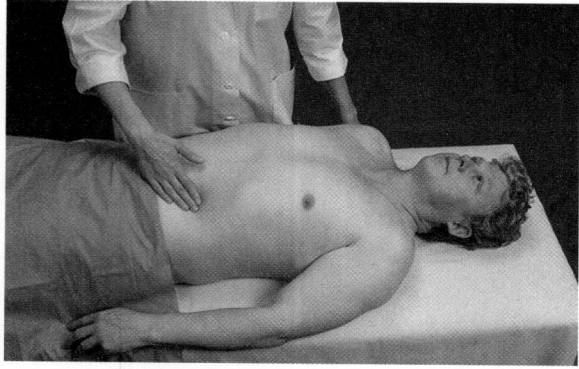

FIGURE 5-10 The medical assistant applies light palpation to the client's abdomen.

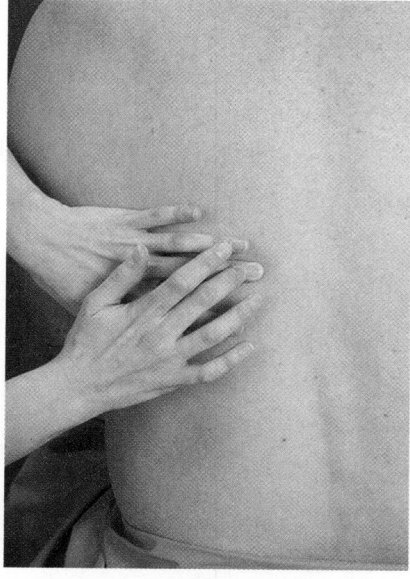

FIGURE 5-11 Apply percussion with your hands.

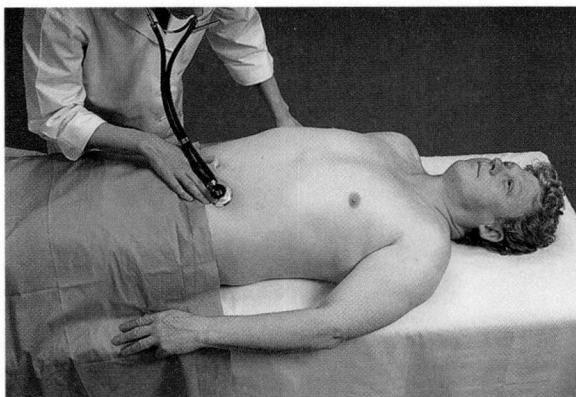

FIGURE 5-12   Auscultation.

stethoscope is placed on the skin surface and the earpieces are placed in the health care provider's ears. The medical assistant uses auscultation to obtain an apical heart rate (see Chapter 4). The medical assistant also uses auscultation to obtain an auscultatory blood pressure reading. The doctor uses auscultation to listen for abnormal heart or lung sounds, such as murmurs, wheezes, or rales. Sounds of movement of air or gas through the intestine, as well as **bruits** (abnormal sounds) can be detected by auscultation.

Positioning the Client for Examination

The medical assistant performs an important role in positioning a client for examination. The medical assistant must be competent in several functions to accomplish this.

Clients are placed in several standard positions for different examinations and procedures. It is up to the medical assistant to:

- Know the procedure
- Correlate or match the procedure with the correct position
- Assist the client to assume that position
- Meet the client's physical needs by ensuring client safety
- Meet the client's emotional needs by providing comfort and easing any fears the client may have about the exam

The position used for any examination is determined by the type of procedure, the preference of the doctor, and the health of the client. Specific positions are commonly used for certain procedures.

Sitting. The client assumes a comfortable sitting position on the examination table, with buttocks and thighs supported and legs hanging freely over the side. This is the most common position for the beginning of a physical examination. Eyes, ears, nose, mouth, throat, and neck are all examined while the client is in the sitting position. The doctor will also listen to the heart and lungs while the client is sitting. Testing of reflexes with a reflex hammer is done with the client in this position.

Fowler's Position. This is the same as the sitting position, with the addition of back support for the client. In the **Fowler's position,** the head of the exam table is lifted to a 90-degree angle or straight up (Figure 5-13). This position is frequently used for the client who can breathe only when sitting straight up (*orthopnea*). It is used when examining the head and neck as well as when listening to the heart and lungs.

Semi-Fowler's Position. The **semi-Fowler's position** is similar to the high Fowler's position, but the head of the table is raised to a 45-degree angle (Figure 5-14). This position is frequently used to support a client who has cardiac or breathing difficulties. It can also help a client

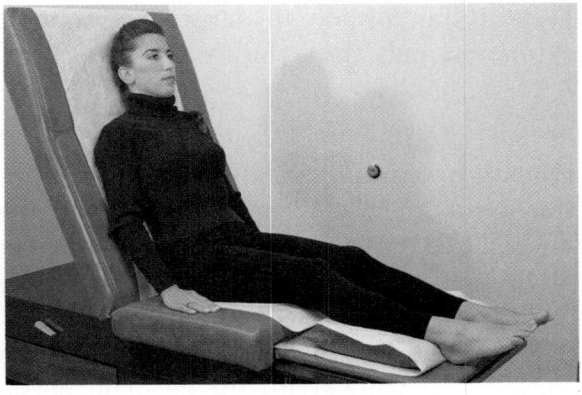

FIGURE 5-13   Client in high Fowler's position.

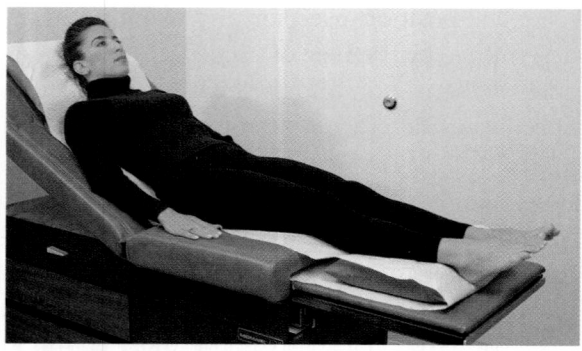

FIGURE 5-14 Client in semi-Fowler's position.

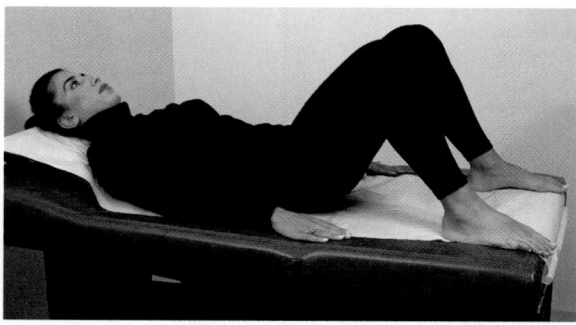

FIGURE 5-16 Client in dorsal recumbent position.

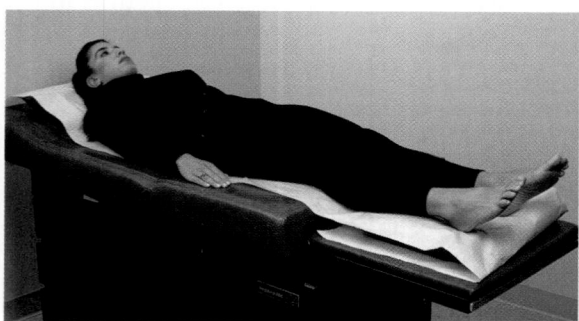

FIGURE 5-15 Client in supine position.

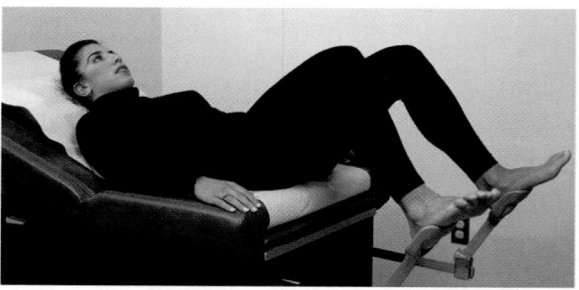

FIGURE 5-17 Client in lithotomy position.

who is weak and unable to sit up for a long period of time. The head, neck, heart, and lungs can be examined with the client in this position. If the client has cardiac or breathing difficulties, partial examination of the abdomen can also be done while the client is in this position.

Supine Position. In the **supine position,** the client lies flat on his back on the examination table. A small pillow can be placed under the client's head for comfort (Figure 5-15). With the client in this position, the doctor can examine the breasts and palpate the abdomen.

Dorsal Recumbent Position. The **dorsal recumbent position** varies from the supine position in that the client lies on his back with the knees flexed (bent) and the soles of the feet flat on the table (Figure 5-16). This position is more comfortable for the client who has back problems. It also eases the stomach muscles if the client is too tense. With the client in dorsal

recumbent position, the physician can examine the breasts and abdomen; he can also do an examination of the genitalia (without instruments) and a rectal exam.

Lithotomy Position. While lying in a supine position with the buttocks at the foot edge of the exam table, the client's feet are placed in **stirrups** (Figure 5-17) for the **lithotomy position.** This provides maximum exposure of the genital area for a pelvic (with instruments) or rectal examination. This position is somewhat uncomfortable, so the medical assistant should help the client on and off the table. Remain with the client during the examination.

Sims' Position. In **Sims' position,** the client lies on the left side with the left leg slightly flexed (bent) and the right leg sharply flexed (bent) (Figure 5-18). The Sims' position is used when obtaining a rectal temperature or administering an enema. The doctor can also examine the rectal area with the client in this position.

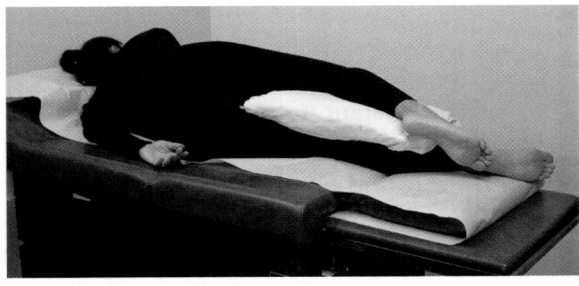

FIGURE 5-18 Client in Sims' position.

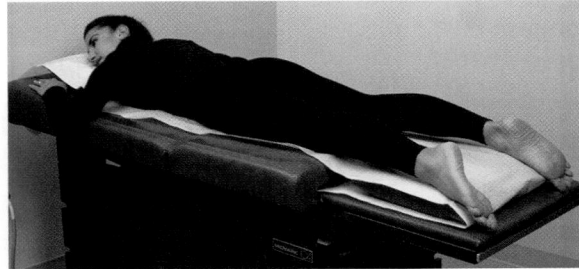

FIGURE 5-19 Client in prone position.

Prone Position. For the **prone position,** the client lies on his abdomen with the face downward (Figure 5-19). The client's arms should be extended so that the head rests on the folded arms. The client can turn the head to the side for comfort and ease in breathing. The doctor can examine the back and check hip extension when the client is in this position.

Knee–Chest Position. To assume the knee-chest posture, the client lies in the prone position, and then lifts up and rests on the knees and chest. The knees should be shoulder-width apart, and the client's back should be straight. Place a small pillow under the client's chest for comfort. Position the client's head to one side. This is an

uncomfortable position to maintain. Do not place the client in this position until the doctor is ready to do the examination or procedure.

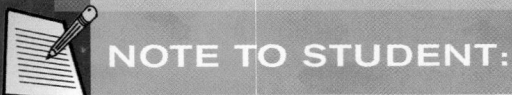

NOTE TO STUDENT:

Some exam tables have parts that can be moved and adjusted to help the client maintain the knee–chest position.

Standing Modified Position. The client stands facing the end of the examination table and bends forward from the waist or hips. The client rests the head, chest, and arms on the examination table. Place a small pillow under the client's head for comfort. This position may also be called the *prostate gland examination position.*

■ ASSISTING WITH EXAMINATIONS

The medical assistant often assists with examinations and procedures. An extremely important part of this role is the communication (both verbal and nonverbal) between the assistant and the client during the examination. Successful completion of the procedure, client outcome, and satisfaction are all aided by positive interaction between the heath care provider and the client. The medical assistant makes a difference by communicating in a professional manner, giving instructions, answering questions, and relieving the client's concerns.

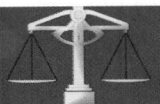

LEGAL/ETHICAL THOUGHTS

Privacy is a critical element of quality client care. Privacy and respect for the dignity of each client must be part of all procedures.

The assistance provided to the doctor is decided by several factors. The medical assistant needs to work within the scope and practice of the profession. State regulations also govern the medical assistant's right to practice. Finally, each health care setting will have its own policies regulating the duties and responsibilities of the medical assistant.

■ SPECIALTY EXAMINATIONS

The medical assistant needs to be aware that specialty examinations may be done. (The medical assistant's role in each of these examinations or procedures is discussed in the chapter on that specialty.) Common specialty examinations are the gynecological or pelvic examination, and the pediatric examination. These procedures are more commonly done in a specialty office, but may be done in the primary care physician's office.

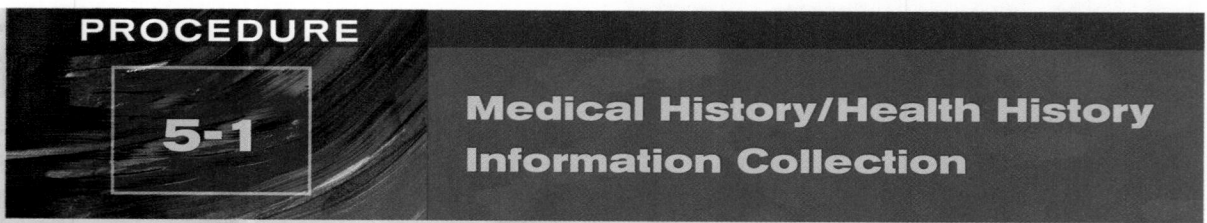

PROCEDURE 5-1

Medical History/Health History Information Collection

Student Competency Objective: The medical assistant student will obtain a medical/health history from a client using the required form.

Items Needed: Medical or health history form, pen, clipboard

Steps:

1. Wash your hands.
2. Get items needed.
3. Review the forms before entering the room with the client.
4. Introduce yourself to the client even if you have seen the client on previous visits to your office. The client may have forgotten your name. This also helps to establish a provider–client relationship, because it shows the client that you want him to know who you are.
5. Identify the client. Ask the client to state his name to establish that this is the right client, and then compare the name given to the name on the chart. Never enter a room and call out a client's name to determine if this person is the correct client. The client may not have heard you clearly and may just nod, smile, or answer yes. Clients almost never question if the medical assistant professional has the right client. It is up to the medical assistant to identify the right client before performing any procedure.
6. Ask the client to sit in a chair rather than on the examination table. This helps to put the client at ease and is much more comfortable than answering questions while sitting on the edge of an examination table.
7. Sit in a chair opposite or next to the client so that you can make eye contact with him.
8. Tell the client, in everyday language, what you are going to do and the purpose of the questions.
9. Speak clearly. When asking questions, look at the client and not down at the clipboard.
10. Give the client time to answer the questions.

(Continues)

PROCEDURE 5-1 (Continued)

11. Repeat the question and use words that the client can understand if he hesitates.
12. When you have completed the medical/health history form, ask if the client has any questions. If he does, give short and simple answers.
13. Thank the client and inform him what will happen next. Tell the client if the doctor will be in or if you need to obtain specimens or prepare the client for an examination.
14. Wash your hands.
15. Sign the form and record information in the client's chart according to office policy.

Charting Example:

> 10/23/20xx   9:30 A.M. Obtained medical/health history from client. Answered questions and prepared client for physical examination by doctor.
>
> *Leslie Atkins, S.M.A.*
>
> Leslie Atkins, S.M.A. (printed name)

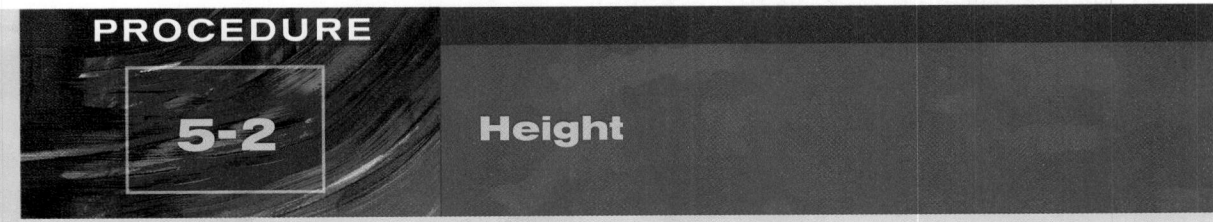

PROCEDURE 5-2 Height

Student Competency Objective: The medical assistant student will measure and record a client's height.

Items Needed: Balance–beam scale, paper, pen or pencil

Steps:
1. Wash your hands.
2. Get items needed.
3. Introduce yourself to the client even if you have seen the client on previous visits to your office. The client may have forgotten your name. This also helps to establish a provider-client relationship, because it shows the client that you want him to know who you are.
4. Identify the client. Ask the client to state his name to establish that this is the right client, and then compare the name given to the name on the chart. Never enter a room and call out a client's name to determine if this person is the correct client. The client may not have heard you clearly and may just nod, smile, or answer yes. Clients almost never question if the medical assistant professional has the right client. It is up to the medical assistant to identify the right client before performing any procedure.
5. Tell the client, in everyday language, what you are going to do.
6. Ask if the client has any questions. If he does, give short and simple answers. Sometimes clients will start (and continue) talking because they are nervous about the procedure.

(Continues)

PROCEDURE 5-2 (Continued)

7. Ask the client to remove his shoes. Shoes and boots vary and can add inches to a person's height.

8. Place a paper towel on the base (flat surfaces) of the balance-beam scale. This keeps the area clean for clients without shoes (Figure 5-20A).

9. With one hand, raise the vertical bar (points up and down). Keep the extension against the vertical bar and raise the bar several inches above the client's head (Figure 5-20B).

10. Help the client to step up onto the scale, facing you and with his back to the scale. The surface of the base moves a little and could cause a client to lose his balance.

11. Always stand close enough to the client and in a body position ready to help if the client becomes unsteady while standing; usually there is nothing on or around the scale to hold for support.

12. Open the extension from the vertical bar. While holding it open, push the bar down until it rests gently on the client's head. The height is not measured where it touches the hair, because styled hair can add several inches. Be careful not to force the bar down too hard, though, or it might hurt the client's head (Figure 5-20C).

13. Help the client off the scale (Figure 5-20D).

14. Offer to help the client put on shoes. A chair should be placed near the scale for client use.

15. Read and record the number shown at the line on the vertical bar (Figure 5-20E).

16. The number will be in inches. To change into feet and inches, divide the number on the scale by 12. For example, the bar reads 63 inches: 63/12 = 5 feet 3 inches.

17. Dispose of the paper towel (from the base of the scale) in a waste container.

18. Wash your hands.

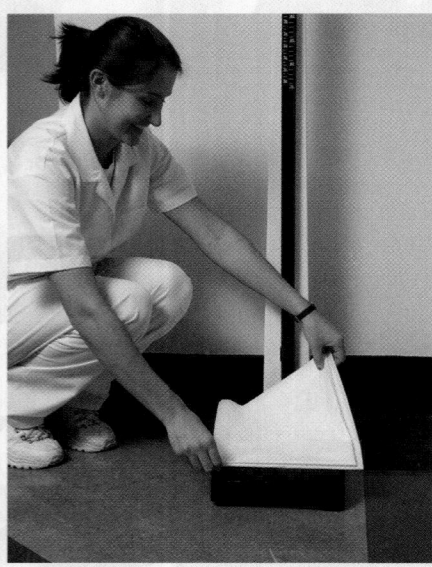

FIGURE 5-20A Place a paper towel on the base of the scale before measuring a client's height. The client takes off his shoes and steps onto the scale.

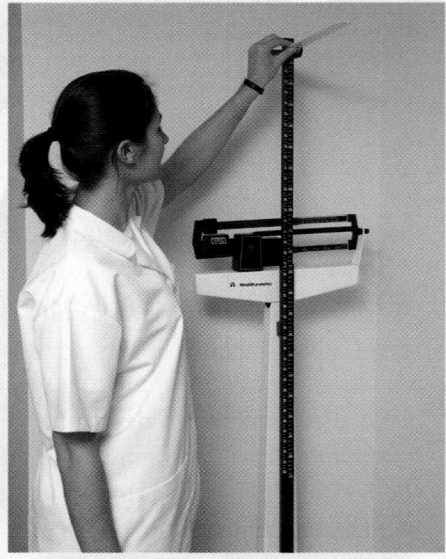

FIGURE 5-20B Raise the vertical bar several inches above the client's head, keeping the extension against the vertical bar.

(Continues)

PROCEDURE 5-2 (Continued)

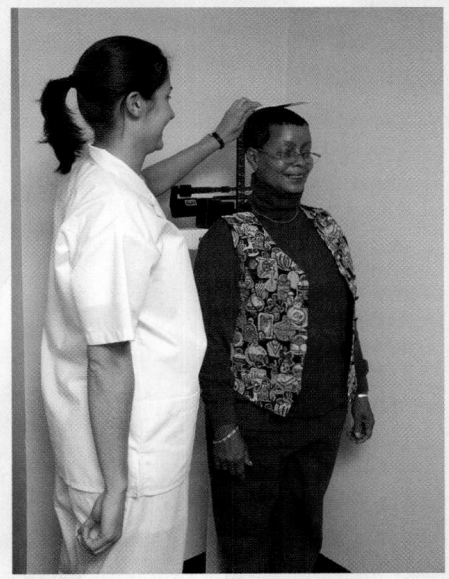

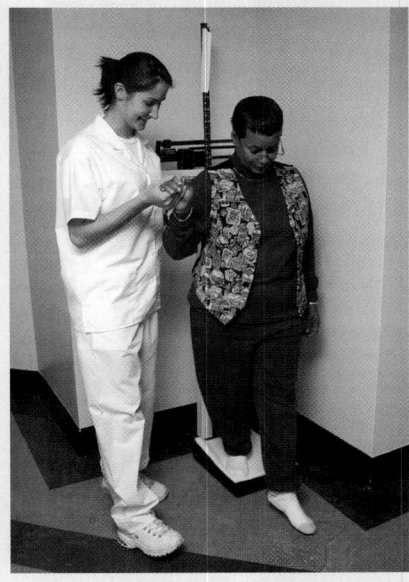

FIGURE 5-20C With the vertical bar extension open, push down until the bar rests gently on the top of the client's head.

FIGURE 5-20D Assist the client to get off the scale.

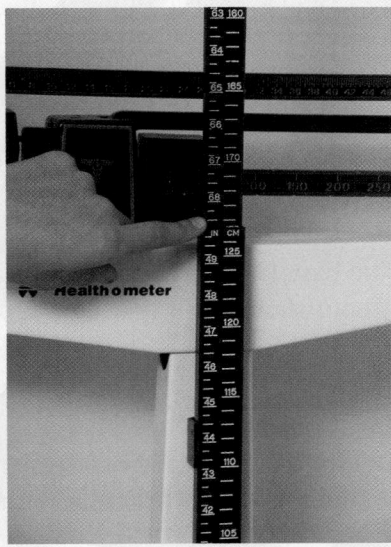

FIGURE 5-20E Read the number shown on the scale bar, and record it in the client's chart.

Charting Example:

The bar reads 63 inches (5 feet 3 inches). You would record the following:

    11/16/20xx   5'3" height without shoes

J. McMullen, S.M.A.

J. McMullen, S.M.A. (printed name)

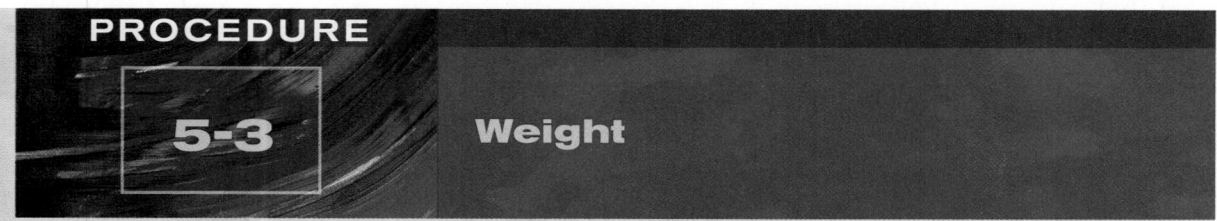

PROCEDURE

5-3   Weight

Student Competency Objective: The medical assistant student will measure and record a client's weight.

Items Needed: Balance-beam scale, paper, pen or pencil

Steps:

1. Wash your hands.
2. Get items needed.
3. Introduce yourself to the client even if you have seen the client on previous visits to your office. The client may have forgotten your name. This also helps to establish a provider-client relationship, because it shows the client that you want him to know who you are.
4. Identify the client. Ask the client to state his name to establish that this is the right client, and then compare the name given to the name on the chart. Never enter a room and call out a client's name to determine if this person is the correct client. The client may not have heard you clearly and may just nod, smile, or answer yes. Clients almost never question if the medical assistant professional has the right client. It is up to the medical assistant to identify the right client before performing any procedure.
5. Tell the client, in everyday language, what you are going to do.
6. Ask if the client has any questions. If he does, give short and simple answers. Sometimes clients will start (and continue) talking because they are nervous about the procedure.
7. Ask the client to remove his shoes. Shoes or boots vary greatly and will add false weight to the measurement.
8. Place a paper towel on the base (flat surfaces) of the balance-beam scale. This keeps the area clean for clients without shoes.
9. Help the client to step up onto the scale with the client's face to the scale and back to the medical assistant. The surface of the base moves a little and could cause a client to lose his balance.
10. Always stand close enough to the client and in a body position ready to help if the client becomes unsteady while standing; usually there is nothing on or around the scale to hold onto for support.
11. Move the large poise (rectangular weight) along the long horizontal bar (the bar that ends in points out to the side). This poise moves in increments of 50 pounds (Figure 5-21A).
12. Move the small poise (smaller rectangular weight) along the upper measuring bar. This bar is marked in increments of pounds or quarter pounds (Figure 5-21B).
13. When the pointed end of the balance beam (at the right side of scale) remains in the middle between the top and bottom, stop moving the poises.

(Continues)

PROCEDURE 5-3 (Continued)

14. Read the number at the large poise.

15. Read the number at the small poise.

16. Add the numbers from the large and small poises. The total is the client's weight. For example, the number at the large poise reads 100 and the number at the small poise reads 40: 100 + 40 = 140; the client's weight is 140 pounds.

17. Often a client's height is measured at the same time as the weight. See Procedure 5-2.

18. Help the client off the scale.

19. Offer to help the client put on shoes. A chair should be placed near the scale for clients.

20. Read and record the weight measurement.

21. Push the poises back to the left. The large one should fit in the notch and the small one against the left side of the scale. (This helps keep the scale functioning accurately.)

22. Dispose of the paper towel (from the base of the scale) in a waste container.

23. Wash your hands.

Charting Example:

The large poise was at the 150 notch and the small poise was at 10. You would record the following:

    11/15/20xx   160 lbs. With clothing on and no shoes

    Susan McMullen, S.M.A.

    Susan McMullen, S.M.A. (printed name)

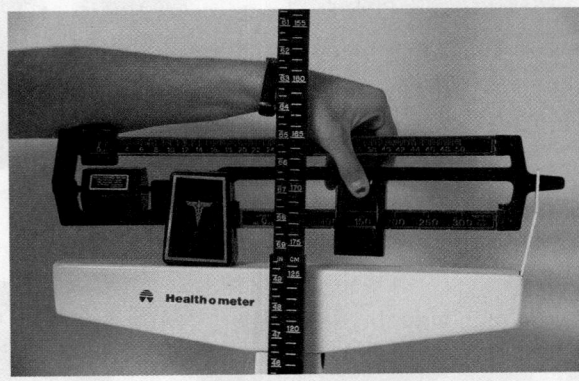

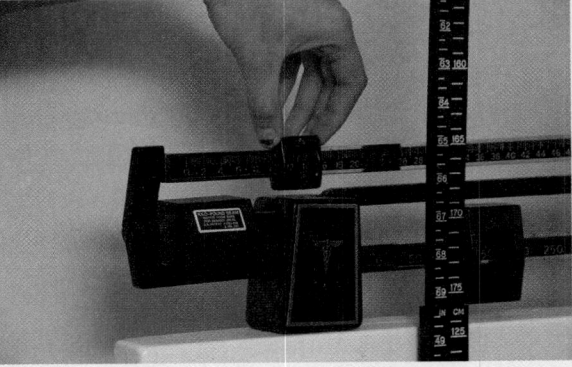

FIGURE 5–21A Stand close to the client, ready to assist if the client loses his balance. Move the large poise of the scale along the long, horizontal scale.

FIGURE 5–21B Move the small poise along the upper bar. The numbers from the large and small poises are added to find the client's weight.

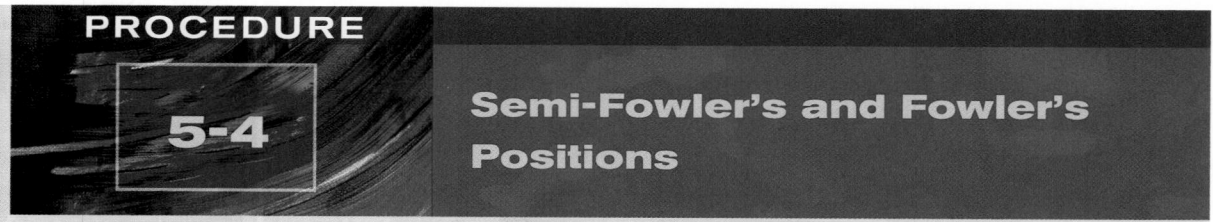

PROCEDURE 5-4

Semi-Fowler's and Fowler's Positions

Student Competency Objective: The medical assistant student will assist the client into the semi-Fowler's or Fowler's position on the examination table.

Items Needed: Examination table with adjustable head or examination table cover, clean paper cover for examination table, pillow

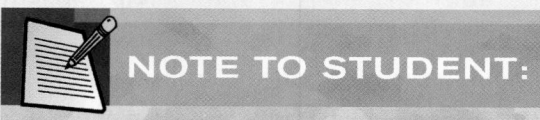

NOTE TO STUDENT:

Before preparing a client for examination, check to see that clean paper is on the examination table and that the room is clean.

Steps:

1. Wash your hands.
2. Get items needed.
3. Introduce yourself to the client even if you have seen the client on previous visits to your office. The client may have forgotten your name. This also helps to establish a provider–client relationship, because it shows the client that you want him to know who you are.
4. Identify the client. Ask the client to state his name to establish that this is the right client, and then compare the name given to the name on the chart. Never enter a room and call out a client's name to determine if this person is the correct client. The client may not have heard you clearly and may just nod, smile, or answer yes. Clients almost never question if the medical assistant professional has the right client. It is up to the medical assistant to identify the right client before performing any procedure.
5. Tell the client, in everyday language, what you are going to do.
6. Ask if the client has any questions. If he does, give short and simple answers. Sometimes clients will start (and continue) talking because they are nervous about the procedure.
7. Ask the client if he needs help undressing and putting on a gown (if a gown is required for this particular examination). Assist as needed.
8. If the client does not need assistance, tell him which way the gown opens (front or back). Provide privacy while the client changes.
9. Move a footstool to the side of the examination table.
10. Standing close to the client, and in a position ready to help as needed for balance, ask the client to step up backward onto the footstool.
11. Ask the client to sit back comfortably on the side of the examination table.
12. Raise the head of examination table to 45 degrees for the semi-Fowler's position or to 90 degrees for the Fowler's position.
13. Ask the client to rest back on the support.
14. Drape the client as needed.
15. Stay with the client and assist the doctor during the examination or procedure, as needed. Remain with the client if he is unsteady or weak.

(Continues)

PROCEDURE 5-4 (Continued)

16. Inform the client before you lower the head of the table. Have the client lean forward before you move the head of the table.

17. Be careful when lowering the head of the table. Sometimes it must be supported while being lowered.

18. After the examination or procedure is completed, ask the client to sit for a minute, with legs over the table edge, before getting off the table. Assist as needed, and then help the client to get off the table.

19. If necessary, assist the client to take off the gown and get dressed.

20. Dispose of the paper table covering, paper covering for the pillow, and gown (if paper) in the appropriate waste container.

21. Clean the table and room according to office policy.

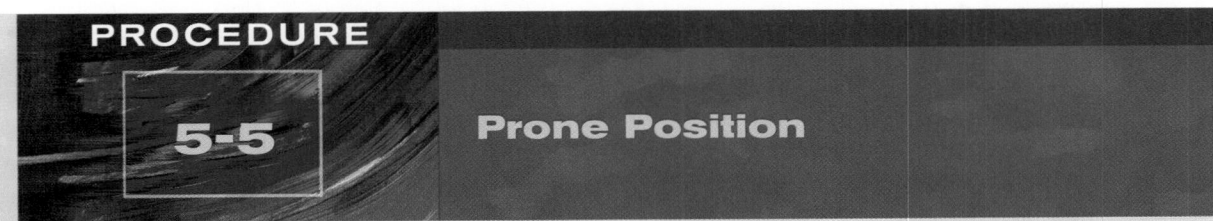

PROCEDURE

5-5   Prone Position

Student Competency Objective: The medical assistant student will assist the client into a prone position on the examination table.

Items Needed: Examination table, clean paper cover for examination table, drape, gown

Steps:

1. Wash your hands.

2. Get items needed.

3. Introduce yourself to the client even if you have seen the client on previous visits to your office. The client may have forgotten your name. This also helps to establish a provider–client relationship, because it shows the client that you want him to know who you are.

4. Identify the client. Ask the client to state his name to establish that this is the right client, and then compare the name given to the name on the chart. Never enter a room and call out a client's name to determine if this person is the correct client. The client may not have heard you clearly and may just nod, smile, or answer yes. Clients almost never question if the medical assistant professional has the right client. It is up to the medical assistant to identify the right client before performing any procedure.

5. Tell the client, in everyday language, what you are going to do.

6. Ask if the client has any questions. If he does, give short and simple answers. Sometimes clients will start (and continue) talking because they are nervous about the procedure.

7. Ask the client if he needs help undressing and putting on a gown (if a gown is required for this particular examination). Assist as needed.

(Continues)

PROCEDURE 5-5 (Continued)

8. If the client does not need assistance, tell him which way the gown opens (front or back). Provide privacy while the client changes.

9. Move a footstool to the side of the examination table.

10. Standing close to the client, and in a position ready to help as needed for balance, ask the client to step up backward onto the footstool.

11. Ask the client to sit back comfortably on the side of the examination table.

12. Pull out the foot extension of the table, if needed.

13. Ask the client to lie on his back.

14. Cover the client with a drape.

15. Standing at the side of the table, ask the client to turn toward you so that he is lying on his stomach. Tell the client to turn slowly, so that he does not fall from the table.

16. Have the client turn his head to the side.

17. Ask the client to bend his arms at the elbow and place his hands near his head.

18. Make sure the client is covered for privacy and modesty.

19. Stay with the client and assist the doctor with the examination or procedure, as needed.

20. After the examination is completed, ask the client to turn on his back. Remain with the client during this movement to make sure he does not fall off the table.

21. Ask the client to sit for a minute, with legs over the table edge, before getting off the table. Assist as needed, and then help the client to get off the table.

22. If necessary, assist the client to take off the gown and get dressed.

23. Dispose of the paper table covering and gown (if paper) in the appropriate waste container.

24. Clean the table and room according to office policy.

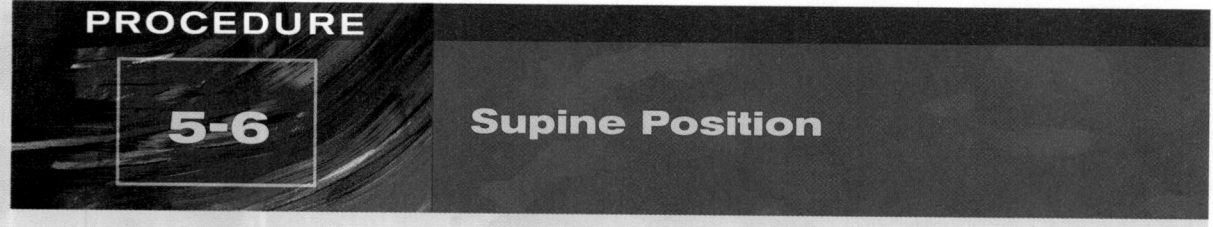

PROCEDURE 5-6   Supine Position

Student Competency Objective: The medical assistant student will assist the client into a supine position on the examination table.

Items Needed: Examination table, paper cover for examination table, pillow, drape, gown

Steps:

1. Wash your hands.

2. Get items needed.

3. Introduce yourself to the client even if you have seen the client on previous visits to your office. The client may have forgotten your name. This also helps to establish a provider–client relationship, because it shows the client that you want him to know who you are.

(Continues)

PROCEDURE 5-6 (Continued)

4. Identify the client. Ask the client to state his name to establish that this is the right client, and then compare the name given to the name on the chart. Never enter a room and call out a client's name to determine if this person is the correct client. The client may not have heard you clearly and may just nod, smile, or answer yes. Clients almost never question if the medical assistant professional has the right client. It is up to the medical assistant to identify the right client before performing any procedure.

5. Tell the client, in everyday language, what you are going to do.

6. Ask if the client has any questions. If he does, give short and simple answers. Sometimes clients will start (and continue) talking because they are nervous about the procedure.

7. Ask the client if he needs help undressing and putting on a gown (if a gown is required for this particular examination). Assist as needed.

8. If the client does not need assistance, tell him which way the gown opens (front or back). Provide privacy while the client changes.

9. Move a footstool to the side of the examination table.

10. Standing close to the client, and in a position ready to help as needed for balance, ask the client to step up backward onto the footstool.

11. Ask the client to sit back comfortably on the side of the examination table.

12. Pull out the foot extension of the table, if needed.

13. Ask the client to lie on his back.

14. Cover the client with a drape.

15. Place a small pillow under the client's head for comfort.

16. Stay with the client and assist the doctor during the examination or procedure, as needed.

17. After the examination or procedure is completed, ask the client to sit for a minute, with legs over the table edge, before getting off the table. Assist as needed, and then help the client to get off the table.

18. If necessary, assist the client to take off the gown and get dressed.

19. Dispose of the paper table covering, paper covering for the pillow, and gown (if paper) in the appropriate waste container.

20. Clean the table and room according to office policy.

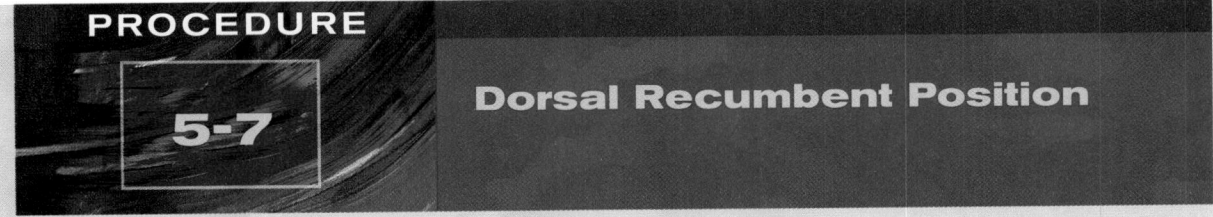

PROCEDURE 5-7   Dorsal Recumbent Position

Student Competency Objective: The medical assistant student will assist the client into a dorsal recumbent position on the examination table.

Items Needed: Examination table, paper cover for examination table, pillow, drape, gown

(Continues)

PROCEDURE 5-7 (Continued)

Steps:

1. Wash your hands.
2. Get items needed.
3. Introduce yourself to the client even if you have seen the client on previous visits to your office. The client may have forgotten your name. This also helps to establish a provider–client relationship, because it shows the client that you want him to know who you are.
4. Identify the client. Ask the client to state his name to establish that this is the right client, and then compare the name given to the name on the chart. Never enter a room and call out a client's name to determine if this person is the correct client. The client may not have heard you clearly and may just nod, smile, or answer yes. Clients almost never question if the medical assistant professional has the right client. It is up to the medical assistant to identify the right client before performing any procedure.
5. Tell the client, in everyday language, what you are going to do.
6. Ask if the client has any questions. If he does, give short and simple answers. Sometimes clients will start (and continue) talking because they are nervous about the procedure.
7. Ask the client if he needs help undressing and putting on a gown (if a gown is required for this particular examination). Assist as needed.
8. If the client does not need assistance, tell him which way the gown opens (front or back). Provide privacy while the client changes.
9. Move a footstool to the side of the examination table.
10. Standing close to the client, and in a position ready to help as needed for balance, ask the client to step up backward onto the footstool.
11. Ask the client to sit back comfortably on the side of the examination table.
12. Pull out the foot extension of the table if needed.
13. Ask the client to bend his knees and put his feet flat on the table.
14. Drape the client.
15. Place a small pillow under the client's head for comfort.
16. Stay with the client and assist the doctor during the examination or procedure, as needed.
17. After the examination or procedure is completed, ask the client to sit for a minute, with legs over the table edge, before getting off the table. Assist as needed, and then help the client to get off the table.
18. If necessary, assist the client to take off the gown and get dressed.
19. Dispose of the paper table covering, paper covering for the pillow, and gown (if paper) in the appropriate waste container.
20. Clean the table and room according to office policy.

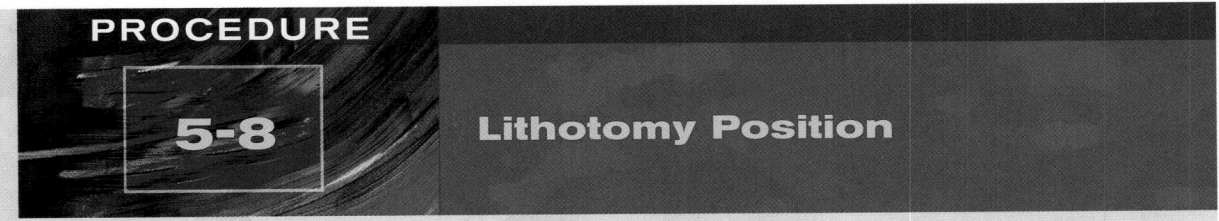

PROCEDURE

5-8   **Lithotomy Position**

Student Competency Objective: The medical assistant student will assist the client into a lithotomy position on the examination table.

Items Needed: Examination table, paper cover for examination table, pillow, drape, gown

Steps:
1. Wash your hands.
2. Get items needed.
3. Introduce yourself to the client even if you have seen the client on previous visits to your office. The client may have forgotten your name. This also helps to establish a provider-client relationship, because it shows the client that you want her to know who you are.
4. Identify the client. Ask the client to state her name to establish that this is the right client, and then compare the name given to the name on the chart. Never enter a room and call out a client's name to determine if this person is the correct client. The client may not have heard you clearly and may just nod, smile, or answer yes. Clients almost never question if the medical assistant professional has the right client. It is up to the medical assistant to identify the right client before performing any procedure.
5. Tell the client, in everyday language, what you are going to do.
6. Ask if the client has any questions. If she does, give short and simple answers. Sometimes clients will start (and continue) talking because they are nervous about the procedure.
7. Ask the client if she needs help undressing and putting on a gown (if a gown is required for this particular examination). Assist as needed.
8. If the client does not need assistance, tell her which way the gown opens (front or back). Provide privacy while the client changes.
9. Move a footstool to the side of the examination table.
10. Standing close to the client, and in a position ready to help as needed for balance, ask the client to step up backward onto the footstool.
11. Ask the client to sit back comfortably on the side of the examination table.
12. Pull out the foot extension of the table, if needed.
13. Ask the client to lie on her back on the examination table.
14. Drape the client.
15. Turn the stirrups away from the table and adjust the height (using the height lever) as needed for client comfort.
16. Ask the client to slide down toward the end of the table. Place the client's feet into the stirrups.
17. Push in the foot extension of the table.
18. Be sure that the footstool and the light are placed correctly for the examiner.

(Continues)

PROCEDURE 5-8 (Continued)

19. The lithotomy position is an uncomfortable position to maintain. Do not put the client in this position until the examiner is ready.
20. Stay with the client and assist the doctor during the examination or procedure, as needed.
21. After the examination or procedure is completed, help the client to lift her feet out of the stirrups.
22. Ask the client to sit for a minute, with legs over the table edge, before getting off the table. Assist as needed, and then help the client to get off the table.
23. If necessary, assist the client to take off the gown and get dressed.
24. Dispose of the paper table covering, paper covering for the pillow, and gown (if paper) in the appropriate waste container.
25. Clean the table and room according to office policy.

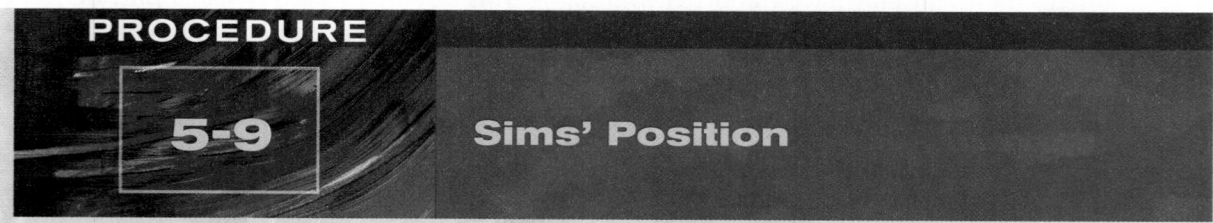

PROCEDURE
5-9   Sims' Position

Student Competency Objective: The medical assistant student will assist the client into the Sims' position on the examination table.

Items Needed: Examination table, paper cover for examination table, pillow, drape, gown

Steps:
1. Wash your hands.
2. Get items needed.
3. Introduce yourself to the client even if you have seen the client on previous visits to your office. The client may have forgotten your name. This also helps to establish a provider-client relationship, because it shows the client that you want him to know who you are.
4. Identify the client. Ask the client to state his name to establish that this is the right client, and then compare the name given to the name on the chart. Never enter a room and call out a client's name to determine if this person is the correct client. The client may not have heard you clearly and may just nod, smile, or answer yes. Clients almost never question if the medical assistant professional has the right client. It is up to the medical assistant to identify the right client before performing any procedure.
5. Tell the client, in everyday language, what you are going to do.
6. Ask if the client has any questions. If he does, give short and simple answers. Sometimes clients will start (and continue) talking because they are nervous about the procedure.
7. Ask the client if he needs help undressing and putting on a gown (if a gown is required for this particular examination). Assist as needed.

(Continues)

PROCEDURE 5-9 (Continued)

8. If the client does not need assistance, tell him which way the gown opens (front or back). Provide privacy while the client changes.

9. Move a footstool to the side of the examination table.

10. Standing close to the client, and in a position ready to help as needed for balance, ask the client to step up backward onto the footstool.

11. Ask the client to sit back comfortably on the side of the examination table.

12. Pull out the foot extension of the table, if needed.

13. Tell the client to lie on his left side. The client may place his left hand on the pillow for comfort.

14. Tell the client to bend his right arm at the elbow, placing the hand near his head.

15. The client's left leg should be flexed or bent slightly and the right leg should be flexed or bent sharply.

16. Place a drape over the client.

17. Stay with the client and assist the doctor during the examination or procedure, as needed.

18. Tell the client to turn onto his back. Stand by the table to prevent the client from falling off the examination table while he turns.

19. After the examination or procedure is completed, ask the client to sit for a minute, with legs over the table edge, before getting off the table. Assist as needed, and then help the client to get off the table.

20. If necessary, assist the client to take off the gown and get dressed.

21. Dispose of the paper table covering, paper covering for the pillow, and gown (if paper) in the appropriate waste container.

22. Clean the table and room according to office policy.

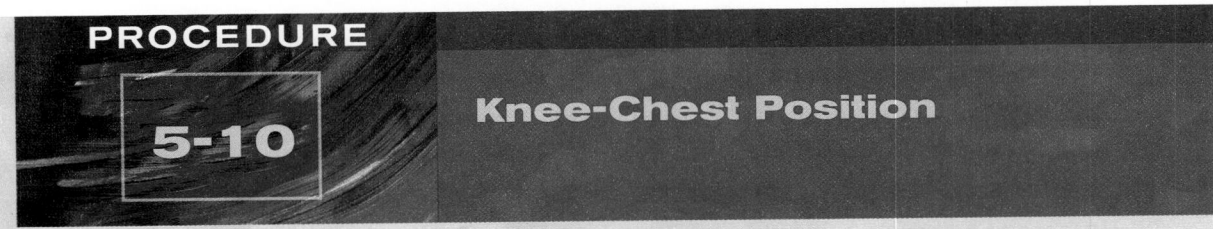

PROCEDURE 5-10

Knee-Chest Position

Student Competency Objective: The medical assistant student will assist the client into a knee-chest position on the examination table.

Items Needed: Examination table, paper cover for examination table, pillow, gown

Steps:

1. Wash your hands.
2. Get items needed.

(Continues)

3. Introduce yourself to the client even if you have seen the client on previous visits to your office. The client may have forgotten your name. This also helps to establish a provider-client relationship, because it shows the client that you want him to know who you are.

4. Identify the client. Ask the client to state his name to establish that this is the right client, and then compare the name given to the name on the chart. Never enter a room and call out a client's name to determine if this person is the correct client. The client may not have heard you clearly and may just nod, smile, or answer yes. Clients almost never question if the medical assistant professional has the right client. It is up to the medical assistant to identify the right client before performing any procedure.

5. Tell the client, in everyday language, what you are going to do.

6. Ask if the client has any questions. If he does, give short and simple answers. Sometimes clients will start (and continue) talking because they are nervous about the procedure.

7. Ask the client if he needs help undressing and putting on a gown (if a gown is required for this particular examination). Assist as needed.

8. If the client does not need assistance, tell him which way the gown opens (front or back). Provide privacy while the client changes.

9. Move a footstool to the side of the examination table.

10. Standing close to the client, and in a position ready to help as needed for balance, ask the client to step up backward onto the footstool.

11. Instruct the client to lie prone (face down) on the exam table.

12. Ask the client to rest on his knees and chest.

13. Tell the client to turn his head to the side.

14. Place a small pillow under the client's chest for comfort.

15. Take sheet and cover back, buttocks, and legs.

16. Tell the client to place an arm above his head or down at the side, whichever is more comfortable for the client.

17. Stay with the client and assist the doctor during the examination or procedure, as needed.

18. After the examination or procedure is completed, ask the client to sit for a minute, with legs over the table edge, before getting off the table. Assist as needed, and then help the client to get off the table.

19. If necessary, assist the client to take off the gown and get dressed.

20. Dispose of the paper table covering, paper covering for the pillow, and gown (if paper) in the appropriate waste container.

21. Clean the table and room according to office policy.

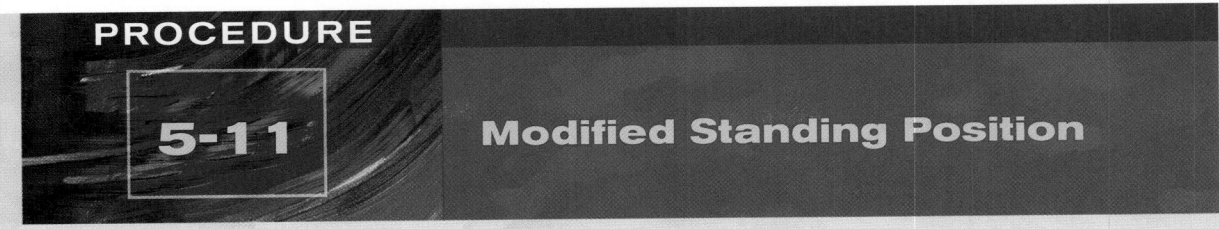

Student Competency Objective: The medical assistant student will assist the client into a modified standing position at the examination table.

Items Needed: Examination table, paper cover for examination table, pillow, gown

Steps:
1. Wash your hands.
2. Get items needed.
3. Introduce yourself to the client even if you have seen the client on previous visits to your office. The client may have forgotten your name. This also helps to establish a provider-client relationship, because it shows the client that you want him to know who you are.
4. Identify the client. Ask the client to state his name to establish that this is the right client, and then compare the name given to the name on the chart. Never enter a room and call out a client's name to determine if this person is the correct client. The client may not have heard you clearly and may just nod, smile, or answer yes. Clients almost never question if the medical assistant professional has the right client. It is up to the medical assistant to identify the right client before performing any procedure.
5. Tell the client, in everyday language, what you are going to do.
6. Ask if the client has any questions. If he does, give short and simple answers. Sometimes clients will start (and continue) talking because they are nervous about the procedure.
7. Ask the client if he needs help undressing and putting on a gown (if a gown is required for this particular examination). Assist as needed.
8. If the client does not need assistance, tell him which way the gown opens (front or back). Provide privacy while the client changes.
9. Ask the client to stand facing the end of the examination table.
10. Cover the client with a drape.
11. Instruct the client to bend forward from the waist or hips.
12. Tell the client to rest his head, chest, and arms on the exam table.
13. Place a small pillow under the client's head for comfort.
14. Stay with the client and assist the doctor during the examination or procedure, as needed.
15. After the examination or procedure is completed, assist the client to take off the gown and get dressed, as needed.
16. Dispose of the paper table covering, paper covering for the pillow, and gown (if paper) in the appropriate waste container.
17. Clean the table and room according to office policy.

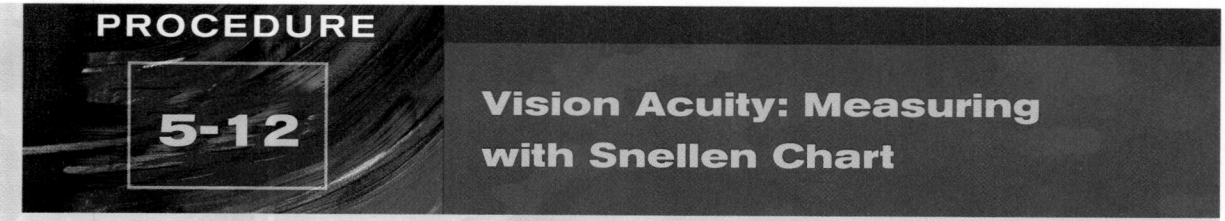

PROCEDURE

5-12

**Vision Acuity: Measuring
with Snellen Chart**

Student Competency Objective: The medical assistant student will measure visual acuity using a Snellen chart.

Items Needed: Snellen chart, paper, pen, eye occluder

Steps:

1. Wash your hands.
2. Get items needed.
3. Introduce yourself to the client even if you have seen the client on previous visits to your office. The client may have forgotten your name. This also helps to establish a provider–client relationship, because it shows the client that you want him to know who you are.
4. Identify the client. Ask the client to state his name to establish that this is the right client, and then compare the name given to the name on the chart. Never enter a room and call out a client's name to determine if this person is the correct client. The client may not have heard you clearly and may just nod, smile, or answer yes. Clients almost never question if the medical assistant professional has the right client. It is up to the medical assistant to identify the right client before performing any procedure.
5. Tell the client, in everyday language, what you are going to do.
6. Ask if the client has any questions. If he does, give short and simple answers. Sometimes clients will start (and continue) talking because they are nervous about the procedure.
7. The client should stand or sit 20 feet from the Snellen chart. Make sure that the chart is at the client's eye level.
8. Identify a line on the chart by pointing to it.
9. Ask the client to read that line with both eyes. If the client wears glasses, he should keep them on for this part of the examination. If the client wears contact lenses, check office policy. Some doctors require that the client not wear contacts for a number of days before the eye examination.
10. Tell the client to cover his left eye with the eye occluder (Figure 5–22A). If the client wears glasses, the procedure is done first with the glasses on, and then without the corrective lenses.
11. Ask the client to keep both eyes open, even though one eye is covered.
12. Observe and record if the client leans forward, squints, or turns his head in an effort to read the lines.
13. The record should state whether each line was read with corrective lenses (glasses), CC; or without corrective lenses, SC.
14. Write down the number by the smallest line that the client can read with his right eye without mistakes (Figure 5–22B).

(Continues)

PROCEDURE 5-12 (Continued)

15. Tell the client to cover his right eye with the occluder. Test the left eye following the same steps 9 through 12.

16. Write down the number by the smallest line that the client can read with his left eye without a mistake.

17. Vision acuity for distance is written as a fraction, such as 20/20; the numerator or top number is the distance or number of feet from the Snellen chart. This is normally 20 feet (20/xx). The denominator or bottom number is the number by the smallest line that the client can read. If the client stood 20 feet away from the Snellen chart and the smallest line that the client could read was numbered 60, the distance visual acuity would be written as 20/60. This means that the client stood 20 feet away and read the line that a client with 20/20 vision would have been able to read at 60 feet away.

18. Record the procedure on the client's medical chart.

Charting Example:

Without glasses, the client read line number 40 with the right eye, line 50 with the left eye, and line 40 with both eyes. No unusual client behavior was necessary to assist in reading in these lines. You would record the following:

> 11/20/20xx Visual acuity with Snellen chart. OD 20/40; OS 20/50; OU 20/40 without correction. No leaning forward or squinting observed.

Tracy Johnson, S. M. A.

Tracy Johnson, S.M.A. (printed name)

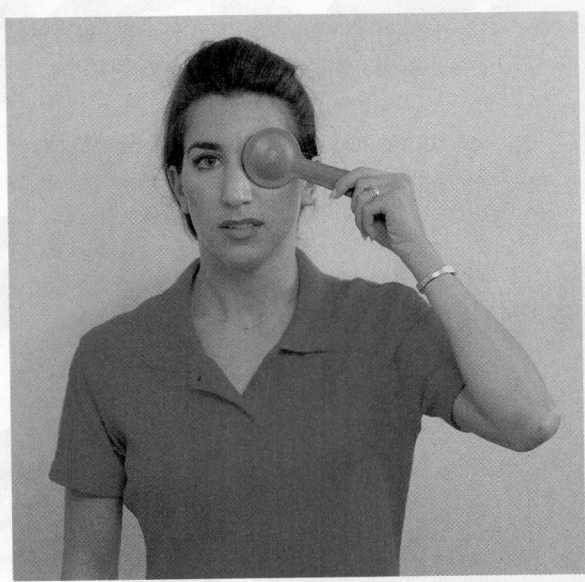

FIGURE 5-22A The client covers her left eye with an occluder, but keeps the eye open beneath it.

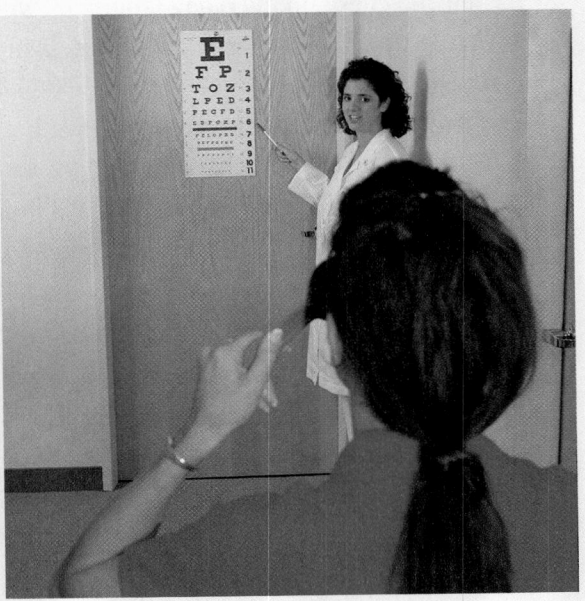

FIGURE 5-22B As the medical assistant points to a line on the Snellen chart, the client attempts to read the line, while keeping the eye covered with an occluder.

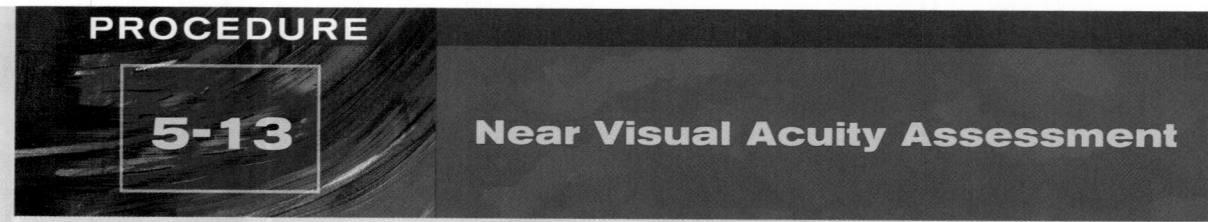

PROCEDURE 5-13 Near Visual Acuity Assessment

Student Competency Objective: The medical assistant student will assess near visual acuity using a Jaeger near visual acuity card.

Items Needed: Jaeger near visual testing card, small gauze pad, paper and pen

Steps:

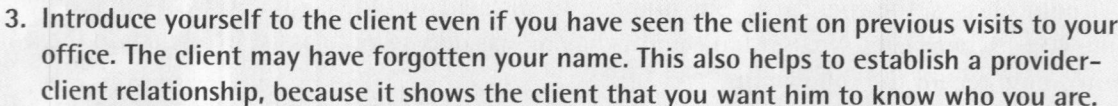

NOTE TO STUDENT:

Another near visual acuity card may be used, but the type selected must be noted when documenting.

1. Wash your hands.
2. Get items needed.
3. Introduce yourself to the client even if you have seen the client on previous visits to your office. The client may have forgotten your name. This also helps to establish a provider-client relationship, because it shows the client that you want him to know who you are.
4. Identify the client. Ask the client to state his name to establish that this is the right client, and then compare the name given to the name on the chart. Never enter a room and call out a client's name to determine if this person is the correct client. The client may not have heard you clearly and may just nod, smile, or answer yes. Clients almost never question if the medical assistant professional has the right client. It is up to the medical assistant to identify the right client before performing any procedure.
5. Tell the client, in everyday language, what you are going to do.
6. Ask if the client has any questions. If he does, give short and simple answers. Sometimes clients will start (and continue) talking because they are nervous about the procedure.
7. Ask the client to sit comfortably.
8. Remind the client to keep both eyes open.
9. Hold the Jaeger card about 15 to 16 inches from the client's face.
10. Position the card at comfortable reading level for the client.
11. Point to a line and instruct the client to begin reading aloud.
12. Note the number by the smallest printed line that the client reads without a mistake.
13. Wipe the card off with a small gauze pad.
14. Discard the gauze pad in an appropriate waste container.
15. Wash your hands.
16. Record the procedure on the client's medical chart.

Charting Example:

The client read up to and including line 6. You would record the following:

> 4/23/20xx   10:30 A.M. Near visual acuity assessed using Jaeger test. Last line correctly read by client—line 6.
>
> *Lindsey Phillips, S.M.A.*
>
> Lindsey Phillips, S.M.A. (printed name)

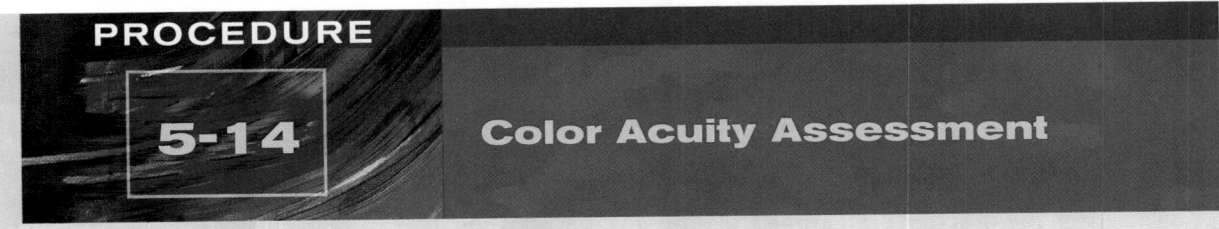

PROCEDURE

5-14

Color Acuity Assessment

Student Competency Objective: The medical assistant student will assess color acuity using the Ishihara testing system.

Items Needed: Ishihara test cards, small gauze pad, paper and pen

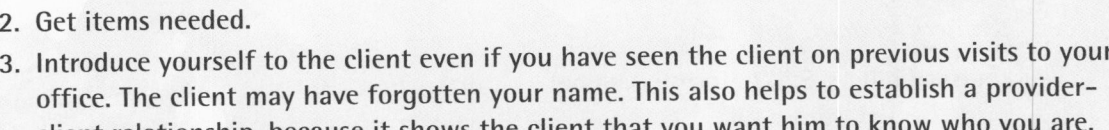

NOTE TO STUDENT:

Another testing system may be used, but the type selected must be documented.

Steps:

1. Wash your hands.
2. Get items needed.
3. Introduce yourself to the client even if you have seen the client on previous visits to your office. The client may have forgotten your name. This also helps to establish a provider–client relationship, because it shows the client that you want him to know who you are.
4. Identify the client. Ask the client to state his name to establish that this is the right client, and then compare the name given to the name on the chart. Never enter a room and call out a client's name to determine if this person is the correct client. The client may not have heard you clearly and may just nod, smile, or answer yes. Clients almost never question if the medical assistant professional has the right client. It is up to the medical assistant to identify the right client before performing any procedure.
5. Tell the client, in everyday language, what you are going to do.
6. Ask if the client has any questions. If he does, give short and simple answers. Sometimes clients will start (and continue) talking because they are nervous about the procedure.
7. Make sure the room has adequate lighting. Natural light is best.
8. Explain the procedure to the client and perform a sample session with a practice card (Figure 5-23).
9. Position the plate or chart at right angles to the client's vision.
10. Hold the chart about 30 inches from the client's face.
11. Instruct the client to keep both eyes open.

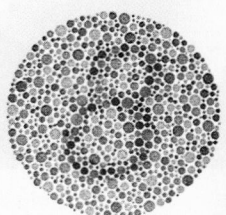 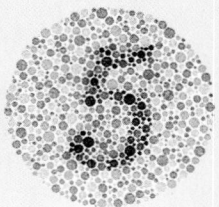

FIGURE 5-23 Ishihara plates are used to determine color acuity.

(Continues)

PROCEDURE 5-14 (Continued)

12. Ask the client to look at the colored dots and tell you what number or symbol he can see in the dots. Plates with colored line trails are available for use with children or adults who cannot read the numbers. The client can show the direction of the line to you.

13. After the practice plate, hold up plate #1 and ask the client to read the number seen.

14. Note if the client read the number correctly.

15. Continue until all the plates or charts have been completed.

16. Clean the plates with a small gauze pad if the charts are laminated.

17. Store the plates properly, away from light that could damage them.

Charting Example:

The client read all plates correctly. You would record the following:

> 4/23/20xx   10:30 A.M. Color acuity assessed using the Ishihara test. Client correctly identified numbers in all the plates. 14/passed.

Lindsey Phillips, S.M.A.

Lindsey Phillips, S.M.A. (printed name)

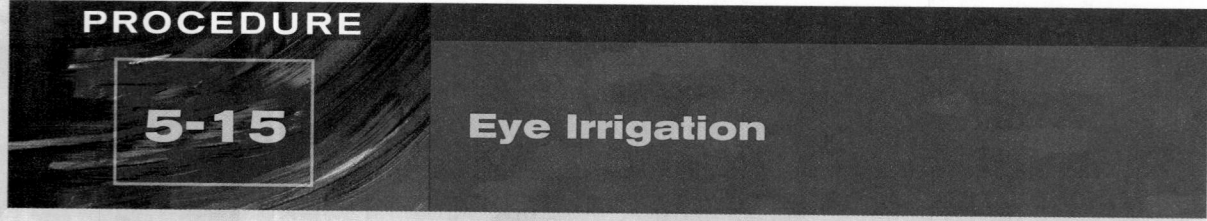

PROCEDURE

5-15   Eye Irrigation

Student Competency Objective: The medical assistant student will irrigate an eye with the ordered ophthalmic solution.

Items Needed: Sterile ophthalmic solution as ordered, sterile container for sterile solution, basin to catch returned solution, sterile gauze or cotton balls, moisture-resistant, absorbent towel, gloves, paper and pen

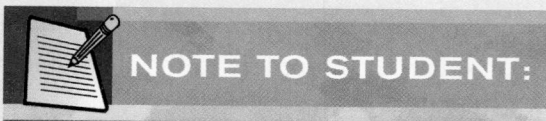

NOTE TO STUDENT:

If both eyes are to be irrigated, you must gather two sets of the items needed.

Steps:

1. Wash your hands.

2. Get items needed.

3. Introduce yourself to the client even if you have seen the client on previous visits to your office. The client may have forgotten your name. This also helps to establish a provider-client relationship, because it shows the client that you want her to know who you are.

(Continues)

PROCEDURE 5-15 (Continued)

4. Identify the client. Ask the client to state his name to establish that this is the right client, and then compare the name given to the name on the chart. Never enter a room and call out a client's name to determine if this person is the correct client. The client may not have heard you clearly and may just nod, smile, or answer yes. Clients almost never question if the medical assistant professional has the right client. It is up to the medical assistant to identify the right client before performing any procedure.

5. Tell the client, in everyday language, what you are going to do.

6. Ask if the client has any questions. If he does, give short and simple answers. Sometimes clients will start (and continue) talking because they are nervous about the procedure.

7. Ask the client to lie on his back on the examination table, unless the client is unable to do this (for example, because of severe asthma, emphysema, or difficulty breathing caused by a cardiac disorder).

8. Drape an absorbent towel over the client's shoulder to prevent the client from getting wet.

9. Ask the client to turn his head toward the affected eye (e.g., if irrigating the right eye, ask the client to turn his head to the right side).

10. Using a moist gauze pad, gently wipe from the inner canthus of the eye (next to the nose) (Figure 5-24A) to the outer canthus of the eye (toward the side of the head) (Figure 24-B) to remove any particles.

11. Place the basin snugly against the side of the client's face (Figure 5-24C).

12. Fill the bulb of a syringe with the ordered solution. Make sure to compare the ophthalmic solution with the doctor's orders, as you would with any medication order.

13. Using your thumb and index finger, gently expose the lower conjunctiva and hold open the client's upper eyelid (Figure 5-24D).

14. Starting at the inner canthus of the eye (next to the nose), hold the syringe 1 inch above the eye and point the flow of solution toward the lower conjunctiva. Do not let the tip of the syringe touch the eye. The cornea of the eye is sensitive and can be hurt (Figure 5-24E).

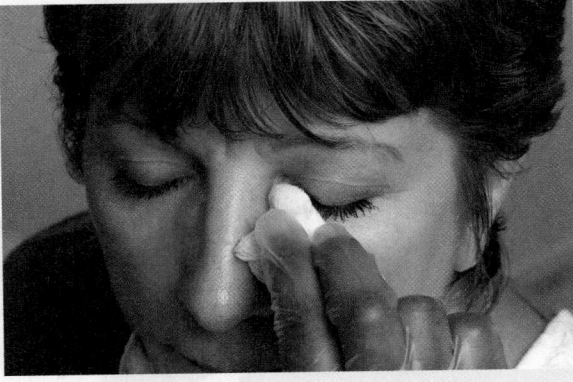

FIGURE 5-24A Wipe the client's face with moist gauze, starting from the inner canthus of the eye.

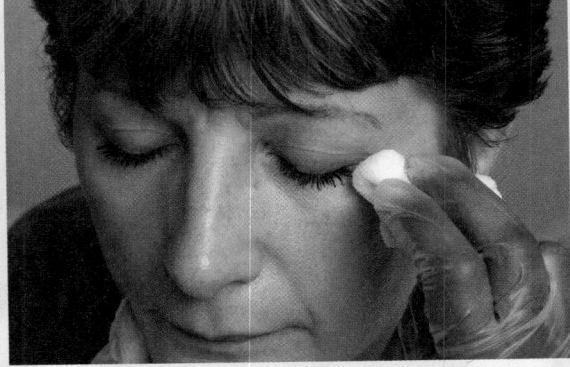

FIGURE 5-24B Wipe to the outer canthus of the eye (toward the ear at the side of the head).

(Continues)

PROCEDURE 5-15 (Continued)

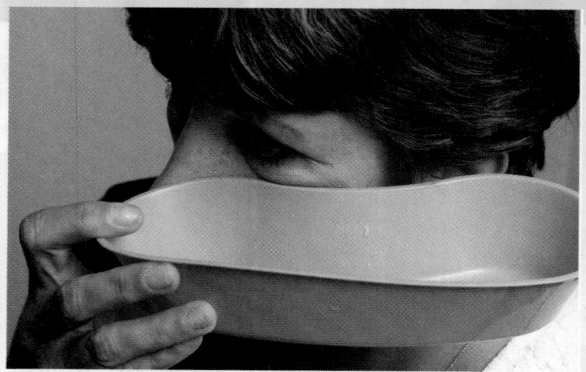

FIGURE 5-24C Place a basin against the side of the client's face, under the affected eye. Drape the client's shoulder with an absorbent towel.

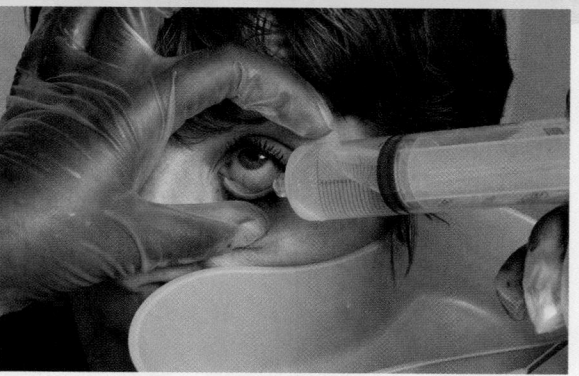

FIGURE 5-24D Using your thumb and index finger, expose the lower conjunctiva while holding the upper eyelid open.

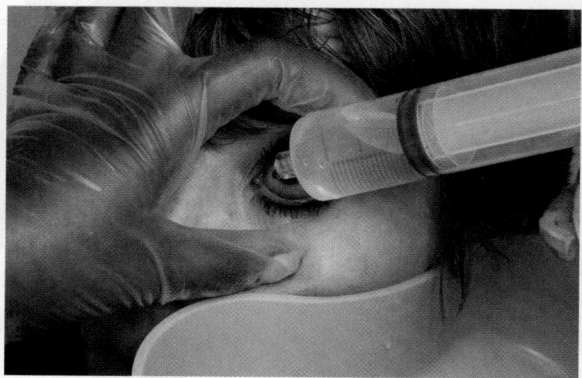

FIGURE 5-24E Hold the syringe containing the ophthalmic solution 1 inch above the eye. Do not let the tip of the syringe touch the eye during the procedure. Starting at the inner canthus of the eye, point the flow of solution toward the lower conjunctiva.

15. When the flow from the syringe is completed, blot excess moisture from the client's eye with sterile gauze or cotton.
16. Observe the returned solution in the basin.
17. Remove the basin, towel, and supplies. Dispose of these items according to office policy.
18. Help the client to an upright sitting position.
19. Remove your gloves and dispose of them properly.
20. Wash your hands.
21. Document the procedure in the client's chart.

(Continues)

PROCEDURE 5-15 (Continued)

Charting Example:

9/27/20xx   4:30 P.M. Irrigated right eye with 100 mL of normal saline sterile ophthalmic solution. Return clear. Client states that he is comfortable and
offered no complaints.

Samantha Smith, S.M.A.

Samantha Smith, S.M.A. (printed name)

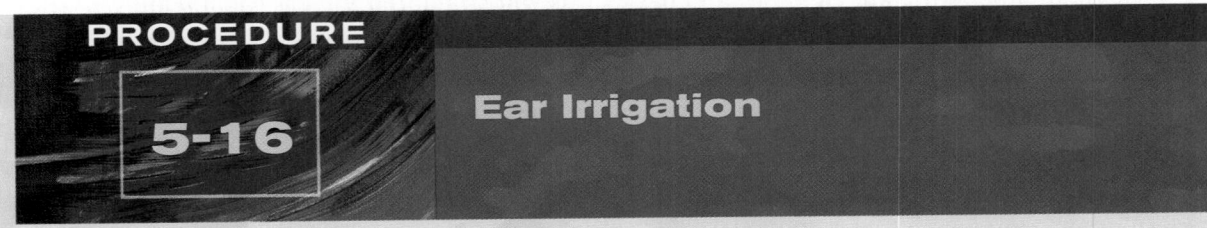

PROCEDURE 5-16

Ear Irrigation

Student Competency Objective: The medical assistant student will irrigate the ear with the ordered otic solution.

Items Needed: Sterile otic solution as ordered by doctor, sterile container, basin to hold return solution, gloves, sterile gauze or cotton balls, absorbent towel, pen and paper

Steps:

1. Wash your hands.
2. Get items needed.
3. Warm the irrigation solution to approximately 100°F. If the solution is too hot or too cold, the client can become uncomfortable and dizzy.
4. Introduce yourself to the client even if you have seen the client on previous visits to your office. The client may have forgotten your name. This also helps to establish a provider-client relationship, because it shows the client that you want him to know who you are.
5. Identify the client. Ask the client to state his name to establish that this is the right client, and then compare the name given to the name on the chart. Never enter a room and call out a client's name to determine if this person is the correct client. The client may not have heard you clearly and may just nod, smile, or answer yes. Clients almost never question if the medical assistant professional has the right client. It is up to the medical assistant to identify the right client before performing any procedure.
6. Tell the client, in everyday language, what you are going to do.
7. Ask if the client has any questions. If he does, give short and simple answers. Sometimes clients will start (and continue) talking because they are nervous about the procedure.
8. Position the client in a comfortable sitting position.
9. Ask the client to bend his head slightly toward the affected ear. (If the left ear is to be irrigated, the client's head should be tilted to the left.)

(Continues)

PROCEDURE 5-16 (Continued)

10. Place an absorbent towel on the client's shoulder.
11. Put on gloves.
12. Wipe the client's outer ear with moist gauze to remove any particles (Figure 5–25A).
13. Ask the client to hold the basin against his ear (Figure 5–25B). If the client is unable to hold the basin steady (for example, because of arthritis in the hands or general weakness), ask another medical assistant to help you.
14. Draw up the ordered solution into a syringe.
15. Gently pull the outer ear (auricle) up and back for an adult client. (In infants and small children, pull the auricle down and back.) This will straighten the ear canal (Figure 5–25C).
16. Place the tip of the syringe into the client's ear canal and point the flow of solution upward toward the roof of the ear canal. Be careful not to push the syringe in straight or too deeply, as this could damage the tympanic membrane (eardrum).
17. Refill the syringe and irrigate again.
18. Wipe the excess moisture from the outer part of the ear with gauze.
19. Observe the returned solution in the basin, noting any cerumen (earwax), and amount and color of any discharge.
20. Remove the basin and towel and dispose of them according to office policy.
21. Allow the client to sit for a few minutes, as he might feel dizzy.
22. Assist client to get off the exam table or out of the chair.
23. Remove your gloves and dispose of them properly.
24. Wash your hands.
25. Document the procedure in the client's chart.

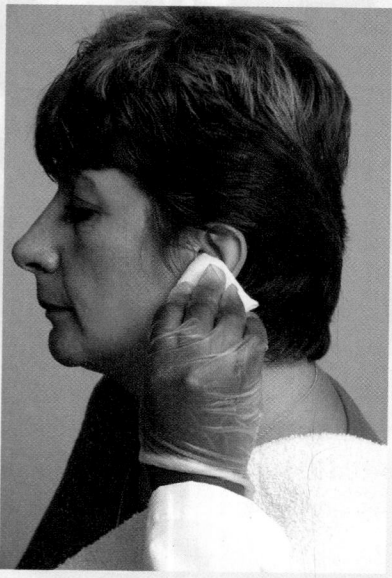

FIGURE 5–25A With the client's head bent toward the affected ear, wipe the outer ear with moist gauze.

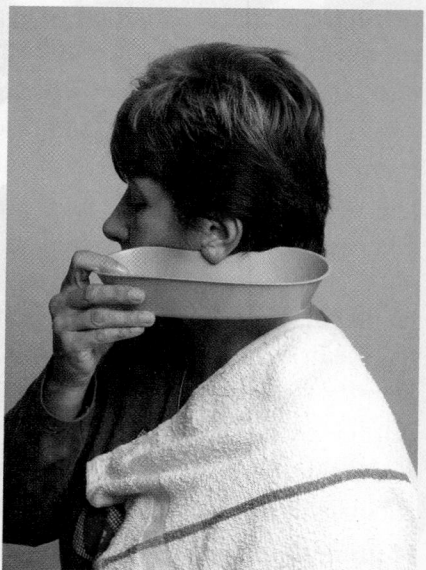

FIGURE 5–25B Ask the client to hold the basin against the ear as you perform the procedure.

(Continues)

PROCEDURE 5-16 (Continued)

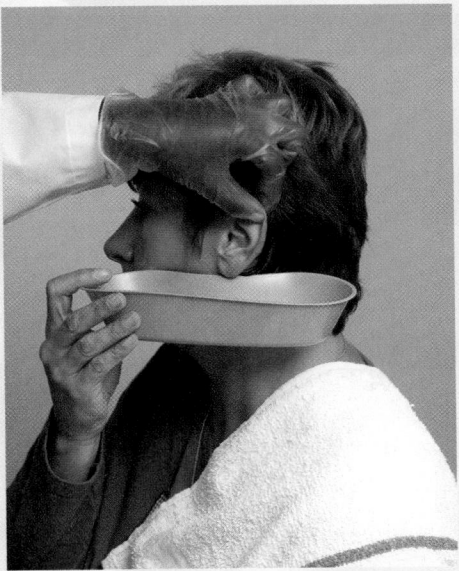

FIGURE 5-25C If the client is an adult, pull the outer ear up and back to straighten the ear canal. For infants and small children, pull the outer ear down and back.

Charting Example:

9/25/20xx   9:30 A.M. Irrigated client's left ear with 200 mL of normal saline as ordered at 100°F. Large amount, four pieces, of cerumen observed in return basin. Client remained for 10 minutes. No complaints of dizziness or light-headedness.

Mary Ellen Pidgeon, S.M.A.

Mary Ellen Pidgeon, S.M.A. (printed name)

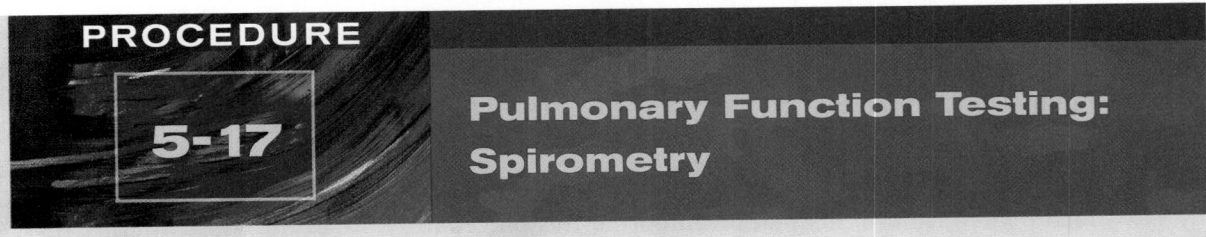

PROCEDURE 5-17

Pulmonary Function Testing: Spirometry

Student Competency Objective: The medical assistant student will administer a pulmonary function test.

Items Needed: Spirometer, nose clip, disposable mouthpiece, alcohol wipe, gloves, biohazardous waste container

(Continues)

PROCEDURE 5-17 (Continued)

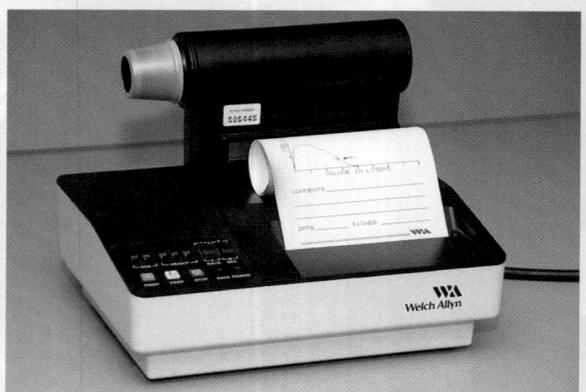

FIGURE 5-26 A spirometer is used to measure pulmonary function.

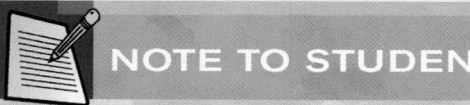

NOTE TO STUDENT:

Some clients may have breathing difficulties that make it difficult for them to stand during this test. Allow the client to sit, but encourage the client to sit as straight as possible. Make sure to inform the doctor and record in the client's chart that the client sat, and why, during the lung function testing.

Steps:

1. Wash your hands.
2. Get items needed.
3. Introduce yourself to the client even if you have seen the client on previous visits to your office. The client may have forgotten your name. This also helps to establish a provider-client relationship, because it shows the client that you want him to know who you are.
4. Identify the client. Ask the client to state his name to establish that this is the right client, and then compare the name given to the name on the chart. Never enter a room and call out a client's name to determine if this person is the correct client. The client may not have heard you clearly and may just nod, smile, or answer yes. Clients almost never question if the medical assistant professional has the right client. It is up to the medical assistant to identify the right client before performing any procedure.
5. Tell the client, in everyday language, what you are going to do.
6. Ask if the client has any questions. If he does, give short and simple answers. Sometimes clients will start (and continue) talking because they are nervous about the procedure.
7. Put in client information on the chart as requested (usually name, age, height, weight, age, gender, race, and smoker/nonsmoker).
8. Ask the client to stand and put on the nose clip. Sometimes, if the client is weak, the doctor will have the client sit down during this procedure. Note in the chart whether the client stands or sits during the procedure.
9. Make sure the correct test is being done.
10. Put on gloves.
11. Instruct the client to put the disposable mouthpiece in his mouth.
12. Tell the client to take a deep breath and blow hard into the mouthpiece.

(Continues)

PROCEDURE 5-17 (Continued)

13. Encourage the client to keep blowing until the machine indicates to stop (for example, you may say, "Keep going . . . keep going" and then "Great" when the client is done).

14. Instruct the client to remove the mouthpiece and relax.

15. Offer suggestions to the client before instructing him to reinsert the mouthpiece.

16. Tell the client again to take a deep breath and blow hard into the mouthpiece. (For accurate measurement, the client should do three best-try attempts.)

17. After the third attempt, tell the client to remove the mouthpiece and nose clip.

18. Dispose of the mouthpiece in the biohazardous waste container.

19. Remove your gloves and dispose of them in the appropriate waste container.

20. Wash your hands.

21. Ask the client if he has any questions; if so, answer them if possible.

22. Print the results of the procedure.

23. Notify the doctor or add the results to the chart per office policy.

Charting Example:

4/23/20xx   10:45 A.M. Pulmonary function test completed. Client sat as per doctor's orders. Three measurements obtained. Answered client's questions. Client states "feeling fine." Doctor notified and test results put in lab report file.

Abigail Hardy, S.M.A.

Abigail Hardy, S.M.A. (printed name)

BRIDGE TO CAAHEP

This chapter, which discusses client examination and the medical assistant's role, provides information and content related to CAAHEP standards for Anatomy and Physiology, Medical Terminology, Medical Law and Ethics, Communication, Medical Assisting Clinical Procedures and Professional Components.

ABHES LINKS

This chapter, which discusses the client examination and the medical assistant's role, links to ABHES course content for medical assisting for Medical Terminology, Medical Law and Ethics, Psychology of Human Relations, Medical Office Business Procedures/Management, Medical Office Clinical Procedures, and Medical Laboratory Procedures.

AAMA AREAS OF COMPETENCE

This chapter, which discusses client examination procedures, provides information or content within several areas listed in the Medical Assistant Role Delineation Study. These areas include: clinical, fundamental principles, patient (client) care, general transdisciplinary, professionalism, communication skills, legal concepts, and instruction.

AMT PATHS

Client examination provides a path to AMT competencies in general medical assisting knowledge, medical terminology, medical law, medical ethics, and human relations and patient (client) education. It also introduces the student to administrative medical assisting in the area of medical/secretarial/receptionist. Clinical medical assisting emphasizing physical examinations is presented.

POINTS OF HIGHLIGHT

- The medical assistant is often the first member of the health care team to interact with a client.
- A fundamental attitude for all health care providers is respect for the client.
- Medical assistants interview clients and collect pertinent client information as part of their responsibilities.
- The chief complaint is the reason that the client came to the medical office for care.
- Past medical history will help to establish a client's baseline health and will be used for comparisons during future visits.
- A family health history of blood relatives gives clues as to possible familial or genetic disorders.
- Questions about lifestyle will help the health care provider to understand the client's health issues and concerns.
- The review of systems is a systematic investigation of each system in the body.
- A client's weight should be measured at each visit. Height should be obtained at the first visit and periodically thereafter.
- Medical assistants can test visual acuity using a Snellen chart.
- The Rinne and the Weber tests are two common methods of testing hearing.
- The degree of mobility can greatly affect the client's ability to perform activities of daily living.
- Four methods used during a physical examination are: (1) inspection, (2) palpation, (3) percussion, and (4) auscultation.
- Common client positions during examinations or procedures are: sitting, Fowler's, semi-Fowler's, supine, dorsal recumbent, lithotomy, and Sims'.

STUDENT PORTFOLIO ACTIVITY

Treating each client with dignity and respect is at the heart of medical assisting. Obtain a copy of the "Creed of Medical Assistants." Discuss how this affects your interactions with others and your professional life. Place a copy of the creed in your portfolio. What does having this document in your portfolio convey to an employer?

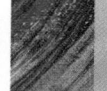

APPLYING YOUR SKILLS

During a routine visit, the client, Mr. Smith, tells you that he has severe painful arthritis in his back. You need to place him in a supine position for the exam. What do you need to know about this client? What do you need to know about the exam? As a medical assistant, what could you do to increase Mr. Smith's physical comfort while still positioning him so that the exam can be performed accurately?

CRITICAL THINKING QUESTIONS

1. How can a medical assistant promote a good provider–client relationship with a new client?

2. You observe a worker speaking with a caregiver and ignoring the developmentally disabled client. What should you do?

3. A client is not satisfied or happy after being seen at your office. What are some possible results in terms of health care outcomes and in terms of your workplace?

4. What are some nonverbal behaviors that the medical assistant can use to communicate a welcoming attitude to a client?

5. List some questions that can help you find out the client's chief complaint.

6. What is included in a social history?

7. Why is it important for the medical assistant to obtain social history information?

8. An elderly client asks why you want to measure his height. What do you tell him?

9. How does the degree of mobility affect a person's activities of daily living?

10. Explain the importance of client preparation to a positive outcome for a procedure or examination.

11. Go back to the beginning of this chapter and review the Anticipatory Statements. Reread each statement and then indicate whether it is true or false. If the statement is false, rewrite it to make it a true statement.

UNIT THREE

Body Systems

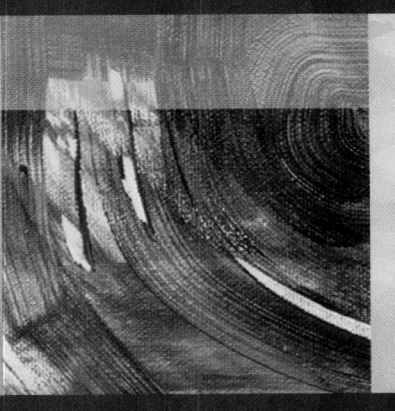

The working of the human body is an example of many smaller systems working together to create a coordinated organism.

To understand disorders and how to give competent care to a client with a specific disorder, you must first know what normal looks like and how each system should work. This unit first introduces you to the human body as a whole. You will learn about the very small parts that constitute successively larger groups that make up complete systems in the body.

The chapters in this unit present the systems that make up the human organism. Each chapter discusses the structure and function of a particular body system. Finding out what is contained in each system and where it is located in the body will make understanding its functions easier. You will find that even very small organs or specialized tissues are vital to the entire system. An overview of how each system works provides you with a basic understanding of the system's functioning.

When you have finished learning about a system, you will be given a situation or problem to solve by using what you have learned in the chapter and applying your critical thinking skills. Finally, for each system, there is a sample client teaching plan that you can change according to the individual client's needs.

CHAPTER 6

Anticipatory Statements

People have different ideas of how the body is organized and how it works. Read and think about the following statements based upon what you believe now. Decide whether you agree or disagree. Write the word **agree** after the statement if you think the statement is true. Write the word **disagree** after the statement if you think the statement is false. Read the chapter to find out if your current beliefs can be supported.

1. Systems of the body depend upon each other to work smoothly.

   _____

2. Only doctors need to know the organization of the body and how it functions.

   _____

3. Using medical terms helps the medical assistant to communicate with other health care professionals.

   _____

4. Organs in the body function on their own.

   _____

5. Knowing anatomical positions and directions helps in describing where a point is on the body.

   _____

Organization of the Human Body

Learning Objectives

Upon completion of this chapter, the medical assistant student should be able to:

- List the four basic units in the body
- State the four types of tissue
- Define each major body system
- Demonstrate the anatomical position
- Identify the main body cavities and the major organs in each
- Point out body directions on an anatomical chart

Key Terms

anatomical Position of the body when standing straight, facing forward, arms down at side with the palms of the hands forward.

cell The basic unit of all living organisms.

cranial cavity Space in the head that contains the brain.

epithelial tissue Tissue that covers structures inside and on the surface of the body, thereby protecting these structures.

organs Groups of tissue(s) that have the same function.

pelvic cavity The space in the body that contains the reproductive organs, urinary bladder, rectum, part of the large intestine, and the appendix.

system A group of organs that work together to perform the same function.

thoracic cavity The space in the body that contains the lungs, heart, trachea, esophagus, thymus gland, and large blood vessels.

tissue A group of cells the function of which is similar.

visceral cavity The space in the body that contains abdominal organs; also called the *abdominal cavity*.

■ INTRODUCTION

The human body is composed of many different systems that work together in a coordinated way. A person's health and life itself depend upon all parts functioning properly. Clients may come to the medical office with a specific system disorder, but the medical assistant needs to know that one system relates to the other systems. That is, a problem in one system can disturb the working of another system. If the medical assistant is to provide competent care, he or she must have a basic understanding of the organization of the body. Learning how the body is organized will make it easier to understand specific systems and what can go wrong with each system.

■ BASIC UNITS OF THE BODY

Four basic units make up the body: cells, tissues, organs, and systems (Figure 6-1).

Cells

Cells are the basic unit or component of all living organisms. All human tissue and matter is made up of cells. Cells divide and multiply. Humans grow and develop because of the increase in the number and specialization of cells. Cells that perform specific tasks are called *specialized.*

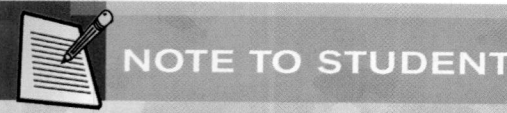

NOTE TO STUDENT:

Matter is composed of even smaller structures than cells, such as atoms, molecules, and organelles. Their structure and activity are explained by chemistry and physics, but are beyond the scope of a basic understanding of human body organization. Cells are the basic starting point for medical assistants' understanding of the body and its functions in relation to giving competent care.

Tissues

There are many kinds of cells. Cells can be grouped by size, shape, outside structure, material inside the cells, and function. Cells that do similar work form a **tissue** that has a definite task or function. Tissues can be separated into four types: epithelial, nervous, muscle, and connective.

Epithelial tissue is outside or covering tissue. The purpose of epithelial tissue is to protect and cover parts of the body. Epithelial tissue is found on all body surfaces, such as the skin. It lines the cavities and passageways in the body. It even lines the blood vessels. Epithelial tissue also secretes various substances, and is found in the glands of the body. Most epithelial tissue lacks blood vessels, and so must get its food and nourishment from underlying tissue, such as connective tissue.

Nervous tissue carries signals or impulses to and from different parts of the body. Cells in nervous tissue found in the skin pick up sensations from the outside world and carry the messages to the brain for interpretation and reaction. Cells in interior nervous tissue can carry impulses or sensations picked up inside the body to the brain and then carry the brain's response to other parts of the body.

Muscle tissue is involved with body movement. These tissues contract and then relax to create movement. The three types of muscle tissue in the body are: skeletal, smooth, and cardiac. Skeletal muscle is connected to bone and is under voluntary control. *Voluntary control* means that the person can start or stop the activity when he or she wants to. Smooth muscle lines the internal organs and is under involuntary control. *Involuntary* means that the activity goes on without any direction from the person; the person usually cannot control how or when the activity occurs. Cardiac muscle, found in the heart, is under involuntary control.

Connective tissue can be divided into several categories or groups based on structure. The functions of all the types are similar, however. Connective tissue can (1) connect other tissues,

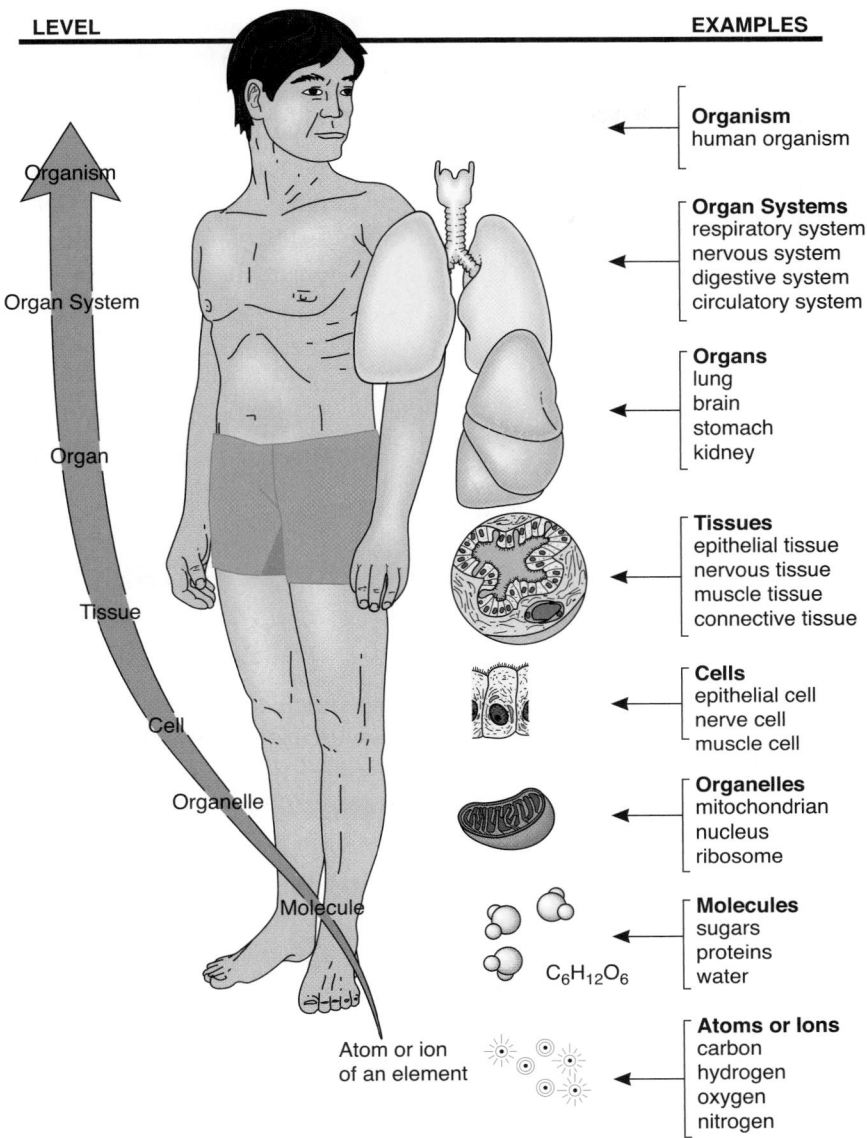

FIGURE 6-1 The formation of the human organism, from atoms and cells to integrated organism.

(2) bring food and carry away waste, (3) store vitamins, and (4) protect organs.

Blood, soft tissue, and hard tissue are the three major groups of connective tissue. Many people do not think of blood as connective tissue. It does have a liquid part—plasma—but it also has a solid or "formed elements" part. It carries nutrients to the cells and takes waste products away from the cells.

Soft connective tissue is generously spread throughout the body. This tissue stretches, giving strength and providing padding between different tissues. For example, skin must stretch to allow movement and to allow food in and waste out. The skin is also the first line of defense; connective tissue gives it strength and allows the other connective tissue, blood, to rush in to fight off any invasion of foreign material through the skin.

The category of hard connective tissue includes bone and cartilage. Bone is the hardest connective tissue in the body. The body's shape, structure, and mobility are due in part to the bone (skeleton) and cartilage.

Organs

Groups of tissues that do the same work become **organs.** Organs are larger than tissues both structurally and functionally. The heart, kidneys, and lungs are just a few of the organs in the body. The skin, which covers the entire body, is the largest organ, as it has the largest surface area.

Systems

Organs do not perform their functions independently. Groups of organs that work together to perform the same job become organized into a **system.** Systems working together combine to form an organism. All the systems of the body are related. How well one works will affect how well the other systems work. If something goes wrong in one system, other systems will try to make up for it to keep the body in balance and functioning.

The major body systems are:

- Integumentary—commonly thought of as the skin, but also includes the hair, nails, and glands in the skin
- Skeletal—made up of bones and joints; gives the body its structural framework
- Muscular—Enables a body to move voluntarily; also performs many involuntary movements to sustain life
- Nervous—coordinates all the body systems by receiving, interpreting, and sending out impulses or messages
- Sensory—receives information or sensations from inside and outside the body
- Endocrine—has glands that secrete chemicals or hormones with specific functions
- Cardiovascular—consists of the strong muscular organ called the heart, and the blood vessels
- Hematologic—the blood, which moves throughout the body
- Lymphatic—made of lymph, which works as a defense system in the body
- Immune—closely related to the lymphatic system; defends against foreign harmful organisms

- Respiratory—structures that take in air (oxygen) from the outside and rid the body of carbon dioxide
- Digestive—receives food; breaks food into various components, absorbs the useful parts, and gets rid of solid waste
- Urinary—filters blood and removes liquid waste from the body
- Male reproductive—organs and structures in the male needed for reproduction of the species
- Female reproductive—organs and structures in the female needed for reproduction of the species

■ BODY POSITION, DIRECTION, AND LOCATION

It is critical for medical assistants to use the same terminology as other health care providers when discussing body location, so that communication will be accurate and understandable. Health care providers use a common point of reference called the **anatomical** position (Figure 6-2). In the anatomical position, the face is front, the arms are down at the sides, and the palms of the hands face forward. This is a front-on view, so the left side of the picture is the right side of the body and the right side of the picture is the left side of the body (Figure 6-3). In other words, left and right are reversed from the viewer's standpoint.

The medical assistant must be able to understand and communicate the location of points on the body. One way to do this is through description of body cavities. *Cavities* are contained spaces. The body is divided into several cavities, and the organs of the body each lie within a specific cavity. The structure of the cavity helps to protect the organs. The names of the cavities correspond to their location (Figure 6-4). Within the dorsal cavity is the **cranial cavity,** containing the brain and the spinal cavity, which protects the spinal cord. Within the ventral cavity are the **thoracic cavity,** containing the heart, lungs, trachea, esophagus, thymus gland, and large blood vessels; and the **visceral cavity** or

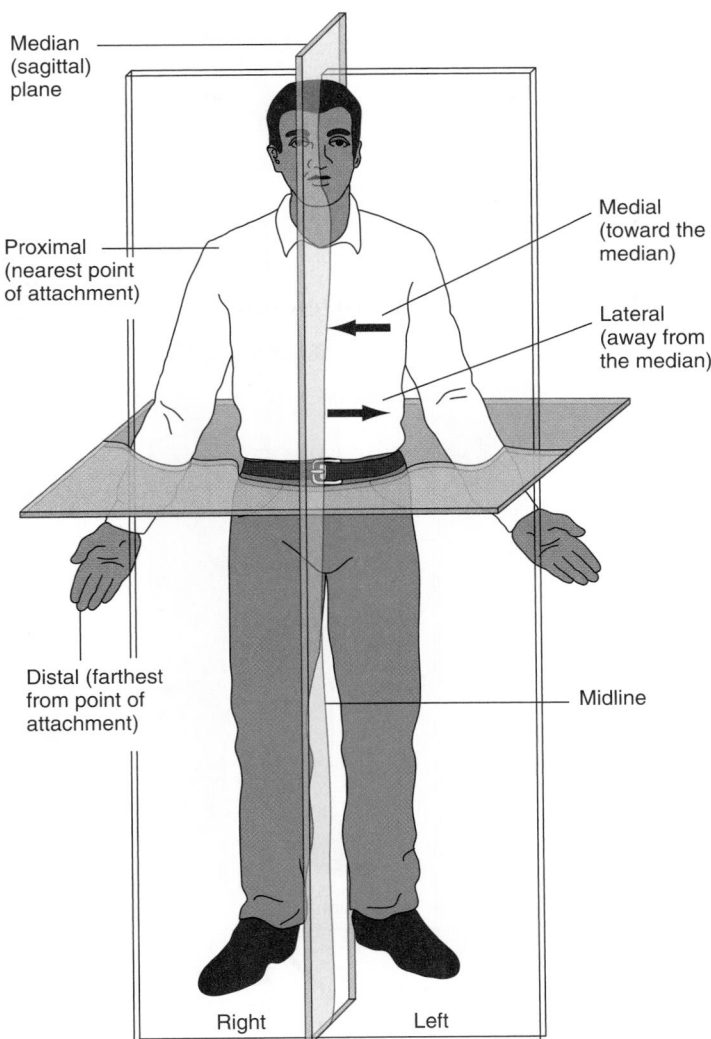

Median (sagittal) plane

Proximal (nearest point of attachment)

Medial (toward the median)

Lateral (away from the median)

Distal (farthest from point of attachment)

Midline

Right   Left

FIGURE 6-2 Anatomical position.

abdominal cavity, containing the stomach, liver, gallbladder, pancreas, spleen, kidneys, adrenal glands, ureters, and most of the intestine. The **pelvic cavity** contains the remainder of the intestines, as well as the urinary bladder, rectum, and internal reproductive organs.

It is important for a health care provider to describe a location on the body in relation to other points. Therefore, the medical assistant needs to know the names of body parts and must be able to describe them in relation to other parts. For example, the foot is below or *inferior* to the knee.

Directional Language

There are basic directional words to use when describing areas of the body in relation to other areas of the body. Table 6-1 lists common directional terms that the medical assistant needs to be familiar with to communicate with other health care providers. Doctors use directional language when writing orders to avoid confusion. For example, chest X-rays are often ordered for "A&P and lateral views," meaning that the X-ray views are from the front *(anterior)*, back *(posterior)*, and side *(lateral)*.

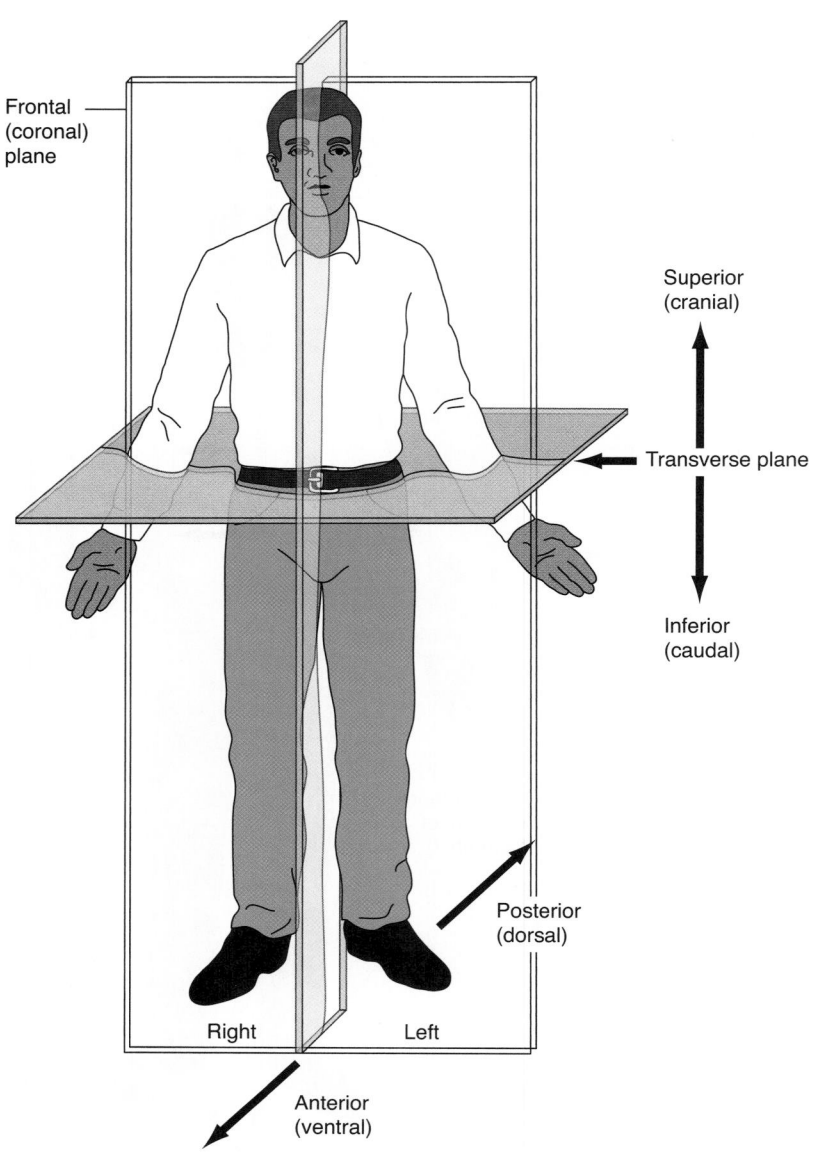

FIGURE 6-3 Anatomical directions.

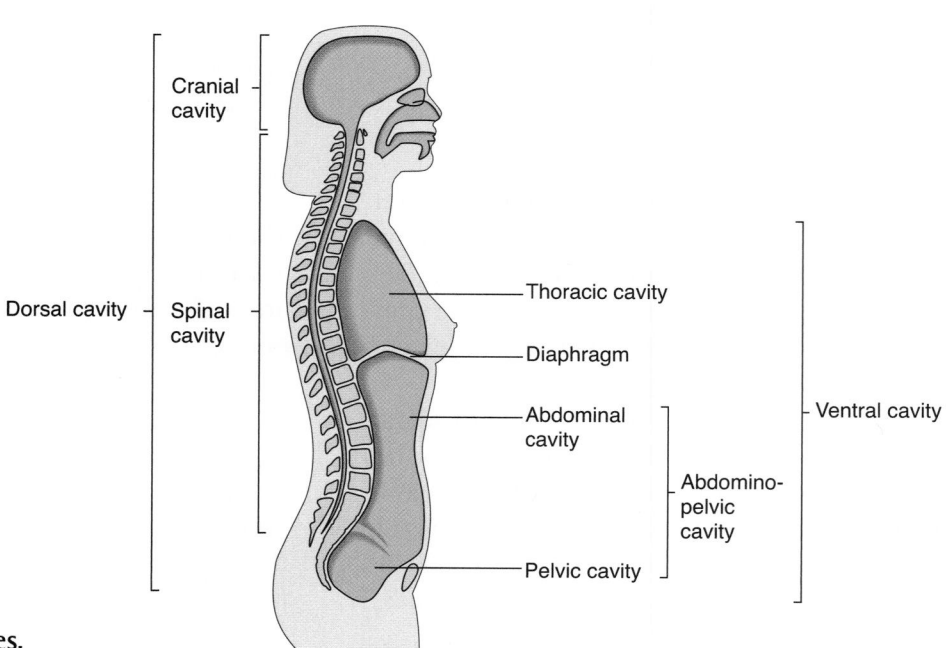

FIGURE 6-4 Body cavities.

TABLE 6-1 Common directional language.

VOCABULARY	MEANING	EXAMPLE
Anterior or ventral	Pertaining to the front	The nose protrudes from the *anterior* surface of the face
Bilateral	Pertaining to two sides	The lungs are found *bilaterally* in the chest
Caudal	Pertaining to the tail	The end of the spinal cord is sometimes called the *caudal* section
Cranial	Pertaining to the skull or head	Swelling in the head causes increased *cranial* pressure
Distal	Pertaining to away	The wrist is *distal* to the elbow
Dorsal	Pertaining to the back	The knuckles are on the *dorsal* surface of the hands
Inferior	Pertaining to below	The feet are *inferior* to the legs
Lateral	Pertaining to a side	A chest X-ray often includes a *lateral* view
Medial	Pertaining to the middle (midline)	The nose is the *medial* point on the face
Posterior	Of or toward the back	The buttocks are on the *posterior* side of the body
Proximal	Toward the trunk of the body	The shoulder is *proximal* to the elbow
Superior	Above	The head is *superior* to the neck
Unilateral	One side only	The numbness and tingling from the injury were *unilateral*

 BRIDGE TO CAAHEP

This chapter, which discusses the organization of the human body, provides information and content related to CAAHEP standards for Anatomy and Physiology and Medical Terminology.

 ABHES LINKS

This chapter, which discusses the organization of the human body, links to ABHES course content for Anatomy and Physiology, Medical Terminology, and Medical Office Clinical Procedures.

 AAMA AREAS OF COMPETENCE

This chapter, which discusses the organization of the human body, provides information or content within several areas listed in the Medical Assistant Role Delineation Study. These areas include: clinical, fundamental principles, diagnostic orders, patient (client) care, general (transdisciplinary) professionalism, communication skills, and instruction.

 AMT PATHS

This chapter, which discusses the organization of the human body, provides a path to AMT competency in general medical assisting knowledge, anatomy and physiology, medical terminology, and patient (client) education.

POINTS OF HIGHLIGHT

- The human body is composed of many body systems working together in a coordinated way. The different systems are interdependent.
- Cells are the basic unit of all living organisms.
- The body is organized from simple to complex. Cells, tissues, organs, and systems are the four fundamental units of the body.
- Epithelial, nervous, muscle, and connective tissue are the four types of tissue.
- Epithelial tissue covers parts of the body.
- Nervous tissue carries signals and messages to and from different parts of the body.
- Muscle tissue helps with body movement.
- Connective tissue connects, transports, stores, and protects.
- Blood is a type of connective tissue composed of a liquid part and a solid part.
- Bone is the hardest connective tissue in the body.
- Specialized groups of tissue are called organs.
- All of the fundamental body units are interrelated, depending on each other for proper function and health.
- Anatomical position is a common point of reference used among health care professionals.
- The body has several cavities, which are contained spaces designed to protect internal organs.

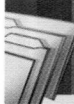

STUDENT PORTFOLIO ACTIVITY

Knowledge of anatomy and physiology is important as a base in clinical medical assisting. Select an objective test on which you earned a good grade and put it in your portfolio to illustrate that you have acquired a basic understanding of anatomy and physiology.

APPLYING YOUR SKILLS

A client comes to the office where you work as a medical assistant. She complains that her "stomach" hurts. You observe that she is bending over and crossing her arms over the area. What questions might you ask to help pinpoint the area and problem? What terms would you use to describe the situation to the doctor? How would you then explain the location of the pain, using the directional and medical terminology you learned in this chapter?

CRITICAL THINKING QUESTIONS

1. What is connective tissue, and what is its function in the body?

2. How would you explain anatomical position to another medical assistant student? What examples could you give her to make your explanation clear?

3. In order from simple to complex, list the four structural units of the human body.

4. Using the correct directional terminology, describe the location of the knee in relation to the hip and foot.

5. Select a body system and describe how the health of that system affects the health or functioning of another system. How could knowing this help you when working with a client who is sick?

6. You hear a medical assistant tell a client that the doctor has ordered an anterior, posterior, and lateral X-ray. The client appears confused. How might the medical assistant have described the X-ray to this client?

7. A client complains that "my stomach hurts" and points to her whole abdomen. What questions could you ask to clarify where the client is experiencing pain?

8. The doctor has finished asking a client many questions about different body systems. The client asks you why the doctor is asking all these questions when she only came in to find relief for her shortness of breath. How would you respond?

9. Another student asks you how learning about the organization of the body relates to medical assistants' work in an office. What would you say?

10. The body can be viewed in many ways, from a simple beginning to a complex interrelated organism. Choose a body system to explain this statement.

11. Go back to the beginning of this chapter and review the Anticipatory Statements. Reread each statement and then indicate whether it is true or false. If the statement is false, rewrite it to make it a true statement.

CHAPTER 7

Anticipatory Statements

People have different ideas about what makes up healthy skin and what can affect the look of the skin. Read and think about the following statements based upon what you believe now. Decide whether you agree or disagree. Write the word **agree** after the statement if you think the statement is true. Write the word **disagree** after the statement if you think the statement is false. Read the chapter to find out if your current beliefs can be supported.

1. The epidermis layer of the skin is composed of dead skin cells.

2. The skin is an organ of the body.

3. Herbal shampoo will increase the rate of hair growth on the scalp.

4. The color of hair is determined by the amount of melanin produced by the melanocytes.

5. Ointments applied to the skin help to form a moisture-proof barrier.

6. Unbroken skin is the body's best defense against infection.

Integumentary System

Learning Objectives

Upon completion of this chapter, the medical assistant student should be able to:

- Define the integumentary system
- List the layers of the skin
- Discuss the accessory structures of the integumentary system
- State the difference between the sebaceous and sudoriferous glands
- Identify at least two functions of the skin
- Describe the purpose of the subcutaneous layer
- Explain reasons for proper handwashing techniques

Key Terms

adipose tissue Fat tissue.

carotene Yellow pigment that is the precursor or forerunner for vitamin A.

conduction Transfer of heat from one object to another.

convection Transfer of heat from an object to cooler air surrounding the object.

dermis True skin.

epidermis Outermost layer of the skin.

evaporation Passing off of moisture in the form of a vapor; as the moisture becomes a gas, it cools the body.

hair follicle Small depression that surrounds the hair shaft; hair receives nourishment in this area.

integumentary Refers to a covering, such as the skin.

keratin A protein that provides a protective shield for the skin.

melanin Pigment that gives the skin, hair, and eyes their color.

metabolism Processing of substances within the body.

precursor Substance out of which another substance is made.

radiation Transfer of heat in the form of waves.

subcutaneous Below the skin.

thermoregulation Regulation of body temperature.

■ INTRODUCTION

The word **integumentary** refers to a covering. The skin and its accessory (supporting) structures, which cover the internal organs and skeleton of the body, make up the body's integumentary system. The skin, which is the largest organ of the body, is made of various specialized tissues.

■ STRUCTURE

The skin is composed of two main layers, the epidermis and the dermis (Figure 7-1). The **epidermis** is the outermost or top layer of the skin. Under the epidermis is the second major layer, the **dermis.** The dermis is sometimes referred to as the *true skin.*

Epidermis

The epidermis is made of layers of scale-like cells called *stratified squamous epithelium.* The epidermis has no blood supply of its own; however, the dermis supplies it with nutrients through diffusion. The epidermal layer can be further divided into five sublayers (Figure 7-2). These five sublayers are grouped in either the stratum germinativum or the stratum corneum.

The *stratum corneum* is the horny top layer of the epidermis. It contains several layers of dead, flattened cells. The body constantly sheds these dead skin cells as new layers of cells push up from the dermis. The dead skin cells fall off daily. Rubbing, friction, washing, and other cosmetic treatments all aid in sloughing off the dead skin cells.

The *stratum germinativum* is the inner sublayer of the epidermis. The cells in this layer divide and replace the dead cells that are sloughed off from the stratum corneum.

Dermis

The second major layer of the skin is the dermis or true skin. It is composed of connective tissue and collagen. Within this layer are blood and capillaries, lymphatic tissues, nerve endings, **hair follicles,** sebaceous (oil) glands and ducts, and sudoriferous (sweat) glands and ducts (Figure 7-3). Receptors for the sensations of touch, pressure, pain, and temperature are also located in the dermal layer of the skin (Figure 7-4).

Subcutaneous Layer

Under the skin is a separate structure called the **subcutaneous** layer or hypodermis (*hypo* meaning "under"). In a diagram of the skin, this may appear to be a third layer of the skin, and in the past it was sometimes referred to as such. The subcutaneous layer secures the skin to the underlying structure to its loose connective tissue. This layer also acts as an insulator against changes in outside temperatures. Insulation is possible because the subcutaneous layer is made of **adipose tissue.** With aging, a person loses subcutaneous tis-

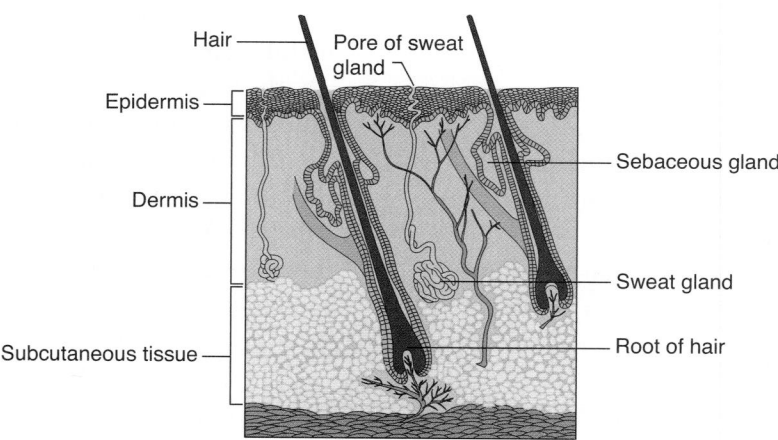

FIGURE 7-1 The layers of the skin.

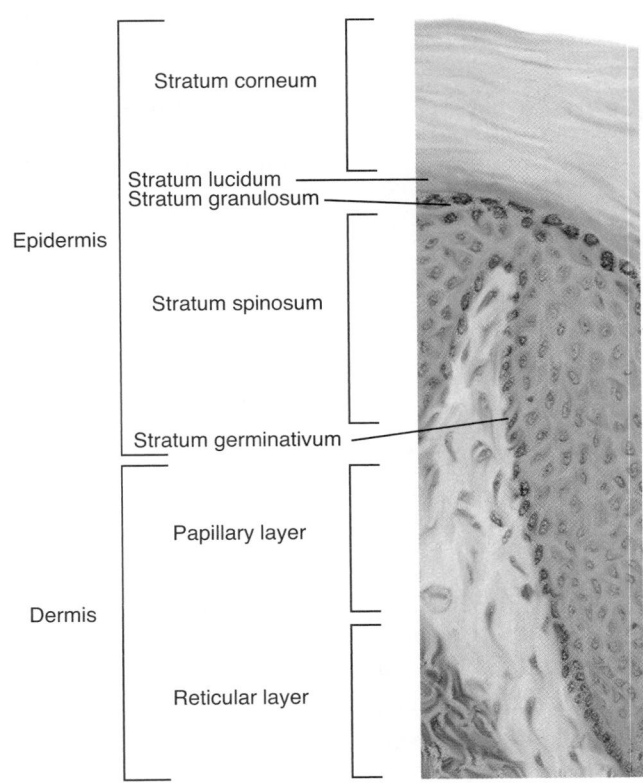

FIGURE 7-2 The epidermis can be divided into five sublayers.

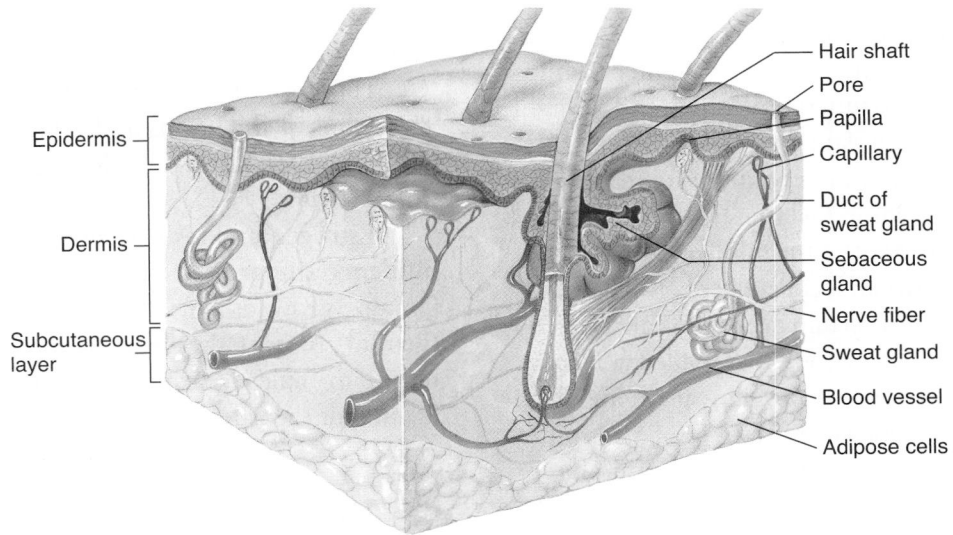

FIGURE 7-3 The structures of the dermis.

sue. As a result, when it is very cold outside, an older person may feel colder than a younger person who has a thicker subcutaneous layer, and will have to dress more warmly than the younger person.

Color

The skin structure as a whole also has a color. To others the skin may appear white, pink, brown, black, or yellow, or as tones of these colors. **Melanin, carotene,** and hemoglobin all

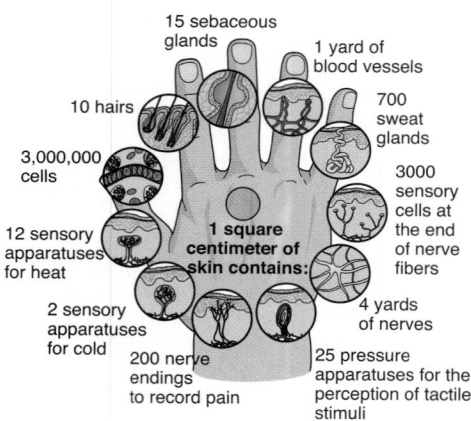

15 sebaceous glands

1 yard of blood vessels

10 hairs

700 sweat glands

3,000,000 cells

3000 sensory cells at the end of nerve fibers

12 sensory apparatuses for heat

1 square centimeter of skin contains:

2 sensory apparatuses for cold

200 nerve endings to record pain

4 yards of nerves

25 pressure apparatuses for the perception of tactile stimuli

FIGURE 7-4 The dermis contains nerve receptors for touch, pressure, pain, and temperature.

contribute to the color and shade of skin. Genetics determines an individual's skin color.

Within the skin are cells called *melanocytes,* which produce the pigment melanin. All people have the same number of melanocytes. What varies is the amount of melanin that the melanocytes produce: The more melanin produced, the darker the skin color. The function of melanin is protection against ultraviolet radiation from sunlight. When a lighter-skinned person spends too much time out in the sunlight without applying sunscreen, the skin either burns or tans. A tan is a result of increased production of melanin as the body attempts to protect itself from the harmful rays of the sun. Freckles are uneven local clusters of melanin. A loss of melanin in certain areas can cause patchy areas of white. This condition is called *vitiligo.*

The body contains a yellow pigment called carotene. Carotene is a **precursor** of vitamin A. The shade from the melanin often dominates or is stronger than the yellow tone from the carotene pigment. People of Asian descent tend to secrete less melanin, and therefore their skin has a yellower tone. A person who has lighter skin may also have a yellow tone. This is seen in people whose diet consists almost exclusively of vegetables with carotene, such as carrots and other yellow vegetables. This happens to young children who insist upon eating only carrots, for example.

Hemoglobin is the iron-containing pigment of red blood cells. People with very light skin produce little melanin, so the hemoglobin in the blood capillaries of the dermis gives a pinkish tint to light skin.

■ ACCESSORY STRUCTURES

Accessory structures support and contribute to the main functioning units of a body system.

Hair

Hair is an accessory structure of the integumentary system. Hair is an outgrowth or shaft of keratinized cells that develops from a hair follicle in the dermis of the skin. A hair shaft and a root are embedded in a hair follicle. The hair shaft has three layers: cuticle, cortex, and medulla. The color of the hair is due to the amount of melanin pigment in the cortex of the hair shaft. As a person ages, the amount produced decreases. With that decrease, some hair will remain pigmented, but some will not; this latter appears as gray hair. White hair is due to the absence of melanin. Red hair is due to an iron compound in the melanin.

Hair is found on most areas of the body. The palms of the hands and soles of the feet do not have hair. The lips, nipples, and penis also do not have hair.

Estrogen and testosterone (sex hormones) influence the growth of hair. Both males and females grow axillary (underarm) and pubic (genital) hair at the onset of puberty. Testosterone in males is responsible for men's heavy facial hair (beard) and hairy chests.

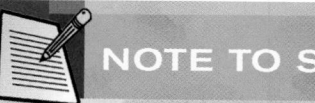

NOTE TO STUDENT:

Hair that is seen is not alive. Hair shampoo and conditioner applied topically to the hair do not affect the growth of hair; rather, these products affect the surface appearance of the hair, making it look shinier and glossier.

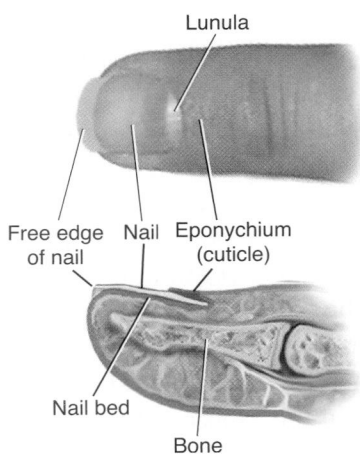

FIGURE 7-5 The structures of the fingernails.

Nails

Nails are found on the dorsal surface of the fingers and toes (Figure 7-5). A nail consists of a body (**keratin**) and a root, which are both on top of the nail bed. The *body* of the nail is the part that can be seen. The root is partially hidden by the nail fold. The *lunula* is the crescent-moon-shaped whitish area near the root. The blood vessels in the dermal layer of the skin cause the pinkish color of the nail.

Glands

Sebaceous (oil) and sudoriferous (sweat) glands are accessory structures of the integumentary system. The sebaceous glands secrete sebum, which is an oily, waxy substance. Most of the sebaceous glands open into hair follicles, and the sebum secreted there works its way to the skin surface. The sebum lubricates the skin and the oily/waxy substances help to waterproof the surface.

The sudoriferous glands, which secrete sweat, are most abundant in the palms of the hands and the soles of the feet. Sudoriferous glands are actually two types of glands. The first type, the *apocrine glands,* are located in the axillary and pubic areas. These glands become active with the onset of puberty. When bacteria interact with the sweat produced by these glands, the result is the familiar odor of perspiration.

The second type of sudoriferous gland is the *eccrine glands,* which are dispersed all over the body. These glands play an important role in helping to regulate body temperature. When exposed to high temperature, the body begins to perspire. Through the process of evaporation, the water vapor on the hot skin is turned into a gas that moves away from the body into the air; this process cools the body.

■ FUNCTIONS OF THE INTEGUMENTARY SYSTEM

The skin and accessory structures perform many essential functions that are critical to an individual's life and the quality of that life. These many functions can be grouped into five categories: protection, **metabolism, thermoregulation,** sensation, and communication.

Protection

A major function of the integumentary system is protection. It is the body's best defense against disease-causing germs (pathogenic microorganisms). Intact or unbroken skin prevents harmful substances from entering the body. Many diseases and infections are transmitted (given to another person) through direct contact. Some bacteria are inevitably contacted in the course of routine activities. If the skin is unbroken, the disease-causing germs cannot get inside the body.

Keeping the skin intact and clean, through good washing techniques, helps to prevent disease. Proper handwashing will help to destroy bacteria picked up during the course of everyday activities. Using the correct water temperature for washing and rinsing will avoid chapping and chafing of the skin. Patting instead of rubbing vigorously will prevent cracking of the skin. After handwashing, apply a cream or lotion to help moisturize the skin. Ointment applied to the skin can help to form a moisture-proof barrier.

The skin also protects against the damaging effects of the sun's ultraviolet rays. The pigment melanin in the skin protects against burns and other harmful effects. A person with more melanin has greater protection from the sun. People with less melanin should make a habit of applying sunscreen to all areas of the skin that are exposed to the sun, including the lips.

The skin and accessory structures act as a barrier against foreign substances such as dirt, chemicals, or insects. The eyebrows and eyelashes prevent dust particles from entering the eyes. These hairs also prevent perspiration (sweat) from getting into the eyes. The hairs in the ears prevent insects from flying or crawling into the ear canal. The hairs and mucous secretions in the nose trap particles and keep them from entering the lungs (respiratory tract).

Finally, the subcutaneous layer of the skin protects by cushioning and securing the delicate internal organs.

Metabolism

Skin uses sunlight in the production and use of vitamin D. Vitamin D is necessary for the body to use calcium effectively. Vitamin D and calcium are important for strong bones. Individuals who are not able to go outdoors into the sunshine prevent the skin from metabolizing vitamin D, and hence will need to supplement with vitamins or foods rich in calcium and vitamin D.

Skin absorbs medication that is applied on the surface (topical application). This is one step in the metabolism of medication.

The subcutaneous layer of the integumentary system provides an area for fat storage. Certain waste products are excreted or gotten rid of through the skin.

Thermoregulation

The integumentary system helps to control a person's body temperature through the four processes of heat production and heat loss: conduction, convection, radiation, and evaporation.

When a cold object comes into direct contact with the skin of a person who is hot, the heat is passed from the hot skin to the cold object. This process is called **conduction.** This helps to cool the person's skin. The reverse is

also true. When a hot object comes into direct contact with cooler skin, the heat passes from the hot object to the cold skin.

The heat from the skin's surface will move to the less densely concentrated, cooler air surrounding the person. This is called **convection.** Outdoors, the process of convection is enhanced by wind, which continuously moves the air around the skin. Indoors, a fan produces a cooling effect by the same action.

When a person is hot, heat is given off as waves from the exposed areas of the skin. This process is called **radiation.** On hot days, when people wear less clothing, more skin is exposed and thus it can radiate more heat. This helps keep the body cool.

Through the process of **evaporation,** perspiration on a person's skin changes to a lighter, less dense gas. This process also helps to cool the body.

The integumentary system helps to maintain body temperature through shivering. The muscle action generates heat internally. When the brain receives a sensation of cold, it instructs the capillaries in the dermis to constrict or get smaller, to prevent any more heat loss. A person then develops little raised areas, called "goosebumps," when the smooth muscles around each hair follicle contract. The raised hairs trap warmer air against the skin, helping to insulate the body.

Sensation

The integumentary system works together with the nervous system and the sensory system to help a person understand and react to the outside world. The skin contains receptors (nerve endings that pick up sensation) for pain, pressure, heat, cold, and touch. These receptors make a person aware of different sensations: "Am I too hot?" "Are the new shoes too tight, causing pressure and discomfort?" "Is another person's touch soft or rough and hard?"

Communication

The skin takes part in the communication of a person's feelings or mood. Through facial

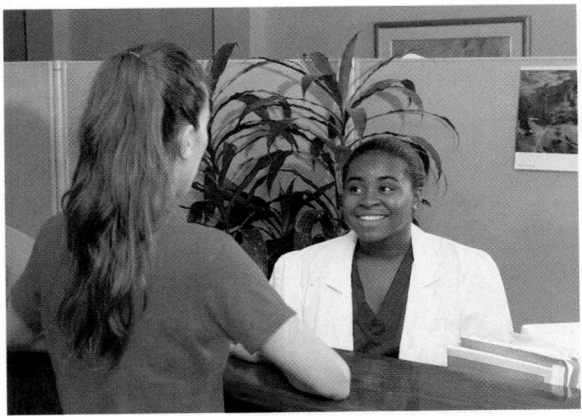

FIGURE 7-6 The medical assistant gives the client a friendly, warm smile.

expressions, moods and emotions are expressed. For example, when a client comes into the office and the medical assistant smiles when greeting that client, the client will understand that the medical assistant is welcoming and glad to see her (Figure 7-6).

Through processes such as perspiration, flushing, or blanching (pallor), a person may display fear, embarrassment, confusion, or anxiety. Skin and hair color also signal sexual and cultural differences to observers.

The skin's general appearance gives clues to personal hygiene, cleanliness, and overall health. It also sends a message about body image. Using observational skills, the medical assistant can note the client's personal hygiene preferences. (The frequency of bathing varies greatly from individual to individual, and also is influenced by a person's cultural group.) In the United States, many skin care services and skin care products are marketed to help

achieve the image that individuals want their skin to project.

 ## BRIDGE TO CAAHEP

This chapter, which discusses the integumentary system, provides information and content related to CAAHEP standards for Anatomy and Physiology, Medical Terminology, Psychology, Communication, Medical Assisting Clinical Procedures, and Professional Components.

 ## ABHES LINKS

This chapter, which discusses the integumentary system, links to ABHES course content for Anatomy and Physiology, Medical Terminology, and Medical Office Clinical Procedures.

 ## AAMA AREAS OF COMPETENCE

This chapter, which discusses the integumentary system, provides information or content within several areas listed in the Medical Assistant Role Delineation Study. These areas include: clinical, fundamental principles, diagnostic orders, patient (client) care, general transdisciplinary, professionalism, communication skills, legal concepts, and instruction.

 ## AMT PATHS

This chapter, which discusses the integumentary system, provides a path to AMT competency in general medical assisting knowledge, anatomy and physiology, medical terminology, and patient (client) education.

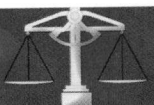
LEGAL/ETHICAL THOUGHTS

Clients who are getting older, or who have health disorders affecting the appearance of the skin, are at risk of becoming victims of unscrupulous marketers. They can be more vulnerable to promises of restoring beauty and youthful skin. Medical assistants should question the effectiveness of products that come with such promises.

POINTS OF HIGHLIGHT

- The skin and accessory structures of hair, nails, and glands make up the integumentary system.
- The skin is the largest organ and covers the entire body.
- Skin can be divided into the epidermis and dermis. A third layer, called the subcutaneous layer or hypodermis, lies underneath the dermis.
- Melanocytes in the skin produce melanin, which is responsible for the color of the skin. The more melanin produced, the darker the skin.
- Melanin also affects hair color. With aging, the amount of melanin decreases and the hair begins to turn gray. The absence of melanin will produce white hair.
- Sebaceous (oil) glands secrete sebum and help lubricate the skin.
- Sudoriferous (sweat) glands secrete sweat to help cool the body.
- The functions of the integumentary system include protection, metabolism, thermoregulation, sensation, and communication.

STUDENT PORTFOLIO ACTIVITY

Unbroken, healthy skin is the body's best defense against infection. Design a handout promoting good skin care that could be given to clients. Keep this handout simple: use common terms, print that is large enough to be read easily, and white or pale-colored paper (fluorescent colors may make a paper easy to find but tough to read, especially for older persons). Be creative! Which characteristics of a medical assistant does this activity correspond with?

APPLYING YOUR SKILLS

A teenage girl comes into the office for a routine visit. During the course of your interaction, she expresses satisfaction with her tan and mentions that she makes weekly visits to the tanning salon. How could this behavior affect this teenager in the future? What does this teenager need to know about skin and the effects of ultraviolet rays? How would you approach the topic of skin protection, and what methods might you use?

CRITICAL THINKING QUESTIONS

1. Why does an older person have gray hair?

2. A young woman tells you about an expensive shampoo and conditioner that she says will make her hair grow well and become thicker. What can you tell her about the effects of these products on her hair?

3. How can skin, which is thin, be called part of the largest organ?

4. Why might an older person feel colder in cold weather that a younger person does?

5. If people have the same number of melanocytes, why is skin color so varied?

6. What is the purpose of the sebaceous glands? How does their functioning affect a person's skin?

7. What causes the odor of perspiration?

8. How do eyelashes and eyebrows protect a person?

9. What is the connection between sunlight and metabolism?

10. On a very hot day, when a person holds a cold container such as a glass of ice-cold water, the person feels cooler. Why? (Explain the process of conduction in your answer.)

11. Go back to the beginning of this chapter and review the Anticipatory Statements. Reread each statement and then indicate whether it is true or false. If the statement is false, rewrite it to make it a true statement.

CLIENT TEACHING PLAN

Handwashing

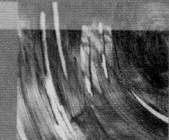

What Is to Be Taught:

- Basic information about clean (aseptic) handwashing and its relation to decreasing the risk of infection.
- How to wash hands using clean aseptic method.

Objectives:

- Client will learn how using the proper handwashing method can decrease the risk of infection.
- Client will wash hands using clean aseptic method.

Preparation Before Teaching:

- Review the infection cycle and the transmission of microorganisms. Remember to put technical medical terms into simple, everyday language that the client will understand.
- Look over the step-by-step handwashing method (even though the medical assistant performs this throughout the course of the day).
- Get together teaching materials, such as pictures of the infection cycle, soap, and paper towels, and a pen and paper for written instructions.
- Make sure that the area is free from distraction while you are teaching.

Steps for the Medical Assistant:

1. Wash your hands.
2. Introduce yourself to the client.
3. Explain what you are going to teach and why.
4. Describe the infection cycle and how bacteria enter the body and are spread by dirty or contaminated hands.
5. Tell the client that he can take part in maintaining his health by following this handwashing method (it decreases the risk of infection).
6. Demonstrate the clean handwashing technique for the client.

7. Ask the client to come to the sink and repeat the steps he has just seen.
8. You will need to cue and prompt the client through the steps.
9. Observe the client for nonverbal cues of confusion or inability to follow the steps in order.
10. Periodically, ask the client if he has any questions.
11. Review any steps or points that the client may have missed.

Special Needs of the Client:

- Look at the client's chart to see if there are any factors that might interfere with the client's ability to practice the proper method of handwashing.
- Ask the client, before and after, if there is anything you need to know that might affect the client's ability to use the aseptic method of handwashing.

Evaluation:

- Client will be able to describe the infection cycle and the role that proper handwashing plays in the infection cycle.
- Client will be able to correctly demonstrate the aseptic method of handwashing.

Further Plans/Teaching:

- Give written instructions, with step-by-step details, and any printed information about the infection cycle to the client, to use as a reference at home.
- Review the information with the client at the next visit.

Follow-up:

- Ask the client if he had any difficulties in practicing this handwashing method.
- Review the steps for proper handwashing.

(Continues)

CLIENT TEACHING PLAN (Continued)

Medical Assistant

Name: _____

Signature: _____

Date : _____

Client

Date: _____

Follow-up Date : _____

CHAPTER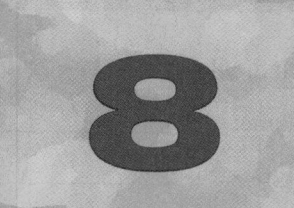

Anticipatory Statements

People have different ideas about what makes up the skeletal system, and about how to keep it healthy. Read and think about the following statements based upon what you believe now. Decide whether you agree or disagree. Write the word **agree** after the statement if you think the statement is true. Write the word **disagree** after the statement if you think the statement is false. Read the chapter to find out if your current beliefs can be supported.

1. The skeleton gives the body its basic shape and form.

   _____

2. The skeleton is made up of hard, dead bone.

   _____

3. Red blood cells are formed in bone marrow.

   _____

4. Cartilage is found only in the nose and the ear.

   _____

5. Joints help the body move into different positions.

   _____

Skeletal System

Learning Objectives

Upon completion of this chapter, the medical assistant student should be able to:

- Define the skeletal system
- List the two divisions of the skeletal system
- State the four shapes of bones and give an example of each
- Identify at least three functions of the skeletal system
- Describe the three types of connection between joints, cartilage, and ligaments
- Explain the main types of movement at synovial joints

Key Terms

appendicular skeleton Bones of arms and legs.

axial skeleton Bones of the trunk of the body.

cartilage Type of connective tissue that helps to absorb shock to the bones and allows smooth movement.

concave Rounded or curved inward.

condyloid Pertaining to a bulge or prominence that is knuckle-like.

convex Rounded or curved out.

joint Point where a part of the skeleton and surrounding structures meet.

ligament Tough, strong band of tissue connecting the ends of bones.

osseous Pertaining to bone or collagen.

pivot Turn.

synovial Relating to the lubricating fluid called synovia.

■ INTRODUCTION

The skeletal system provides a framework that supports and gives a shape to the human body. Bones, joints, cartilage, and ligaments make up the skeletal system. The system protects structures inside the body, stores calcium and other minerals, and produces red blood cells. Along with the muscular system, it enable a person to move about and flex in many ways. An understanding of the structure and normal functioning of the skeletal system allows the medical assistant to recognize disorders and be aware of how these disorders can affect a client's everyday activities.

■ BONES

The skeletal system is made up of bones (the skeleton), joints, cartilage, and ligaments. The skeletal framework as a whole contains 206 bones. The skeleton can be further divided into the **axial skeleton** and the **appendicular skeleton.** In the axial skeleton of the body, there are 80 bones. In the appendicular skeleton, there are 120 bones (Figure 8-1). Sometimes people think of the skeleton as a group of dead bones. However, this is not true: Bones are living material consisting of specialized, thick, connective tissue called **osseous** tissue. Of all the connective tissue, bone tissue is the hardest.

Compact bone makes up the outer layer of bone and the shaft of the long bone. Spongy, porous bone makes up the inner part (Figure 8-2). Additionally, short, flat, and irregular bones and the ends of the long bones are composed mostly of spongy bone. Compact bone contributes strength. Spongy bone is lighter, decreases weight while still giving structure, and contains red bone marrow.

Bones can be grouped according to shape. The four shapes of bone are: long, short, flat, and irregular (Figure 8-3). Long bones are found in the arms and legs. Short bones, found

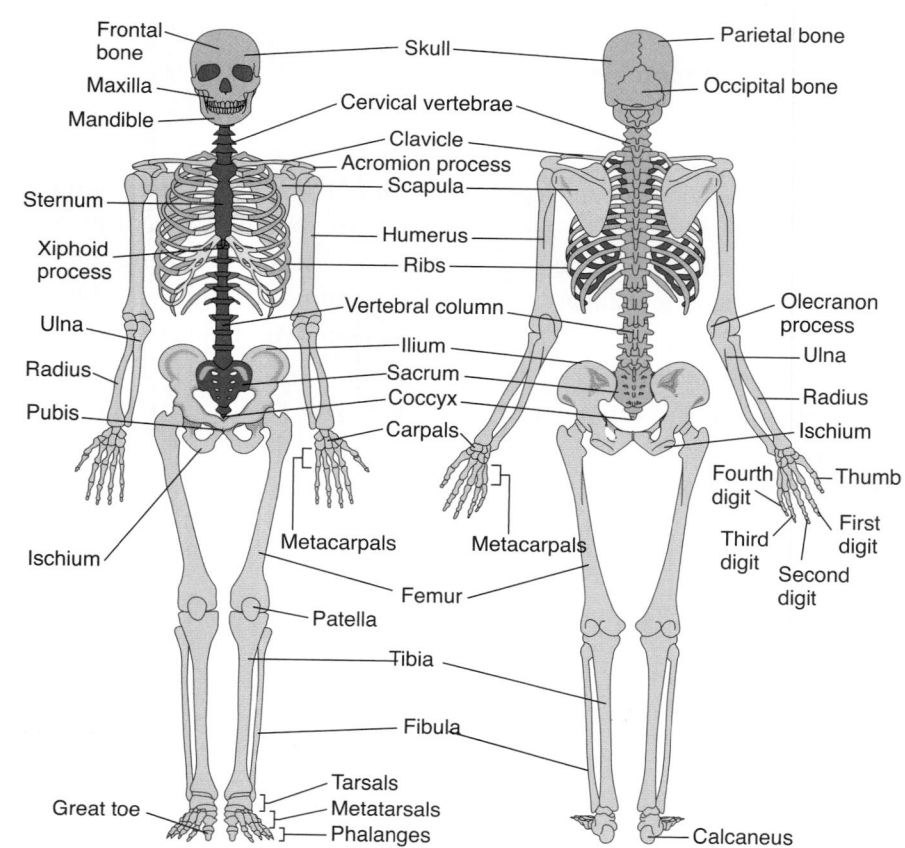

FIGURE 8-1 Axial and appendicular skeletons.

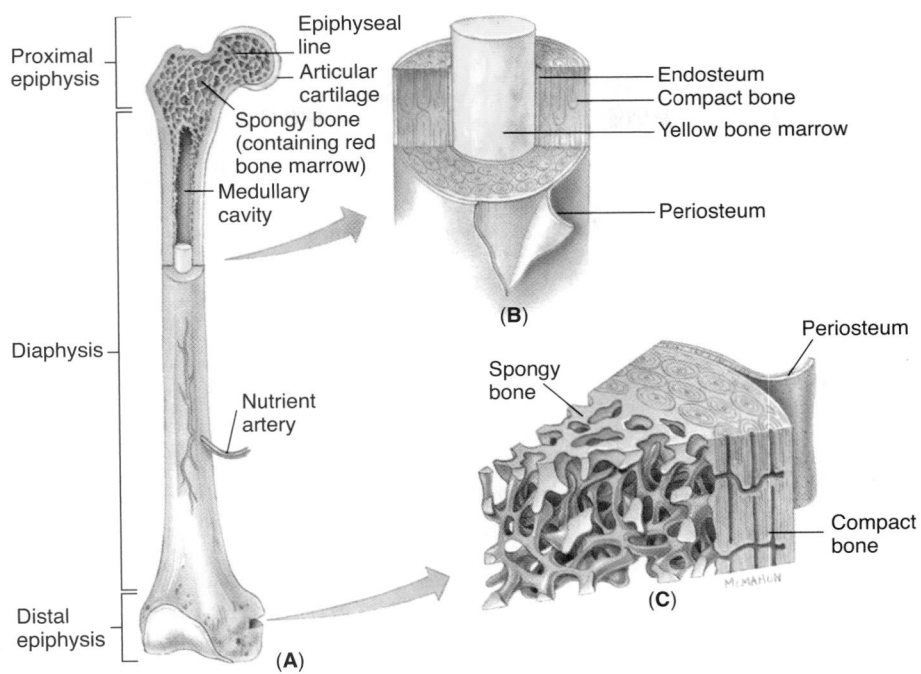

FIGURE 8-2 Structure of long bone, showing compact bone and spongy bone.

in the wrists and ankles, look like cubes. The skull, ribs, and sternum contain flat bones which, in addition to being flat, are thin and curved. Bones that do not belong in any of the first three categories are termed *irregular*. The vertebrae, hip bones, and some bones in the skull are examples of irregular bones.

Joints

A **joint** is a place where bones come together. Joints are composed of dense connective tissue and cartilage. Joints are grouped according to structure and function (Figure 8-4). They can be classified as: immovable, slightly movable, freely movable, or **synovial.**

Joints help the body to move into different positions, and so are grouped according to movement (Figure 8-5). The major movement groups are: ball and socket, hinge, pivot, condyloid, gliding, and saddle.

In a *ball and socket joint*, the head (end) of one bone fits into a rounded cavity or hole of another bone. Examples of ball and socket joints are the hips and shoulders. A *hinge joint* allows movement of a part on a stationary or immoveable frame. The elbow is a hinge joint.

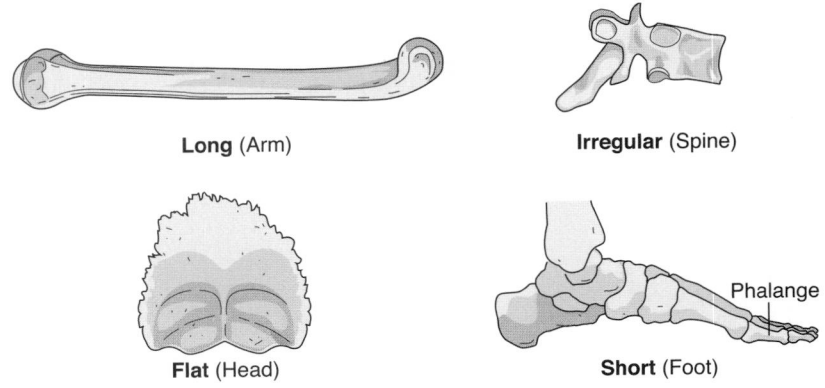

Long (Arm)

Irregular (Spine)

Flat (Head)

Short (Foot)

FIGURE 8-3 Shapes of bones.

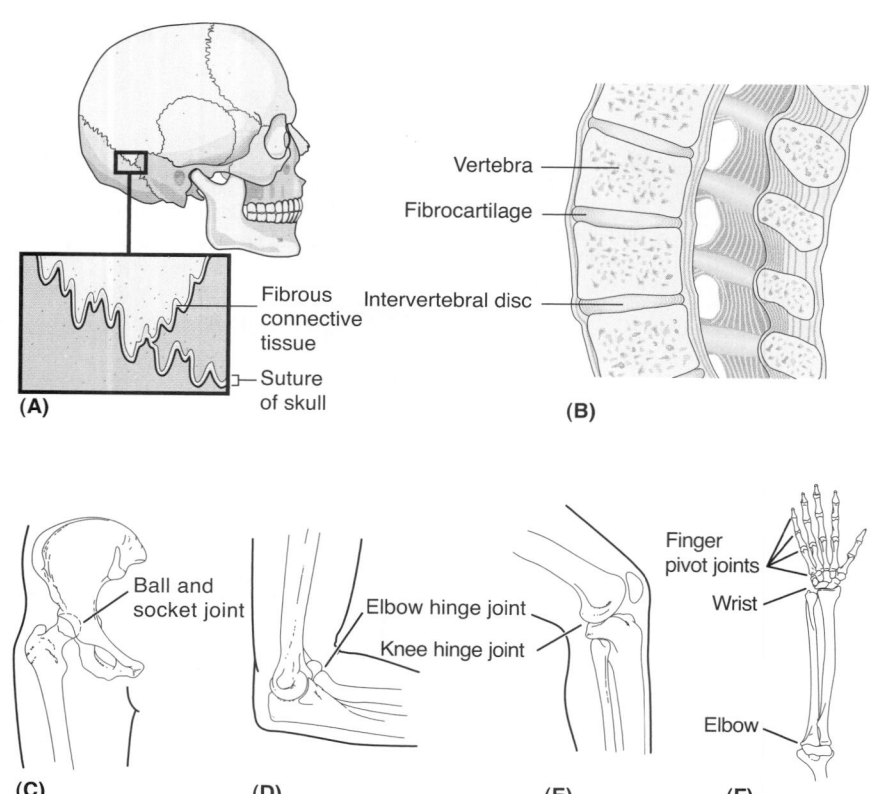

FIGURE 8-4 Types of joints.

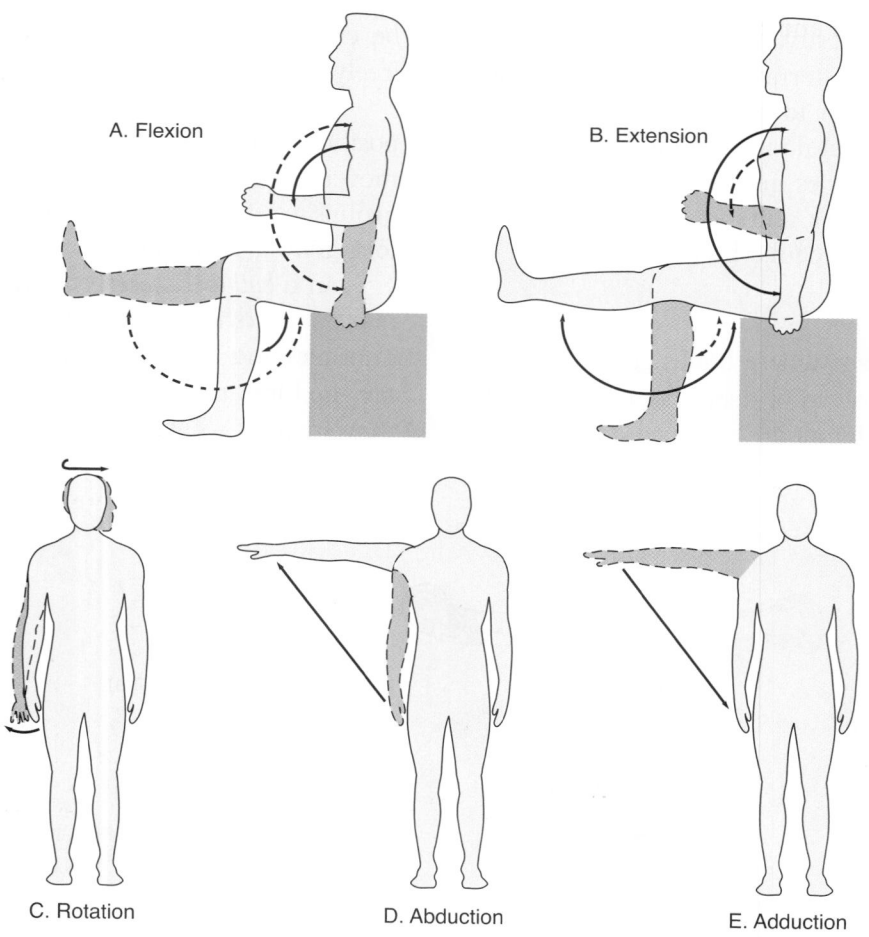

FIGURE 8-5 Joint movements.

A **pivot** joint allows rotation, which is a circling, swinging motion. The head's turning side to side, as if to say no, is an example of a pivot movement.

A **condyloid** joint is a rounded prominence at the end of a bone. The jaw and the knuckles of the hands are examples of condyloid joints.

A *gliding joint* moves in a smooth, seemingly effortless way. The carpal bones in the wrist have gliding joints.

A *saddle joint* consists of two bones at right angles (90 degrees) to each other. Each has a **convex** and a **concave** side. The thumb is a saddle joint.

Cartilage is firm connective tissue, which is found mainly in joints, parts of the air passages, and the ears. Most of the fetal skeleton is cartilage, which slowly is replaced by bone as the child grows.

Ligaments are fibrous tissues that join bones or cartilage. Ligaments hold them together, and can both assist and constrain movement.

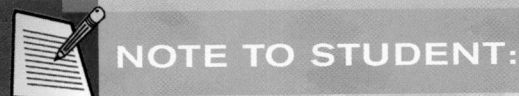

NOTE TO STUDENT:

The working of the skeletal system depends on bone health. People can do much to ensure that their bones stay healthy for a lifetime. Healthful eating, with enough calcium in the diet, and doing weight-bearing exercises (such as running, walking, and bicycling) will help the skeletal system stay in good working order.

■ FUNCTIONS OF THE SKELETAL SYSTEM

The skeletal system performs five functions: support, protection, movement, mineral storage, and red blood cell production.

Support

The human skeleton gives the body its basic shape and framework. There are some varia-tions among people, depending on the size and density of the bone (commonly referred to as small-boned or large-boned). The skeleton provides support for the entire human organism. The structure of the human skeleton, especially the spine, supports the normal upright position.

Protection

The skeletal system provides protection for the internal organs, keeping them safe from injury. For example, the hard cranium (skull) safeguards the brain. The rib cage protects the heart and lungs.

Movement

The skeletal system, in conjunction with the muscular system, enables a person to move about. The joints permit smooth, flexible movements. For example, if the knees, which are hinge joints, become unable to function properly, the walking movement will be stiff and the person will walk with a leg that is unable to bend.

Mineral Storage

Bones can store minerals. Calcium and phosphorus are two important minerals stored in the bones. If an individual does not ingest enough calcium (in an absorbable form), the body will draw upon (deplete) the calcium that is stored in the bones. A person continues to "lay down" new bone while young, so it is critical that young people consume enough calcium to build strong, healthy, dense bone. Even when a person is elderly, it is important to get calcium in the diet, to preserve the bone mass. Dairy products such as milk and cheese are excellent sources of calcium. Vitamin supplements can also add calcium; however, calcium from natural food sources is metabolized and used more efficiently than calcium found in supplements.

Red Blood Cell Production

Red blood cells are formed in the bone marrow. This takes place mainly in the vertebrae, sternum, ribs, part of the cranial bones, humerus (bone in upper arm), and femur (thigh). An important factor for the correct and adequate formation of red blood cells is healthy bone marrow.

BRIDGE TO CAAHEP

This chapter, which discusses the skeletal system, provides information and content related to CAAHEP standards for Anatomy and Physiology, Medical Terminology, Communication, Medical Law and Ethics, Medical Assisting Clinical Procedures, and Professional Components.

ABHES LINKS

This chapter, which discusses the skeletal system, links to ABHES course content for medical assistants for Anatomy and Physiology, Medical Terminology, and Medical Office Clinical Procedures.

AAMA AREAS OF COMPETENCE

This chapter, which discusses the skeletal system, provides information or content within several areas listed in the Medical Assistant Role Delineation Study. These areas include: clinical procedures, fundamental principles, diagnostic orders, patient (client) care, general transdisciplinary, professionalism, communication skills, legal concepts, and instruction.

AMT PATHS

This chapter, which discusses the skeletal system, provides a path to RMA competency in general medical assisting knowledge, anatomy and physiology, medical terminology, and patient (client) education.

POINTS OF HIGHLIGHT

- Bones, joints, cartilage, and ligaments make up the skeletal system.
- The two divisions of the skeletal system are the axial skeleton and the appendicular skeleton.
- Bone tissue is the hardest of all connective tissue.
- The outer layer of bone and the shafts of long bones are composed of compact bone.
- Short, flat, and irregular bones, and the ends of the long bones, are made of spongy bone.
- Bones are grouped according to their shape.
- A joint is made up of dense tissue and cartilage. Joints join bones together and allow movement.
- Joints can be immovable, slightly movable, freely movable, or synovial.
- Joints classified by major movement groups are: ball and socket, hinge, pivot, condyloid, gliding, and saddle.
- The five major functions of the skeletal system are: support, protection, movement, mineral storage, and red blood cell production.
- The skeleton gives the body its framework and protects the internal organs.
- The skeletal system works with the muscular system to enable mobility (movement).
- Minerals such as calcium and phosphorus are stored in the bones.
- The bone marrow forms red blood cells, mainly in the vertebrae, sternum, ribs, parts of the cranial bones, humerus, and femur.

STUDENT PORTFOLIO ACTIVITY

Back injuries can cause long-term problems for people, with large costs in terms of pain, suffering, and loss of employment. They also cost employers much in terms of lost productivity. For your own health and the protection of others, taking care of your back is critical.

Draw a map that looks like a spider. Label the center circle "Back Care." Label the legs coming off the back-care circle with ways to maintain a healthy back. Think of preventive steps you can take to ensure that your back stays healthy and strong. Employers want to know that employees understand the importance of body mechanics and value their own health and the health of others whom they work with or care for.

APPLYING YOUR SKILLS

How do the joints help a person to perform different activities? Select a specific joint and explain how that joint works together with the bones. What type of movement does this joint allow a person to do? What would happen to that part of the skeleton if the joint did not work properly? What do you expect to see in a client who has a problem with the joint that you chose to discuss?

CRITICAL THINKING QUESTIONS

1. What is the relationship between bones and the storing of minerals such as calcium? How does a person's diet affect this function of the skeletal system?

2. Spongy bone and compact bone work together. What does each part contribute to the overall bone function?

3. How would you explain to a client what is meant by a hinge joint? (For example-elbow)

4. What does the position of the vertebrae (back) allow a human to do?

5. Choose a part of the skeleton and tell how that bone protects. What organs inside the body are protected from injury?

6. Bones store minerals. Why are minerals stored? Does the body use the stored minerals and if so when are the stored minerals used?

7. How do red blood cells depend upon healthy bones?

8. How does the health of a person's bones affect the person's muscles?

9. Why is it incorrect when people refer to the skeleton as a "bunch of dead bones"? How would you explain to a client the concept that the skeleton is living matter?

10. Go back to the beginning of this chapter and review the Anticipatory Statements. Reread each statement and then indicate whether it is true or false. If the statement is false, rewrite it to make it a true statement.

CLIENT TEACHING PLAN

Bicycle Safety

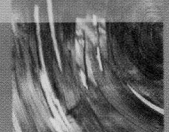

■ What Is to Be Taught:

- Steps for safe bicycle riding; how to reduce risk when riding a bicycle.

■ Objectives:

- Client will be able to list and explain steps for safe bicycle riding.

■ Preparation Before Teaching:

- Review information about safety issues and guidelines regarding equipment and bike helmet safety.
- Gather appropriate printed material regarding bike safety.
- Have paper and pen available.
- Get a sample bicycle helmet that meets safety regulations and samples of reflective tape or a reflective vest.

■ Steps for the Medical Assistant:

1. Wash your hands.
2. Introduce yourself to the client.
3. Explain what you are going to teach and why.
4. Show the client a bicycle helmet that meets or exceeds the safety standards.
5. Demonstrate what the client should look for in a safety helmet. It should fit snugly and not slip around. The helmet should sit on the head with the front one inch above the eyebrows. The chin strap should be adjusted so that the helmet fits snugly.
6. Show the client samples of reflective vests or tape, telling her also to wear bright or fluorescent clothing when riding, whether during the day or night. The purpose is to be highly visible to motorists.
7. Remind the client to keep the bicycle in good working order, including making sure that the tires are inflated to the correct pressure and that the brakes work.
8. Instruct the client to install reflectors on the bike, as well as a headlight if she is going to ride at night.
9. Inform the client to keep her hands on the handlebars so that she always has control of the bicycle; any items taken along on the ride should be in a carrier or backpack.
10. A bicycle is a vehicle, so tell the client that she must obey the rules of the road. The rules include:
    a. Ride with the flow of traffic, never against it.
    b. Obey signals, traffic signs, and any markings on the road.
    c. Signal when turning. This is courteous as well as a safety measure. Watch for turning traffic.
    d. Ride so that others can see you. Avoid drivers' blind spots.
    e. Stay as far away from parked cars as possible, in case they suddenly pull out or the car door is opened.
    f. Observe for any obstacles on the road that could tip or trap the bike, such as potholes or wet leaves.
    g. Above all else, STAY ALERT.
11. Write this information down and hand the paper to the client unless there is preprinted material for you to give to clients.

■ Special Needs of the Client:

- Check the client's chart to see if there are any factors that might interfere with the way you plan to do your teaching.
- Ask the client, before and after, if there is anything you need to know that might affect her ability to comply with your teaching.

■ Evaluation:

- Client is able to identify and do safety preparations before riding a bicycle.
- Client can list the safety rules for bicycling.

(Continues)

CLIENT TEACHING PLAN (Continued)

▪ Further Plans/Teaching:

- Ask the client if she has any questions or if she would like any additional information.

▪ Follow-up:

- Call the client at home after one or two weeks. Ask her if she is experiencing any difficulties in getting a bicycle helmet, reflective tape, or reflective vest.
- Ask the client which safety rules she has been able to incorporate into her riding.

Medical Assistant

Name: _____

Signature: _____

Date: _____

Client

Date: _____

Follow-up Date : _____

Anticipatory Statements

People have different ideas about the muscular system and how muscles work. Read and think about the following statements based upon what you believe now. Decide whether you agree or disagree. Write the word **agree** after the statement if you think the statement is true. Write the word **disagree** after the statement if you think the statement is false. Read the chapter to find out if your current beliefs can be supported.

1. Bodybuilders use only isotonic exercises to tone muscles. _____

2. The body's center of gravity is the head. _____

3. A person's body shape depends on the amount of physical activity he or she gets and which muscles are used. _____

4. Body mechanics involves thinking of the body as a machine. _____

5. A narrow base of support will cause instability. _____

Muscular System

Learning Objectives

Upon completion of this chapter, the medical assistant student should be able to:

- Define skeletal muscle and give an example
- Define smooth muscle and give an example
- Define cardiac muscle and give an example
- State the difference between isometric and isotonic exercises
- Explain what is meant by body mechanics
- Develop a teaching plan to teach a client the benefits to muscles of exercise

Key Terms

body mechanics Use of the body based on a view of the body as a machine. A person must keep the body in good alignment and use the correct muscles when moving and lifting to prevent injury to the body.

cardiac muscle A type of involuntary muscle found only in the heart.

conductivity The ability to send impulses or messages.

contractibility The ability to shrink or get smaller in size.

elasticity The ability to return to original shape after being stretched or pulled.

irritability The ability to quickly react to something, such as a stimulus.

isometric exercises Exercises that involve muscular contractions with sharp increase in muscle tone and very little shortening of muscle fibers.

isotonic exercises Exercises that involve muscular contractions with very little increase in muscle tone and much shortening of muscle fibers.

skeletal muscle Voluntary muscles that connect to the skeleton and allow movement of the body.

smooth muscle A type of muscle that is involuntary; found in the internal organs.

■ INTRODUCTION

The muscular system is the system that moves part or all of the body. Sometimes it is considered to be combined with the skeletal system, and is called the *musculoskeletal* system. However, it is a separate system even though the muscular system is interdependent with the skeletal system (that is, they need each other to work properly). All systems in the body are interdependent; if there is a problem in one system, the other body systems will also be affected.

■ MUSCLES

Muscles make up the muscular system (Figures 9-1 and 9-2). Muscle is tissue that has the ability to contract or shorten, which is called **contractibility.** This is its major feature. Muscles

also have **irritability** (sensitivity), **conductivity** (ability to transmit messages), and **elasticity** (stretchiness and springiness). A muscle consists of a thick middle part with two ends called *attachments.* One attachment is joined to a solid point; this is the *origin* of the muscle. The other attachment is joined to a moveable part called the *insertion* of the muscle.

Muscles are grouped according to type. The three types of muscle are smooth, skeletal, and cardiac (Figure 9-3). **Smooth muscle** is also called *involuntary* because the movement of this muscle type is not under conscious control. Smooth muscle tissue is under the control of the autonomic nervous system. Smooth muscle is found in the internal (inside the body) organs. The respiratory tract, the walls of blood vessels, the urinary bladder, and genital ducts all contain smooth muscle tissue. **Skeletal muscle**, or

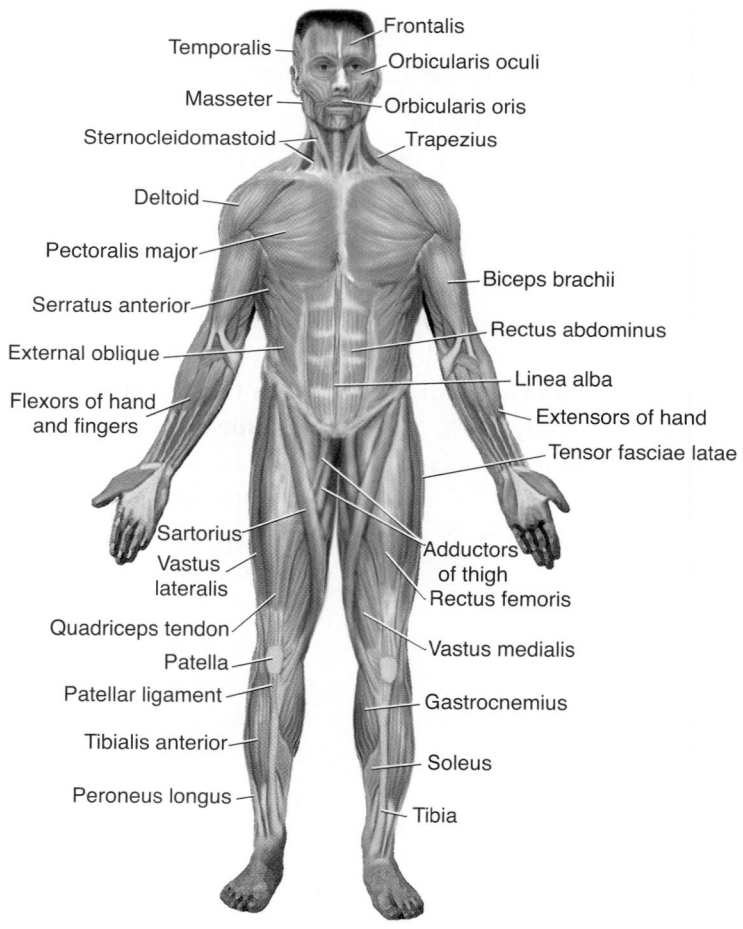

FIGURE 9–1 Anterior view of muscles.

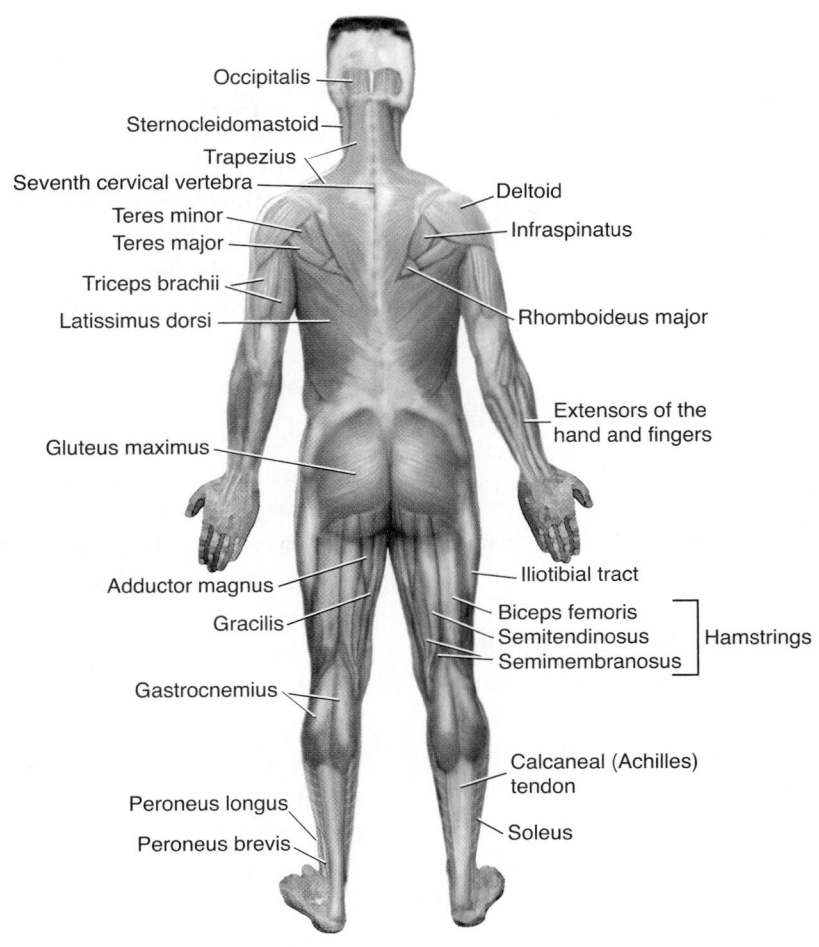

FIGURE 9–2 Posterior view of muscles.

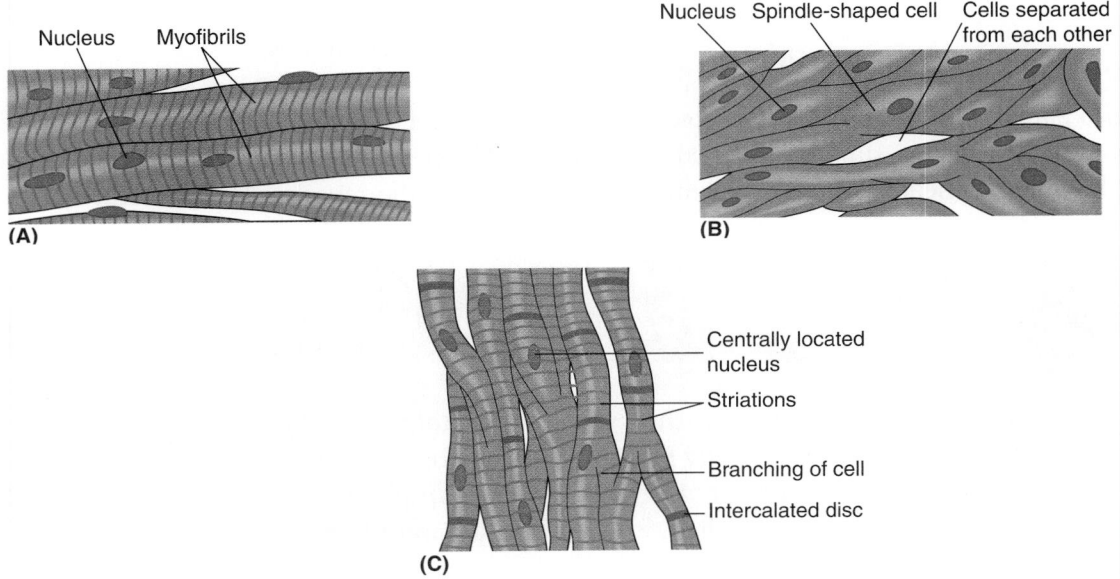

FIGURE 9–3 Three types of muscle: (A) Skeletal, (B) Cardiac, (C) Smooth.

striated muscle, is also called *voluntary* because the person can control the movement of muscles of this type. The tongue, pharynx (throat), and the top part of the esophagus contain voluntary muscle. The third type of muscle, called **cardiac muscle**, is found in the heart or cardium. The automatic nervous system controls the working of the cardiac muscle.

■ WORK OF MUSCLES

Muscles perform many tasks, such as thermoregulation, movement, support, protection, and appearance. In addition, the muscular system as a whole has important functions.

Thermoregulation

The work of the muscles helps to keep the body warm. In cold weather, a person who keeps moving and is doing physical activity does not feel the cold as much, as the contractions of the muscles produce heat. If the surrounding air is warm and a person is doing heavy physical activity, the person may become overheated because of the production of heat by the working muscles.

Movement

Without working muscles, a person could not move. The muscular system acts with the skeletal system to make movement possible.

Support and Protection

Muscles also play a role in support and protection. The muscles help to support the body, including holding the head and neck upright.

The muscles of newborn babies are not yet developed or strong enough for them to hold their heads up. Similarly, it takes time for muscles to develop enough to allow a baby to stand and walk. When disorders attack the muscular system, the result often is an inability to walk or move freely. Muscles protect the internal organs of the body by providing cushioning that absorbs or deflects potentially injurious forces.

Shape

Muscles give shape to the body's framework, giving it a distinctive form. Heredity plays a role in how people look, but a person's shape will also vary depending upon physical activity and which muscles are used. Weightlifters have strong, developed chest and arm muscles, making their chests and arms appear more muscular. Runners and ballet dancers have muscular legs; swimmers have muscular arms.

Physical fitness centers often advertise by encouraging people to work out and keep muscles toned. *Muscle tone* means that some cells in the muscles always remain partially contracted. Some contract while others relax. Muscle tone allows a person to continue a task or activity without fatigue. A person who has well-toned muscles has more endurance then someone who does not. Prolonged bedrest puts a person at risk of losing muscle tone. When a person becomes deconditioned, even slight physical activity will cause fatigue.

Isotonic/Isometric Exercises. Different actions work different muscle groups and different characteristics of the muscles. *Isotonic* contractions

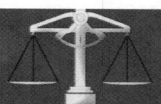

LEGAL/ETHICAL THOUGHTS

The medical assistant will work with clients to maintain mobility and independence in activities of daily living. While performing these tasks, medical assistants gain access to protected health information (PHI). Health care providers have a legal responsibility, in addition to a moral and ethical obligation, to maintain client confidentiality.

occur when the tension or tone of the muscle does not change, but the muscle becomes shorter and thicker. This happens when a person lifts objects. *Isometric* contractions occur when the muscle length does not change, but the muscle tension increases. Exercises can be either isotonic, isometric, or a combination of the two. Many physical exercises involve both. **Isometric exercises** use muscle contraction without movement, whereas **isotonic exercises** use muscle contraction with movement. For example, standing by a wall and pushing both hands equally against it involves muscle contraction but no movement, and so would be considered isometric. Running or walking are isotonic exercises, because the muscles contract and movement is involved.

■ BODY MECHANICS

Body mechanics is based on thinking of the body as if it were a machine. It is important to use the machine safely and efficiently to keep it in good working order. Use of the body in a safe, efficient manner is use of good body mechanics.

    Three points form the core of body mechanics: center of gravity, line of gravity, and base of support. The center of gravity is the pelvic area. This imaginary line divides the body's weight in half. Keeping the back straight and the body in good alignment maintains the center of gravity of the pelvic area over the feet, thus enhancing a person's stability (Figure 9-4).

    The base of support is the feet. If the base of any object is wide, it has more stability; that is, it will stay in position and not fall over. The same idea applies to people. The wider the base, the greater the stability. (If the feet are spread out too far, though, the line of gravity will not be centered and the person will lose balance.) For greatest stability, place one foot slightly ahead of the other, to avoid falling forward or backward. The weight must be kept on both feet equally. The knees should be slightly bent and not locked. When moving a person or object, the feet must turn (Figure 9-5).

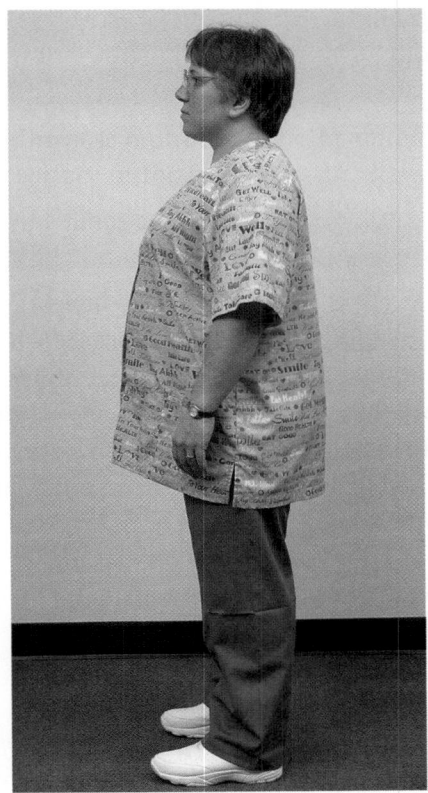

FIGURE 9-4 Good body mechanics can prevent back injuries.

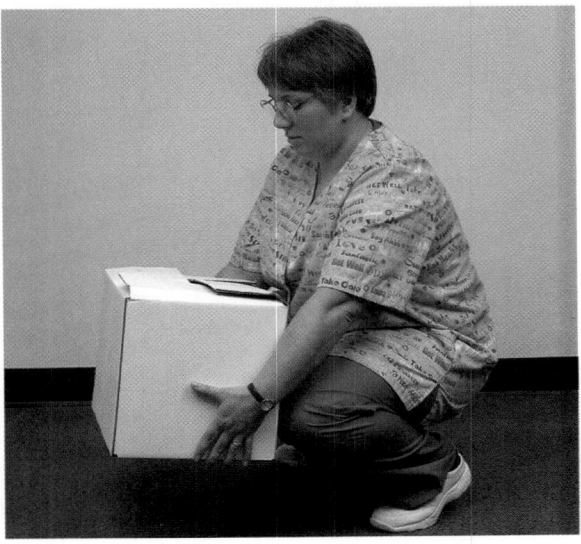

FIGURE 9-5 Establish a good base of support by keeping the back straight and the feet apart.

NOTE TO STUDENT:

Never twist your body when moving a client or object. Twisting motions can result in muscle, vertebral, or other back injury.

The line of gravity goes vertically from the top of the head through the base. For the body to work best, the line of gravity should be straight. For this to happen, the person must keep the back straight, the head erect, and the abdomen somewhat toned or tight.

NOTE TO STUDENT:

Using proper body mechanics will be easier for the medical assistant if the body is kept in alignment during all activities. Stand tall and use good posture, with head erect, back straight, abdomen in, and weight evenly divided between the feet. When the medical assistant remembers to do this, all the muscles of the body work safely together as the medical assistant performs the necessary tasks.

BRIDGE TO CAAHEP

This chapter, which describes the muscular system, provides information and content related to CAAHEP standards for Anatomy and Physiology, Medical Terminology, Medical Law and Ethics Communication, Medical Assisting Clinical Procedures, and Professional Components.

ABHES LINKS

This chapter, which discusses the muscular system, links to ABHES course content for medical assisting for Anatomy and Physiology, Medical Terminology, Medical Law and Ethics, and Medical Office Clinical Procedures.

AAMA AREAS OF COMPETENCE

This chapter, which discusses the muscular system, provides information or content within several areas listed in the Medical Assistant Role Delineation Study. These areas include: clinical, fundamental principles, diagnostic orders, patient (client) care, general transdisciplinary, professionalism, communication skills, legal concepts, and instruction.

AMT PATHS

This chapter, which discusses the muscular system, provides a path to AMT competence in general medical assisting knowledge, anatomy and physiology, medical terminology, and patient (client) education.

POINTS OF HIGHLIGHT

- Muscle is tissue that has the ability to contract or shorten.
- Muscles have four characteristics: irritability (sensitivity), contractility, conductivity, and elasticity.
- Muscles have a thick middle part.
- Muscles have two ends called attachments. One attachment, joined with a solid point, is the origin of the muscle. The other attachment, joined to a moveable part, is called the insertion of the muscle.
- The three types of muscle are: smooth, skeletal, and cardiac.
- Smooth muscle is found inside the internal organs.
- Skeletal muscle is also called striated muscle or voluntary muscle (controlled by person). The movement of this muscle type is under conscious, voluntary control.
- Cardiac muscle is found in the heart.
- Isotonic and isometric exercises help to build and maintain muscle tone.
- To prevent injury and keep the muscles in good working condition, it is important to use good body mechanics.
- Awareness of the center of gravity, base of support, and line of gravity will help the medical assistant to use correct body mechanics throughout the course of the day.

STUDENT PORTFOLIO ACTIVITY

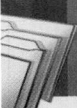

Attend a physical therapy session. You can accompany a client as part of your externship experience or make an appointment to observe at a local physical therapy clinic. Write an observational experience report and ask the physical therapist to add comments and sign your report.

APPLYING YOUR SKILLS

A client whose broken arm has been healing comes in for an examination. When you try to move his arm into different positions, he complains of stiffness and pain. When asked if he is doing the prescribed exercises at home, he replies that he is waiting until his arm does not hurt anymore and is completely healed. What should this client know about muscles and their use and disuse?

CRITICAL THINKING QUESTIONS

1. As part of the exam, a young female client states that she takes extra calcium, so she is sure that she has good, strong bones. When you ask about physical activity, though, she says she hates exercising. As a medical assistant, what can you explain about the relationship between strong, well-toned muscles and healthy bones?

2. How does moving around (physical activity) keep a person warm while outdoors in cold weather?

3. Why are newborn babies unable to hold their heads up?

4. What is the relationship between fatigue (extreme tiredness) and muscle condition?

5. You observe another medical assistant student picking a heavy object off the floor by bending from the waist while keeping her legs straight. What would you say to this student?

6. Before attempting to transfer (move) a client, how should you position your feet? Why?

7. Thinking of your body as a machine and using good body mechanics is critical to maintaining a healthy back. What does this statement mean?

8. Why is skeletal muscle considered voluntary muscle?

9. Why is it important for you, as a medical assistant, to encourage clients to include exercise in their daily activities? What effect does exercise have on the muscular system?

10. Go back to the beginning of this chapter and review the Anticipatory Statements. Reread each statement and then indicate whether it is true or false. If the statement is false, rewrite it to make it a true statement.

CLIENT TEACHING PLAN

Active Range-of-Motion Exercises (AROM)

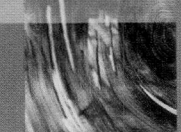

■ What Is to Be Taught:

- Active range-of-motion exercises for the client's left wrist and fingers.

■ Objectives:

- Client will perform active range-of-motion exercises for the wrist and fingers.

■ Preparation Before Teaching:

- Review AROM exercises and the rationale and reasons for performing them. Make sure to put technical medical terms into words that the client will understand.

■ Steps for the Medical Assistant:

1. Introduce yourself to the client.
2. Explain what you are going to teach and why.
3. Inform the client that the wrist and fingers must be exercised to maintain strength and flexibility. If they are not exercised, the muscles will contract and the client will lose function of the wrist and fingers. Performing these exercises is something the client can do to take part in his own health care.
4. Wash your hands.
5. Ask the client to sit or lie down in a comfortable position.
6. Tell the client that you will be gentle, but if the movements cause pain or discomfort, the client should tell you and you will stop.
7. Watch for nonverbal cues or signs of pain, especially if the client has difficulty speaking.
8. While supporting the client's left arm, bend and then straighten the left wrist.
9. Repeat this three times.
10. Do not force this movement if you feel resistance in the muscles.
11. Turn the wrist away from the center of the body, then return it to neutral or straight center. Next, turn the wrist toward the center

of the body and then return it to neutral or straight center.
12. Repeat this three times.
13. Do not force the movement if you feel resistance in the muscles.
14. While supporting the client's wrist, bend and straighten each finger individually.
15. Repeat this three times on each finger.
16. Do not force this movement on any finger if you feel resistance.
17. Move each finger away from the center and then toward the center.
18. Repeat this three times for each finger.
19. Do not force this movement on any finger if you feel resistance.
20. Move the thumb in a circle.
21. Repeat this three times.
22. Do not force this movement if you feel resistance in the thumb.
23. Ask the client if he has any questions or concerns.
24. Tell the client to use his right hand to bend and then straighten the left wrist. He should do this motion three times.
25. Remind the client to stop the movement if he feels any pain or resistance.
26. Ask the client to use his right hand to bend and straighten each finger on the left hand individually. He should do this motion three times for each finger.
27. Remind the client to stop the movement if he feels any pain or resistance.
28. Ask the client to use his right hand to turn the left wrist away from the center of the body and then return it to neutral or straight center. He should do this motion three times.
29. Ask the client to move each finger away from the center and then toward the center. Have him repeat this three times with each finger.
30. Remind the client to stop the movement if he feels any pain or resistance.

(Continues)

CLIENT TEACHING PLAN (Continued)

31. Tell the client to move the thumb in a circle. He should do this motion three times.

32. Remind the client to stop the movement if he feels any pain or resistance.

Special Needs of the Client:

- Look at the client's chart to see if there are any factors that might interfere with the client's ability to perform the exercises.
- Ask the client, before and after, if there is anything you need to know that might affect the client's ability to follow through on doing these exercises.

Evaluation:

- Client will be able to list the steps for doing the specific active range-of-motion exercises.
- Client will be able to demonstrate the AROM exercises on the right wrist and fingers.

Further Plans/Teaching:

- Give written instructions to the client to use as a reference when doing these exercises at home.

- At a follow-up visit, review the teaching plan for the AROM exercises. Make any changes necessary to meet the client's current health needs.

Follow-up:

- Call the client within one week to see if he has any concerns or problems.
- At a follow-up visit, review the teaching plan for the AROM exercises. Make any changes necessary to meet the client's current health needs.

Medical Assistant

Name: _____

Signature: _____

Date: _____

Client

Date: _____

Follow-up Date : _____

CHAPTER 10

Anticipatory Statements

People have many different levels of understanding about the nervous system, how it works, and how it is related to the senses. Read and think about the following statements based upon what you believe now. Decide whether you agree or disagree. Write the word **agree** after the statement if you think the statement is true. Write the word **disagree** after the statement if you think the statement is false. Read the chapter to find out if your current beliefs can be supported.

1. The brain and spinal cord make up the peripheral nervous system. _____

2. The picture that the eye sees is interpreted by the brain. _____

3. During stress, the sympathetic nervous system slows the heart rate. _____

4. Bones in the ear vibrate when sound waves come into the ear. _____

5. The brainstem part of the brain looks like a stem on a plant. _____

Learning Objectives

Upon completion of this chapter, the medical assistant student should be able to:

- Define the nervous system
- Name the two divisions of the nervous system
- Explain the difference between the sympathetic and parasympathetic nervous systems

Nervous System and Sensory System

- Describe the main functions of the nervous system
- Define the sensory system
- Identify the special senses
- Explain the role of the eye in vision
- Explain the role of the ear in hearing and equilibrium
- Describe the sense of taste
- Describe the sense of touch
- Describe the sense of smell
- Explain how the nervous system and the sensory system are connected

Key Terms

autonomic nervous system The part of the nervous system that controls involuntary muscles and actions.

axon The part of a neuron that carries impulses away from the cell body.

cerebellum The second largest part of the brain; concerned with coordination and movement.

cerebrum The largest part of the brain.

cornea Tough outer covering of the eyeball.

cranial Pertaining to the skull (from which the *cranial* nerves originate).

dendrite A part of the neuron that carries impulses to the cell body.

diencephalon The part of the brain that contains the thalamus and hypothalamus.

medulla oblongata The part of the brainstem that controls vital life processes.

neuroglia Nerve cells that support the neurons; the "glue" of the nervous system.

neuron Working or functional cell of the nervous system that transmits impulses.

parasympathetic nervous system The part of the autonomic nervous system that controls digestion and takes over body functions during times of rest.

peduncles Bands of fibers that connect parts of the brain; they look like stalks of a plant.

peripheral nervous system The part of the nervous system outside of the central nervous system; consists of the cranial nerves and spinal nerves.

sympathetic nervous system The part of the autonomic nervous system that becomes active in "fight or flight" situations.

■ INTRODUCTION

The brain can be compared to an air traffic controller who is constantly receiving many different bits of information from inside and outside sources. This information, as in the case of the brain, is taken in, checked, and acted upon constantly to maintain all the bodily functions necessary to support life and the health of the brain, even during sleep, while the body rests. If an emergency develops, the brain, like the air traffic controller, focuses on that problem to prevent a disaster, all the while keeping the other functions properly maintained and thus preventing, or at least keeping to a minimum the problem. Small changes are responded to promptly, without a dramatic emergency response, thus allowing for stable functioning as in the case of the air traffic controller who is responsible for a smooth takeoff and safe landing.

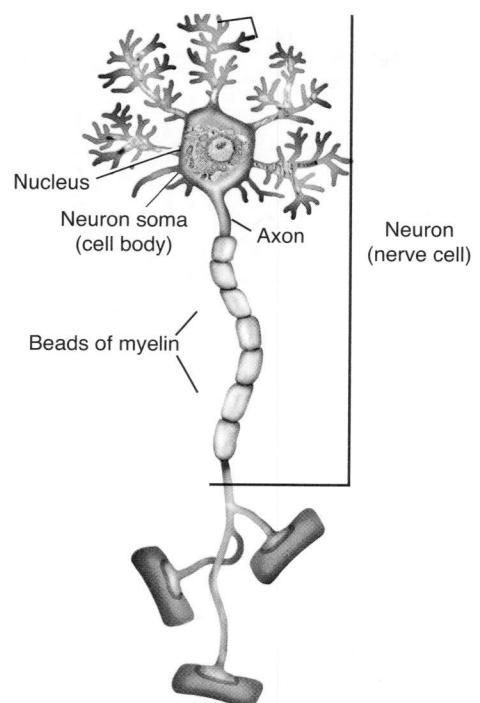

FIGURE 10-1 A neuron.

■ THE NERVOUS SYSTEM

Two types of cells make up the nervous system: neurons and neuroglia. The **neuron** is the functional unit or working part of the nervous system (Figure 10-1). The neurons react to both physical and chemical stimuli. These cells can initiate (start), conduct, and transmit or transfer messages. The neuron is made up of a cell body, an axon, and one or more dendrites. The **axon** conducts electrical impulses or waves of excitement away from the cell body. **Dendrites** (usually more than one per cell) conduct impulses to the cell body. The *cell body* is the center part of the neuron.

The **neuroglia** are the second type of nervous system cell. There are many more neuroglia than neurons in the body. The purpose of neuroglia is to act as "glue" for the neurons, holding the neurons in place. Neuroglia also protect the neurons from injury or infection. They do not transmit impulses.

The nervous system is divided into the central nervous system (CNS) and the peripheral nervous system (PNS).

■ CENTRAL NERVOUS SYSTEM

The central nervous system (CNS) is composed of the brain and spinal cord. The brain is a mass of nervous tissue enclosed in the cranium (skull) (Figure 10-2). Neurons and the supporting neuroglia make up the brain's gray and white matter. The gray is mostly composed of neuron cell bodies, whereas the white matter is

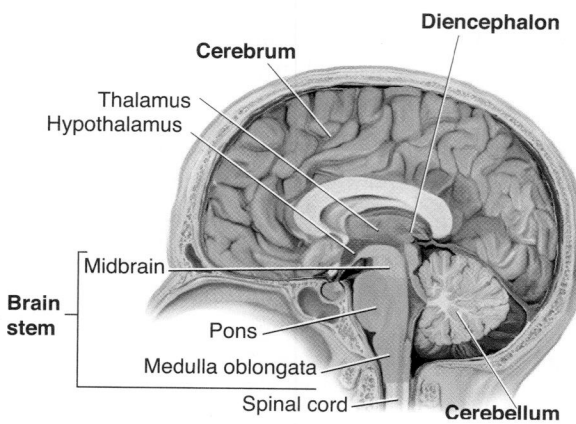

FIGURE 10-2 The main parts of the brain are the cerebrum, cerebellum, diencephalon, and brainstem.

the axons. The brain has four main parts: the cerebrum, the diencephalon, the cerebellum, and the brainstem.

Cerebrum

The **cerebrum**, which is the largest part of the brain, has two hemispheres (halves) separated by a deep groove or fissure called the *corpus callosum*. The surface of the hemispheres appears bumpy because of its many folds.

The cerebrum has four lobes: the frontal, parietal, occipital, and temporal (Figure 10-3). The frontal lobe, found toward the front of the head, initiates voluntary skeletal muscle movement. The parietal lobe, found on top and in the central part of the head, is concerned with taste and sensations on the skin. The temporal lobe, found on the side of the head, is connected to the sense of hearing and the sense of smell. The occipital lobe, in the back of the head, is central to the sense of vision.

The cerebral part of the brain controls memory, intelligence, and emotions. It is also critical to a person's ability to learn new things, reason or figure out ideas, and apply judgment. The cerebrum also interprets sensory impulses and guides voluntary muscular activities.

Cerebellum

The second largest part of the brain is the **cerebellum.** It is connected to the brainstem by

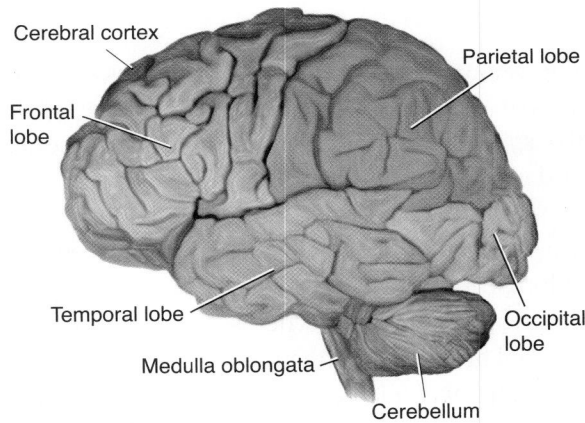

FIGURE 10-3 The cerebrum consists of the frontal lobe, parietal lobe, temporal lobe, and occipital lobe.

three pairs of fiber bundles called **peduncles.** The cerebellum controls and coordinates both voluntary and some involuntary movements such as maintaining posture and balance. It does not begin the movements, but it maintains and carries them out. Walking, running, and smooth movements of the eye are under the control of the cerebellum. The ability to perform fine motor movements necessary for activities of daily living depends on the cerebellum (Figure 10-4). These activities of daily living include: eating (forks, spoons, other utensils), dressing (buttons, zippers, clasps, shoelaces), writing (pens, pencils), and even playing instruments (piano, violin).

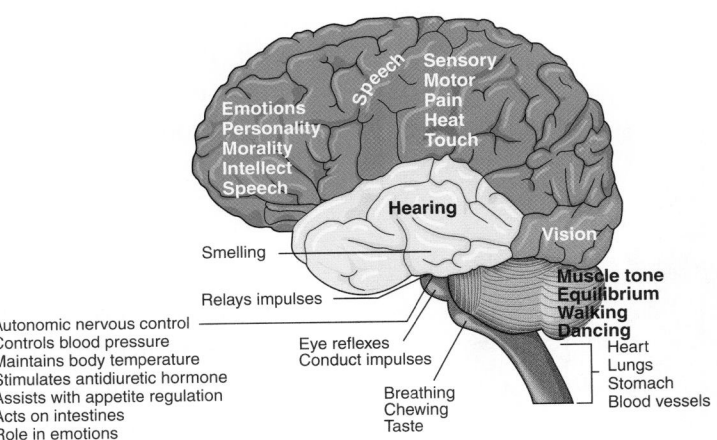

FIGURE 10-4 Cerebral functions. The cerebellum is responsible for the movements necessary for activities of daily living (voluntary activities); the cerebrum processes sensory information and creates emotions.

Brainstem

The brainstem, which looks like a thick stem of a plant, connects the cerebral hemispheres with the spinal cord. The medulla oblongata, pons, and midbrain are all part of the brainstem.

Pons means bridge, and this structure acts as a bridge-like connector between the medulla oblongata, the cerebellum, and the upper portions of the brain. It helps to maintain the normal breathing pattern.

The *midbrain* connects the pons and cerebellum with the cerebrum. When visual (seeing) and auditory (hearing) stimuli, such as a bright flashlight or a sharp crack, are received the eyes and head move in response. This movement is controlled by the midbrain.

The lowest part of the brainstem is the **medulla oblongata.** This part controls the vital processes of life. Breathing, heart rate, blood pressure, and the essential reflexes of coughing, sneezing, swallowing, and vomiting all depend on the proper working of the medulla oblongata.

Small Essential Parts of the Brain

Smaller parts within the brain also play vital roles in the functioning of the nervous system. These important structures—the limbic system, reticular activating system, and basal nuclei—overlap in some areas of the brain. The limbic system affects a person's emotions and motivated behavior (Figure 10-5). The reticular

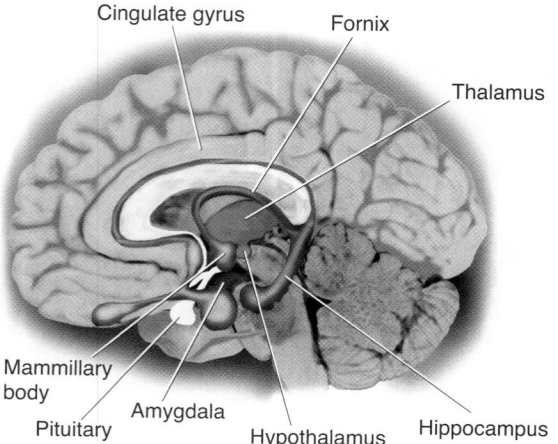

Cingulate gyrus   Fornix

Thalamus

Mammillary body

Pituitary   Amygdala   Hypothalamus   Hippocampus

FIGURE 10-5 The limbic system.

activating system starts and continues wakefulness and creates the ability to pay attention. Drugs that calm or sedate a person slow down activity in this area of the brain for a time.

Diencephalon

Under the cerebrum and above the brainstem lies the **diencephalon.** The diencephalon includes the thalamus and the hypothalamus. Most sensory information that will eventually go to the cerebrum is relayed and processed in the thalamus. The hypothalamus is found below the thalamus (*hypo* means "below" or "under"). It organizes the autonomic nervous system, regulating body temperature, metabolism, and water balance. Happiness (enjoyment), fright, thirst, appetite, and sexual feelings are all regulated by the hypothalamus. The hypothalamus produces both hormones and hormone-releasing or -inhibiting secretions, thus controlling the pituitary gland and other endocrine functions.

Spinal Cord

The spinal cord, which is mostly encased in the spinal canal, is the second major part of the central nervous system. It starts at the medulla and continues to the second lumbar vertebra (L2). It is surrounded by bone (the vertebrae of the spine). This is the pathway for sensory impulses going to the brain and for motor impulses coming from the brain.

The spinal cord is a major reflex center. For example, when a person touches a hand to a hot object, the hand is automatically pulled away, without conscious thought. The impulse for that reflex action comes directly from the spinal cord.

How the Central Nervous System Is Protected

The central nervous system (brain and spinal cord) is protected in four ways: by bone, meninges, cerebrospinal fluids, and the blood-brain barrier. The brain is located in the hard, bony cranium (skull). The vertebral column (spine or backbone) protects the spinal cord. The connective tissue of the meninges has three layers: the dura mater, the arachnoid, and the pia mater. The *dura mater* (the name translates as "hard or strong mother") is the outer, thick connective tissue. The middle membrane layer is the arachnoid. *Arachnoid* means "spider-like," and this layer does look like a spider web. The third layer of protection is the *pia mater* ("internal or soft mother"). Blood vessels in this membrane supply the brain with blood. Between the second and third layers of protection is a space called the *subarachnoid* ("below the arachnoid") space. It acts as a cushion for the brain and spinal cord.

The third way of protecting the brain and spinal cord is through cerebrospinal fluid. This clear liquid is formed from blood in the ventricles of the brain. This liquid cushions and protects the delicate brain tissue.

The fourth layer of protection is the blood-brain barrier, which keeps foreign, harmful substances out through its network of cells. The blood-brain barrier is not totally effective, however; for example, alcohol can pass through it, so the brain is not protected from the harmful effects of alcohol. Sometimes the blood-brain barrier keeps out foreign substances that would be helpful. For example, it can be difficult to administer medications for a brain infection, because the blood-brain barrier keeps out some kinds of antibiotics (depending on the antibiotic's chemical makeup).

■ PERIPHERAL NERVOUS SYSTEM

The **peripheral nervous system** is the part of the nervous system that is outside the central nervous system. Twelve pairs of **cranial** nerves and 31 pairs of spinal nerves make up this system (Figure 10-6).

The cranial nerves connect the brain directly with the sense organs (Figure 10-7): the eyes, ears, tongue, skin, and nose. The purpose of the cranial nerves is to carry sensory and motor function information. The cranial nerves are numbered with Roman numerals in the order in which the nerves leave the brain, from front to back. Except for the vagus nerve (X), the

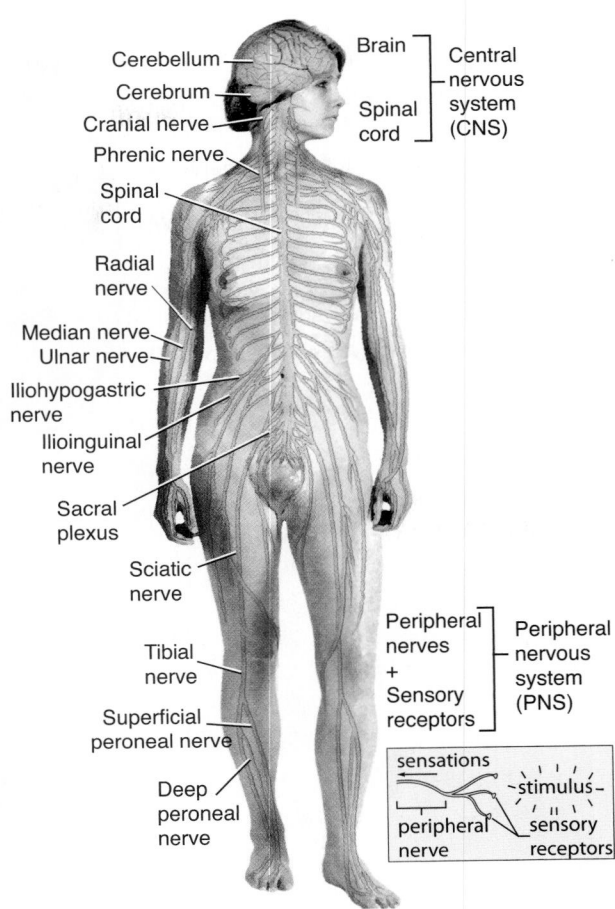

FIGURE 10-6 The peripheral nervous system.

cranial nerves "leave" the head and neck area, radiating into the rest of the body.

The 31 pairs of *spinal nerves* are numbered and named according to where they start in the spinal cord (Figure 10-8). There are 5 pairs of cervical nerves, 12 pairs of thoracic nerves, 5 pairs of lumbar nerves, 5 pairs of sacral nerves, and 1 pair of coccygeal nerves. These spinal nerves stimulate different and specific areas of the body.

Autonomic Nervous System

The **autonomic nervous system** is within the peripheral nervous system. It controls involuntary bodily functions. Motor nerves go to the smooth muscle and cardiac muscle. This is how the salivary glands, sweat glands, and adrenal medulla are stimulated. As a result, the autonomic nervous system affects a person's breathing, heart rate, and digestion.

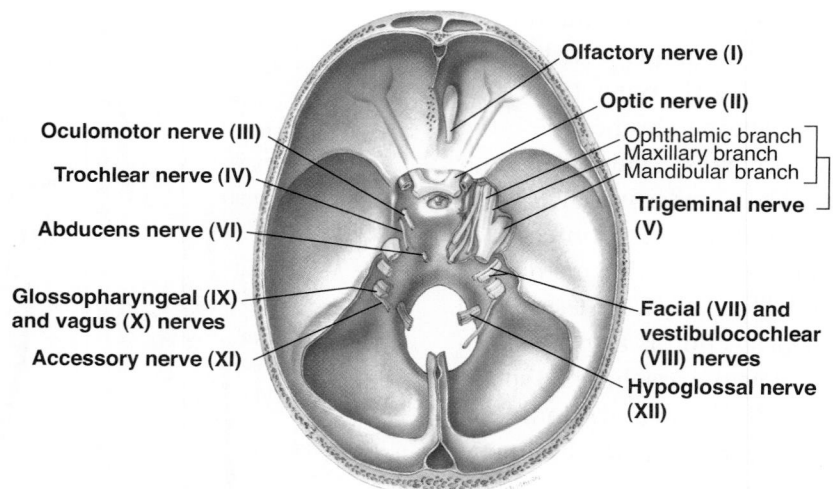

FIGURE 10-7 Cranial nerves.

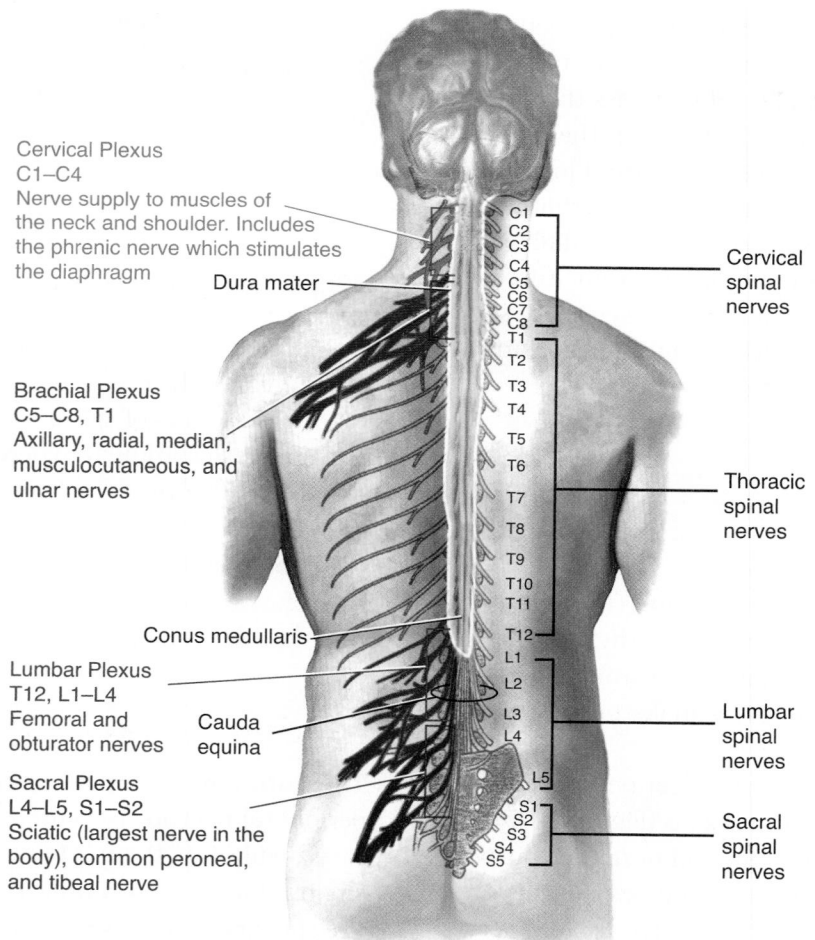

FIGURE 10-8 Spinal nerves.

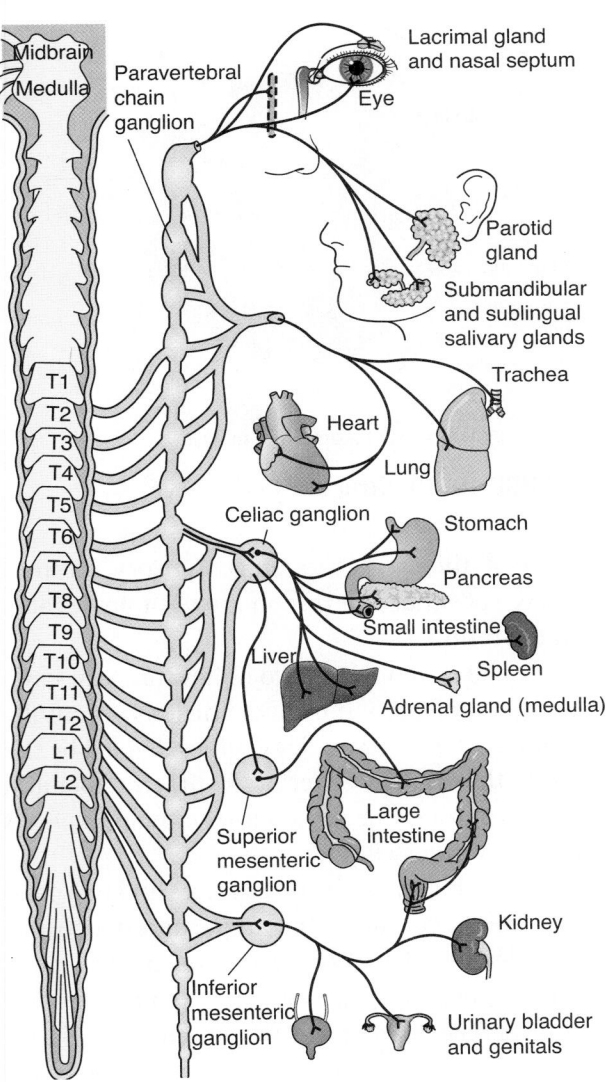

FIGURE 10–9A The sympathetic division of the autonomic nervous system.

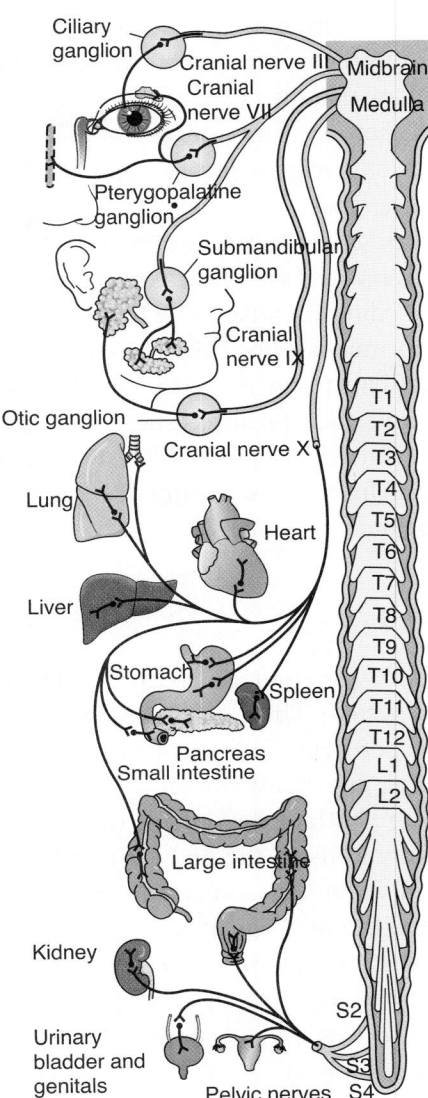

FIGURE 10–9B The parasympathetic division of the autonomic nervous system.

The autonomic nervous system is divided into the sympathetic and parasympathetic nervous systems (Figures 10-9A and 10-9B). The **sympathetic nervous system** springs into action during stressful situations. It is often called the "fight- or -flight" system. During times of stress, the actions of the sympathetic nervous system cause several responses in the body. The heart rate increases; the bronchioles in the lungs open up and become larger, and the blood vessels to the skeletal muscles open up or dilate. Vasoconstriction occurs in the skin. Sweat glands increase the production of sweat. Glycogen or stored energy is

changed to glucose and released for use in energy production. The pupils of the eyes become more open and the hair stands on end (gooseflesh). These responses all assist the person in fighting or running away from danger. Other bodily activities, such as digestion, which are relatively unimportant during the time of perceived danger, slow down.

These responses and activities are critical in times of crisis. Humans' survival often depended on their ability to run away from or fight off danger, and these reflexes are still an integral part of the human system. Sympathetic nervous system action still takes place today, even though the choices of running away or fighting are usually not available or appropriate. Trauma, severe illness, or even a near-miss car accident can trigger the sympathetic nervous system response.

During nonstressful times, the **parasympathetic nervous system** takes over, causing several bodily responses. The heart rate returns to the normal baseline rate. The diameter of the lungs returns to normal size. The skeletal muscles resume their prestress status. The pupils of the eyes constrict to normal size. Finally, gastric secretions increase to resume the regular pace of digestion.

■ SENSORY SYSTEM

The sensory system is closely related to the nervous system. Through the use of the senses, a person perceives and interacts with the world outside her own body. The senses allow a person to be aware both of the outside world and what is happening inside the body. When the senses receive a stimulus (something that causes a response), the message of perception is sent by way of the sensory nerves to the brain, where the information is interpreted. Through knowledge of the sensory system and the five special senses, the medical assistant will begin to recognize the close relationship between the senses and a client's well-being.

Sight

The organ of sight (vision) is the eye. Perception of light, color, shape, and differences between objects being viewed is made possible through coordination of the eye and the nervous system.

Three layers compose the eyeball (Figure 10-10). A tough outer layer of connective tissue called the *sclera* covers the eyeball. The sclera layer becomes clear or transparent where it passes over the front of the eyeball. This clear part is called the **cornea.** The middle layer of the eye is the *choroid.* This layer nourishes or feeds the eye through its blood vessels. The innermost

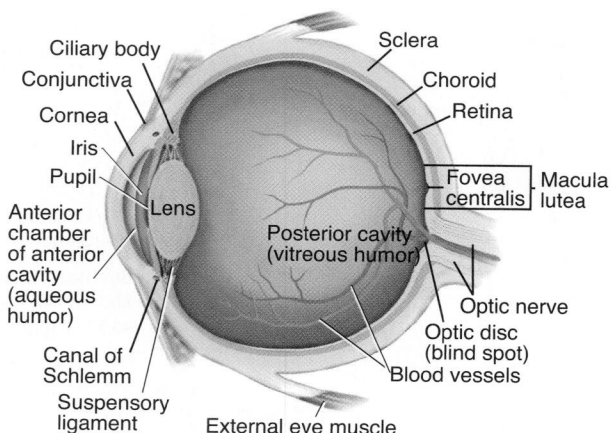

FIGURE 10–10 Structures of the eye.

layer of the eye is the *retina.* Sensory receptor nerve cells that can respond to light are located in the retina.

The eye contains two hollow areas or cavities. A small area in front of the lens is actually composed of two smaller cavities divided by the iris of the eye. The anterior (front) chamber and the posterior (back) chamber hold *aqueous humor,* a watery liquid.

In addition to the three layers and two cavities, the eye contains other important structures. The clear *lens* lies between the iris and the vitreous humor. The iris is an expandable and contractible membrane whose change in size controls the size of the pupil. A person's eye color, which is determined genetically, is the color of the iris. The pupil, which appears to be black, is actually an opening. The two eyelids are folds of skin that can cover the exposed area of the eye.

The eye is often compared to a camera. The front of the eye structure is the lens, and at the back of the eye is the retina, which acts as a screen. Light enters the eye and travels through the cornea, pupil, lens, and vitreous body until it is focused on the retina. Specialized cells in the retina then change the light into nerve impulses to the optic nerve, which sends these impulses to the brain. The optic nerve is a direct extension of the brain. The brain is critical to the sense of sight because it is the brain that receives the separate images from the eye and interprets them into a continuous visual experience. The brain first interprets visual sensations, and then

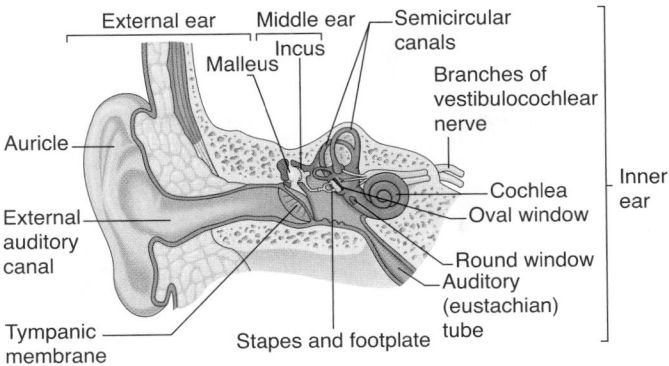

FIGURE 10–11   Structures of the ear.

stores, organizes, and compares them with other, previously stored visual experiences. Thus, people can "see" pictures in their minds even with the eyes closed.

Hearing

The organ of hearing is the ear (Figure 10-11). The ear has three main parts: the external ear, the middle ear, and the inner ear. The external ear consists of the auricle and external auditory canal. The outer ear—the part not contained inside the skull—is called the *auricle* or *pinna*. The external auditory canal is the passageway leading from the outside to the tympanic membrane (eardrum). The tympanic membrane separates the external ear from the middle ear. Cerumen (earwax) lubricates the auditory canal and protects the ear.

The area from the tympanic membrane to the internal ear is the middle ear. Within the middle ear space are three connected small bones: the malleus, incus, and stapes. The *malleus* looks like a hammer, the *incus* like an anvil, and the stapes like a *stirrup.* As sound waves traveling through the ear meet the tympanic membrane, these bones vibrate, further transmitting the motion of the sound waves. In addition to hearing, the middle ear helps in maintaining balance (equilibrium) by keeping the air pressure in the ear the same as the outside air pressure. The middle ear connects to the nasopharynx (nose and throat) through the eustachian tubes.

The inner ear contains the receptors for hearing, as well as receptors for equilibrium and

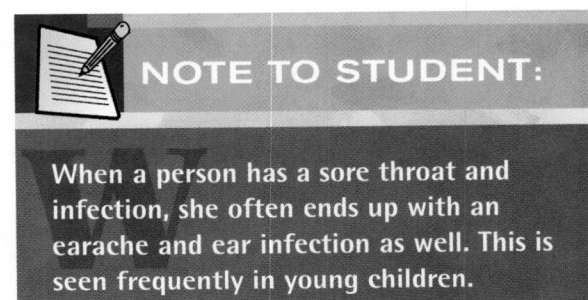

NOTE TO STUDENT:

When a person has a sore throat and infection, she often ends up with an earache and ear infection as well. This is seen frequently in young children.

balance. The snail-shaped *cochlea* contains the receptor for hearing, which is the *organ of Corti.* The sound waves go through the cochlear branch of the vestibulocochlear nerve (cranial nerve VIII) to the brain (Figure 10-12). The semicircular canal contains the receptors for equilibrium and balance. The vestibular branch of the vestibulocochlear nerve or VIII cranial nerve conducts the impulses to the cerebellum.

Taste and Smell

The organ of taste is the tongue. The sense of taste allows a person to perceive the sweet, sour, salty, and bitter qualities of substances taken into the mouth (Figure 10-13). The taste buds found on the tongue help to distinguish between these qualities. The facial nerve (cranial nerve VII) and the glossopharyngeal nerve (cranial nerve IX) carry the information from the taste buds to the brain. The taste bud cells constantly deteriorate, die, and are replaced.

The sense of taste is closely related to the sense of smell, and the sensation of taste is affected by a person's ability to smell. Sensory

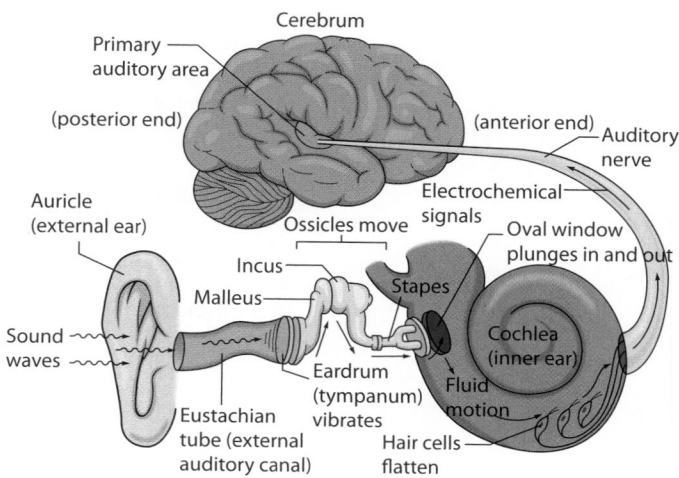

FIGURE 10-12 The pathway of hearing.

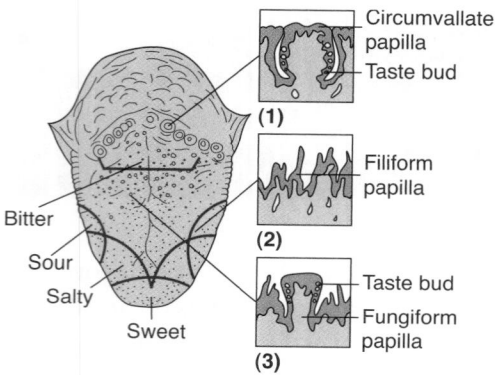

FIGURE 10-13 The tongue distinguishes between bitter, sour, salty, and sweet tastes.

cells in the nose react to odors inhaled through the nose and dissolved in the mucus of the nose. The message of perception then travels to the olfactory center in the brain. The olfactory center, which is the oldest part of the brain, is connected to the memory centers in the brain. Even very young babies are able to identify their mothers by smell.

Touch

The sense of touch can be called both a special sense and a general sense. The skin is the organ of the special sense of touch. The nervous system, working with the sensory system, makes it possible for a person to experience many different sensations as the skin receives stimuli from the environment. Hardness, softness, warmth, pricking, and pressure are all perceived in this way. However, the sense of touch is influenced by memory and past experiences.

The sense of touch also has a protective function. Pain alerts a person to contact that is harmful to the body.

BRIDGE TO CAAHEP

This chapter, which discusses the nervous and sensory systems, provides information and content related to CAAHEP standards for Anatomy and Physiology, Medical Terminology, Communication, Patient (Client) Care, and Professional Components.

ABHES LINKS

This chapter, which discusses the nervous and sensory systems, links to ABHES course content for Anatomy and Physiology, Medical Terminology, and Medical Office Clinical Procedures.

AAMA AREAS OF COMPETENCE

This chapter, which discusses the nervous and sensory systems, provides information or content within several areas listed in the Medical Assistant Role Delineation Study. These areas include: clinical, fundamental principles of

POINTS OF HIGHLIGHT

- The nervous system can be divided into the central nervous system and the peripheral nervous system.
- The brain and the spinal cord make up the central nervous system.
- Neurons and neuroglia are the two types of cells in the nervous system. Neurons are the functional or working unit and the neuroglia is the glue that holds the neurons in place.
- The cerebrum is the largest part of the brain. It is critical to enable a person to learn new skills, reason, and use judgment.
- The cerebellum controls and coordinates voluntary movements.
- The sensory system helps a person to be aware of his surroundings and to respond to that environment.
- The eye is often compared to a camera in its functioning.
- Interpretation by the brain allows a person to have a visual experience from the images seen by the eye.
- The ear functions to hear sounds and to maintain balance.
- Taste and smell are closely linked.
- Touch is both a special sense and a general sense.

diagnostic orders, patient (client) care, general transdisciplinary, communication, legal concepts, and instruction.

STUDENT PORTFOLIO ACTIVITY

Rehabilitation helps an individual return to the highest functioning possible for that individual. Rehabilitation is often needed when the nervous system is damaged or fails to work effectively. Find out what rehabilitation services are available in your community. Make a list of day and residential resources. Select a few and make an appointment to visit and observe. The medical assistant's knowledge of related community services is beneficial to clients who may develop a need for these services. Be prepared to share your knowledge and interests with prospective employers.

 ## AMT PATHS

This chapter, which discusses the nervous and sensory systems, provides a path to AMT competency in general medical assisting knowledge, anatomy and physiology, medical terminology, and patient (client) education.

APPLYING YOUR SKILLS

You are preparing a client for a procedure. You observe that the client is perspiring, breathing fast, talking quickly, and in general appears jittery. What part of the client's nervous system is responsible for what you are observing? How could this affect client care? What can you as a medical assistant do?

CRITICAL THINKING QUESTIONS

1. A client comes to the office complaining that she cannot taste food anymore. Why does the doctor question and test for the sense of smell?

2. If an injury occurred to a client's cerebellum, what activities would the client have difficulty performing?

3. What other health professionals might be able to help the client who has an injury to the cerebrum?

4. A client becomes very afraid and nervous about all medical procedures. As a medical assistant, you need to obtain her vital signs and prepare her for a procedure. How might her vitals signs be affected? What would cause this to happen?

5. How is the sense of sight related to the brain?

6. How do the three small bones in the middle ear (the malleus, incus, and stapes) aid in the process of hearing?

7. What part of the brain controls the vital processes of breathing, heart rate, and blood pressure? What happens if a person holds her breath? Can she die from holding her breath?

8. What would you say to a client who states that she cannot get rid of all her earwax? As a medical assistant, what should you explain about the purpose of earwax (cerumen)?

9. Touch is more than a physical sensation. What role does the brain play in a person's experience of touch?

10. Describe a situation in which the spinal cord, acting as a major reflex center, protects a person from injury.

11. Go back to the beginning of this chapter and review the Anticipatory Statements. Reread each statement and then indicate whether it is true or false. If the statement is false, rewrite it to make it a true statement.

CLIENT TEACHING PLAN

Instillation of Eye Ointment

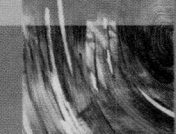

▣ What Is to Be Taught:

- Instillation of eye ointment.

▣ Objectives:

- Client will instill eye ointment into affected eye as directed.

▣ Preparation Before Teaching:

- Review any medication precautions for the eye ointment prescribed.
- Get a sample eye ointment tube to use for teaching and paper and pen for written instructions.

▣ Steps for the Medical Assistant:

1. Introduce yourself to the client.
2. Explain what you are going to teach and why.
3. Demonstrate proper handwashing technique.
4. Ask the client to wash her hands in the same way.
5. Show the client how to remove the cap from the ointment tube. Lay the cap on a clean area or ask the client to hold it in her hand to avoid contamination.
6. Ask the client to look up.
7. Tell the client to gently pull down on the lower lid of the eye in which the ointment will be instilled (put in).
8. Instruct the client to line up the tip of the ointment tube by the inner canthus of the eye (the part nearest the nose).
9. Guide the client to gently squeeze the tube and direct the ointment into the lower lid from the inner canthus of the eye part to the outer canthus (the part farthest away from the nose). Never let the tip of the tube touch the eye.
10. When the client reaches the outside edge of the eyelid, instruct the client to twist her wrist to break off the string of ointment.
11. Have the client replace the cap on the ointment tube.
12. Ask the client to close the medicated eye gently to allow absorption of the medicine.

13. Remind the client that her vision might be blurry for a few minutes until the medication is completely absorbed.

▣ Special Needs of the Client:

- Look at the client's chart to see if there is any factor that might interfere with the client's ability to instill ointment into her own eye.
- Ask the client, before and after, if there is anything you need to know that might affect the client's performance of the procedure as directed.

▣ Evaluation:

- Client will be able to state the steps of the procedure and the precautions necessary to avoid contamination.
- Client will be able to instill the eye ointment (with the help of the medical assistant if necessary).

▣ Further Plans/Teaching:

- Write the instillation instructions on paper and give the paper to the client for use at home.
- Give the client the office number and your extension and instruct her to call if she has any questions or concerns.

▣ Follow-up:

- Call the client at home the next day and ask if she had any problems instilling the eye ointment.

Medical Assistant

Name: _____

Signature: _____

Date: _____

Client

Date: _____

Follow-up Date : _____

Anticipatory Statements

People have various levels of understanding about the endocrine system. Some of their ideas are accurate, some are not. Read and think about the following statements based upon what you believe now. Decide whether you agree or disagree. Write the word **agree** after the statement if you think the statement is true. Write the word **disagree** after the statement if you think the statement is false. Read the chapter to find out if your current beliefs can be supported.

1. Sweat is produced by a person's skin.   _____

2. A person's rate of metabolism is supported by the thyroid gland.   _____

3. Hormones are responsible for the secondary sex characteristics in males and females.   _____

4. Hormones have no effect on a person's blood pressure.   _____

5. Humans are the only animals that secrete tears in response to emotion.   _____

Endocrine System

Learning Objectives

Upon completion of this chapter, the medical assistant student should be able to:

- Explain the functions of the endocrine system
- Compare the endocrine and exocrine glands
- Describe how the pituitary gland and the hypothalamus work together
- Name two major glands
- Explain how each major gland acts on the body system

Key Terms

adrenal cortex Outer part of the adrenal gland; these glands are found above the kidneys.

adrenal medulla Inner part of the adrenal gland; these glands are located above the kidneys.

endocrine glands Ductless glands that secrete hormones directly into the bloodstream.

exocrine glands Glands that secrete hormones into ducts, which then open onto a body surface.

gonad Reproduction or sex organ (testes in the male, ovaries in the female).

hormone Chemical released by endocrine glands.

hypothalamus Part of the diencephalon of the brain; part of the nervous system that regulates the pituitary gland.

insulin Hormone released by the pancreas; involved in carbohydrate metabolism.

islets of Langerhans Cells in the pancreas that secrete glucagons and insulin.

lacrimal gland Gland that makes tears; located in the eye.

pancreas Organ that has both endocrine and exocrine functions.

parathyroid One of four glands that secrete hormones to regulate levels of calcium in the blood.

pineal gland Small gland in the brain that secretes melatonin.

pituitary gland Small gland in the brain that has an anterior (front) and posterior (back) area; involved in many bodily functions.

progesterone Hormone released by the ovaries.

testosterone Hormone released by the testes.

thymus gland Gland found in the chest area.

thyroid Gland found in the front part of the neck; plays a major role in metabolism.

■ INTRODUCTION

Body functions are affected by the release of hormones from many glands in the body. These various glands, taken together, and the hormones they secrete are collectively called the *endocrine system*. Glands can have an endocrine function, an exocrine function, or both. **Endocrine glands** secrete **hormones** directly into the bloodstream. These hormones then travel through the bloodstream to various parts of the body. When a hormone reaches its target area, that body area or tissue then increases or decreases its own activity or stimulates or inhibits the release of additional hormones. Secretion of hormones, and the specific responses of the targeted tissues directed by the hormones, is the function of the endocrine system. In contrast, **exocrine glands** release hormones to an epithelial surface, either directly or by means of a duct or channel (Figure 11-1).

■ MAJOR ENDOCRINE GLANDS

There are many endocrine glands scattered throughout the body (Figure 11-2). One way to study them is by location—that is, by where they are found in the body. A logical way to organize a study of the glands is to start at the head and go down through the body.

Pineal Gland

The **pineal gland,** found in the brain, looks like a pinecone that is approximately 5 to 8 millimeters long and 3 to 5 millimeters wide. The pineal gland produces melatonin, which affects the sleep-wake cycle and body rhythms (circadian). Melatonin can soothe or calm a person.

Pituitary Gland

The **pituitary gland** is found the near the **hypothalamus** of the brain (Figure 11-3). It is a

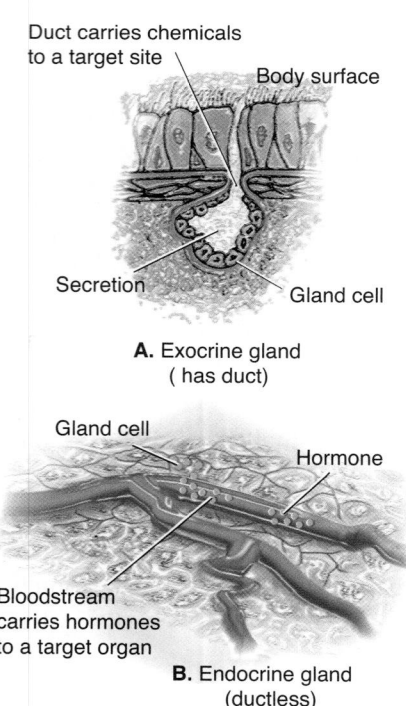

FIGURE 11-1 (a) Exocrine gland (B) Endocrine gland.

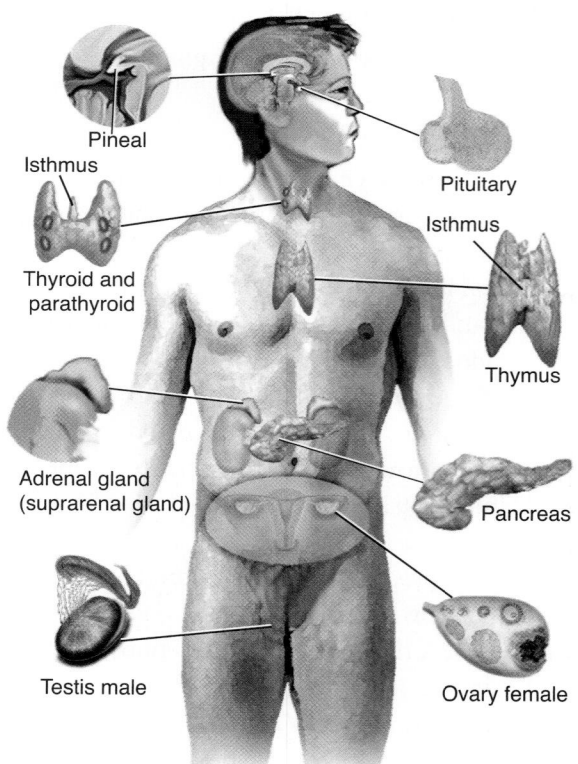

FIGURE 11-2 The endocrine system.

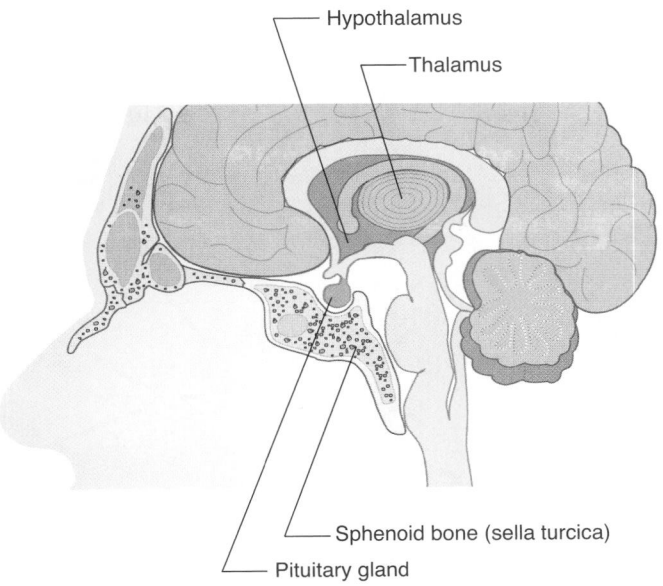

FIGURE 11-3 Position of the pituitary gland in relation to the brain.

major endocrine gland whose functioning affects many parts of the body. Because of its wide-reaching effects on so many different systems, it used to be called the "master gland." However, research has shown that the hypothalamus of the brain actually controls the pituitary gland. The pituitary releases hormones from both its anterior (front) portion and its posterior (back or behind) portion.

The anterior portion of the pituitary gland has six functions. First, it releases growth hormone (somatotropic hormone), which regulates the processes responsible for growth. Second, it secretes adrenocorticotropic hormone (ACTH), which controls the activities of a part of another gland—the **adrenal cortex.** Third, the pituitary releases thyrotropin (also called thyroid-stimulating hormone or TSH), which signals the thyroid gland. Fourth, it releases certain gonadotropic hormones (Figure 11-4), which act on the female ovaries or the male testes. Fifth, in males, follicle-stimulating hormone (FSH) from the pituitary gland sets in motion spermatogenesis (creation of functioning spermatozoa). In females, FSH stimulates the follicles of the ovaries and production of estrogen. Sixth, in males, luteinizing hormone (LH) and interstitial

cell-stimulation hormone (ICSH) secreted by the pituitary increase the production of testosterone. In females, LH and FSH stimulate ovulation (ripening and discharge of an egg from the ovary) and the release of estrogen and **progesterone.** Also, in adult females, the pituitary hormone prolactin triggers the release of milk from the mammary glands.

The posterior portion of the pituitary gland releases two important hormones. Antidiuretic hormone (ADH) increases blood pressure by constricting blood vessels. It stimulates the kidneys to reabsorb water. The posterior part of the pituitary also releases oxytocin, which acts on the uterus and mammary glands. During childbirth, the uterus contracts, and stays that way after delivery of the baby to keep the mother from bleeding excessively. Shortly after delivery, the new mother's breasts will release milk in response to the action of oxytocin.

Thyroid Gland and Parathyroid Gland

The **thyroid** gland is found in the neck. It is in front of and partially circles around the thyroid

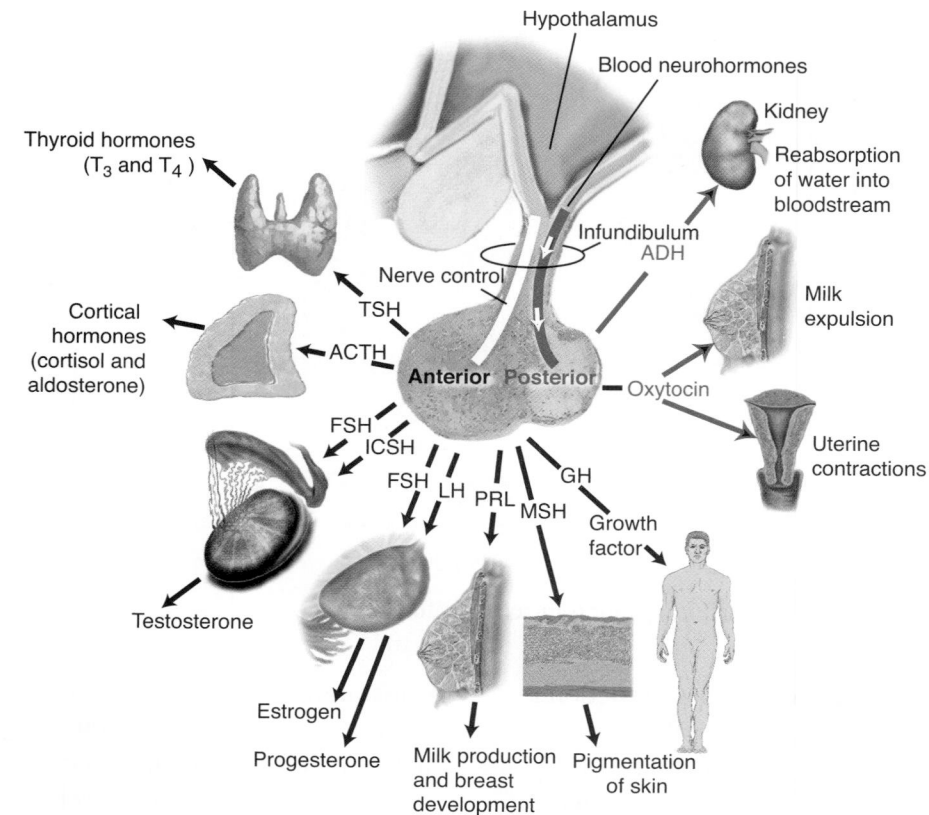

FIGURE 11-4 Hormonal secretions of the pituitary gland.

cartilage and upper circles of the trachea (commonly referred to as the *windpipe*) (Figure 11-5). This gland sends out thyroid hormones T3 and T4. These hormones support the metabolic rate and control growth and development of the body, and are important for the correct working of the central nervous system.

The **parathyroid gland** is actually four or more small glands close to the thyroid gland.

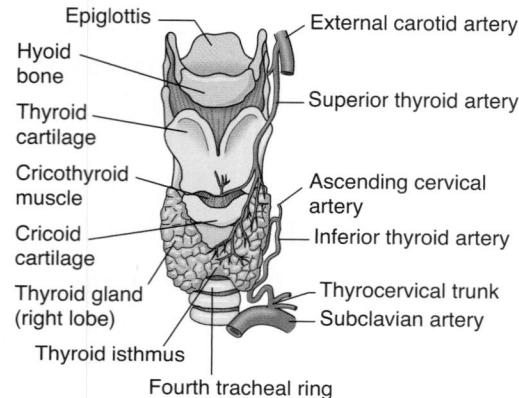

FIGURE 11-5 Thyroid gland.

The parathyroid gland secretes parathyroid hormone, which affects metabolism of calcium and phosphorus.

Thymus Gland

The **thymus gland** is found in front of and above the heart. It has many lobes, each of which consists of an outer part or *cortex* and an inner part or *medulla*. The thymus grows until the person reaches puberty (adolescence). At that point the thymus begins to shrink. The decrease in size is most likely related to the work of the thymus: The purpose of the hormone from this gland is to stimulate maturation of the T-lymphocytes necessary for immune system responses.

Adrenal Glands

The adrenal glands are located on the superior (top) surface of each kidney (Figure 11-6). Because of this positioning, the adrenal glands

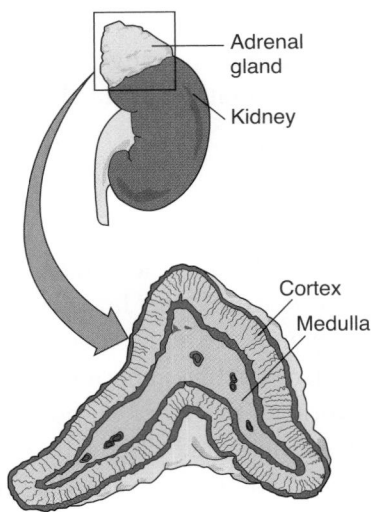

FIGURE 11-6 Adrenal or suprarenal glands.

are sometimes referred to as the *suprarenals* (*super* meaning "top" and *renal* meaning "kidney"). The adrenals also have a medulla and a cortex.

Hormones from the Adrenal Medulla. The medulla releases the hormones epinephrine and norepinephrine. When the sympathetic nervous system is stimulated, the **adrenal medulla** responds by releasing mostly epinephrine. The effects of this hormone mirror the effects of the sympathetic nervous system (see Chapter 10), creating the "fight-or-flight" response. When a person is in a stressful situation, epinephrine helps the person to become a survivor, which was necessary in ancient times on a daily basis. It is referred to as the fight-or-flight response. Epinephrine helps to keep the airways open, increase the heart rate, and dilate pupils to see the danger. Blood pressure increases to maintain blood circulation to all vital areas during the perceived danger or emergency. The vessels to the skeletal muscles are dilated to enhance the ability to run. The blood glucose levels rise to give needed energy.

This primitive response may occur frequently or for a prolonged time in situations in which neither fight nor flight is appropriate or possible. For example, a person who works under very stressful conditions, and is always under pressure to complete tasks quickly (hospitals,

emergency room workers), or must always be on the alert for danger (police, security officers, military personnel), may respond with a near-continuous epinephrine release. Constant high production and blood levels of these hormones can be unhealthy, so individuals who are often subjected to stressful situations need to learn ways to decrease stress, increase relaxation, or otherwise manage their bodily responses.

Hormones from the Adrenal Cortex. The outside part of the adrenal glands, the cortex, releases several hormones. These include glucocorticoids, mineralocorticoids, and sex hormones.

Glucocorticoids help to organize carbohydrate metabolism and, to a lesser degree, protein and fat metabolism. Blood glucose levels increase in response to release of this group of hormones, especially during times of stress. *Mineralocorticoids* act directly on the kidneys, stimulating the kidneys to keep sodium and get rid of potassium. The body's fluid (water) levels and electrolytes are kept in balance by the mineralocorticoid hormones.

The *sex hormones* include androgens, estrogens, and progestins. These are important in reproduction. Also, secondary sex characteristics in both males and females develop in response to these hormones. Together, the hormones secreted by the adrenal glands affect almost every system in the body.

Pancreas

The **pancreas** is found in the upper part of the abdominal cavity, lying in front of the first and second lumbar vertebrae and behind the stomach. This gland has both endocrine and exocrine functions.

The exocrine function of the pancreas aids in the digestion of food, through the release of digestive enzymes. These secretions travel to the small intestine where most digestion takes place.

Hormone-secreting cells called the **islets of Langerhans** perform the endocrine functions of the pancreas. The islets of Langerhans contain two kinds of cells, alpha and beta. The alpha cells send out glucagons and the beta cells send

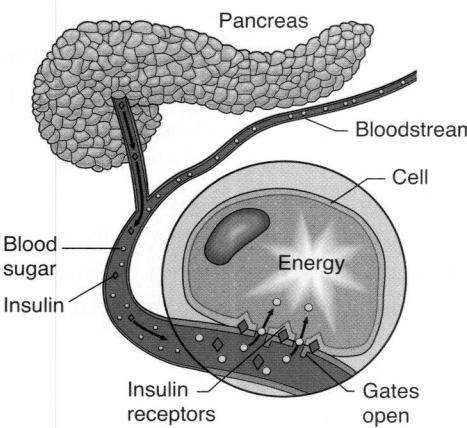

Pancreas

Bloodstream

Cell

Blood sugar

Energy

Insulin

Insulin receptors

Gates open

FIGURE 11-7 Insulin lowers blood glucose levels.

out **insulin.** The purpose of glucagons is to raise blood glucose levels. Insulin lowers blood glucose through the regulation of carbohydrate, fat, and protein metabolism (Figure 11-7). Both the alpha and beta cells target the liver, muscles, and adipose tissue.

Gonads

The **gonads,** or reproductive organs (in both the male and the female), release hormones that affect the reproductive system. In the male, the gonads are the *testes.* The testes, which are found in the scrotum, produce **testosterone.** This in turn acts on the skin, muscles, and sex organs of the male. Sperm and male sex characteristics develop because of the action of testosterone. In the female, the gonad is the *ovary.* The two ovaries are found in the pelvic cavity, attached to the uterus by ligaments close to the fallopian tubes. The ovaries produce estrogen and progesterone, which in turn act on the skin, bones, muscles, and sex organs of the female. Ova (eggs) and female sex characteristics develop because of the action of estrogen and progesterone.

■ MAJOR EXOCRINE GLANDS

Major exocrine glands are the sweat glands, tear glands, mammary glands, and salivary glands. Substances released from the exocrine glands go through ducts and are deposited directly into external or internal coverings. Generally, exocrine glands have either protective or specific functions.

Sweat Glands

The sweat glands or *sudoriferous glands* are found in the dermis (true layer of the skin). Some sweat glands are active throughout a person's life. Others, such as apocrine sweat glands, begin to work at the start of puberty. These glands are also activated when a person experiences extreme emotions. Sweating cools the body and helps regulate body temperature.

Lacrimal Glands

The **lacrimal glands** or *tear glands* are found at the outer edges of the eyes. The purpose of the lacrimal gland is to secrete the tears that lubricate and protect the eyes from infection and foreign bodies. When the eye comes into contact with any substance that irritates it, the lacrimal gland increases the amount of tears it produces. Humans are the only animals that secrete tears in response to emotion.

Mammary Glands

The mammary glands are found in the breasts. The ducts from the mammary glands open up into the nipple, thus stimulating the release of milk during lactation.

Salivary Glands

The salivary glands are located in and around the mouth. Pairs of *sublingual* (below the tongue), *submandibular* (below the lower jaw), and *parotid* (cheek) glands comprise the salivary glands. These glands all release their secretions into the mouth. Nervous system reflexes control the action of these glands: A stimulus sends a message to the nervous system, which in turn stimulates the salivary glands to begin secretion. This can also happen as a result of a conditioned reflex, such as when a person thinks about some delicious food.

NOTE TO STUDENT:

The endocrine system is a clear example of how the body components work together as a team to maintain a balance. If one part of the team (glands) secretes too little of a hormone, the other parts of the team (other glands) produce more to maintain proper body functioning. How well the entire team (endocrine system) works directly affects the functioning of the other body systems.

■ ADDITIONAL HORMONE-RELEASING BODY AREAS

During pregnancy, the placenta, which supplies nourishment and oxygen to the fetus, acts as an endocrine gland. The placenta releases hormones that help maintain the pregnancy and aid in supplying nourishment to the growing and developing baby.

During digestion of food, some parts of the digestive system secrete hormones. Gastrin from the stomach walls stimulates the gastric glands to secrete gastric juices.

Pancreozymin and secretions from the small intestine stimulate the pancreas to secrete pancreatic juices. Cholecystokinin from the small intestine causes the gallbladder to contract and release bile.

The hormone renin, which helps to maintain blood pressure, is produced within the kidney. An adult kidney also produces erythropoietin, which increases red cell production. In a child, this process takes place in the liver.

The heart also produces a hormone that helps to control blood pressure, thus easing pressure on the heart.

BRIDGE TO CAAHEP

This chapter, which discusses the endocrine system, provides information and content related to CAAHEP standards for Anatomy and Physiology, Medical Terminology, Communication, Medical Assisting Clinical Procedures, and Professional Components.

ABHES LINKS

This chapter, which discusses the endocrine system, links to ABHES course content for medical terminology, medical law and ethics, psychology of human relations, and medical office clinical procedures.

AAMA AREAS OF COMPETENCE

This chapter, which discusses the endocrine system, provides information or content within several areas listed in the Medical Assistant Role Delineation Study. These areas include: clinical, patient (client) care, general professionalism, communication, legal concepts, and instruction.

AMT PATHS

This chapter, which discusses the endocrine system, provides a path to AMT competency in general medical assisting knowledge, anatomy and physiology, medical terminology, medical ethics, human relations, and patient (client) education.

POINTS OF HIGHLIGHT

- The endocrine system affects many bodily functions through the secretion of hormones from its component glands.
- Endocrine glands secrete hormones directly into the bloodstream; exocrine glands secrete hormones to a surface either directly or through a duct or channel.
- The sleep-wake cycle is affected by the pineal gland, which is located in the brain.
- The pituitary gland has an anterior and a posterior part, both of which have many important functions.
- Through secretion of various hormones, the anterior part of the pituitary helps to regulate growth, control the adrenal cortex, regulate the thyroid, release hormones that affect the reproductive system, and stimulate the release of milk from the mammary glands.
- The posterior part of the pituitary releases antidiuretic hormone, which raises the blood pressure, and oxytocin, which acts on the uterus and mammary glands.
- The thyroid gland affects the metabolic rate and growth and development of the body.
- The parathyroid glands, found close to the thyroid, affect calcium and phosphorus metabolism.
- The purpose of the thymus is to mature T-lymphocytes, which are necessary for the immune system response.
- On the top surface of each kidney lies an adrenal gland.
- The medulla or inner part of the adrenal gland is closely related to the working of the sympathetic nervous system.
- The cortex or outer part of the adrenal gland releases glucocorticoids, mineralocorticoids, and sex hormones.
- The pancreas functions as both an endocrine and an exocrine gland.
- The male gonads, the testes, release testosterone.
- The female gonads, the ovaries, release estrogen and progesterone.
- The major exocrine glands are the sweat glands, tear glands, mammary glands, and salivary glands.

STUDENT PORTFOLIO ACTIVITY

Time management is an important issue for employers in health care settings. Your classes are helping you develop that skill. Learning anatomy and physiology involves not only attending classes, but also finding the time to study, complete assignments for other courses, and attend to family and work responsibilities. Using a calendar, plan a weekly or monthly schedule for your activities. Make sure to include classes, laboratory sessions, clinicals, study time, and other activities. Follow the schedule, but make changes as needed. What competencies does this organizational activity illustrate to employers?

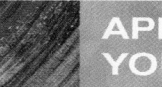

APPLYING YOUR SKILLS

The doctor has prescribed eyedrops for a client with a condition commonly known as dry eye. The client complains of dry, itchy eyes and a gritty feeling in the eyes. What can you tell this client about the function of the lacrimal glands? Why is tear production important?

CRITICAL THINKING QUESTIONS

1. Where is the pituitary gland found in the body? How is it related to the hypothalamus of the brain?

2. What is the difference between an endocrine gland and an exocrine gland? Are they the same in any way?

3. Can an endocrine gland also be an exocrine gland? If so, give an example and explain how a gland can function as both.

4. A person is involved in a car accident. How do the adrenal glands help that person survive in this situation?

5. Explain how the functioning of the endocrine system affects the different body systems.

6. How can the sudoriferous glands affect a client's body temperature?

7. In what ways do the lacrimal glands protect the eyes?

8. What hormone helps to raise the blood pressure? What organ secretes this hormone?

9. If the pancreas does not secrete enough insulin, what effect will this have on the client's metabolism?

10. A client feels that the cause of her obesity is her "thyroid." As a medical assistant, what would you explain about the relationship between the thyroid and a person's weight?

11. Go back to the beginning of this chapter and review the Anticipatory Statements. Reread each statement and then indicate whether it is true or false. If the statement is false, rewrite it to make it a true statement.

CLIENT TEACHING PLAN

Self-Examination of Neck

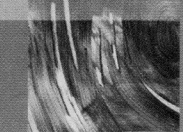

■ **What Is to Be Taught:**

- How to check the neck to feel for the thyroid gland.

■ **Objectives:**

- Client will be able to check her neck for anything unusual in the thyroid area.

■ **Preparation Before Teaching:**

- Review information about the thyroid gland and some common disorders of this gland: nodules, enlargements, cancer, and so on. Make sure to put technical medical terms into everyday language that the client will understand.
- Gather supplies: a glass of water, a handheld mirror, pen and paper.

■ **Steps for the Medical Assistant:**

1. Wash your hands.
2. Introduce yourself to the client.
3. Explain what you are going to teach and why.
4. Tell the client that by performing a few quick steps, she can take an active part in caring for her own health.
5. Demonstrate on yourself the steps for performing a thyroid neck check.
6. Focus a handheld mirror on the area just below the Adam's apple on the neck and above the clavicle or collarbone.
7. Tip your head back while continuing to look into the mirror.
8. Take the glass of water and swallow a mouthful while continuing to look into the mirror.
9. While swallowing, see if the neck bulges or sticks out in any particular spot.
10. Repeat the preceding step if necessary.
11. Give the mirror to the client and ask her to focus the mirror on the thyroid area, below the

Adam's apple and above the clavicle or collarbone.
12. Hand the client a glass of water.
13. Tell the client to tip her head back and swallow a mouthful of water.
14. Remind the client to continue to look at the thyroid area of the neck while she is swallowing, and note if the thyroid area bulges out.
15. Tell the client to repeat the swallowing step if necessary.
16. Instruct the client that if she notices any bulges or prominences in the area, she should call the doctor for an appointment.
17. Give written instructions to the client to use as a reference at home.

■ **Special Needs of the Client:**

- Check the client's chart for any factors that might interfere with the client's ability to perform a thyroid check.
- Ask the client, before and after, if there is anything you should know that might affect her ability to perform this activity.

■ **Evaluation:**

- Client is able to state the purpose of the thyroid check.
- Client is able to demonstrate the steps of the thyroid check, in the correct order, after observing you.

■ **Further Plans/Teaching:**

- Ask the client if she has any questions or needs any additional information.

■ **Follow-up:**

- At the next office visit, review the examination steps with the client.
- Ask the client to demonstrate the steps.

(Continues)

CLIENT TEACHING PLAN (Continued)

Medical Assistant

Name: _____

Signature: _____

Date: _____

Client

Date: _____

Follow-up Date : _____

Anticipatory Statements

People have different ideas about the working of the heart and what makes a healthy heart. Read and think about the following statements based upon what you believe now. Decide whether you agree or disagree. Write the word **agree** after the statement if you think the statement is true. Write the word **disagree** after the statement if you think the statement is false. Read the chapter to find out if your current beliefs can be supported.

1. A person's heart is in the right side of the chest cavity.

   _____

2. Heart valves act like faucets guiding the flow of blood through the heart.

   _____

3. The pulmonary arteries carry oxygen-rich blood.

   _____

4. The heart has an electrical signal that starts and then coordinates the heartbeat.

   _____

5. The bicuspid valve in the heart has three cusps or flaps.

   _____

Cardiovascular System

Learning Objectives

Upon completion of this chapter, the medical assistant student should be able to:

- Find the chambers of the heart and its major vessels on an anatomical model
- List the layers of the heart
- Trace the pathway of blood through the heart
- Trace the pathway of an electrical impulse through the conduction system of the heart
- Explain the functions of the cardiovascular system
- Describe the purpose of the coronary blood vessels
- Describe the parts of the systemic blood vessels

Key Terms

aorta The largest artery in the body.

arteries Thick-walled blood vessels that carry blood away from the heart.

bicuspid valve Valve found between the left atrium and the left ventricle of the heart.

capillary The smallest type of blood vessel.

coronary Relating to the heart.

endocardium Inner layer of the heart.

epicardium Outermost layer of the heart.

mitral valve Also called the bicuspid valve.

myocardium Middle layer of the heart.

pulmonary valve Valve found between the right ventricle and the pulmonary artery.

Purkinje fibers Heart fibers found in the walls of the ventricles of the heart.

semilunar valves Two valves found at the point where the blood leaves the ventricles.

tricuspid valve Valve found between the right atrium and the right ventricle; has three flaps.

■ INTRODUCTION

The heart and the blood vessels that lead to and from the heart make up the cardiovascular system. The heart acts as a muscular pump that sends blood through the vessels. The blood vessels are long, round tubes that carry the blood. The arteries, capillaries, and veins are all types of blood vessels. The **arteries** are stretchy tubes that carry oxygen-rich blood from the heart to the body. (The only exception is the pulmonary artery.) The veins carry deoxygenated blood to the heart. (The only exception is the pulmonary veins.) The **capillaries** are very small vessels. Because the blood moves through them slowly, the nutrients carried in the blood have a chance to pass through the capillary walls to reach other cells.

If the heart is strong and in good working order, and the blood vessels are open and elastic, the cardiovascular system will keep the other body systems sufficiently supplied with essential nutrients and oxygen. An understanding of what the cardiovascular system is and what it does is important to the medical assistant's work with clients. Clients can make choices to keep their hearts healthy. The medical assistant often works with the client in making these decisions, so knowledge in this area is essential.

■ HEART

The heart is found in the middle of the chest cavity, a little to the left (Figure 12-1). It is protected by the breastbone or sternum. The heart is a hollow, muscular organ that acts as a pump for the cardiovascular system, to keep blood circulating throughout the body. The wall of the heart has three layers (Figure 12-2). The outside layer is the **epicardium** (*epi* means "covering"). The middle layer of cardiac muscle is the **myocardium** (*myo* means "muscle"). The innermost layer of the heart is the **endocardium** (*endo* means "within"). This endocardium not only lines the heart, but also covers the valves.

Chambers

The heart has four chambers or compartments. There are two upper chambers, the right atrium and the left atrium. The two lower chambers are

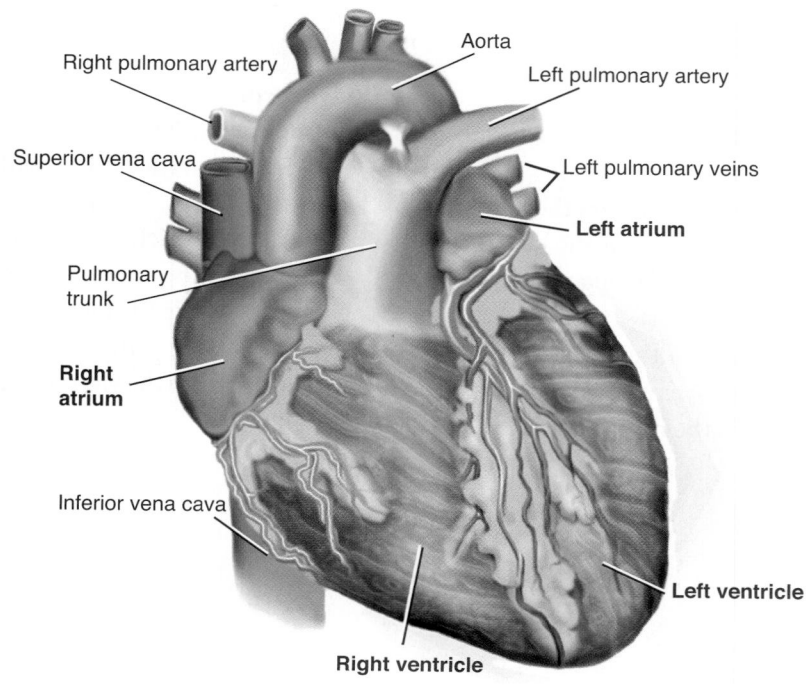

FIGURE 12-1 The heart and valves.

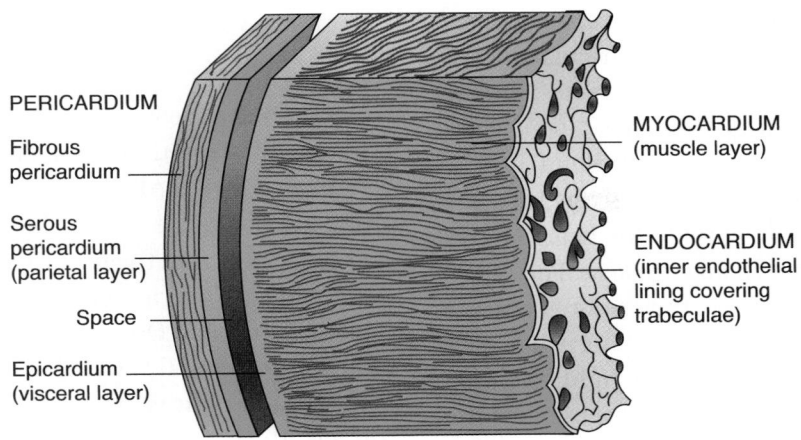

FIGURE 12-2 Layers of pericardial sac and layers of the walls of the heart.

the right ventricle and the left ventricle. The thin-walled atria receive blood. The ventricles, which pump blood out of the heart, are of necessity thick-walled. Within the heart itself are four major valves, which act like faucets to control the direction of blood flow. When working properly, the valves close periodically to keep the blood flowing in one direction only (Figure 12-3). Large blood vessels attached to the atria and ventricles carry blood to and from the heart.

Valves

The heart valves control the flow of blood in the heart. They allow the blood to flow in one direction only. The atrioventricular valves, which are normally just called the AV valves, are found between the atria and the ventricles, as the name suggests. The AV valves keep the blood flowing from the atria to the ventricles and prevent it from flowing backward into the atria.

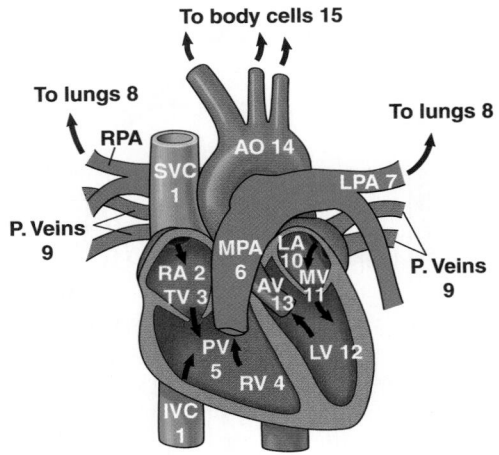

AO — Aorta
AV — Aortic valve
IVC — Inferior vena cava
LA — Left atrium
LPA — Left pulmonary artery
LV — Left ventricle
MPA — Main pulmonary artery
MV — Mitral valve
PV — Pulmonary valve
P.VEINS — Pulmonary veins
RA — Right atrium
RPA — Right pulmonary artery
RV — Right ventricle
SVC — Superior vena cava
TV — Tricuspid valve

1. Blood reaches heart through superior vena cava (SVC) and interior vena cava (IVC)
2. To right atrium
3. To tricuspid valve
4. To right ventricle
5. To pulmonary valve (semilunar)
6. To main pulmonary artery
7. To left pulmonary artery and right pulmonary artery
8. To lungs—blood receives O_2
9. From lungs to pulmonary veins
10. To left atrium
11. To mitral (bicuspid) valve
12. To left ventricle
13. To aortic valve (semilunar veins)
14. To aorta (largest artery in the body)
15. Blood with oxygen then goes to all cells of the body

FIGURE 12-3 The workings of the heart.

The AV valves can be further distinguished as right and left. The right atrioventricular valve is called the **tricuspid valve.** The name *tricuspid* describes the structure of the valve, which has three cusps or flaps that aid in controlling the flow of blood in the heart. The edges of the tricuspid valve are connected to parts of the heart muscle by special fibers called *chordae tendinae.* The tricuspid valve closes when the right ventricle contracts, so that the heart's pumping action does not force blood backward into the right atrium.

The left atrioventricular valve is called the **bicuspid valve.** The name *bicuspid* describes the structure of this valve, which has two cusps or flaps that aid in controlling the flow of blood in the heart. The bicuspid valve closes when the left ventricle contracts, so that the force of the heart's pumping action does not push blood backward into the left atrium. The bicuspid valve is also called the **mitral valve** because it looks like a mitre (a hat worn by a bishop). The two names are used interchangeably.

The **semilunar valves** guide the flow of blood as it leaves the ventricles. The prefix *semi* means "half" and the word *lunar* refers to "moon." The flaps of these valves look like half-moons. The right semilunar valve is found between the right ventricle and the pulmonary artery. This valve is more frequently called the **pulmonary valve** because of its location at the pulmonary artery. The pulmonary valve closes when the right ventricle relaxes, so that blood will not flow backward from the pulmonary artery into the right ventricle. The left semilunar valve, also called the *aortic valve,* is found between the left ventricle and the **aorta.**

■ PATHWAY OF BLOOD THROUGH THE HEART

Blood that is deoxygenated (lacking oxygen or having decreased oxygen content) enters the right atrium of the heart by means of the superior and inferior venae cavae. The superior vena cava drains blood from the upper part of the body and the inferior vena cava drains blood from the lower part of the body. Once the blood enters the right atrium, it travels through the tricuspid valve on its way to the right ventricle. When the heart contracts, the blood travels through the pulmonary valve to the pulmonary artery and lungs. After the blood has exchanged gases (taking in oxygen and shedding carbon dioxide), the newly oxygenated blood travels to the left atrium by means of the pulmonary veins. Once the blood enters the left atrium, it travels through the mitral or bicuspid valve on its way to the left ventricle. When the heart contracts, the blood is pushed through the aortic valve into the aorta, which is the largest artery in the body. The blood then enters the body or systemic circulation (Figure 12-4).

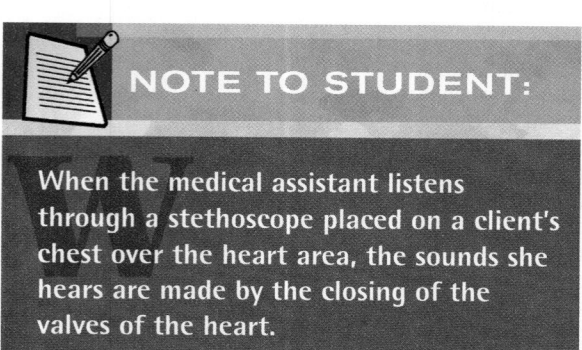

NOTE TO STUDENT:

When the medical assistant listens through a stethoscope placed on a client's chest over the heart area, the sounds she hears are made by the closing of the valves of the heart.

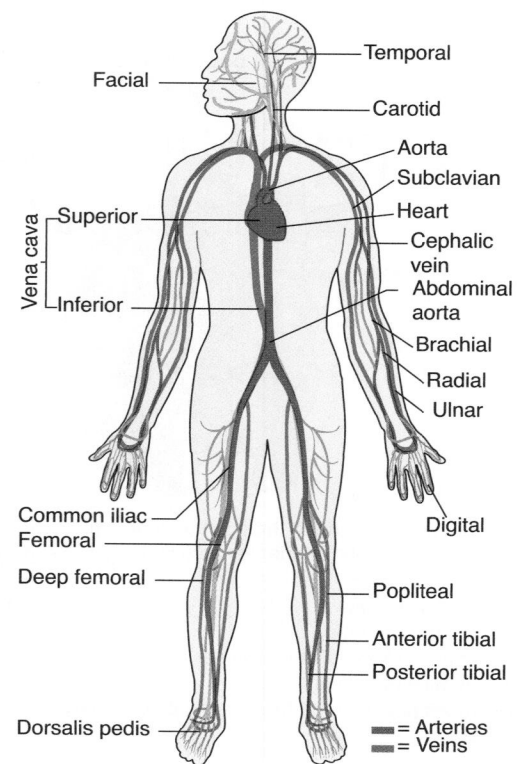

FIGURE 12-4 Systemic circulation.

NOTE TO STUDENT:

The pulmonary veins are the only veins in the body that transport oxygenated blood. The pulmonary arteries are the only arteries in the body that transport deoxygenated blood.

■ PATHWAY OF ELECTRICAL IMPULSES OF THE HEART

The heart has an electrical signal that starts and then coordinates the heart action. It stimulates the heart muscle to contract and then coordinates the chambers (atria and ventricles) so that they act together in a rhythmical pattern.

Within the upper wall of the right atrium is the sinoatrial (SA) node. Because the heartbeat starts in the SA node, the SA node is often called the *pacemaker.* It sets the pace or rhythm of a person's heart cycle. In the average adult, the heart normally beats 60 to 100 times per minute. The signal that comes from the SA node spreads throughout the atria in the conducting fibers, causing the atria to contract or depolarize. This impulse then travels to the atrioventricular (AV) node, which is found on the bottom of the atria. The atrioventricular node is not the same as the atrioventricular valve. A *node* is a group or bunch of fibers close together. These specialized heart muscle fibers slow the electrical impulse as it travels through the heart, thereby delaying the contraction of the ventricles. The ventricles need this time to fill with the blood from the contraction of the atria. The impulse then travels to the bundle of His, a structure that further divides into a left bundle branch and a right bundle branch. The bundle fibers lead into the muscles of the ventricles and then into the **Purkinje fibers.** The Purkinje fibers send the impulse quickly through the ventricles, causing both ventricles to contract at the same time. The Purkinje fibers are the last part of the conduction system of the heart. After completion of this part of the cycle, the heart relaxes and repolarizes, and then the whole cycle begins again with a new impulse.

■ THE HEART'S BLOOD SUPPLY

The heart muscle acts as a pump, sending nourishing blood throughout the body. However, this pump also needs its own supply of oxygen and nutrients from the blood. The blood that flows through the heart is not used to nourish the heart muscle.

The heart muscle receives its blood supply from the right and left **coronary** arteries. The word *coronary* means "crown" or "circle," and is used because the coronary arteries appear to be encircling the heart. The right and left coronary arteries branch off the ascending aorta. The right side of the heart receives nourishment from the right coronary artery. The left side of the heart receives nourishment from the left coronary artery, which is divided into the left anterior descending artery and the circumflex artery. The blood that nourishes the heart is then picked up by the coronary veins, which take it to the coronary sinus (vessel). From there the blood flows into the right atrium. The heart muscle needs a constant flow of oxygen-rich blood. Any lessening or stoppage, even for a short time, can cause serious damage to the heart (see Chapter 24).

 BRIDGE TO CAAHEP

This chapter, which discusses the cardiovascular system, provides information and content related to CAAHEP standards for Anatomy and Physiology, Medical Terminology, Communication, Medical Assisting Clinical Procedures, Patient (Client) Care, and Professional Components.

 ABHES LINKS

This chapter, which discusses the cardiovascular system, links to ABHES course content for Anatomy and Physiology, Medical Terminology, and Medical Office Clinical Procedures.

POINTS OF HIGHLIGHT

- A healthy cardiovascular system keeps the rest of the body supplied with essential nutrients and oxygen.
- The three layers of the heart are the epicardium, myocardium, and endocardium.
- The heart has two upper chambers, called the right atrium and the left atrium, and two lower chambers, called the right ventricle and the left ventricle.
- Valves in the heart allow the blood to flow in one direction only. They keep the blood from flowing backward.
- The tricuspid valve prevents the backflow of blood into the right atrium; the bicuspid valve prevents the backflow of blood into the left atrium.
- The right semilunar valve prevents the backward flow of blood from the pulmonary artery into the right ventricle.
- The medical assistant can hear the sounds made by the action of the heart valves by listening with a stethoscope placed on the client's chest.
- The heart has a system of electrical impulses that starts and then coordinates the heartbeat and heart actions.
- The coronary vessels keep the heart muscle furnished with its own supply of oxygen and nutrients.
- Medical assistants can work with clients in practicing heart-healthy behaviors.

AAMA AREAS OF COMPETENCE

This chapter, which discusses the cardiovascular system, provides information or content within several areas listed in the Medical Assistant Role Delineation Study. These areas include: clinical patient (client) care, general transdisciplinary, communication, legal concepts, and instruction.

AMT PATHS

This chapter, which discusses the cardiovascular system, provides a path to AMT competency in general medical assisting knowledge, anatomy and physiology, medical terminology, and patient (client) education.

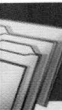

STUDENT PORTFOLIO ACTIVITY

Exercise is important for physical and mental health. It can relieve tension and contribute to strong bones and toned muscles, which in turn lessen the chance of injury while working. If you belong to a gym, attend exercise classes, or participate in a sport, make sure to include this information as part of your portfolio. If you do not participate in formal, organized exercise, but you regularly take walks, run, swim, or ride a bicycle, remember to include this as well. It lets the employer know that striving for wellness and taking care of yourself are important to you. This shows that you will be an employee who maintains a balance in life.

APPLYING YOUR SKILLS

In your client teaching, you explain that the heart is a muscle. What are two ways to keep this muscle in good working condition?

CRITICAL THINKING QUESTIONS

1. What happens when the coronary vessels get clogged? What effects does this clogging have on the heart? What are some symptoms that a client whose vessels are clogged might experience?

2. When you listen to the heart with a stethoscope, what are you hearing?

3. Why is the sinoatrial node called the pacemaker of the heart? How is its function related to the pulse rate and rhythm?

4. From where does the heart muscle receive its blood supply?

5. What is unusual about the pulmonary arteries and pulmonary veins?

6. What role do the heart valves play in the flow of blood?

7. Why is the heart called a pump?

8. Trace the path of the blood flow, from where blood enters the heart to where it leaves the heart.

9. As a medical assistant who teaches clients, how would you explain the role of exercise in maintaining a healthy heart?

10. The valves of the heart can be compared to faucets. How can you explain the function of the heart's valves to a client? What happens if the valves leak?

11. Describe what can happen to the heart if the right coronary artery becomes clogged or blocked. Which other areas would be affected, and how?

12. A well-conditioned athlete comes to the office for a physical. You are asked to obtain her vital signs. What would you expect to find in terms of rate, rhythm, and volume of the pulse? Why?

13. Go back to the beginning of this chapter and review the Anticipatory Statements. Reread each statement and then indicate whether it is true or false. If the statement is false, rewrite it to make it a true statement.

CLIENT TEACHING PLAN

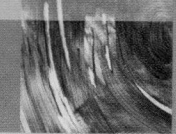

Heart-Healthy Behaviors for Women

■ **What Is to Be Taught:**

• Behaviors to promote heart health in women.

■ **Objectives:**

• Client will become aware of and begin to practice behaviors for a healthy heart.

■ **Preparation Before Teaching:**

• Review information about women and heart disease. Look at risk factors and practices to prevent cardiovascular disorders.
• Gather printed materials, such as pictures and diagrams of the heart and vessels, to help illustrate what you will be teaching.
• Have paper and pen available for notes and instructions.
• Make sure the area is free from distractions while you are teaching.

■ **Steps for the Medical Assistant:**

1. Wash your hands.
2. Introduce yourself to the client.
3. Explain what you are going to teach and why.
4. Tell the client that the signs and symptoms of heart problems, such as disease and heart attack, are different for women than for men. Heart disease is the leading cause of death in women, but the client can take an active role in keeping her heart healthy.
5. Inform the client that symptoms of heart problems in women include: unusual fatigue or feeling very tired; general weakness; shortness of breath; weak, heavy feeling in the arms; dizziness; cold sweats; and pain in the back, especially near the shoulder blades or scapula.
6. Tell the client that there are steps she can take to help keep her heart healthy. For example, to promote a healthy heart:

a. Be active—ride less and walk more. Moderate exercise helps to keep the heart beating and the blood flowing.
b. Eat heart-healthy foods such as whole grains, fresh fruits and vegetables, and wild salmon.
c. Do not smoke, and do not stay near someone who does smoke.
d. Reduce bad stress by maintaining a healthful lifestyle and getting adequate amounts of sleep, meditation, and relaxation.
e. Keep the waist measurement to less than 35 inches.
7. Work with client as to decide how these steps can be worked into her daily routine.
8. Compose a form with the client so she can keep a diary of her heart-healthy behaviors for a month.

■ **Special Needs of the Client:**

• Check the client's chart to see if there are any factors that might interfere with the client's ability to incorporate these steps into her daily routine.
• Ask the client if there is anything you should know that would affect her ability to adopt these practices.

■ **Evaluation:**

• Client suggests which practices she can put into her daily routine for a month.

■ **Further Plans/Teaching:**

• Review information with the client regarding women and risks for heart disorders.
• Restate practices that promote heart health.

■ **Follow-up:**

• Call the client after one week to see if she has been able to incorporate any heart-healthy practices.

(Continues)

CLIENT TEACHING PLAN (Continued)

- Encourage the client to continue.
- Ask the client if she has any questions or if she has encountered any problems.

Medical Assistant

Name: _____

Signature: _____

Date: _____

Client

Date: _____

Follow-up Date : _____

CHAPTER 13

Anticipatory Statements

People have varying ideas about the blood and what it does in the body. Read and think about the following statements based upon what you believe now. Decide whether you agree or disagree. Write the word **agree** after the statement if you think the statement is true. Write the word **disagree** after the statement if you think the statement is false. Read the chapter to find out if your current beliefs can be supported.

1. The major part of the hematologic system is the blood.   _____

2. Blood is only liquid.   _____

3. Type AB blood is called the universal donor.   _____

4. Tonsils have no role in the lymphatic system.   _____

5. A person cannot live without a spleen.   _____

Learning Objectives

Upon completion of this chapter, the medical assistant student should be able to:

- Explain three functions of the hematologic system
- Describe the liquid and formed elements of blood
- Name the types of white blood cells
- Identify the major parts of the lymphatic system
- Explain the functions of the lymphatic system
- List the four blood groups
- Explain the importance of the Rh factor
- Develop a teaching plan and teach another person

Hematologic and Lymphatic Systems

Key Terms

agglutination Clumping of red blood cells.

agranular White blood cells that do not have granules in the cytoplasm.

albumin The smallest of the plasma proteins.

basophil A type of white blood cell; sends out histamine and heparin to initiate and promote inflammation.

eosinophil A type of white blood cell important in allergic reactions.

erythrocytes Red blood cells.

fibrinogen Plasma protein involved in blood clotting.

globulin Plasma protein that protects the body from infection.

hemoglobin Oxygen-carrying part of the blood cell.

leukocytes White blood cells.

lymph Pale, watery fluid important in immunity and defense.

lymphocyte A type of white blood cell concerned with immunity.

monocyte A type of white blood cell; helps to kill some bacteria and viruses and neutralize toxins.

neutrophils Most numerous of the white blood cells.

phagocytosis Process by which cells surround and destroy bacteria.

plasma The liquid part of the blood.

prothrombin Plasma protein involved in the clotting process.

serum Liquid part of the blood remaining after a clot forms.

spleen Vascular organ found in the upper left region of the abdominal cavity.

thrombocytes Platelets; involved in the clotting of blood.

thymus Gland found in the thoracic area.

tonsils Found in the oral cavity and pharynx; protect against invasion by bacteria.

■ INTRODUCTION

The main functions of the hematologic and lymphatic systems are transportation and protection. Although they are different systems, they work together and so are presented in this one chapter. The blood, with its smaller components, and the bone marrow make up the hematologic system. The lymphatic tissues and vessels make up the lymphatic system. The spleen, liver, and kidneys also work with these two systems.

■ MAJOR PARTS OF THE HEMATOLOGIC SYSTEM

Blood is the major part of the hematologic system. Most people think of blood as a fluid, but it is actually connective tissue. The connective tissue cells are contained in the liquid portion of the blood. Blood has both a liquid component and a formed-element component (often called a solid part).

Plasma

The liquid part of the blood is called **plasma.** It makes up more than half (55%) of the volume of blood (Figure 13-1). Plasma is about 90% water; the remaining 10% is mostly proteins. Since water makes up most of the plasma, plasma is normally colorless or very light yellow. Within plasma are proteins, gases, salts, hormones, enzymes, and waste products. The plasma carries substances to and away from body tissues. Each part of the plasma has a specific task.

Plasma contains four important proteins: albumin, globulin, fibrinogen, and prothrombin. **Albumin** helps to maintain blood pressure and fluid volume by stopping the loss of plasma from the capillaries. It thickens the blood. **Globulin** acts to protect the body from infection, by giving immunity against certain infectious diseases. **Fibrinogen** and **prothrombin** are important in the process of blood clotting. When fibrinogen is subtracted from the plasma, the liquid that is left is called **serum.** All the components of plasma, taken together, assist in three general tasks: protection from infection, maintenance of fluid balance, and prevention of blood loss from injury.

Formed Elements

The formed elements are also referred to as the *solid part* of the blood. This blood component contains: red blood cells, white blood cells, and platelets (Figure 13-2). The formed elements make up 45% of the volume of blood.

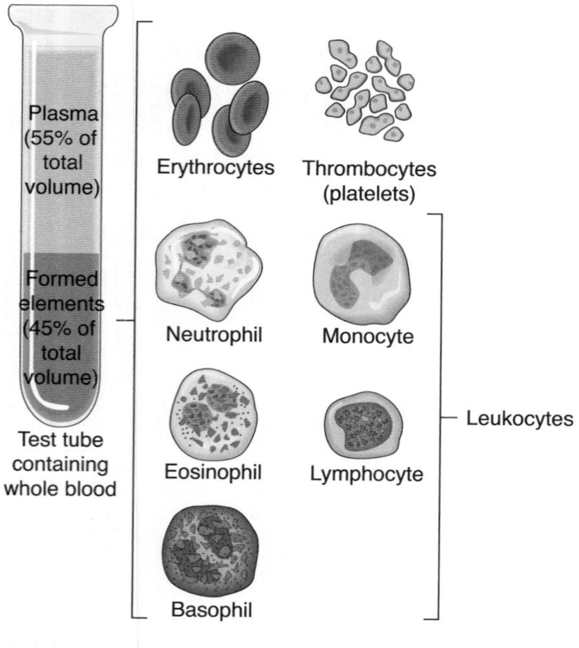

FIGURE 13-1 Major components of blood.

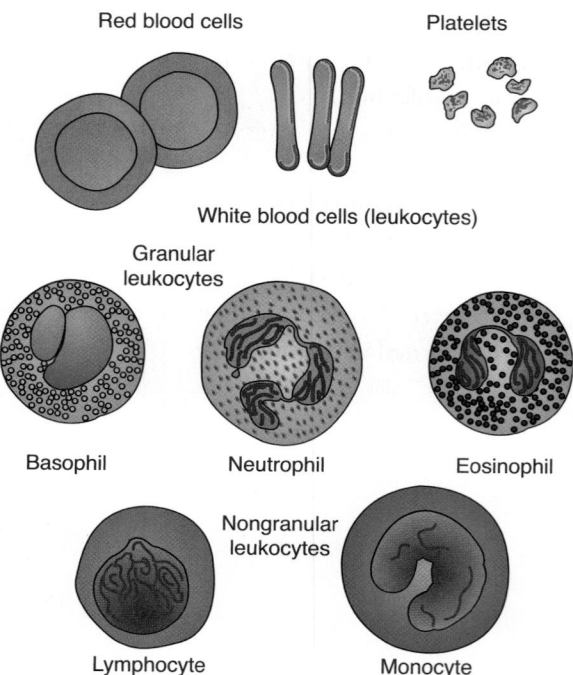

FIGURE 13-2 Classification of blood cells.

Red Blood Cells. The red blood cells (RBCs or **eryth-rocytes**) are the most numerous blood cells. Red blood cells contain **hemoglobin.** As the blood travels to the lungs, the hemoglobin picks up oxygen. The blood cells deliver this oxygen to other cells in the body and exchange it for carbon dioxide. Oxygen-rich blood looks bright red and oxygen-poor blood looks dark red. A red blood cell has a short life span of only about four months. The liver and **spleen** get rid of the old red blood cells (Figure 13-3).

White Blood Cells. The white blood cells (WBCs) are also called **leukocytes.** The purpose of the white blood cells is to protect against infections and toxins. White blood cells may be either granular or **agranular** (nongranular).

Blood cell	Life span in blood	Function
Erythrocyte	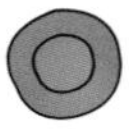 120 days	O_2 and CO_2 transport
Neutrophil	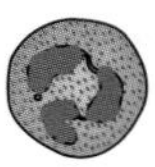 7-12 hours	Immune defenses
Eosinophil	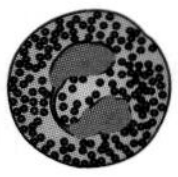 Unknown	Defense against parasites
Basophil	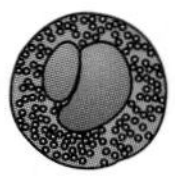 Unknown	Inflammatory response
Monocyte	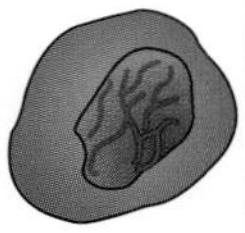 3 days-years	Immune surveillance (precursor of tissue macrophage)
B Lymphocyte	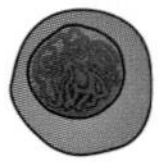 Unknown	Antibody production (precursor of plasma cells)
T Lymphocyte	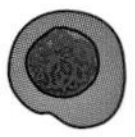 Unknown	Cellular immune response
Platelets	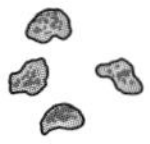 7-8 days	Blood clotting

FIGURE 13-3 Work of blood cells.

Granular white blood cells can be further divided into three kinds: neutrophils, eosinophils and basophils. **Basophils** contain chemicals that are released when a foreign chemical enters the body. This begins an allergic or inflammatory response. The client may experience the typical symptoms of an allergic response: itching, swelling of tissues, and sometimes breathing problems. **Eosinophils** are also called into action during an allergic response. The most numerous white blood cells are the **neutrophils.** These are most important in the fight against invading bacteria. Neutrophils increase in number, travel to the site of the infection, and engulf or surround the bacteria, essentially "eating" them. This process is called **phagocytosis.** Neutrophils have a very short life span and so, during times of infection, new ones have to be produced. These new, immature cells appear as bands in a blood analysis. If a client has an infection, the medical assistant would notice that the blood work from the laboratory reports an increase in the number of these cells.

Monocytes and **lymphocytes** are both agranular white blood cells. During an inflammatory process, the monocytes become active. A client's monocyte level will be high if he has an infection, tuberculosis, or certain chronic diseases. There are two kinds of lymphocytes, B lymphocytes and T lymphocytes, both of which are an important part of the immune response. During a viral infection or the active stage of an autoimmune disease, the numbers of these lymphocytes will increase.

Platelets. Platelets are also called **thrombo-cytes.** They are critical to the clotting of blood. When a person injures himself, the platelets go to work to stop the bleeding and prevent hemorrhaging. A *hemorrhage* is a large loss of blood. Blood loss may occur inside the body (internal hemorrhage, in which the blood stays within the body), or outside the body (external hemorrhage, in which the blood is lost to the outside environment). Without the clotting mechanism of the thrombocytes, even a small injury would become a hemorrhage, because the person would not stop bleeding.

■ BLOOD GROUPS

Every person inherits one of four specific blood types or groups: A, B, AB, or O in the ABO blood-typing system. The blood type is determined by the presence or absence of specific antigens and antibodies. Blood type A has A antigen. Blood type B has B antigen. Blood type AB has both A and B antigens. Type O has neither A nor B antigen. Each blood type produces specific antibodies. The plasma in type A blood has the B antibody. The plasma in type B has the A antibody. The plasma in type AB blood has neither A nor B antibodies. The plasma in type O blood has both A and B antibodies.

Only certain blood groups are compatible—that is, the blood can be interchanged without harm—with each other. Type O blood is called the universal donor because it can be given to any person in an emergency. Persons with type O blood can only receive type O blood. Type AB persons can receive blood from any blood group in an emergency. This is most critical when a client needs a blood transfusion or an organ transplant. If blood is mixed with blood from an incompatible group, the blood will clump or stick together. This clumping or sticking together is called **agglutination.** The client with a transfusion reaction may experience a serious or life-threatening situation.

A second way to categorize blood groups is by the Rh factor. This system is named after the rhesus monkeys used in Dr. Landsteiner's pio-neer work of the 1940s. The Rh factor is an antigen. Among the several antigens, antigen D is the one most likely to cause a problem if not matched correctly. If a person has the Rh factor D, he is said to be *Rh positive* (Rh+). If a person does not have the Rh factor D, he is said to be *Rh negative* (Rh−). The majority of people are Rh+. The Rh factor must be tested before any blood transfusion is given. A problem may also arise if an Rh- mother is pregnant with a baby who has the opposite Rh factor (in the example, an Rh+ baby). Women need to be tested and treated if the situation exists. The pregnant woman's body will produce antibodies against the developing baby because of the difference in the blood. The mother's body recognizes the baby's blood as different and foreign and fights against it as if it were an infection. The developing fetus will die if this condition is not recognized and treated.

■ MAJOR PARTS OF THE LYMPHATIC SYSTEM

The lymphatic system is closely related to the hematologic system. **Lymph,** which is a clear, watery substance, derives from plasma. Lymph carries fluid away from the tissues. It is a one-way system (Figure 13-4). When lymph cells grow to a certain size, they are called lymphatics. At various spots along the length of the lymphatic system are little oval structures known as *lymph nodes* (Fig-

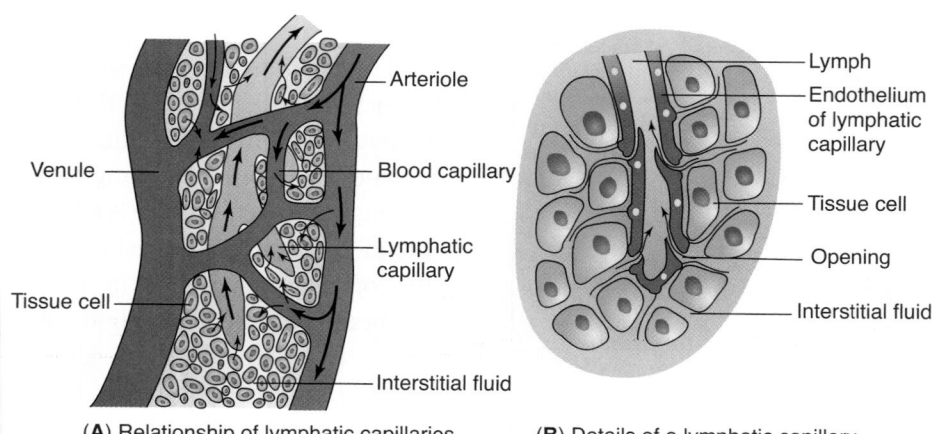

(**A**) Relationship of lymphatic capillaries to tissue cells and blood vessels

(**B**) Details of a lymphatic capillary

FIGURE 13–4 Lymph circulation.

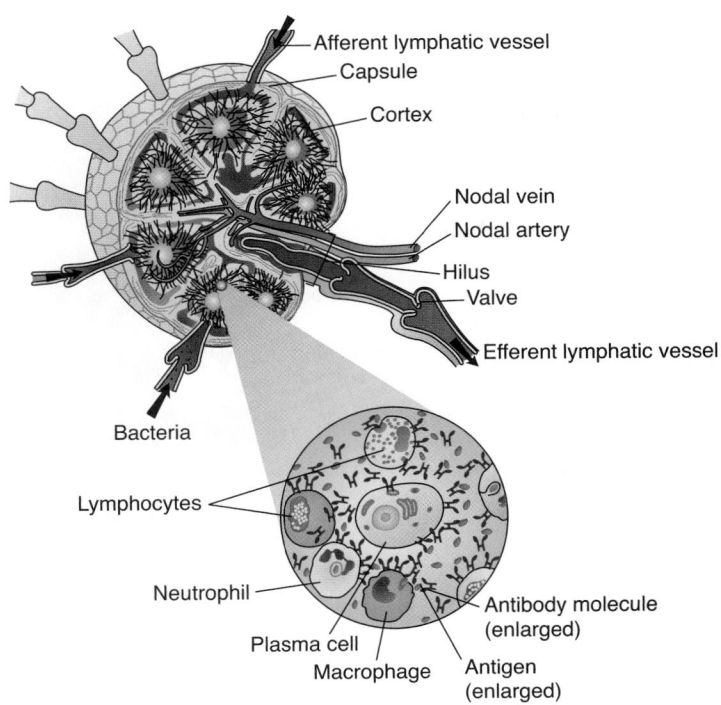

FIGURE 13-5A Lymph nodes become enlarged when fighting bacteria.

ures 13-5A and 13-5B). The lymph nodes may also be called *lymph glands.* The lymph nodes fight infection. Sometimes, when they are working very hard to get rid of invading bacteria, they become enlarged or swollen. A client who has an infection may complain of "swollen glands." The medical assistant may feel swollen nodes in the client's neck, groin, or armpits (Figure 13-6). They may be soft and tender to the touch.

The major structures associated with the lymphatic system are the tonsils, the spleen, and the thymus gland. They work a little differently than the lymph vessels and nodes. The **tonsils**

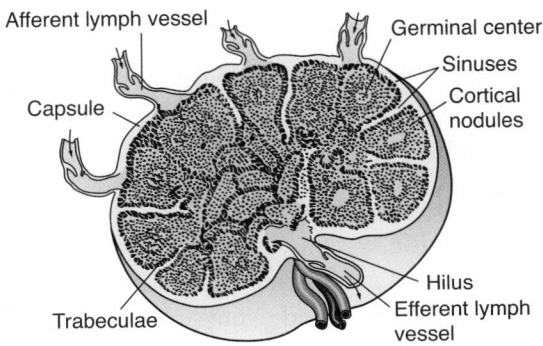

FIGURE 13-5B Internal view of a lymph node

are found in the throat area, around the pharynx. They protect against bacteria that may try to enter the body through the respiratory tract. Sometimes the tonsils are surgically removed if they become very enlarged or the client has had repeated problems with them. This surgery, which used to be routine, is now done much less frequently than in the past.

The **spleen** (Figure 13-7) acts as part of the lymphatic system by filtering blood. The spleen is found behind the stomach, in the left upper part of the abdominal cavity. It is the largest mass of lymphoid tissue in the body, and has important functions. It filters the blood. It helps to fight off bacteria. It gets rid of old red blood cells. It can also store blood for use in an emergency. The spleen holds monocytes, which help to engulf and destroy bacteria. It produces lymphocytes, which are important in the immune response. However, a person can live without a spleen.

The **thymus** is a small gland found in the upper chest. It is a place where lymphocytes can be made and grow to maturity. The thymus is most active in children. It begins to shrink at puberty and gets quite small thereafter.

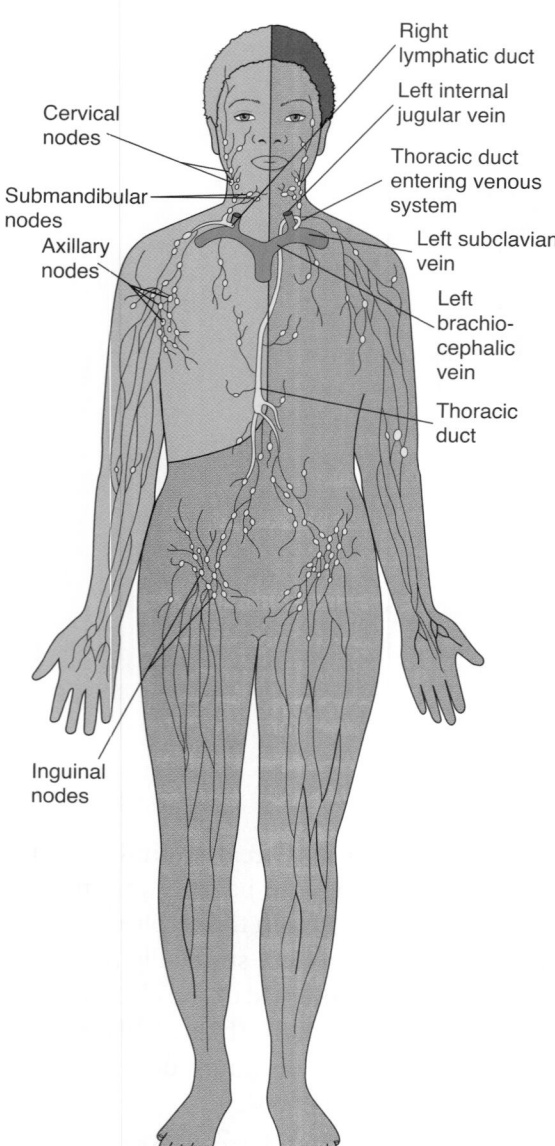

FIGURE 13-6 Lymph nodes are located alone or grouped in various places along the lymph vessels throughout the body.

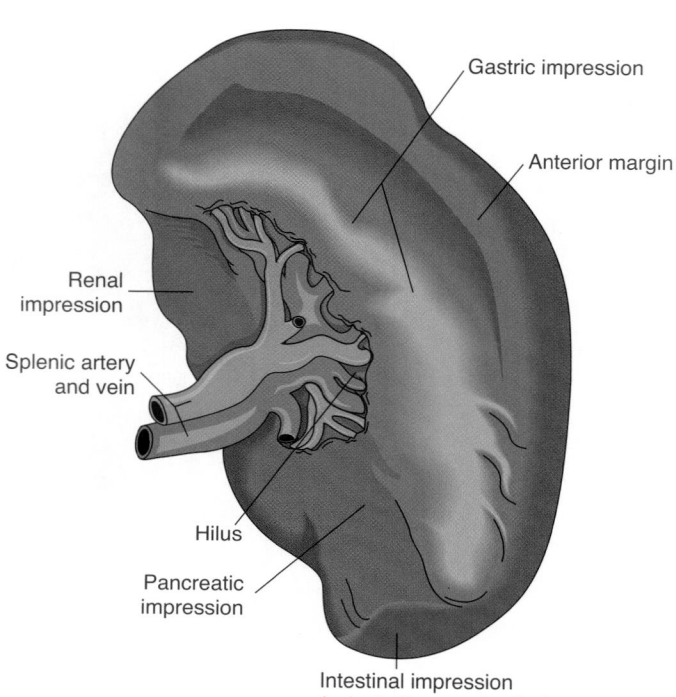

FIGURE 13-7 The spleen.

 ABHES LINKS

This chapter, which discusses the hematologic and lymphatic systems, links to ABHES course content for Anatomy and Physiology, Medical Terminology, and Medical Office Clinical Procedures.

 AAMA AREAS OF COMPETENCE

This chapter, which discusses the hematologic and lymphatic systems, provides information or content within several areas listed in the Medical Assistant Role Delineation Study. These areas include: clinical, fundamental principles, patient (client) care, general transdisciplinary, communication, legal concepts, and instruction.

 AMT PATHS

This chapter, which discusses the hematologic and lymphatic systems, provides a path to AMT competency in general medical assisting knowledge, anatomy and physiology, medical terminology, and patient (client) education.

 BRIDGE TO CAAHEP

This chapter, which discusses the hematologic and lymphatic systems, provides information and content related to CAAHEP standards for Anatomy and Physiology, Medical Terminology, Communication, Medical Assisting Clinical Procedures, and, Professional Components.

POINTS OF HIGHLIGHT

- The hematologic system is comprised of the blood and the bone marrow.
- The lymphatic system is comprised of lymphatic tissues and vessels.
- Blood is connective tissue with both a liquid and a solid part.
- Plasma, which is the liquid portion of blood, is 90% water.
- The solid part of the blood contains red blood cells, white blood cells, and platelets. The red blood cells are concerned with supplying the cells with oxygen and nutrients; the white blood cells protect the body against infection and toxins; the platelets are critical for blood clotting.
- The ABO blood types are A, B, AB, and O. Type O is the universal donor; in an emergency, it can be given to anyone. Type AB is the universal recipient; in an emergency, a person with type AB blood can receive blood from any of the other groups.
- The lymph glands and nodes filter the blood and help fight off infection.
- The tonsils, spleen, and thymus gland are the major structures of the lymphatic system.

STUDENT PORTFOLIO ACTIVITY

Medical assistants work with clients from diverse cultural groups. It is important to understand all clients' values and beliefs. Choose a cultural group and find background information on their major beliefs about health and health care. Make a list of "Points to Remember" for medical assistants who work with individuals from that cultural group. This list could take the form of a small paper to share with others. The cultural-diversity paper is an example of your awareness and respect for cultural diversity in health care settings.

APPLYING YOUR SKILLS

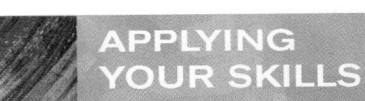

A client is scheduled for a surgical procedure next month. The doctor has ordered blood-type testing, in addition to other tests. The client asks you to explain the importance of knowing the blood type. What is the reason for this test, and how do you explain it in everyday terms?

CRITICAL THINKING QUESTIONS

1. Why is it important to know if a pregnant woman is Rh negative? What could happen?

2. When reviewing a lab report, what types of white blood cells would you expect to see at higher-than-normal levels if the client has had an allergic reaction?

3. What is the function of the red blood cells? How is their function related to the respiratory system?

4. Why is the type O blood group called the universal donor?

5. The client who has a sore throat complains of swollen glands. What would you as a medical assistant expect to see? What is happening when the lymph nodes or glands are enlarged and swollen? How would you explain this to the client?

6. What explains the almost colorless appearance of plasma?

7. Why does some blood look bright red and other blood look dark red?

8. A client is very concerned that he might have to have his spleen removed. What can you say to this client?

9. What might you expect to see in a client with a low number of platelets who has fallen and has cuts and abrasions?

10. When looking at the lab report for a client who was diagnosed with an infection, why might you expect to see a large number of neutrophil bands?

11. Go back to the beginning of this chapter and review the Anticipatory Statements. Reread each statement and then indicate whether it is true or false. If the statement is false, rewrite it to make it a true statement.

CLIENT TEACHING PLAN

Application and Use of Anti-Embolic Stockings

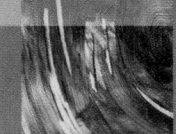

■ What Is to Be Taught:

• The application and use of anti-embolic stockings to promote venous return (good circulation) and prevent clot, thrombus, or embolus.

■ Objectives:

• Client will be able to put on and remove anti-embolic stockings and to care for them.

■ Preparation Before Teaching:

• Review the pathway of blood and the circulation process. Look over the factors that assist circulation and help to prevent clots. Make sure to put technical medical terms into everyday language.
• Gather supplies, such as a sample pair of anti-embolic stockings and pen and paper for writing instructions.
• Make sure the area is free from distractions while you are teaching.

■ Steps for the Medical Assistant:

1. Introduce yourself to the client.
2. Explain what you are going to teach and why.
3. Describe the flow of blood, and explain that muscular activity or leg support helps to prevent clot formation by promoting venous return.
4. Show the client a sample pair of anti-embolic stockings.
5. Wash your hands.
6. Ask the client to remove his socks.
7. Remind the client to make sure that his feet are clean and dry before putting on anti-embolism stockings.
8. Instruct the client that the stockings should always go on before he gets out of bed in the morning. If he waits until after he has been up for awhile, blood will have pooled in the lower part of the legs and feet. The stockings should be kept where they can be reached.

9. Take one stocking and gather it so that it is folded down to the toe part.
10. Using both hands, fit the toe part of the stocking over the client's toes. Work the stocking over the heel. Warn the client that this may take some effort. However, the stockings must fit tightly over the foot if they are to accomplish their purpose.
11. Work the stocking up the leg. When you reach the end, take both hands and run them up the leg, starting at the toes, to smooth all parts of the stocking.
12. Take the other stocking.
13. Ask the client to put this stocking on his other foot. Assist the client with prompts or cues if he is hesitant or cannot remember.
14. Remind the client that the fit will be snug. He will be measured from the doctor's prescription.
15. Tell the client that having two pairs will be more convenient. If he has only the one pair, remind him to wash the stockings by hand at night and make sure that they will be dry before morning.
16. Give the client written instructions that he can refer to at home.
17. Tell the client to call if he has any questions or concerns. Make sure that you give him the telephone number and extension.

■ Special Needs of the Client:

• Review the client's chart to see if there is any factor that might interfere with his ability to perform this task.
• Ask the client if there is anything you need to know about his ability to perform this task or that would help you to assist him.

■ Evaluation:

• Client is able to state the purpose of anti-embolic stockings.
• Client can put on anti-embolic stockings correctly after observing your demonstration.

(Continues)

CLIENT TEACHING PLAN (Continued)

■ Further Plans/Teaching:

- Give written instructions to the client.
- Ask the client if he has any questions or if he needs more information.

■ Follow–up:

- Call the client at home at the end of the week and ask if he has any questions.
- Ask the client if he encountered problems in putting on, taking off, or caring for the anti-embolic stockings.

Medical Assistant

Name: _____

Signature: _____

Date: _____

Client

Date: _____

Follow-up Date : _____

CHAPTER 14

Anticipatory Statements

People have different ideas about the working of the body's immune system. Read and think about the following statements based upon what you believe now. Decide whether you agree or disagree. Write the word **agree** after the statement if you think the statement is true. Write the word **disagree** after the statement if you think the statement is false. Read the chapter to find out if your current beliefs can be supported.

1. The immune system protects a person from infection. _____

2. A person's body tries to fight off disease-causing organisms or foreign bodies. _____

3. The immune system has special cells that can remember or recognize a foreign substance the second time that same foreign substance tries to attack. _____

4. The immune system only fights harmful foreign substances. _____

5. The spleen plays a role in the immune system. _____

Immune System

Learning Objectives

Upon completion of this chapter, the medical assistant student should be able to:

- State the difference between specific immunity and nonspecific immunity
- Identify examples of nonspecific immunity
- Identify examples of specific immunity
- Discuss the role of lymphocytes in the immune system
- Explain the action of antibodies on antigens
- Describe what happens during an allergic reaction
- Explain the functions of the immune system
- Talk about the relationship between vaccination, immunization, and diseases

Key Terms

antibodies Produced by the body to fight off foreign proteins and other substances.

antigen Protein or foreign substance, the entry of which into the body causes the body to respond by producing antibodies.

interferon Protein whose actions fight against viruses.

lymphocyte A type of white blood cell concerned with immunity.

nonspecific immunity The body's defense against invasion by all types of foreign substances.

pathogen Disease-causing microorganisms.

specific immunity The body's memory of a response to a particular foreign substance or organism.

vaccination Process of giving a vaccine, usually by injection, to make an individual resistant to or protected against a disease.

■ INTRODUCTION

This chapter introduces the medical assistant to the immune system. It explains the vital role of the immune system in the functioning of the other body systems, and in the general health of the person.

To maintain life, the body must always protect itself from harm by foreign attackers such as pathogenic organisms and foreign proteins. It is the job of the immune system to be always ready, keeping a lookout or surveillance for any foreign invaders. When an intrusion is noted, the immune system resists, defends against, and counterattacks the foreign substance. The immune system has two ways of protecting the body. There is a nonspecific defense, which is sometimes called *nonspecific immunity*. This protects against any invaders that try to come into the body. The second line of defense is specific defense or *specific immunity*, which guards against a particular or specific invader.

■ LYMPHOCYTES

Many factors work together to provide protection for the body. The foundation of the immune system is the **lymphocytes,** a cell grouping that becomes specialized. The two most important kinds of lymphocytes are the B lymphocytes and the T lymphocytes, called *B cells* and *T cells*. B cells produce **antibodies.** T cells protect the body from viral infections and cancer.

■ NONSPECIFIC IMMUNITY

In **nonspecific immunity,** the defense is not targeted to a certain type of invader; rather, it works to guard against any invasion (Figure 14-1). The skin is the body's first line of defense. Unbroken skin provides a physical wall or barrier that keeps out invaders. Some chemicals present on the skin also ward off **pathogens** (see Chapter 7). Tears wash out any invading organisms or particles out of the eyes. The mucous membranes that line the respiratory tract have cilia and

mucus-producing cells that trap and remove particles. For nonspecific immunity, it does not matter what the particles are; the cells just know that it is foreign. The digestive system, through the release of hydrochloric acid in the stomach, kills off some disease-causing organisms. If the unwanted organisms pass through the digestive tract, they may simply be expelled from the body in the feces. Bacteria may also pass out of the body in urine. In some instances, the body can protect itself by vomiting to get rid of foreign organisms.

During an infection, the body responds with an inflammatory process that includes a fever. Fever increases the action of **interferon,** a protein that tries to slow down virus production. Neutrophils and monocytes entrap and devour bacteria (see Chapter 13).

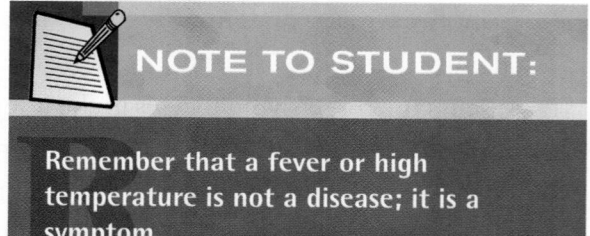

NOTE TO STUDENT:

Remember that a fever or high temperature is not a disease; it is a symptom.

If the attackers get by the nonspecific line of defense, it is up to **specific immunity** to protect the body. Specific immunity watches and keeps activity under surveillance. It recognizes earlier invaders and reacts to known pathogens. In other words, this type of immunity has a memory.

■ SPECIFIC IMMUNITY

Specific immunity may be either inborn or acquired. *Inborn immunity* is immunity or protection that a person is born with. It may be present in a single individual, or it may be common to a group of people. An acquired immunity is based on the body's previous encounter(s) with a pathogen. Acquired immunity may be natural or artificially acquired; artificially acquired immunity can be either actively or passively acquired.

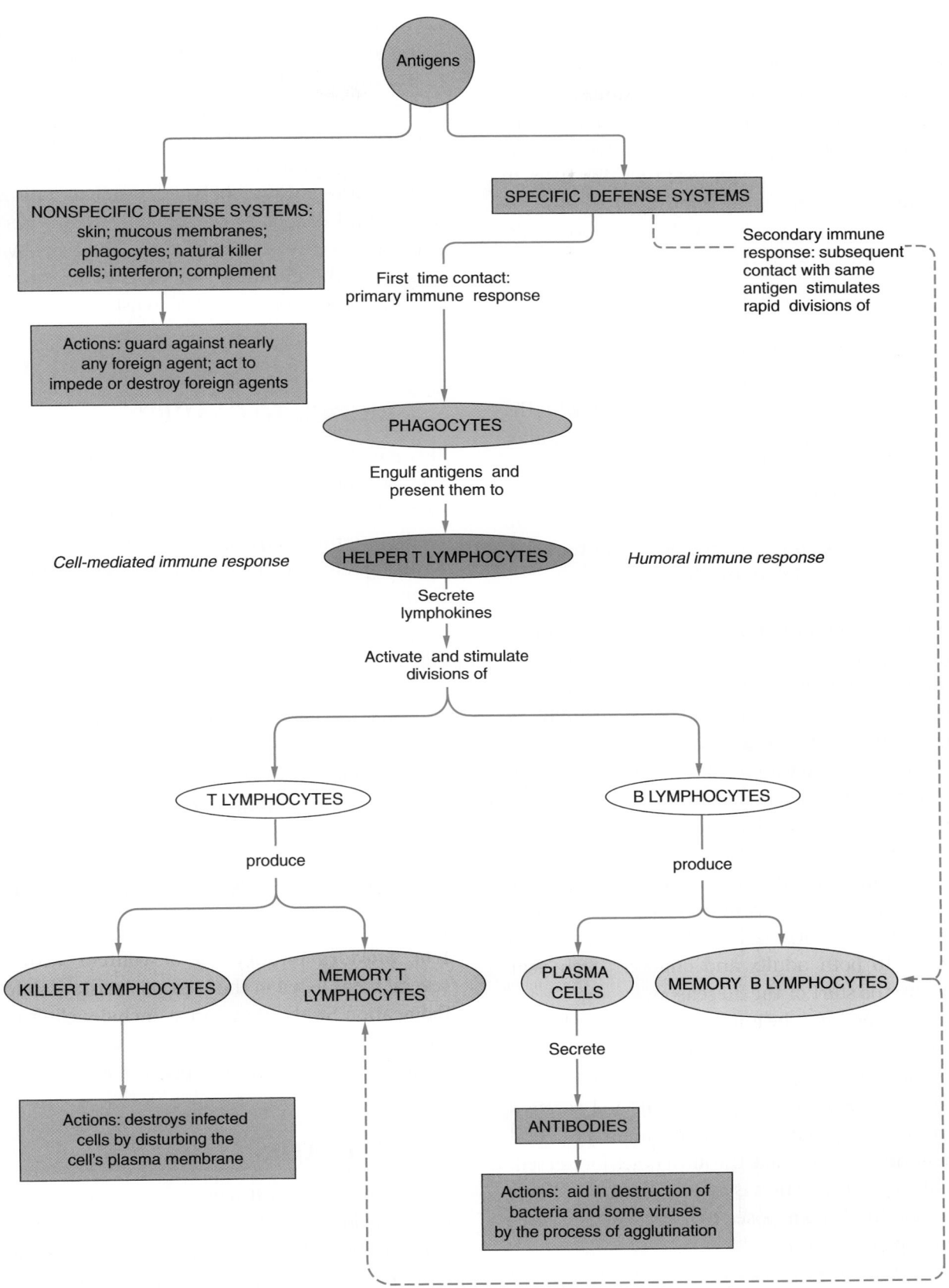

FIGURE 14–1 Overview of body's defense mechanisms.

Inborn Immunity

An infant receives naturally acquired passive immunity when protection is passed from the mother to the fetus through the placenta. An infant can also receive this protection in the breast milk. This transmitted immunity helps to protect the infant for several months until the baby's own immune system develops more fully.

Acquired Immunity

A person who has been exposed to a disease may build up an immunity to that disease. Sometimes the person actually becomes sick with the disease, and is thus rendered immune to it after recovery, as was the case for many children before the vaccine for chickenpox was developed. Other times, the protection builds up gradually over time and the person never actually comes down with the disease.

Artificially acquired immunity is similar to naturally acquired immunity in that it can be actively or passively obtained. **Vaccination** or immunization is an example of artificial active immunity. The person is exposed, usually by injection, to the **antigen** that causes a disease. Of course, the pathogen used for immunization is purposely weakened, so that the person does not actively get the disease from the immunization. Examples are vaccinations for diseases such as measles, mumps, rubella, and pertussis. Children are routinely immunized against these diseases. Flu vaccinations (flu shots) are often given to both adults and children each year before the start of the flu season.

Sometimes the antibodies produced by one individual are injected into another person. The resulting protection is called *artificially acquired passive immunity.* The person injected receives short-term protection against a disease, and does not have to make the antibodies for herself. This type of injection is frequently given after a person has been exposed to a disease or disease-causing organism.

All these processes, taken together, form the body's immune system. Most of these processes

take place inside the body without the person being aware of them. An immune system that is working smoothly and effectively allows the person to interact with the environment and not worry much about catching a disease. The medical assistant can also teach clients to practice immune-boosting behaviors such as eating a healthful diet, keeping the body clean, and getting the right amount of sleep. These behaviors assist the immune system to do its job of keeping the person safe from invasion by harmful organisms.

 BRIDGE TO CAAHEP

This chapter, which discusses the immune system, provides information and content related to CAAHEP standards for Anatomy and Physiology, Medical Terminology, Communication, Medical Assisting Clinical Procedures, and Professional Components.

 ABHES LINKS

This chapter, which discusses the immune system, links to ABHES course content for Anatomy and Physiology, Medical Terminology, and Medical Office Clinical Procedures.

 AAMA AREAS OF COMPETENCE

This chapter, which discusses the immune system, provides information or content within several areas listed in the Medical Assistant Role Delineation Study. These areas include: clinical, patient (client) care, general transdisciplinary, communication, legal concepts, and instruction.

 AMT PATHS

This chapter, which discusses the immune system, provides a path to AMT competency in general medical assisting knowledge, anatomy and physiology, medical terminology, and patient (client) education.

POINTS OF HIGHLIGHT

- The body must constantly protect itself from pathogenic organisms and foreign proteins. The immune system performs this function.
- The immune system resists, defends against, and counterattacks invading foreign organisms.
- The foundation of the immune system is the lymphocytes.
- B lymphocytes produce antibodies.
- T lymphocytes protect the body from viral infections and cancer.
- The skin is the body's first line of defense in nonspecific immunity.
- Specific immunity can be inborn or acquired.
- Inborn immunity is protection that a person is born with.
- Acquired immunity can be obtained either naturally or artificially.
- An immune system that is working well allows a person to interact freely with the environment, without excessive worry about infection.

STUDENT PORTFOLIO ACTIVITY

Look at completed homework assignments that demonstrate your problem-solving ability in client situations. Place a good example of your problem-solving skills in your portfolio. Medical assistants need to solve problems every day, and this skill will be valuable in the work setting.

APPLYING YOUR SKILLS

As a medical assistant, you come into contact with many potentially harmful microorganisms during your work. Therefore, it is important that you keep your immune system healthy. How does a system that is working smoothly allow you to interact with the environment free from getting or having to worry about getting infections?

CRITICAL THINKING QUESTIONS

1. Even when the body does not recognize a specific invader, the immune system still tries to defend against potential harm. In what ways does the body protect itself?

2. How can a newborn infant be protected against disease?

3. If a person is exposed to a disease or disease-causing organism, what can she do to protect herself?

4. What type of immunity does a person receive from a flu vaccine or flu shot?

5. What steps can a medical assistant teach a client to help the immune system do its job?

6. If a client has a low number of T lymphocytes, what would she be susceptible to?

7. A client has an infection. Why is it actually a positive sign that the client has a fever?

8. What is meant by the statement that the immune system has a surveillance role?

9. A client who has no chronic disorders, and is in excellent general health, confides to you that she is hesitant to go to community functions because she is afraid of "catching something." What could you tell her about the working of a healthy immune system and disease?

10. A new first-grade teacher comes to the office complaining about having "another cold." She mentions that another first-grade teacher, who has been at the school for years, never seems to get sick. What might explain this situation?

11. Go back to the beginning of this chapter and review the Anticipatory Statements. Reread each statement and then indicate whether it is true or false. If the statement is false, rewrite it to make it a true statement.

CLIENT TEACHING PLAN

Food Allergy—Peanut Avoidance

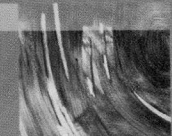

■ What Is to Be Taught:

• How to avoid a food allergen (peanuts) to prevent a severe allergic reaction.

■ Objectives:

• Client will be able to identify and avoid foods with peanuts and thus prevent a severe allergic reaction.

■ Preparation Before Teaching:

• Review the working of the immune system and how it protects against antigens and foreign invaders. Make sure to put technical medical terms into everyday language that the client can easily understand (Chapter 14 and Chapter 22).
• Get together teaching materials, such as pictures of common items containing peanuts, sample food labels, information about Medic Alert bracelets, and paper and pen for written information.
• Make sure that the area is free from distractions while you are teaching.

■ Steps for the Medical Assistant:

1. Wash your hands.
2. Introduce yourself to the client.
3. Explain what you are going to teach and why.
4. Inform the client that by understanding allergies and taking safety precautions, she can take an active role in staying healthy.
5. Describe what is meant by a hypersensitivity. Explain that the hypersensitive person's immune system reacts to a normally harmless substance as if that substance were an enemy.
6. Discuss what goes on in the client's body when she comes into contact with peanuts in any amount or form.
7. Show the client the pictures of common sources of peanuts and foods that may contain

peanuts or peanut oil. For example, many foods are cooked in peanut oil, and many ethnic foods contain peanuts. Bakeries or other places that prepare food by hand (rather than machine processing) are often a source of accidental peanut contamination. Candies that are not supposed to contain peanuts may in fact do so because the same machines or utensils were used to prepare both peanut-containing food and non-peanut food. Cross-contamination from handling is a frequent source of peanut contamination.

8. Demonstrate to the client how to read a whole food label—not just the nutritional information part. Allow the client to follow along with a copy. Show the client the disclaimer, found on many labels, stating that the food was manufactured in a factory that processes peanuts. Stress to the client that although she may believe there most likely are no peanuts in such a product, she should never, ever take that chance.
9. Hand the client another food label and ask her to check for information about peanuts.
10. Give the client written information about the Medic Alert system. The identification bracelets from this organization inform others that the client has a severe allergy.
11. Remind the client that if she should accidentally come into contact with or ingest peanuts, she should immediately follow the prescribed First Aid steps; do not wait. (Most likely, these emergency steps will include injecting epinephrine and taking oral antihistamines, if possible.) The client should also seek emergency care through an emergency department and doctor.
12. Hand the client written instructions prescribed by the doctor. Make sure that the client has the telephone numbers to call if there is any question or problem.

(Continues)

CLIENT TEACHING PLAN (Continued)

■ Special Needs of the Client:

- Check the client's chart to see if there are any factors that might interfere with the client's ability to remember and follow instructions to avoid a severe allergic reaction.
- Ask the client, before and after, if there is anything you should know that might affect her ability to implement what she has learned.

■ Evaluation:

- Client is able to state what happens when the immune system is hypersensitive.
- Client can demonstrate how to read a food label to check for peanut ingredients.
- Client can list safety precautions to avoid an allergic reaction.

■ Further Plans/Teaching:

- Ask the client if she has any questions or needs any additional information.

■ Follow-up:

- Call the client at home after one week. Ask if she has had difficulty in reading food labels or finding out which foods contain peanuts or peanut products.
- At the next office visit, review the information with the client.

Medical Assistant

Name: _____

Signature: _____

Date: _____

Client

Date: _____

Follow-up Date : _____

CHAPTER

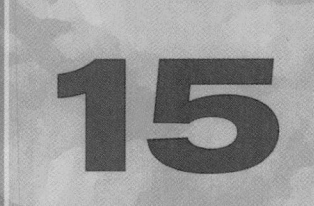

15

Anticipatory Statements

People have different ideas about the respiratory system and the mechanics of breathing. Read and think about the following statements based upon what you believe now. Decide whether you agree or disagree. Write the word **agree** after the statement if you think the statement is true. Write the word **disagree** after the statement if you think the statement is false. Read the chapter to find out if your current beliefs can be supported.

1. Oxygen and carbon dioxide are exchanged in the alveoli of the lungs.   _____

2. In cold weather, a person should breathe through the mouth to warm the air.   _____

3. The larynx is sometimes called the voice box.   _____

4. During inhalation, the diaphragm rises.   _____

5. Involuntary respiration is controlled by the lungs.   _____

Respiratory System

Learning Objectives

Upon completion of this chapter, the medical assistant student should be able to:

- List the structures of the respiratory system
- Trace the flow of air from where it enters the body until it reaches the alveoli
- Explain the functions of the respiratory system
- Describe the process of mechanical breathing or respiration
- Identify the respiratory control center
- Define internal respiration
- Define external respiration

Key Terms

alveoli Small sacs at the end of the bronchial tree. Alveoli look like a bunch of grapes.

bronchus Tube-like structure that extends from the trachea to the lung. There is a left and a right bronchus.

epiglottis Flap of tissue that prevents food and liquids from entering the larynx when swallowing.

larynx Voice box.

pharynx Throat.

respiration Inhalation (taking in of air) and exhalation (letting out of air).

sinus Cavity or hollow space.

trachea Also called windpipe; a tube-like structure that divides into a left and right bronchus.

■ INTRODUCTION

The simple act of breathing in and breathing out, repeated several times a minute, is part of the respiratory system's function of maintaining life. In most cases, breathing occurs without the person even being aware of it.

The respiratory system structures can be grouped into the upper respiratory tract and the lower respiratory tract. All the structures of the respiratory system work together to supply the cells with the oxygen necessary for life. The respiratory system works closely with the cardiovascular system to deliver this oxygen to the cells. In addition to exchanging oxygen and carbon dioxide, the respiratory system also plays a role in protection of the body, allows speech, and has a minor role in elimination.

■ UPPER RESPIRATORY TRACT

The parts of the upper respiratory system are the nose, sinuses, pharynx, larynx, and trachea (Figure 15-1).

The *nose* is the passageway where incoming air begin its journey through the respiratory system. The nose warms the inhaled air. When the surrounding air is very cold, it is important to remember to breathe in through the nose rather than the mouth. In addition to warming the air, the nose filters and traps particulate matter and some organisms. The nose contains hair to help trap these particles. The moist, sticky mucous membranes lining the nose warm the air and also act as a barrier to unwanted particles.

Sinuses or cavities are found in the head. *Cavities* are spaces within or enclosed by bone. A sinus is named according to the bone near which it is located. The sinuses make the skull lighter and give a resonant tone or quality to the voice. The medical assistant may notice that a client who has a respiratory infection sounds different. Fluid or congestion in the sinuses can cause this different sound. The sinuses drain into the nasal tract, so an infection in one area can easily travel to the other.

Most people call the **pharynx** the throat. Both air and food travel through this passageway (Figure 15-2). The muscular passageway of the pharynx is lined with mucous membranes. The pharynx has three parts: the nasopharynx, the oropharynx, and the laryngopharynx. The

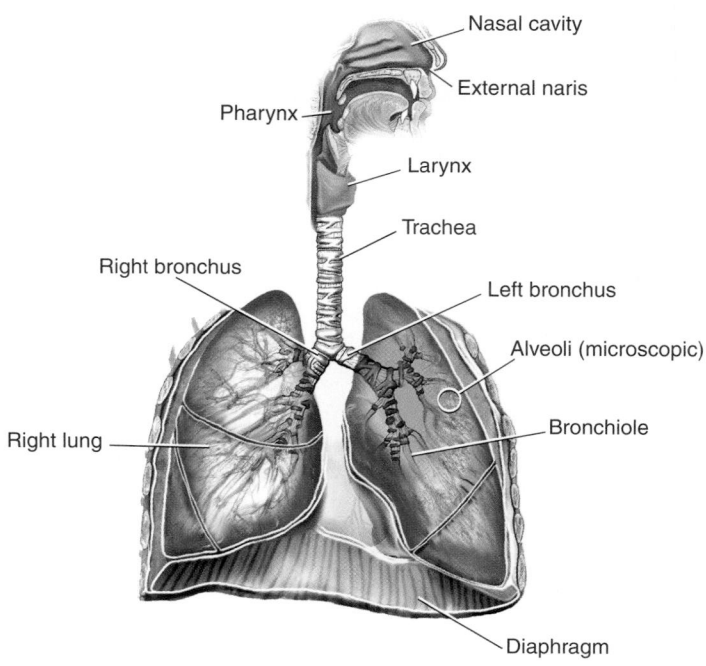

FIGURE 15-1 Organs of the respiratory system.

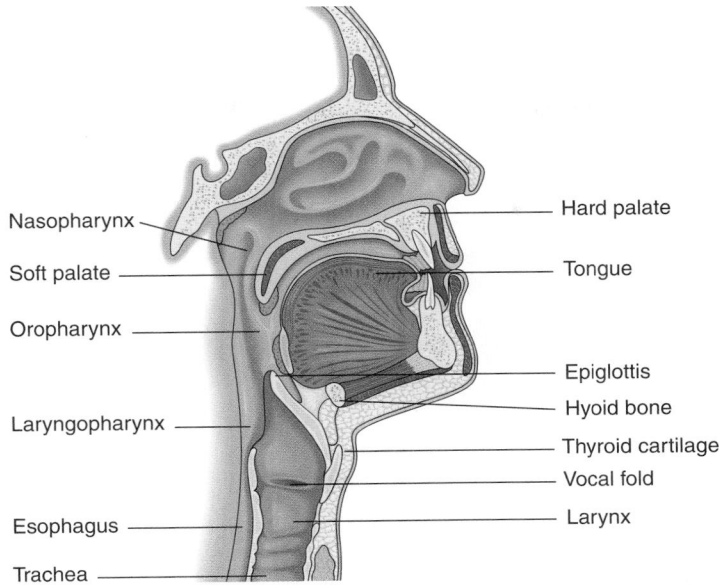

FIGURE 15-2 Pathway of air through the face and neck.

nasopharynx connects with the nasal tract (nose). The *oropharynx* connects with the oral cavity (mouth). The *laryngopharynx* connects with the larynx.

The **larynx** is commonly called the voice box. The larynx connects the pharynx and the trachea (Figure 15-3). This passageway, which is made of rings of cartilage, is for air only. The **epiglottis** ensures that food stays out. The epiglottal cartilage acts as a flap or cover that closes when a person swallows. If food accidentally gets caught in the "wrong tube," the person will involuntarily cough to dislodge the

foreign matter (see Chapter 39). The thyroid cartilage is the biggest piece of cartilage in the larynx. It is sometimes called the Adam's apple. It is larger and more easily seen in males than in females.

The vocal cords are also found in the larynx. The larger size of this structure in males is responsible for men's deeper voices. When a person breathes out, air passes through the vocal cords, which vibrate and produce sound waves. The amount of pressure that a person uses affects the sound. The more pressure, the louder the sound; the less pressure, the softer the sound. The pitch of a person's voice is related to how fast the vocal cords vibrate. Due to the stretch of cords, men's cords generally vibrate more slowly and have a lower pitch. Women's cords vibrate more quickly and therefore give women's voices a higher pitch.

Many people refer to the **trachea** as the windpipe. This passageway extends from the larynx down into the chest, eventually branching into the right **bronchus** and the left bronchus (Figure 15-4). Mucous membranes and cilia in the trachea help to keep particles out of the trachea. The trachea remains open at all times because of the stiffness of the cartilage. The trachea is considered the end of the upper respiratory tract.

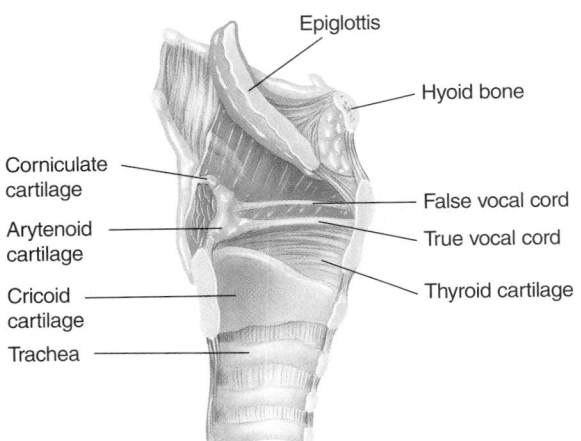

FIGURE 15-3 The larynx.

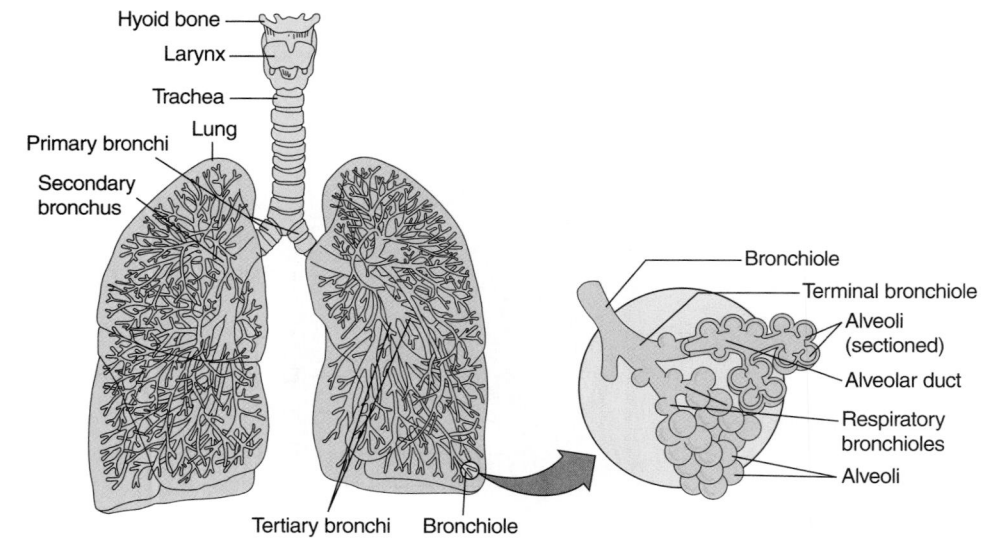

FIGURE 15-4 Trachea, bronchi, and bronchioles.

LOWER RESPIRATORY TRACT

As noted, the trachea branches into the right and left bronchi. The lower respiratory tract consists of the right and left bronchi and the lungs. The right bronchus goes to the right lung and the left bronchus goes to the left lung. There they branch many times into smaller networks. This subdivision looks like the branches and twigs of a tree and so is sometimes called the bronchial tree. The right lung has three lobes and the left lung has two lobes. The smaller, thinner bronchial divisions are called *bronchioles.* The bronchioles go into the alveolar ducts and then become alveolar sacs. These sacs look like little spheres or grapes. It is in the **alveoli** that the exchange of gases takes place. Cells in the alveoli of the lungs secrete surfactant that helps keep the lungs elastic.

MECHANICS OF BREATHING

The act of breathing, or *ventilation,* takes air from the outside and gets it to the lungs. One inhalation (taking in of air or breath) and one exhalation (letting out of air or breath) is called

one **respiration** (Figure 15-5). This is important for the medical assistant to remember, because the medical assistant is responsible for counting the client's respirations when obtaining vital signs. When a person inhales, the diaphragm moves down, allowing the lungs to expand to take in the air. When a person exhales, the diaphragm moves up, allowing the lungs to return to their previous size and position. When the air reaches the alveoli in the lungs, an exchange of gases takes place: oxygen goes into the blood and carbon dioxide comes out of the blood. This is called *external respiration.* At the cellular level, the transport of oxygen to the cells and use of oxygen within the cells is called *internal respiration.*

A person has some voluntary control over respiration; however, the major control comes from the medulla oblongata in the brain. A buildup of carbon dioxide triggers the respiratory response.

To summarize, air enters the nose, goes through the pharynx, larynx, and trachea, enters the lungs through the bronchi and bronchioles, and finally ends up in the alveoli of the lungs, where gases are exchanged (Figure 15-6). The major function of the respiratory system is to take in oxygen for the cells and pick up waste carbon dioxide to expel it from the body.

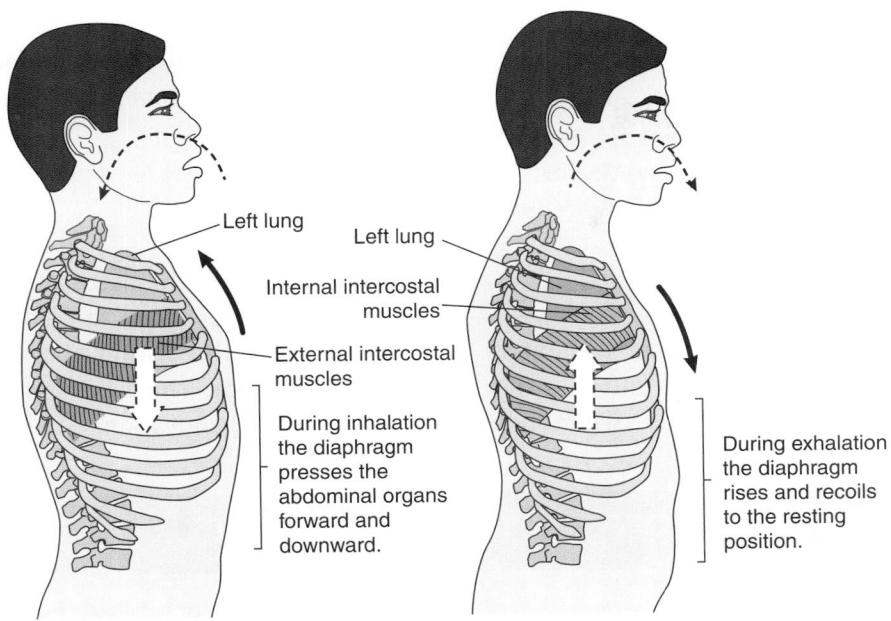

FIGURE 15-5 Respiration.

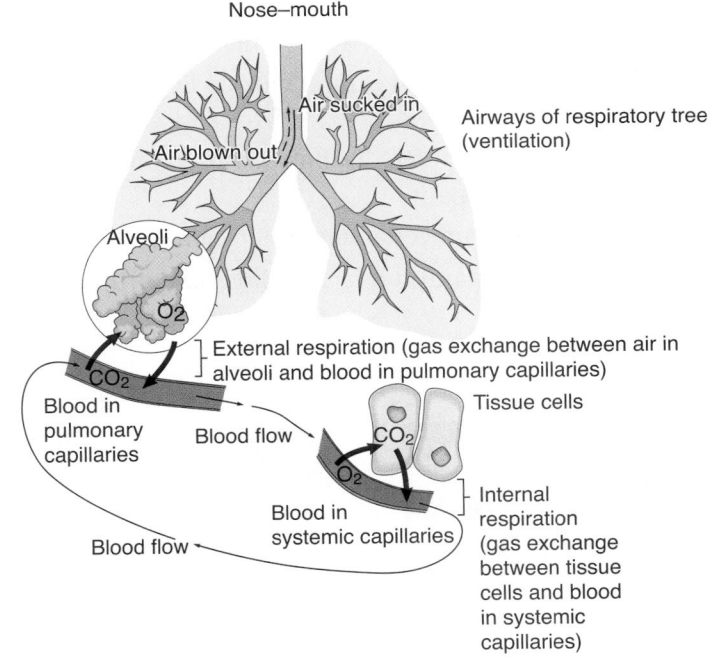

FIGURE 15-6 Mechanics of breathing.

 BRIDGE TO CAAHEP

This chapter, which discusses the respiratory system, provides information and content related to CAAHEP standards for Anatomy and Physiology, Medical Terminology, Communication, Medical Assisting Clinical Procedures, and Professional Components.

ABHES LINKS

This chapter, which discusses the respiratory system, links to ABHES course content for Anatomy and Physiology, Medical Terminology, Medical Law and Ethics, and Medical Office Clinical Procedures.

AAMA AREAS OF COMPETENCE

This chapter, which discusses the respiratory system, provides information or content within several areas listed in the Medical Assistant Role Delineation Study. These areas include: clinical, patient (client) care, professionalism, general transdisciplinary, communication, legal concepts, and instruction.

AMT PATHS

This chapter, which discusses the respiratory system, provides a path to AMT competence in general medical assisting knowledge, anatomy and physiology, medical terminology, and patient (client) education.

POINTS OF HIGHLIGHT

- The respiratory system brings in vital oxygen for transport to the body's cells and gets rid of carbon dioxide.
- The respiratory system is divided into the upper and lower respiratory tracts.
- Nose, sinus, larynx, pharynx, and trachea make up the upper respiratory tract. The lower respiratory tract consists of the right and left bronchi and lungs.
- In the alveoli of the lungs, oxygen and carbon dioxide are exchanged. This is called external respiration.
- The term mechanics of breathing refers to the act of breathing air in (inhalation) and letting air out of the lungs (exhalation).
- One inhalation and one exhalation equal one respiration.
- Most respiration occurs involuntarily, under the direction of the medulla oblongata in the brain.

STUDENT PORTFOLIO ACTIVITY

Clients use the Internet as a source of health information. Begin to explore Web sites for health information. Keep a list of sites you have explored and note which yield useful health information. The medical assistant should be aware of the major health information resources used by many clients. Your list demonstrates to an employer that you are staying current with available resources and will be able to work with and respond to clients' knowledge base.

APPLYING YOUR SKILLS

A client complains to you that in cold weather, he always starts coughing after being outside for a few minutes. What questions would you, as a medical assistant, ask this client? What would you explain about the mechanics of breathing? What steps could the client take to lessen his coughing when he is outdoors in the cold weather?

CRITICAL THINKING QUESTIONS

1. How are the cardiovascular system and nervous system related to the respiratory system?

2. Why is the larynx called the voice box? How is sound produced?

3. How does the respiratory system keep food out of the larynx?

4. Explain the mechanics of breathing.

5. When a person has a respiratory infection, why might his voice sound different?

6. Explain the difference between internal and external respiration. Where does each take place?

7. The respiratory and cardiovascular systems are closely related. If a client has difficulty exchanging carbon dioxide and oxygen in the alveoli of the lungs, how will this affect the cardiovascular system?

8. What role does the diaphragm have in respiration?

9. If a client has an upper respiratory infection, why do the sinuses often become involved?

10. Why do females usually have higher-pitched voices than men?

11. Explain the statement that respiration is both a voluntary and an involuntary activity.

12. Go back to the beginning of this chapter and review the Anticipatory Statements. Reread each statement and then indicate whether it is true or false. If the statement is false, rewrite it to make it a true statement.

CLIENT TEACHING PLAN

Measurement of Peak Flow

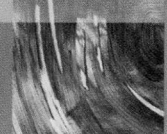

What Is to Be Taught:

- Measurement of peak expiratory flow rate (PEFR); measures the speed at which air can be expelled from the lungs after a deep breath is taken.

Objectives:

- Client will measure his own peak flow using a home monitoring instrument.

Preparation Before Teaching:

- Review lung function and how it relates to the breathing process and common client disorders. Remember to put technical medical terms into everyday language.
- Get a peak flow meter to use for teaching purposes, along with paper, pen, and printed materials or pictures of the lungs to aid in teaching about lung function.

Steps for the Medical Assistant:

1. Wash your hands.
2. Introduce yourself to the client.
3. Explain what you are going to teach and why.
4. Inform the client that good lung function is critical to a healthy respiratory system. Many factors, including allergic reactions, air or environmental pollutants, or an impending asthma attack, can affect breathing.
5. Explain to the client that by learning to use a peak flow meter at home, he can participate in his own health care.
6. Inform the client that even small changes in lung function can be picked up by the meter, often before they are noticed by the person.
7. Show the meter to the client. Demonstrate how the mouthpiece fits on and what the numbers on the side mean.
8. Move the small sliding indicator button to the bottom of the scale. It must always be in this position before the instrument is used.

9. Show the client how to hold the meter. The fingers should not be on the sliding indicator button, because they will keep the sliding button from moving. The fingers must also not block the opening.
10. Ask the client to stand.
11. Tell the client to inhale as deeply as possible, put the mouthpiece into the mouth (farther in than the teeth), and form a tight seal with the lips around the mouthpiece. The client should not bite down on the mouthpiece.
12. Instruct the client to blow out air as fast and as hard as possible. This should be quite a strong action. The sliding indicator will move down the scale.
13. Ask the client to take the meter out of his mouth.
14. Read the number where the sliding indicator button stopped. Write this number on a piece of paper.
15. Rest one minute.
16. Repeat the steps.
17. Read the number where the sliding indicator button stopped on the second attempt. Write this number on the paper.
18. Ask the client to keep a record of the results of use of the peak flow meter. Note the date and time and breathing symptoms, if any. Record the highest number obtained.
19. Instruct the client to keep a record of the peak flows. This will help the doctor and client to respond to any changes.
20. Instruct the client that if he has any breathing difficulties, such as coughing, wheezing, or tightness in the chest, call the doctor even if the numbers have not gone down.
21. Ask the client if he has any questions.

Special Needs of the Client:

- Check the client's chart to see if there are any factors that might interfere with his ability to perform this procedure and follow directions.

(Continues)

CLIENT TEACHING PLAN (Continued)

- Ask the client if there is anything you should know that might affect his ability to perform this activity.

▪ Evaluation:

- Client will be able to explain the purpose of measuring peak flow.
- Client will be able to correctly demonstrate the steps for using the meter.

▪ Further Plans/Teaching:

- Give written instructions to the client for use at home.
- Write down the telephone number of the medical office and tell the client to call if he has any questions or problems.

▪ Follow-up:

- Call the client at home in a few days and ask if he has any concerns.

- Ask the client to read to you the numbers that he recorded for the last few days.
- Inform the doctor of the client's peak flow readings.

Medical Assistant

Name: _____

Signature: _____

Date: _____

Client

Date: _____

Follow-up Date : _____

CHAPTER 16

Anticipatory Statements

People have different ideas about how the digestive system functions and what happens in each part of the system. Read and think about the following statements based upon what you believe now. Decide whether you agree or disagree. Write the word **agree** after the statement if you think the statement is true. Write the word **disagree** after the statement if you think the statement is false. Read the chapter to find out if your current beliefs can be supported.

1. Digestion begins in the mouth. _____

2. Healthy teeth and gums are not important to the process of digestion. _____

3. Most materials are absorbed in the small intestine. _____

4. Water is absorbed from the solid waste material in the large intestine. _____

5. It is important to have a bowel movement every day. _____

Learning Objectives

Upon completion of this chapter, the medical assistant student should be able to:

- Identify the organs of the digestive system
- Identify the accessory organs of the digestive system
- Trace the path of food from its entry into the digestive system to the elimination of waste products
- List five functions of the liver
- Describe what takes place in the small intestine
- Describe what takes place in the large intestine

Digestive System

- Define metabolism
- State five factors that affect metabolism
- Explain the functions of the digestive system
- Teach another person steps to prevent constipation

Key Terms

absorption Process by which a substance is taken in and used.

colon Part of the large intestine that extends from the cecum to the rectum.

digestion Process of breaking down food into smaller and simpler parts that can be used by the body.

elimination Act of releasing or getting rid of waste products from the body.

esophagus Connects the pharynx (throat) to the stomach.

gallbladder Organ found underneath the liver; stores bile.

hydrochloric acid Secreted in the stomach; aids in the digestion of protein and kills bacteria.

large intestine Extends from the small intestine to the outside of the body at the anus.

liver Organ found in the upper right part of the abdominal cavity; has many vital functions.

metabolism Process of chemical changes in the body as energy is used and new material is taken in and broken down for use as fuel for the body.

pancreas Gland that has both endocrine and exocrine functions.

salivary gland Releases saliva.

stomach Organ found in the upper left part of the abdominal cavity; receives food, helps to break it down, and moves it to the small intestine.

tongue Muscle that takes part in digestion; has taste buds and is critical for speech.

■ INTRODUCTION

The digestive system is responsible for completing an activity that takes place several times a day: namely, eating and drinking. Eating and drinking are important *activities of daily living* (ADLs). ADLs are conscious activities that a person must do to sustain life. If a person cannot do ADLs by herself, others must help. Eating is not merely an activity to sustain life, though. It also plays a part in religion, culture, and society. Each of these influences what a person eats or the way in which it is eaten. The type and amount of food and drink affect an individual's health. Intake and nutrition also affect the outcome of health disorders.

A medical assistant will work with clients regarding eating and its effect on health. For a medical assistant to be able to do this, she must first understand the functions of the organs and the digestive system as a whole.

■ ORGANS OF THE DIGESTIVE SYSTEM

Several organs and accessory or helper organs, working together, provide for smooth functioning of the digestive system. Anything that affects one organ will in turn affect the other organs. The major parts of the digestive system are: mouth, teeth, tongue, salivary glands, pharynx, esophagus, stomach, small intestine, and large intestine (Figure 16-1). The liver, gallbladder, and pancreas are the vital accessory organs.

Mouth, Teeth, and Tongue

The mouth is the first part of the digestive system. Within the mouth are the teeth and a **tongue** (Figure 16-2). When a person takes food or drink and puts it in the mouth, the person experiences several sensations. She notices the consistency, or thickness, of the food or drink: Is the liquid like water, or is it thick, like a milkshake? Is the soup thin, like a broth, or thick, like a creamy soup? She notices the texture of food. When a baby is introduced to new foods, the baby often needs time to develop a liking for

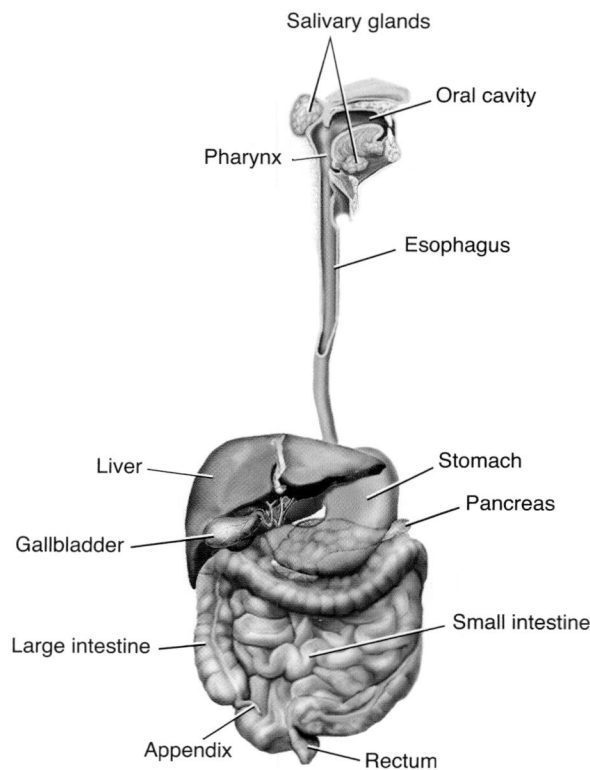

FIGURE 16-1 Structures of the digestive system.

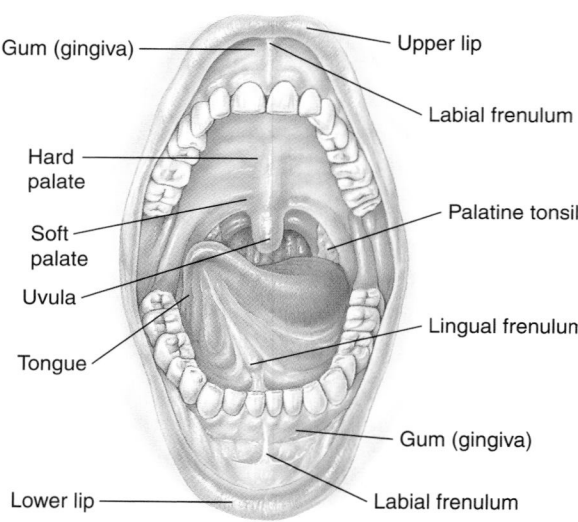

FIGURE 16-2 The mouth and surrounding structures.

certain textures, and might resist a new food for a while.

People can also tell how food tastes. They are able to tell the difference between sweet, sour, salty, and bitter. This is possible because of the taste buds on the tongue. The taste buds contain receptors to pick up tastes. The tip of the tongue notes sweet. Sour is tasted on both sides of the tongue, whereas salty can be perceived on both sides as well as the tip. Bitterness is most notable on the back of the tongue. A person's perception of food and willingness to eat are often based on these sensations. As a person ages, the sensitivity of the taste buds decreases. The sensation of taste is also affected by the sensation of smell. If a client has a cold, the senses of smell and taste are likely to be diminished. The client who has a sinus infection sometimes complains of a "bad taste."

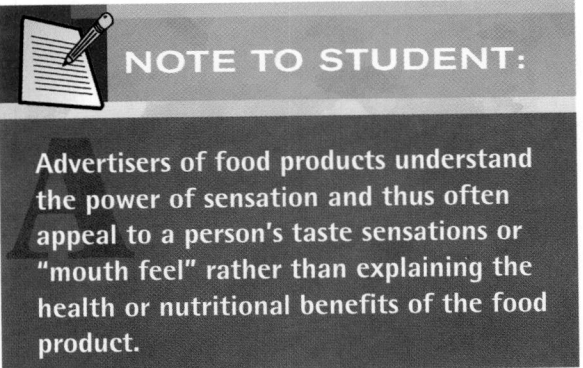

NOTE TO STUDENT:

Advertisers of food products understand the power of sensation and thus often appeal to a person's taste sensations or "mouth feel" rather than explaining the health or nutritional benefits of the food product.

The teeth help in the process of **digestion** by enabling us to break the food down into smaller parts, thus allowing it to continue on its way through the digestive tract. The teeth are supported and protected by the gums, also called *gingivae.* Good oral hygiene is essential to keep the gums healthy. Without healthy gums, the teeth will deteriorate. Gum disease (also called *gingivitis* or *periodontal disease*) is one of the most common reasons for loss of teeth in the older person.

Salivary Glands

Salivary glands are found in the mouth (Figure 16-3). The three major pairs of glands are the parotid, sublingual, and submandibular glands. The *parotid glands* are found below the ear. The *sublingual glands* are found below the tongue (*sub* means "below"). The *submandibular glands* are found below the mandible (jaw). The salivary glands secrete saliva that contains mucus and enzymes. The enzymes are chemicals that aid in the breakdown of food for digestion.

Pharynx, Esophagus

The *pharynx* or throat is the common passageway for air and food. The mouth swallows food, and the pharynx helps to propel the food (drives the food onward) further through the digestive

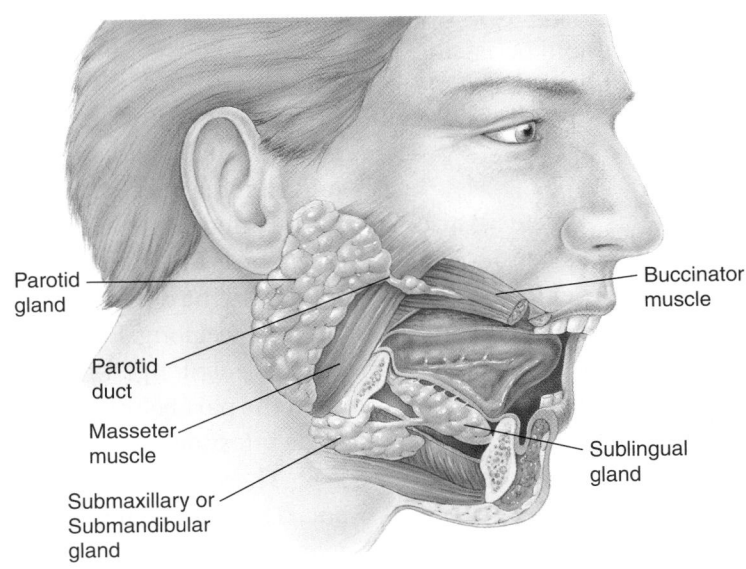

Parotid gland
Parotid duct
Masseter muscle
Submaxillary or Submandibular gland
Buccinator muscle
Sublingual gland

FIGURE 16-3 The salivary glands.

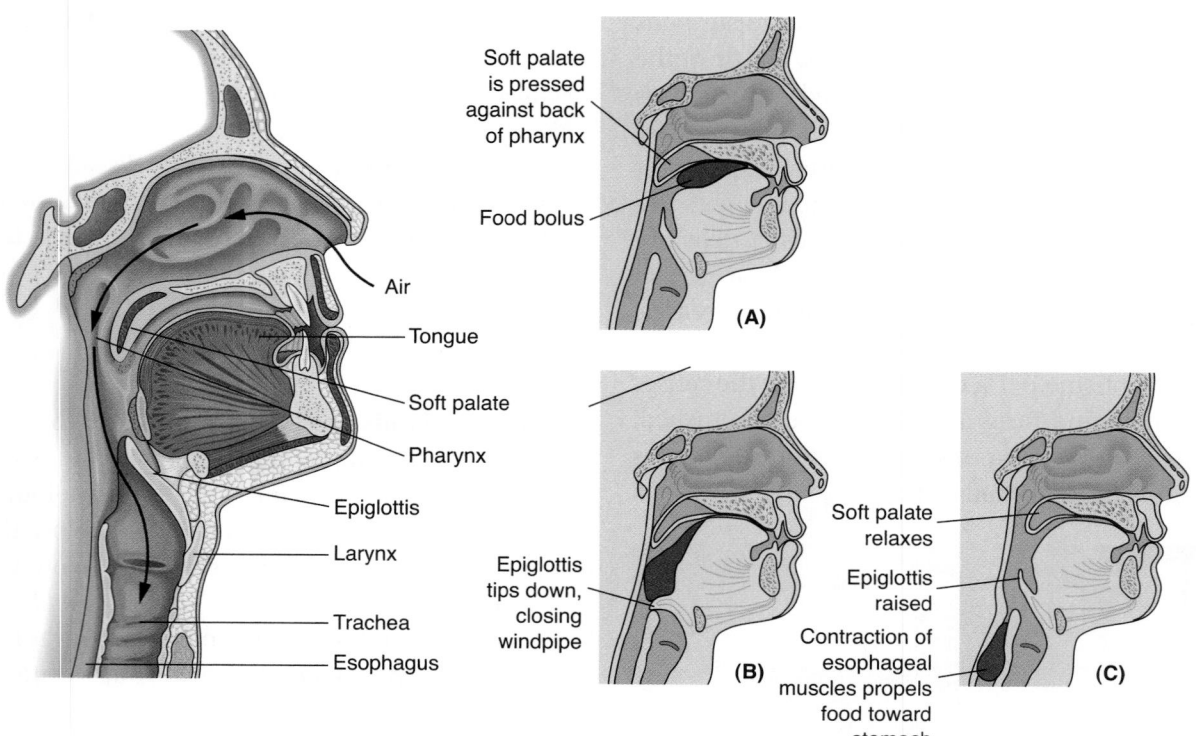

Soft palate is pressed against back of pharynx

Food bolus

(A)

Air

Tongue

Soft palate

Pharynx

Epiglottis

Larynx

Trachea

Esophagus

Epiglottis tips down, closing windpipe

(B)

Soft palate relaxes

Epiglottis raised

Contraction of esophageal muscles propels food toward stomach

(C)

FIGURE 16–4 Steps in swallowing.

tract (Figure 16-4). The **esophagus,** a muscular tube about 12 inches long, ends at the upper portion of the stomach, called the *cardiac portion* of the stomach. This upper part of the stomach is found near the end of the sternum at the xiphoid process. The esophagus produces propelling waves called *peristalsis,* which move the food onward toward the stomach. A person is not consciously aware of this propulsion; peristaltic waves are under involuntary control.

Stomach

In the **stomach,** gastric glands secrete gastric juice. Chemical substances such as pepsinogen are secreted, in addition to **hydrochloric acid.** Mucous cells in the stomach secrete mucus. All of these secretions aid in the process of digestion. The stomach acts as a holding place while these forces are at work, and then the stomach gradually empties. Hormonal secretions and nervous system controls are responsible for the movement of food from the stomach into the small intestine. Very little digestion or absorp-

tion actually takes place within the stomach. However, water and alcohol are absorbed at this point.

Small Intestine

The next part of the journey of food along the digestive tract is the small intestine. The small intestine can be divided into three parts. The first part is the *duodenum,* which is from 8 to 11 inches long. The common bile duct brings bile from the gallbladder, secretions from the liver, and pancreatic juices from the pancreas to enter at the duodenum. The second part of the small intestine is the *jejunum,* which is about nine feet long. The third part is the *ileum,* which is more than 13 feet long. Each part of the intestine gets successively longer; that, is each part is longer than the part before it. The ileum opens into the large intestine.

The small intestine is lined with folds of tissue. These folds increase the surface area that can absorb the end products of digestion. These folds end in projections that look like fingers and are called *villi*. Each villus has capillaries that absorb the end products of digestion, such as amino acids, fatty acids, glycerol, vitamins, minerals, and water. **Absorption** of nutrients from food, and the movement of matter along to the large intestine, are the major activities of the small intestine. Most digestion and absorption of nutrients takes place here.

Large Intestine

The **large intestine** goes from the ileum of the small intestine to the anus. The *anus* is the opening to the outside of the body. The large intestine is about five feet in length. The purpose of the large intestine is to absorb water, some minerals, and some vitamins; it also helps to move along and get rid of waste material from the process of digestion. It does this through the process of *defecation*.

The large intestine can be divided into parts (Figure 16-5). The first part, the cecum, is where the ileum enters. The ascending **colon** extends

from the cecum, goes under the liver, then turns left and becomes transverse. *Transverse* means "horizontal," and this part of the large intestine travels across, and then turns down. When it turns downward, it becomes the part called the *descending colon*. The descending colon ends in an S-shaped portion, which is called the *sigmoid colon*. The straight part of the intestine at the end of the sigmoid colon is called the *rectum*. The rectum is four to five inches long. The last inch is called the *anal canal*, which opens into the anus.

The Anal Canal. The anal canal is the last part of the large intestine, and opens into the anus. Within the anal canal is an internal (inside) sphincter of muscle. There is also an external sphincter of voluntary muscle. Both of these muscles aid in the process of defecation, which is the **elimination** of solid wastes. In other words, the process gets the waste products out of the body. Defecation is both a voluntary and an involuntary process. People may call the act of defecation "having a bowel movement." When

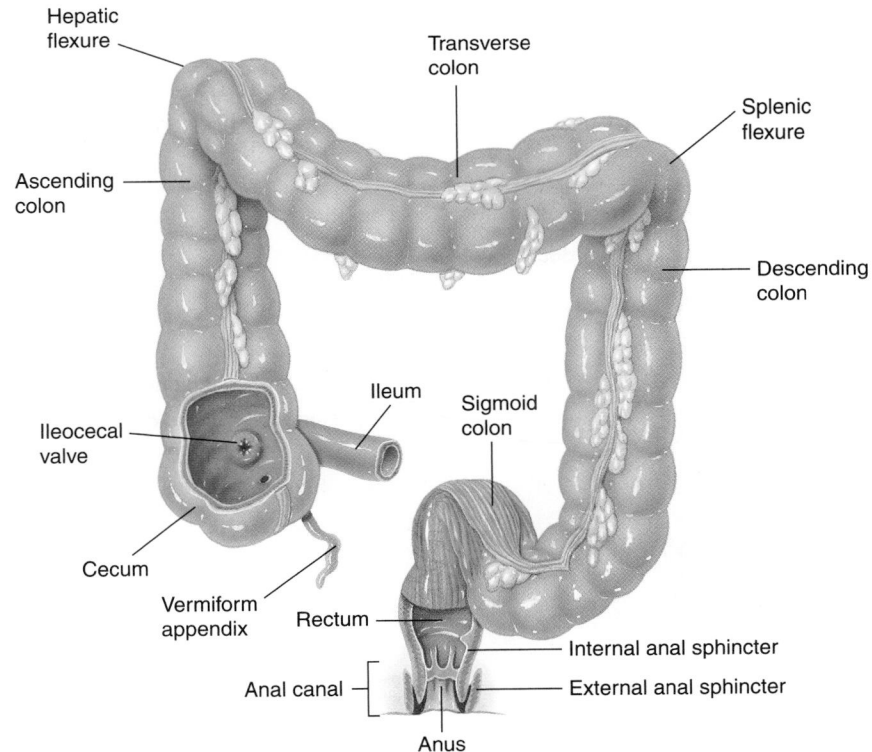

FIGURE 16-5 The large intestine.

the rectum becomes distended, a reflex is triggered. The impulse travels to the spine, then the spinal cord sends an impulse to the rectal area. In response to this signal, the rectal muscles contract and the internal sphincter relaxes and the fecal matter or waste material comes out. To allow this, the external sphincter must also relax. The external sphincter is under voluntary control, so a person can delay the bowel movement. The act of having a bowel movement is thus both an involuntary and a voluntary act.

■ ACCESSORY ORGANS

The accessory organs of the pancreas, liver, and gallbladder play a vital role in the digestion of food (Figure 16-6). The **pancreas** secretes digestive juices, which travel through the pancreatic duct to enter the duodenum of the small intestine. The powerful enzymes of the liver help to digest all food types, while the gallbladder releases bile.

Liver

The **liver** is the largest solid organ in the body (Figure 16-7). The liver, which is necessary for life, performs many vital functions. Among these functions is the production of bile, which

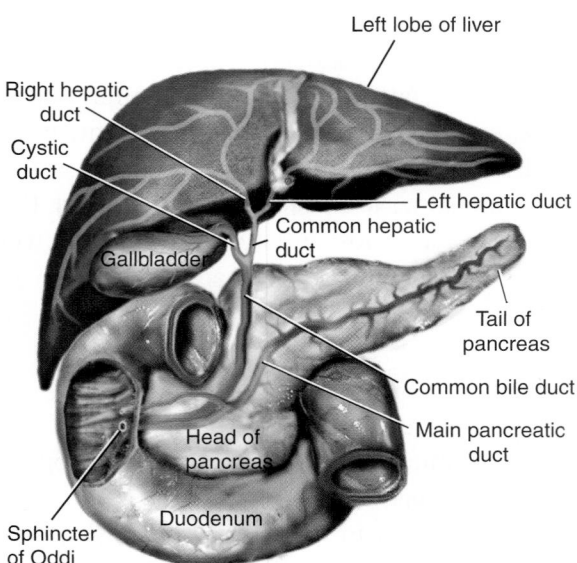

FIGURE 16–6 The liver, gallbladder, and pancreas.

is necessary to digest fats. The bile contains salts, pigments, bilirubin, cholesterol, and some electrolytes. The hepatic bile duct combines with the cystic duct in the gallbladder to form the common bile duct. This common bile duct carries bile from both organs to the small intestine through the duodenum. The liver also stores glycogen, which is a form of glucose, for use when the body requires it.

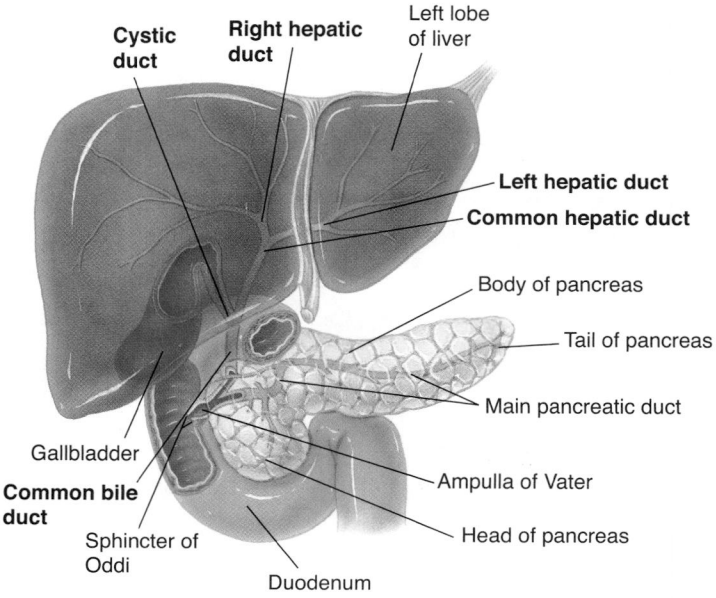

FIGURE 16–7 The anatomy of the liver.

The liver manufactures proteins that are critical for blood clotting: heparin, fibrogen, prothrombin, thrombin, and globulin. Thrombin maintains the fluid balance in the body. Globulin is critical for the body's immunity and its defenses against infection. The breakdown of amino acids results in waste products, such as ammonia. The liver also helps to produce urea, which is the chief waste product from the breakdown of amino acids from protein metabolism. The liver also stores minerals and fat-soluble vitamins (A, D, E, and K, as well as the B complex vitamins). Red blood cells and white blood cells that are no longer viable are phagocytosed or eaten by cells in the liver.

Gallbladder

The gallbladder is found on the right lobe of the liver. The gallbladder stores bile that has come from the liver. The cystic duct from the gallbladder lines up with the hepatic duct and from there the bile empties into the duodenum. When food enters the small intestine, the **gallbladder** releases the stored bile that is needed for digestion.

■ METABOLISM

Metabolism is the term for the physical and chemical changes in the body. During the process of metabolism, energy is produced for activities of the body, and new matter is gained. The two parts of metabolism are catabolism and anabolism. During *catabolism*, food is broken down into useable forms. Water, heat, carbon dioxide, and energy are produced by this breakdown. The products of catabolism are used to build and repair the cells of the body. This process is called *anabolism*. The basal metabolism (*basal* means "base" or "basic") of a person is the amount of energy the person uses at rest.

 BRIDGE TO CAAHEP

This chapter, which discusses the digestive system, provides information and content related to CAAHEP standards for Anatomy and Physiology, Medical Terminology, Communication, Medical Assisting Clinical Procedures, and Professional Components.

POINTS OF HIGHLIGHT

- The major functions of the digestive system are digestion, absorption, and elimination.
- The mouth, teeth, tongue, salivary glands, pharynx, esophagus, stomach, small intestine, and large intestine are the major parts of the digestive system.
- The pancreas, liver, and gallbladder are accessory organs of digestion.
- Food enters at the mouth, where it is broken down into smaller parts and begins to be changed into a useable form.
- The pharynx is the common passageway for food and air.
- Most digestion and absorption of nutrients takes place in the small intestine.
- The large intestine absorbs water and gets waste material (stool, fecal matter) ready for elimination from the body.
- Defecation (elimination of waste) is both a voluntary and involuntary process.
- Medical assistants work with clients to promote good digestion through teaching of healthful eating behaviors.

ABHES LINKS

This chapter, which discusses the digestive system, links to ABHES course content for Anatomy and Physiology, Medical Terminology, Medical Law and Ethics, and Medical Office Clinical Procedures.

AAMA AREAS OF COMPETENCE

This chapter, which discusses the digestive system, provides information or content within several areas listed in the Medical Assistant Role Delineation Study. These areas include: clinical, fundamental principles, patient (client) care, general transdisciplinary, communication, legal concepts, and instruction.

AMT PATHS

This chapter, which discusses the digestive system, provides a path to AMT competency in general medical assisting knowledge, anatomy and physiology, medical terminology, and patient (client) education.

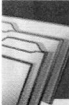
STUDENT PORTFOLIO ACTIVITY

Leadership is a criterion for medical assistants above the entry level, on the way to advanced-level medical assisting. As a student, you can develop leadership potential. Join a school organization. If there is a club for medical assisting students on the school campus, check it out! Explore student government or other college groups as a way to become a leader. A person who is active in student organizations is more likely to use these skills in the workplace.

APPLYING YOUR SKILLS

As part of your interaction with a client, you ask about dental care and visits to the dentist. The client states that teeth are not important; she will just get dentures eventually and not worry about it. What questions would you ask? What can you explain about the role of the mouth, teeth, and gums in the entire digestive process and in the client's health?

CRITICAL THINKING QUESTIONS

1. What is the role of teeth in mechanical digestion, and how do the teeth affect the ability to eat?

2. Why is it important for a client to practice good oral hygiene? What effect will this have on digestion?

3. The liver is a helper organ for digestion. Explain the important functions of the liver and how they are essential to life.

4. Explain how the act of defecation is both an involuntary and voluntary process.

5. Why are the liver, gallbladder, and pancreas all called accessory organs? How do they aid in the process of digestion?

6. Explain the role of the large intestine in the digestive process.

7. How does the large intestine help to rid the body of waste products?

8. How is the small intestine vital to deriving nutritional benefits from food?

9. What happens to food once it reaches the stomach?

10. What is peristalsis, and why is it critical to the digestion of food?

11. Go back to the beginning of this chapter and review the Anticipatory Statements. Reread each statement and then indicate whether it is true or false. If the statement is false, rewrite it to make it a true statement.

CLIENT TEACHING PLAN

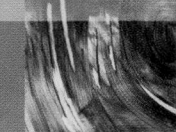

Prevention of Chronic Constipation

▪ What Is to Be Taught:

- Ways to encourage healthy bowel habits.

▪ Objectives:

- Client will take steps to practice healthy bowel habits and prevent chronic constipation.

▪ Preparation Before Teaching:

- Review information about the causes of constipation and ways to promote healthy bowel habits.
- Get together printed material about healthy food choices and exercises; find diagrams of the digestive system to help illustrate your teaching.
- Make sure the area is free from distractions while you are teaching.

▪ Steps for the Medical Assistant:

1. Wash your hands.
2. Get supplies needed.
3. Introduce yourself to the client.
4. Explain what you are going to teach and why.
5. Tell the client about the digestive system, using simple words. (For example, "Food is taken in and broken down into useable parts. The body uses what it needs, stores some for future use, and gets rid of solid wastes through a bowel movement. The solid waste is called *feces* or *stool*.")
6. Tell the client that she can take steps to help this bodily function work smoothly.
7. Using printed material, if available, share the following information with the client:
   a. Drink plenty of water (at least eight glasses per day). This will add water to the intestine and help prevent hard stools.
   b. Add fiber to the diet, especially whole grains such as oatmeal and whole-grain bread.
   c. Eat fresh fruits and vegetables daily.
   d. Exercise. Any activity, even just increasing one's everyday activity level a little, will help normal activity of the digestive system and move waste materials along.
8. Give the client a form to be used as a diet and activity diary.
9. Review with the client how to complete the form and what is to be included on it.
10. Ask the client to fill in the parts of the form that she is able to complete.
11. Ask questions about what you have taught regarding the digestive system, food, and activities. Help the client as needed. Remember, you do not want the client to perceive this as a test. Rather, you are trying to assist the client to assume a role in her own health care.

▪ Special Needs of the Client:

- Check the client's chart to see if there are any factors that might interfere with her ability to implement and carry out the plan.

▪ Evaluation:

- Client is able to list the types of food to include in a diet to promote digestive health.
- Client is able to suggest ways of increasing her activity level in her everyday life.

▪ Further Plans/Teaching:

- Give written information to the client to refer to at home.
- Remind the client to call if she has any questions or concerns. Make sure that the client has the phone number and your extension.

▪ Follow-up:

- Call the client at the end of a week and ask what parts of the teaching she has been able to fit into her daily life.
- Give encouragement even if the client has been able to do only a small amount.
- Review the diary with the client at the next office visit.

(Continues)

CLIENT TEACHING PLAN (Continued)

Medical Assistant

Name: _____

Signature: _____

Date: _____

Client

Date: _____

Follow-up Date : _____

CHAPTER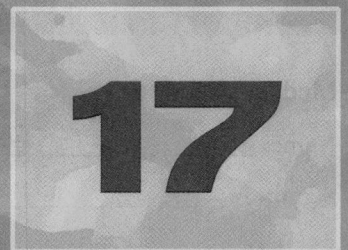

Anticipatory Statements

People have various levels of understanding about the urinary system. Read and think about the following statements based upon what you believe now. Decide whether you agree or disagree. Write the word **agree** after the statement if you think the statement is true. Write the word **disagree** after the statement if you think the statement is false. Read the chapter to find out if your current beliefs can be supported.

1. A person cannot live with only one working kidney.   _____

2. In the male, the urethra's only function is to carry urine to the outside of the body.   _____

3. Drinking lots of water will make the urine look dark yellow.   _____

4. The kidneys are bean-shaped organs found toward the back of the body on either side of the vertebral column.   _____

5. On a hot day, when a person perspires heavily, less urine will be expelled.   _____

Urinary System

Learning Objectives

Upon completion of this chapter, the medical assistant student should be able to:

- List the structures of the urinary system
- Explain the functions of the urinary system
- Describe the urinary bladder and its purpose
- Identify the role of the kidneys in blood pressure control
- Explain how urine is formed
- Describe the normal characteristics of urine
- Trace the pathway of urine from formation to elimination from the body

Key Terms

bladder Hollow, muscular organ that holds urine until the urine is released from the body.

glomerular filtration Action of the kidneys that strains or filters blood.

kidneys Organs important in waste removal, in the production of urine, and in the maintenance of homeostasis.

nephron Functional or working part of the kidneys.

pubic symphysis Also called *pelvic girdle;* place where the bones come together at the front of the pelvic region.

tubular reabsorption Return of blood to the general circulation after filtration by the kidneys.

tubular secretion Addition of material into the urine after filtration and maximum reabsorption.

ureter Narrow tube that carries urine from the kidneys to the bladder. There are two ureters.

urethra Tube that carries urine to the outside of the body.

urinary meatus Opening that allows urine to exit the body from the urethra.

void To release urine from the body.

■ INTRODUCTION

The urinary system is the body system that filters the blood, regulates fluid and electrolyte balance, and rids the body of liquid waste material, in the form of urine. The urinary system works with other systems. The respiratory system functions for elimination of waste material primarily ridding the body of carbon dioxide, although some water and nitrogenous wastes are also gotten rid of during respiration. The integumentary system assists in waste removal through perspiration. The digestive system rids the body of solid waste material after digestion. However, the urinary system plays the major role in filtration and waste removal.

■ PARTS OF THE URINARY SYSTEM

The structure of the urinary system is relatively simple, with only four main parts: two kidneys, two ureters, the urinary bladder, and the urethra (Figure 17-1).

Kidney

The body has two **kidneys.** Each is shaped like a kidney bean, and they are found in the back of the body on either side of the vertebral col-

umn, just below the waist. The kidneys lie against the deep muscles of the back. Connective tissue holds the kidneys in place, and surrounding adipose (fat) tissue protects the kidneys from damage that might occur from a strike, blow, or trauma to the person's back. The kidneys are only a few inches wide and four to five inches long—about the size of an adult's fist.

The lateral (away from the middle) side of this bean-shaped organ is *convex,* meaning that it bulges out. The medial (near the middle) side of the kidney is *concave,* meaning that it bends in. The outer part of the kidney is called the *cortex;* the inner part is called the *medulla* (Figure 17-2).

Blood, lymph, nerves, and ureters connect with the kidneys in the concave medial side of the kidneys. The kidneys are supplied with blood by the renal arteries. Each minute, about 1,200 mL of blood goes into the renal arteries. This large amount is nearly 25% of the total cardiac output. Cardiovascular functioning and kidney functioning are interdependent, affecting not only the filtration of blood but also the blood pressure.

Each kidney contains approximately 1 million functional units called **nephrons** (Figure 17-3). Not all the nephrons work at the same time. If one kidney stops functioning, additional nephrons in the other kidney can take over.

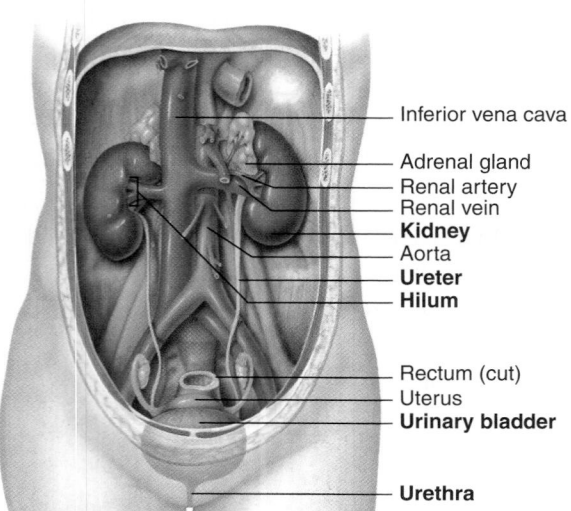

FIGURE 17-1 The organs of the urinary system.

Labels: Inferior vena cava; Adrenal gland; Renal artery; Renal vein; **Kidney**; Aorta; **Ureter**; **Hilum**; Rectum (cut); Uterus; **Urinary bladder**; **Urethra**

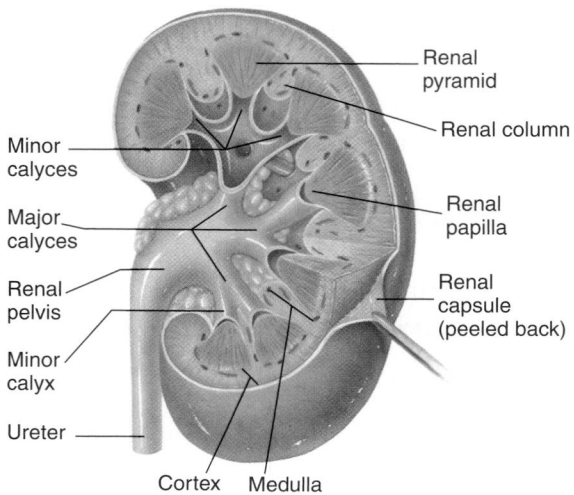

FIGURE 17-2 Internal structure of a kidney.

Labels: Renal pyramid; Renal column; Renal papilla; Renal capsule (peeled back); Minor calyces; Major calyces; Renal pelvis; Minor calyx; Ureter; Cortex; Medulla

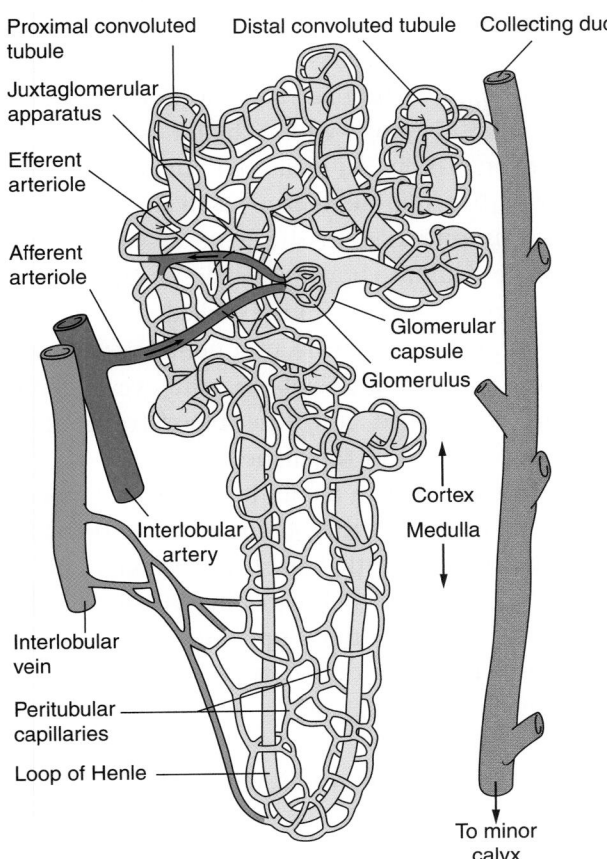

Proximal convoluted tubule
Distal convoluted tubule
Collecting duct
Juxtaglomerular apparatus
Efferent arteriole
Afferent arteriole
Glomerular capsule
Glomerulus
Cortex
Medulla
Interlobular artery
Interlobular vein
Peritubular capillaries
Loop of Henle
To minor calyx

FIGURE 17-3 The structure of a nephron.

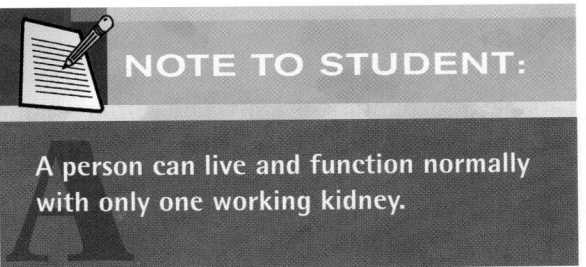

NOTE TO STUDENT:

A person can live and function normally with only one working kidney.

Ureters

The body contains two **ureters**. Each ureter is attached at the top end to a kidney and at the other end to the urinary bladder (Figure 17-4). Each ureter is a hollow, tube-like organ about 12 inches long, with a diameter of about half an inch. The ureters are the passageway through which urine travels from the kidneys to the urinary bladder. The ureter assists gravity by propelling the urine toward its destination with muscular contractions called *peristaltic waves*. A membrane flap at the entrance to the bladder permits urine to enter the bladder but not to flow backward. This is similar to the valves in the heart, which allow blood to flow in only one direction.

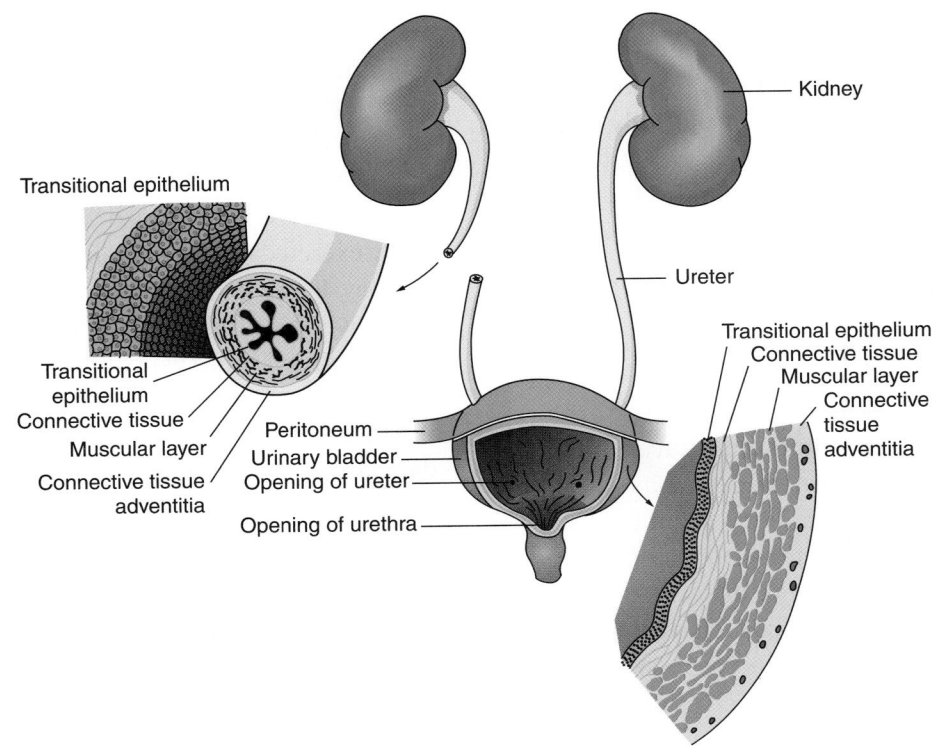

Transitional epithelium
Transitional epithelium
Connective tissue
Muscular layer
Connective tissue adventitia
Kidney
Ureter
Transitional epithelium
Connective tissue
Muscular layer
Connective tissue adventitia
Peritoneum
Urinary bladder
Opening of ureter
Opening of urethra

FIGURE 17-4 Ureters are connected to the kidney and urinary bladder.

Urinary Bladder

The urinary **bladder** is a hollow, muscular sac capable of expanding greatly. The urinary bladder is found behind the **pubic symphysis.** When the bladder is distended (filled or overfilled), it can be felt by placing the pads of the fingers on the lower abdominal wall just above the pubic hairline. The bladder has many folds or wrinkles, which smooth out as it fills with fluid. The purpose of the urinary bladder is to store the urine until the urine is expelled from the body. An adult usually feels the urge to **void** (urinate) when the bladder holds 200 mL of urine. It is possible for the bladder of an adult to hold as much as 800 to 1,000 mL of urine. However, the bladder would be quite distended at this point and the client would be uncomfortable.

Urethra

The **urethra** is a tube connected to the urinary bladder that extends to the outside of the body. The endpoint of the urethra, which opens at the outside of the body, is called the **urinary meatus.** Smooth muscle and mucous membranes line the urethral tube. In females, the urethra is about 1 1/2 inches long, and its only purpose is to carry urine to the outside of the body. In males, the urethra is about 8 inches long. It too carries urine to the outside of the body, but it is also part of the male reproductive system and carries semen as well. Special muscles prevent semen and urine from traveling through the urethra at the same time.

■ PRODUCTION OF URINE

To assist clients in maintaining healthy urinary systems, medical assistant must have an understanding of urine formation and its pathway through the body before elimination.

Urine contains water, waste products, and electrolytes. The majority of urine (90%) is composed of water. Waste products make up the remaining 10%. The waste products found in urine include urea, uric acid, creatinine, ammonia, sodium, chloride, calcium, magnesium, potassium, phosphate, and sulfate.

The production of urine is a process with three steps: glomerular filtration, tubular reabsorption, and tubular secretion. **Glomerular filtration** begins when blood enters the nephron. The blood is filtered during this step. During the **tubular reabsorption** step, cleansed blood is returned to the general circulation. There is a limit to how much can be reabsorbed; anything over this limit is expelled in the urine. The final step in urine production is **tubular secretion.** During this phase, whatever has not been reabsorbed into the bloodstream gets excreted as part of the urine.

Urine flows in a definite pathway. Urine is formed in the kidneys. It then travels through the two ureters until it reaches the urinary bladder. Urine is stored in the urinary bladder until a certain amount builds up. The urine is then released into the urethra, where it travels to the outside of the body.

Factors That Influence the Amount of Urine

An adult voids from 700 to 2,000 mL of urine each day. Certain factors can increase or decrease the amount a person voids each day. How much fluid a person drinks will affect the amount. The more fluids a person takes in, the more urine will be voided. Some medications, such as diuretics, also increase the amount of urine expelled. The amount of urine excreted also depends on how much water and waste are being excreted through other systems. On a very hot day, if the person is perspiring heavily, less urine will be produced and eliminated. Rapid breathing will cause water vapor to exit through the lungs, and thus reduce the amount of urine. Fever, vomiting, and diarrhea will all cause a decrease in the amount of urine expelled.

Appearance

Normal urine has a range of yellow color. Whatever the shade, from almost colorless to light straw, to straw to light amber, to amber to dark amber, normal urine is clear, with no cloudiness, mucus, or particles in it. Freshly voided urine has a slight odor. Strong odor, cloudiness, or a color other than a tone of yellow all indicate a possible abnormality (see Chapter 41).

■ OTHER FUNCTIONS OF THE URINARY SYSTEM

In addition to the production of urine and waste removal, the urinary system performs other functions. It works with other body systems to maintain blood volume, concentration, and pH (acid) balance. This balance is called *homeostasis*. The kidneys produce renin, an enzyme that helps to keep blood pressure within a normal range. Through the production of erythropoietin, the making of red blood cells is encouraged. Vitamin D is also activated by these other functions of the kidneys.

To summarize, the urinary system plays a vital role in many life processes. It rids the body of excess water and waste in the form of urine. It helps to maintain homeostasis or balance. Blood pressure maintenance is supported and regulated in part by the urinary system. Through an understanding of the components of the urinary system and how they work, the medical assistant can help the client with urinary health.

The medical assistant can teach and aid the client in practicing healthy behaviors, which will help the urinary system to function smoothly. Some healthy behaviors are relatively easy to include in a daily routine. Drinking an adequate amount of water can keep the body well hydrated; the amount needed depends partially on the amount of activity and surrounding temperature. Water is critical, because it is used as the kidneys filter the blood and get rid of toxins. A person should not try to hold the urine for a long time. Retention (allowing the urine to remain in the bladder for an extended period) puts a person at risk of infection.

BRIDGE TO CAAHEP

This chapter, which discusses the urinary system and the production of urine, provides information and content related to CAAHEP standards for Anatomy and Physiology, Medical Terminology, Communication, Medical Assisting Clinical Procedures, and Professional Components.

POINTS OF HIGHLIGHT

- The kidneys, ureters, urinary bladder, and urethra are the main structures of the urinary system.
- 25% of the total cardiac output filters through the kidneys each minute.
- Kidney function and cardiovascular function are closely linked, affecting both the filtration of blood and the blood pressure.
- Two ureters are the passageway through which urine travels from the kidneys to the bladder.
- The urinary bladder stores the urine until it is expelled. The bladder expands and is capable of holding up to 1,000 mL of urine.
- The urethra carries urine to the outside of the body. In the male, the urethra is also part of the reproductive system, and carries semen.
- Normal urine is clear, with a yellow color range and a slight odor.
- Urine formation is a three-step process, consisting of glomerular filtration, tubular reabsorption, and tubular secretion.
- The urinary system rids the body of waste and excess water in the form of urine, maintains homeostasis, and plays a role in maintaining blood pressure.

ABHES LINKS

This chapter, which discusses the urinary system and the production of urine, links to ABHES course content for Anatomy and Physiology, Medical Terminology, Medical Law and Ethics, and Medical Office Clinical Procedures.

 ## AAMA AREAS OF COMPETENCE

This chapter, which discusses the urinary system and the production of urine, provides information or content within several areas listed in the Medical Assistant Role Delineation Study. These areas include: clinical, fundamental principles, patient (client) care, general transdisciplinary, professionalism, communication skills, legal concepts, and instruction.

 ## AMT PATHS

This chapter, which discusses the urinary system and the production of urine, provides a path to AMT competency in general medical assisting knowledge, anatomy and physiology, medical terminology, and patient (client) education.

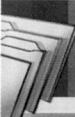 ### STUDENT PORTFOLIO ACTIVITY

Some of the technical skills that you learn in the classroom today will become obsolete in a few years. Medical assistants must keep up to date with new knowledge and technology. Attend a conference or inservice related to medical assisting or an aspect of health care. Be sure to sign in and receive a certificate of attendance to place in your portfolio as proof of professional development and continuing education.

 ### APPLYING YOUR SKILLS

The doctor asks you to teach a client some behaviors to encourage urinary health. The doctor has determined that the client does not have an infection or disorder. However, he has recently begun to notice that his urine is dark and has a strong odor. The client states that he drinks very little water, because he dislikes the taste. What would you tell this client about the working of the kidneys and the amount of water taken in? How would you encourage him to increase his daily intake of water?

CRITICAL THINKING QUESTIONS

1. What is the purpose of fat tissue around the kidneys? Briefly describe a situation in which these tissues would be helpful.

2. How is the working of the heart related to the working of the kidneys?

3. How does normal urine appear? What might alert you to a possible problem when you look at a urine sample?

4. What happens when one of a person's kidneys does not function?

5. What factors influence the amount of urine that a person voids each day? How do these factors affect the amount?

6. How does urine get from the kidneys to the urinary bladder?

7. What is the purpose of the urethra in the female? What is its purpose in the male?

8. Trace the steps involved in the formation of urine.

9. What is meant by the word filtration as it relates to the formation of urine?

10. What is the role of the kidneys in maintaining blood pressure?

11. Go back to the beginning of this chapter and review the Anticipatory Statements. Reread each statement and then indicate whether it is true or false. If the statement is false, rewrite it to make it a true statement.

CLIENT TEACHING PLAN

Bladder Control for Urinary Health

■ What Is to Be Taught:

- Steps to maintain bladder control for urinary health.

■ Objectives:

- Client will be able to state and follow steps to maintain bladder control for urinary health.

■ Preparation Before Teaching:

- Review information about the structure and working of the urinary system.
- Review factors that can affect the urinary bladder.
- Assemble teaching materials, such as a diagram of the urinary system, and paper and pen for written instructions.
- Make sure that the area is free from distractions while you are teaching.

■ Steps for the Medical Assistant:

1. Wash your hands.
2. Get together supplies needed.
3. Introduce yourself to the client.
4. Explain what you are going to teach and why.
5. Suggest to the client that she can participate in her own health care by following some steps for urinary health.
6. Show the client the diagram of the urinary system and trace the flow of urine from the kidneys where it is made, down through the ureters to the urinary bladder, where the urine is stored until it is expelled through the urethra to the outside of the body.
7. Tell the client that many factors, such as certain foods and drinks, smoking, and exercise, can all affect bladder control.
8. Inform the client that spicy foods and citrus foods, such as tomatoes and fruit juices, can irritate the bladder. Caffeine (found in coffee, tea, colas, and chocolate) and alcohol both act

as diuretics (causes the body to make and get rid of more urine). This means that the client has to go to the bathroom to void more frequently.

9. Explain how extra weight can put pressure on the bladder area and add to the feeling of need to urinate frequently. Suggest some ways to help keep a healthy weight through good eating habits and increase of physical activity.
10. Describe how smoking can affect bladder control. Nicotine causes bladder spasms, which signal the need to urinate to the body. Secondly, the cough that goes along with smoking weakens the pelvic muscles that support the internal structures, including the bladder.
11. Suggest to the client that she might be able to maintain a satisfactory interval between bathroom stops by slightly increasing the time between. If the client urinates every hour or hour and a half, maybe she could try to lengthen the time to one and a half to two hours. The client can do this very gradually, perhaps increasing the time by only 15 minutes. She should not make such a big increase as to cause worry about making it to the bathroom or having an "accident."
12. Tell the client to write in a little notebook each day whether she was able to increase urination interval time. Write in the times, whether successful or not.
13. Ask the client to bring the notebook to the next visit.
14. While both the client and the medical assistant are sitting down, instruct the client to imagine urinating and then to squeeze as if trying to stop the urine flow. The muscles felt are the ones the client should exercise, to help strengthen for better bladder control. (Do not squeeze the leg muscles or the stomach.)
15. Instruct the client to squeeze these muscles again and hold them tight, if she can, for

(Continues)

CLIENT TEACHING PLAN (Continued)

10 seconds. Ask her then to relax for 10 seconds. Instruct the client to do these exercises 10 times, at least three times a day. Inform her that these can be done while sitting anywhere.

16. Give written instructions to the client to use as a reference at home.

Special Needs of the Client:

- Check the client's chart to see if there are any factors that might interfere with the client's ability to follow these instructions for urinary health.
- Ask the client, before and after the teaching, if there is anything you should know that might affect her ability to perform these activities.

Evaluation:

- Client is able to tell you factors that affect bladder control and, as a result, urinary health.
- Client is able to perform the exercises.

Further Plans/Teaching:

- Ask the client if she has any questions or needs any additional information.

Follow-up:

- Call the client at home in a few days to see if she has any questions and if she has been able to put some of these activities into her daily routine.
- At the next office visit, review these teaching points with the client.
- Look at the client's notebook. Offer suggestions if the client has not been successful in increasing the interval time and encourage her to continue with the plan.

Medical Assistant

Name: _____

Signature: _____

Date: _____

Client

Date: _____

Follow-up Date : _____

CHAPTER 18

Anticipatory Statements

People hold different beliefs about the male reproductive system. Read and think about the following statements based upon what you believe now. Decide whether you agree or disagree. Write the word **agree** after the statement if you think the statement is true. Write the word **disagree** after the statement if you think the statement is false. Read the chapter to find out if your current beliefs can be supported.

1. The penis and the scrotum are the internal structures of the male reproductive system.

   _____

2. The foreskin is loose skin that covers the head of the penis.

   _____

3. Secondary sex characteristics in a male include chest hair and a low voice.

   _____

4. Sperm cells mature in the ejaculatory duct.

   _____

5. Male hormones and sperm need to stay at higher temperatures than the rest of the body.

   _____

Male Reproductive System

Learning Objectives

Upon completion of this chapter, the medical assistant student should be able to:

- List the structures of the male reproductive system
- Explain the role of the accessory glands
- Identify the effects of the hormone testosterone
- Explain the function of the male reproductive system
- Trace the movement of sperm through the reproductive system

Key Terms

bulbourethral glands Small glands found on either side of the urethra in males.

ductal system Stores and carries sperm.

epididymis Small, tubelike organ next to the testis; holds sperm during maturation.

penis Organ of copulation (sexual intercourse).

prostate gland Gland that encircles the upper end of the urethra in males, just below the bladder.

scrotum Saclike structure that holds the testes.

semen Thick, sticky fluid in which sperm cells move and are transported.

seminal vesicles Glands that make more than half the volume of semen.

spermatazoa (sperm) Male gamete or germ cell.

testis Male gonad (sex organ).

testosterone Hormone made by the testes.

vas deferens Also called *ductus deferens*; carries sperm from the epididymis to the ejaculatory duct.

■ INTRODUCTION

Working together, the male and female reproductive systems allow perpetuation (continuation) of the human species. A male's ability to reproduce begins with puberty. The male reproductive role is to fertilize the egg from a female. Some structures in the male have both urinary and reproductive functions. Medical assistants need to have an understanding of the structure and functioning of this system in preparation for clinical medical assisting.

■ THE MALE REPRODUCTIVE SYSTEM

The male reproductive system contains organs, structures, and hormones necessary for the production of children and perpetuation of the species (Figure 18-1). The reproductive system has both external and internal structures. The penis and the scrotum are the external structures. Internal structures include the testes, epididymis, vas deferens, urethra, seminal vesicles, bulbourethral glands, and prostate gland.

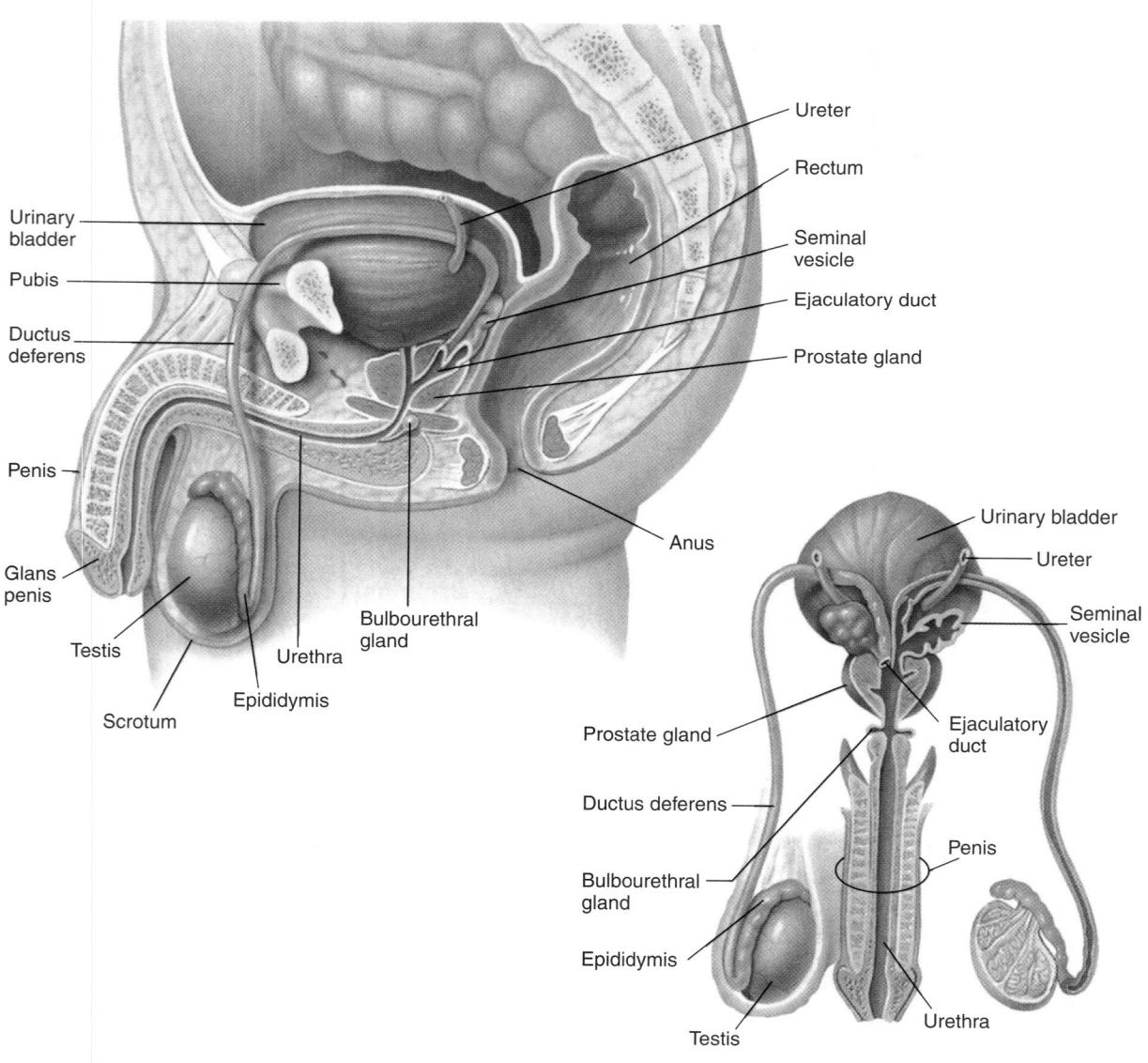

FIGURE 18-1 Organs and structures of the male reproductive system.

External Structures

The **scrotum** is a pouch or sac that contains the testes. It is made mainly of skin and fascia. On the outside it is a pouch with a distinct ridge or line that appears to divide it into two pouches. There is one testis in each half of the sac. Male hormones and sperm need to stay at a lower temperature than the rest of the body. On warm days, the scrotum hangs somewhat lower to get away from the warm body. In very cold temperatures, the sac raises slightly to get closer to the warm body.

The **penis** is a structure that contains erectile tissue and blood vessels as well as the urethra. The urethra carries urine to the outside of the body, but it also performs a second role in males, which is to carry **semen**. Semen is a thick, sticky fluid that helps the sperm to swim while they are being transported; it also makes the male urethral and female vaginal environments less acidic. The blood vessels in the penis dilate during sexual arousal. This dilation makes the penis stiff and hard, to enable sexual intercourse. The main part of the penis looks like a shaft or cylindrical tube. At the end of the shaft the penis enlarges. This part, called the *head* or *glans penis,* looks somewhat like an acorn. The head of the penis is covered by the *prepuce* or foreskin, essentially a loose skin hood. *Circumcision* is surgical removal of the foreskin. Some males are circumcised; others are not. Cultural beliefs and traditions play a large role in the decision on whether to circumcise. In uncircumcised males, the foreskin should be pushed back gently when cleansing the area.

Internal Structures

The **testis** is the male gonad. It is also called the *testicle.* A male has a pair of gonads, called *testes* in the plural form, which are located in the scrotum. The testes produce **spermatozoa** (**sperm** or male reproductive cells), the male hormone **testosterone,** and other hormones. Testosterone is responsible for the changes that occur during puberty and for the secondary sex characteristics in males. One of these male characteristics is body hair patterns, such as chest hair. The thyroid cartilage becomes bigger, causing the male's visible "Adam's apple." The male voice takes on a lower pitch. Testosterone also encourages bone growth, resulting in the characteristic broad shoulders and narrow hips of the male, and encourages sperm cells to mature.

Attached to the testes is the **epididymis,** a duct-like organ that extends to the vas deferens. Sperm are kept in the epididymis while they continue to mature. It takes about three weeks until the sperm cells move to the next part of the reproductive system. Peristaltic (contraction) waves move the sperm along. The **vas deferens** is a duct that is actually a continuation of the epididymis. The vas deferens leads to the ejaculatory duct. The ejaculatory duct ejects sperm into the urethra. The urethra acts as the last duct of the male reproductive system. These structures are part of the ductal system whose purpose is to store and carry sperm.

Accessory Glands

The accessory glands of the male reproductive system are the seminal vesicles, the prostate gland, and the bulbourethral glands. The **seminal vesicles** look like sacs and are located behind the urinary bladder. The vesicles secrete semen, which is the sticky fluid that sperm move in. The **prostate gland** is shaped like a doughnut and surrounds the upper part of the urethra just below the bladder and anterior to the rectum. The prostate gland secretes fluid to help the sperm to swim. The gland performs two tasks in the male reproductive system. It releases sperm and secretions that help the sperm to move and, during ejaculation, contracts to help the sperm leave the body.

The **bulbourethral glands** are a pair of very small glands found under the prostate gland; they are also called the *Cowper's glands.* The bulbourethral glands also secrete fluid that becomes part of the semen. This fluid provides lubrication, helps to wash out any acidic matter in the male urethra, and neutralizes the acidic environment of the vagina.

The structure and working of the male reproductive system are very different from the female reproductive system. Nevertheless, these structures and hormones all work together to produce and transport the sperm necessary for continuation of the species.

BRIDGE TO CAAHEP

This chapter, which discusses the male reproductive system, provides information and content related to CAAHEP standards for Anatomy and Physiology, Medical Terminology, Communication, and Clinical Medical Assisting Procedures, and Professional Components.

ABHES LINKS

This chapter, which discusses the male reproductive system, links to ABHES course content for Anatomy and Physiology, Medical Terminology, Medical Law and Ethics, and Medical Office Clinical Procedures.

AAMA AREAS OF COMPETENCE

This chapter, which discusses the male reproductive system, provides information or content within several areas listed in the Medical Assistant Role Delineation Study. These areas include: clinical, fundamental principles, patient (client) care, general transdisciplinary professionalism, communication skills, legal concepts, and instruction.

AMT PATHS

This chapter, which discusses the male reproductive system, provides a path to AMT competency in general medical assisting knowledge, anatomy and physiology, medical terminology, and patient (client) education.

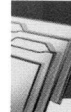

STUDENT PORTFOLIO ACTIVITY

Become involved in your community. Find out the needs in your area. Think of ways that you could become an active member. Medical assistants who take an interest in the community can transfer this concern for others to the clients they serve. This illustrates a caring attitude critical in a health provider.

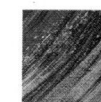

APPLYING YOUR SKILLS

A teenaged boy comes to the office for a routine examination. What are some of the changes you would observe in this client at puberty? What is responsible for these changes?

POINTS OF HIGHLIGHT

- The testis is the male gonad.
- The penis contains erectile tissue and blood vessels as well as the urethra.
- The urethra performs two functions in the male. It carries urine to the outside of the body and also transports sperm.
- Testosterone, which is the male hormone, is responsible for the development of secondary sex characteristics in the male.
- The seminal vesicles, prostate gland, and bulbourethral glands are the accessory glands of the male reproductive system.

CRITICAL THINKING QUESTIONS

1. What is the male hormone responsible for the development of male secondary sex characteristics? Identify at least three of the male secondary sex characteristics.

2. What is the purpose of semen?

3. What is the role of the prostate gland?

4. What are the external structures of the male reproductive system, and what role do these structures play?

5. Explain the two roles of the male urethra.

6. Why does the scrotum hang slightly lower on warm days? Why is this important?

7. Why is it important for men to have a prostate examination performed on a regular basis?

8. What is important for a male to remember about personal hygiene and the penis?

9. A man who is thinking of beginning a family tells you that he doesn't have to worry, because only the mother's health behaviors determine if the baby will be healthy. How do you respond as a medical assistant?

10. From statements made by a young male client, you realize that he has misconceptions about the male reproductive system. Why is it important for this young man to understand the male reproductive system? What should be included in talking about male reproductive health?

11. Go back to the beginning of this chapter and review the Anticipatory Statements. Reread each statement and then indicate whether it is true or false. If the statement is false, rewrite it to make it a true statement.

C H A P T E R 19

Anticipatory Statements

People have various ideas about how the female reproductive system works. Read and think about the following statements based upon what you believe now. Decide whether you agree or disagree. Write the word **agree** after the statement if you think the statement is true. Write the word **disagree** after the statement if you think the statement is false. Read the chapter to find out if your current beliefs can be supported.

1. Estrogen is important to the female reproductive system. _____

2. An ovary releases an egg to be fertilized every day of the month. _____

3. A woman can become pregnant throughout her life after puberty. _____

4. Fertilization of the egg or conception takes place in the uterus. _____

5. Special instruments are needed to see internal parts of the female reproductive system. _____

Female Reproductive System

Learning Objectives

Upon completion of this chapter, the medical assistant student should be able to:

- List the structures of the female reproductive system
- Define menarche
- Describe the menstrual cycle
- Explain the effects of estrogen and progesterone
- Explain the function of the female reproductive system
- Define menopause and what takes place during it

Key Terms

estrogen Hormone produced by the ovaries; important in the menstrual cycle and responsible for secondary sex characteristics in the female.

fallopian tubes Tubes that carry eggs from the ovaries to the uterus.

mammary glands Glands in the breast; in females, secrete milk after childbirth.

menopause The cessation of the menstrual cycle; signals the end of a female's reproductive years.

ovary Female reproductive organ.

ovum Female reproductive cell.

progesterone Hormone secreted by the ovaries.

uterus Hollow, muscular organ in which a fetus grows and develops.

vagina Tube that extends from the uterus to the vulva.

vulva External structure of the female genitalia.

■ INTRODUCTION

The female and male reproductive systems, working together, allow perpetuation (continuation) of the human species. The female reproductive system releases eggs (*ova*) for possible fertilization by sperm from the male. If conception takes place, the organs of the female reproductive system then nourish the growth and development of the baby inside the uterus. The reproductive ability of the female is time limited. It begins with puberty and the onset of the menstrual cycle and ends with menopause and the stoppage of the menstrual cycle.

■ THE FEMALE REPRODUCTIVE SYSTEM

The female reproductive system consists of several organs and accessory structures. The internal female reproductive organs are found in the pelvic cavity (Figure 19-1A). Special instruments, such as a vaginal speculum or a laparoscope, are needed to see these structures. The female reproductive system includes the ovaries, fallopian tubes, uterus, and vagina (Figure 19-1B). The external structures, which can be seen during a physical examination, are the mons pubis, labia majora, labia minora, clitoris, and vaginal opening. This area is often referred to as the **vulva.** The urethral meatus is also located in this region, above the vaginal orifice. The vagina connects the external and internal structures. The breasts are accessory structures.

External Structures

The mons pubis consists of tissue that serves as protection for the vulvar region. During puberty, hair grows and covers the area. Within the vulvar region are the clitoris, the urethral meatus (opening), and the opening of the vagina. The *clitoris* is spongy tissue that

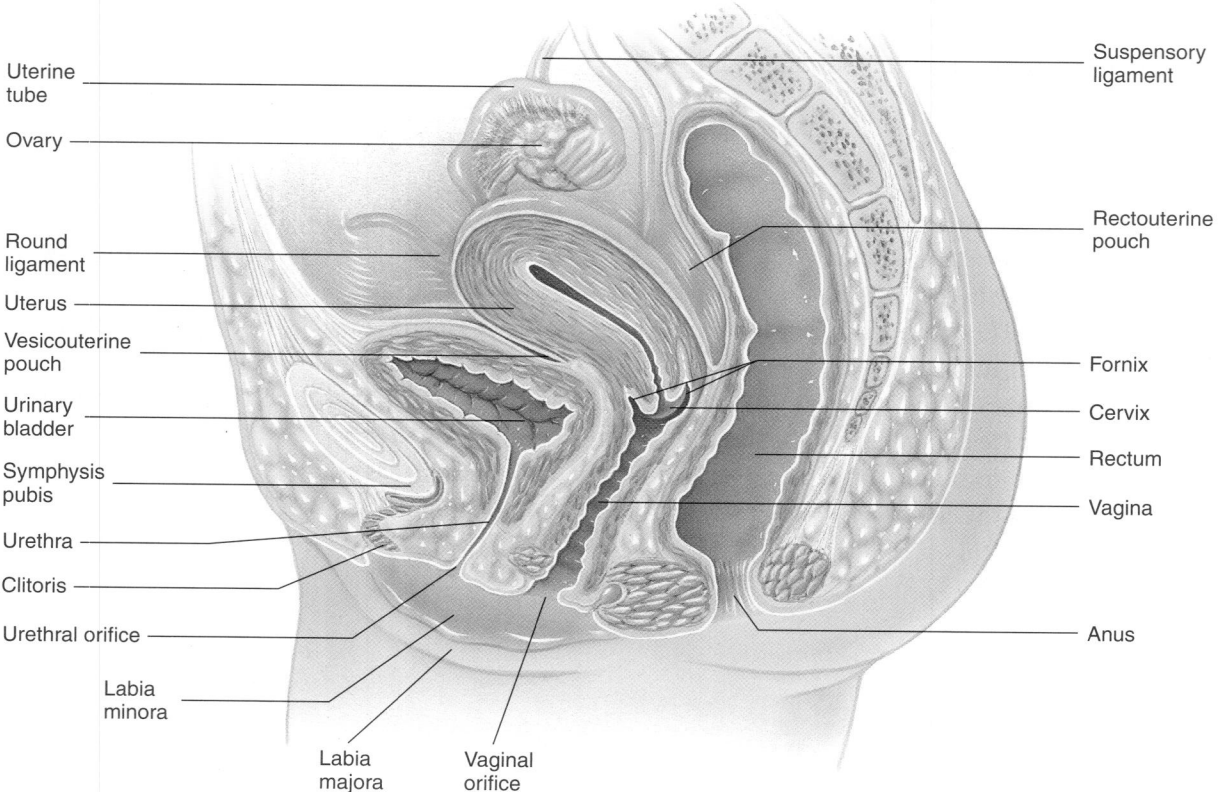

FIGURE 19-1A Organs and their positions in the female reproductive system.

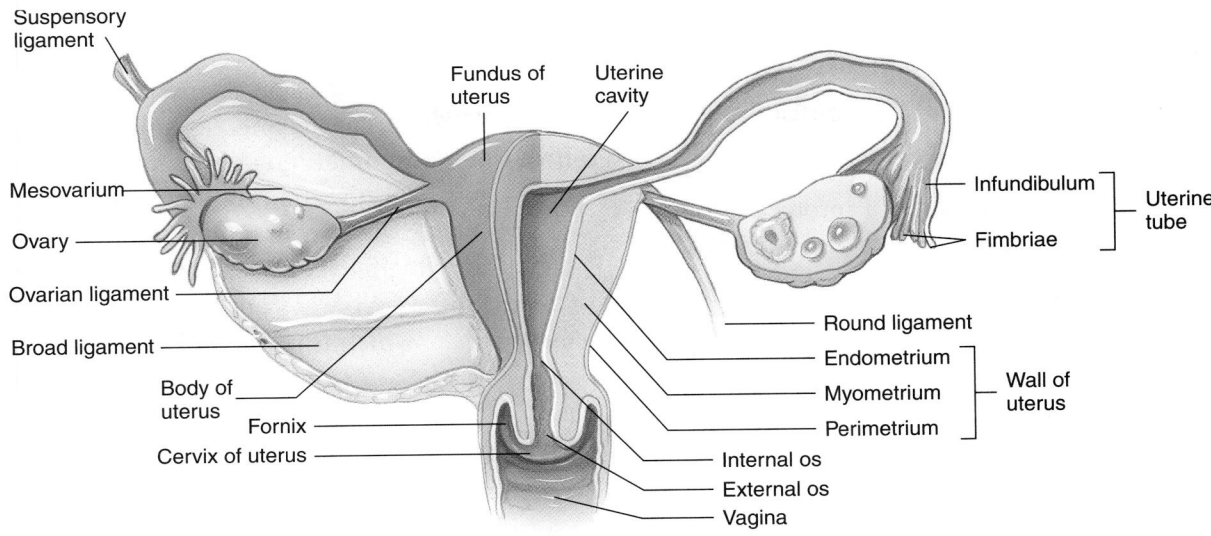

FIGURE 19-1B The ovaries, uterine tube, uterus, and vagina.

becomes swollen during sexual arousal. The clitoris is extremely sensitive and is protected by a prepuce or foreskin that partially covers it. The urinary meatus (opening for release of urine) is found below the clitoris. Below the urinary meatus is the opening of the vagina, which allows the flow of menstrual blood and serves as the passageway for the birth of a baby. The urinary meatus and the vaginal opening are protected by two sets of tissue that resemble lips (Figure 19-2). The inner lips are called the *labia minora* and the outer lips are called the *labia majora*.

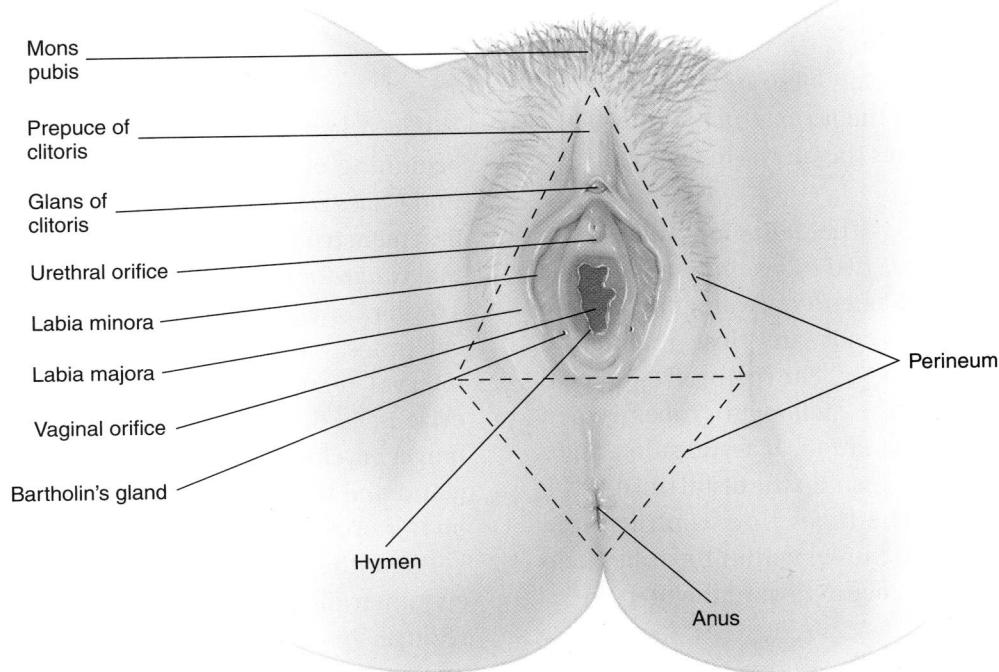

FIGURE 19-2 External genitalia of the female reproductive system.

Internal Structures

The vagina, uterus, fallopian tubes, and ovaries are the internal structures of the female reproductive system. These structures work together to produce ova or eggs, carry them for possible fertilization, and provide a protected place where the fertilized egg and the fetus that it develops into can grow. Hormones secreted in the brain and reproductive system begin and maintain this process, and also produce the secondary sex characteristics of the female.

Vagina. The **vagina** connects the internal structures with the exterior of the body. In addition to being a passageway for menstrual blood and a birth canal, the vagina also serves as a structure for sexual pleasure. The vagina receives the male's penis during intercourse (*coitus*). The upper portion of the vagina, which is inside the body, is called the *neck* of the uterus or *cervix*. The muscles in the cervix control the opening into the uterus.

Uterus. The **uterus** is a pear-shaped, hollow, muscular organ. The uterus has three layers. The innermost layer, which is called the *endometrial layer*, sloughs off during menstruation. The *myometrium*, which is the middle muscular layer, contracts during labor or childbirth. The outer layer, called the *perimetrium*, protects the uterus and attaches the uterus to ligaments.

Fallopian Tubes. The **fallopian tubes**, also called oviducts, are two tubes that are attached to the uterus and extend outward, ending in a fringed area. The ends are close to but not attached to the ovaries. The matured eggs (ova) travel through the fallopian tubes when released during ovulation. If fertilization takes place, it usually happens in the distal third of the fallopian tubes. The tubes then contract, and cilia (hair-like structures) within the tubes help move the fertilized ovum toward the uterus.

Ovaries. Ligaments attach two almond-shaped organs called **ovaries** to the uterus. The ovaries are the gonads of the female reproductive system. They produce eggs and send the ova out for possible fertilization. The ovaries also secrete **estrogen** and **progesterone,** hormones that are necessary for maintaining a pregnancy and for developing and maintaining female secondary sex characteristics. From puberty until the end of the reproductive years, each ovary is about 1½ inches long, 1 inch wide, and 1 inch thick. After **menopause,** which is the end of the reproductive years, the ovaries shrink and are not usually palpable during a physical examination.

Mammary Glands

The **mammary glands** in the female breasts are an accessory structure of the female reproductive system. Hormones cause the mammary glands to increase in size during puberty. Lobules or compartments within the mammary glands hold milk-secreting cells called *alveoli*. The milk passes into the mammary ducts and eventually leaves the breast through the nipples during *lactation,* for breastfeeding of a baby. The size of the breasts is not related to the ability to breastfeed. The difference in women's breast sizes is due to the amount of adipose tissue in the breast.

■ THE MENSTRUAL CYCLE

When a female reaches puberty, which is the beginning of her reproductive years, her body undergoes many changes. The beginning of the first menstrual cycle is called *menarche.* The normal range for the time of menarche is from 9 to 16 years of age. Menstruation is a normal cyclical process that happens at a fairly regular interval (Figure 19-3). Although the average cycle is 28 days, many women have shorter or longer cycles. Hormones from the pituitary gland and the ovaries are the primary controls on this cycle.

At the end of the menstrual flow, the endometrial layer of the uterus begins to change in case a fertilized **ovum** (egg) is implanted. Estrogen and other hormones are released at this time, and an egg in an ovary

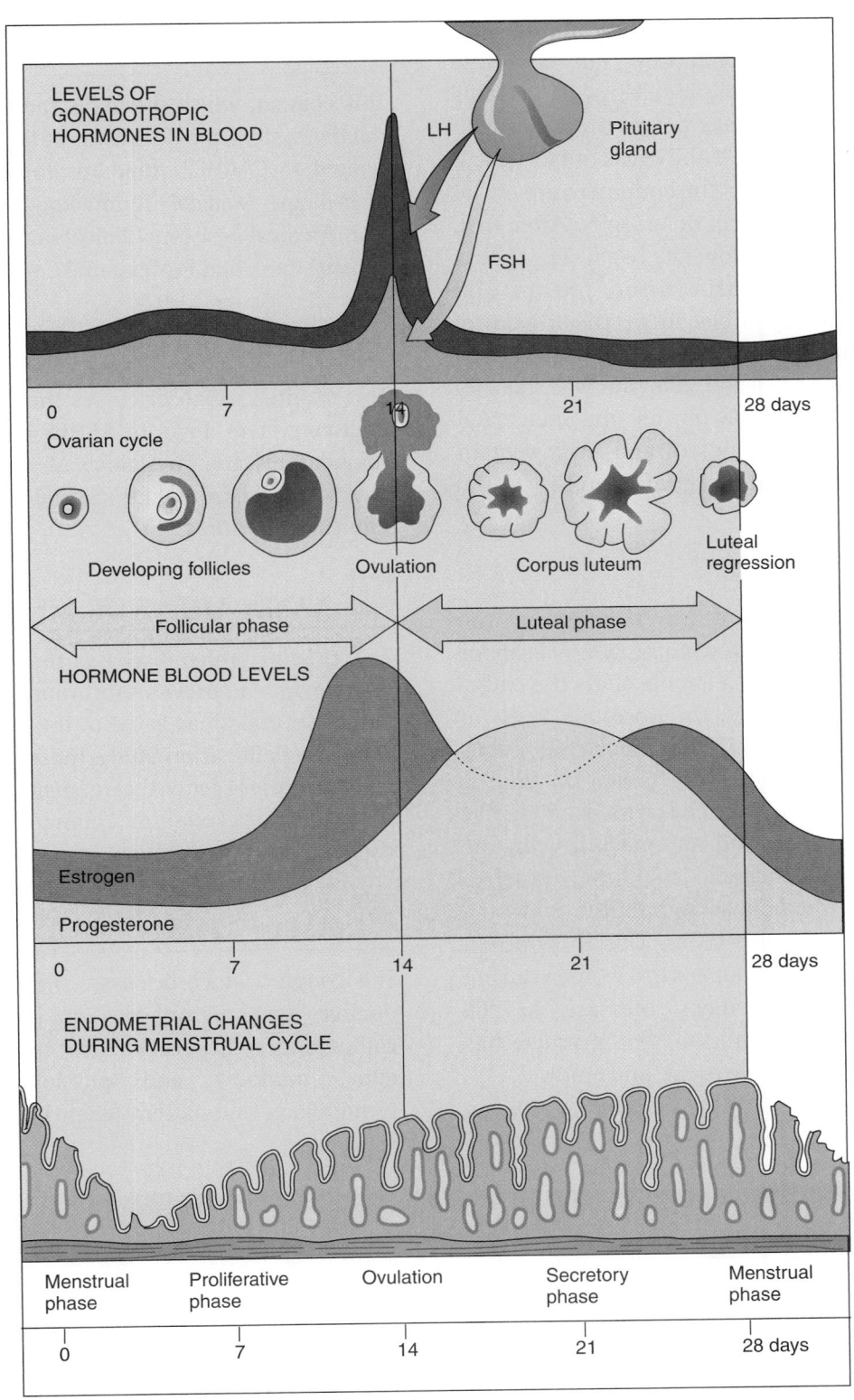

FIGURE 19-3 The menstrual cycle.

begins to mature or ripen. When mature, the ovum enters the fallopian tubes. This discharge of a ovum from the ovary is called *ovulation.* This occurs about two weeks before the menstrual flow or menstruation. If the egg is not fertilized, it will not implant, and the endometrium of the uterus begins to shrink or atrophy. After this, the menstrual blood flow will begin. The flow is made up of endometrial tissue, mucus, and blood. The first day of bleeding is the first day of the menstrual cycle. If conception (fertilization) took place, and the fertilized ovum was successfully implanted in the uterus, the menstrual cycle will be interrupted and will remain stopped until after the pregnancy ends.

■ MENOPAUSE

Menstrual cycles continue throughout the reproductive years of a woman, which is about 30 to 35 years. When a female nears the end of her reproductive years, the hormone levels in her body change and the menstrual cycles become less frequent. This period of time is called *perimenopause.* When the menstrual cycle has completely stopped for one full year, the woman is considered to have reached **menopause.** Menopause signals the end of a woman's reproductive years. This is a normal process that usually happens to a woman during her fifties. With today's increase in life expectancy, a woman, on the average has another third of her life to live and enjoy.

BRIDGE TO CAAHEP

This chapter, which discusses the female reproductive system, provides information and content related to CAAHEP standards for Anatomy and Physiology, Medical Terminology, Communication, Medical Assisting Clinical Procedure, Patient (Client) Care, and Professional Components.

ABHES LINKS

This chapter, which discusses the female reproductive system, links to ABHES course content for Anatomy and Physiology, Medical Terminology, Medical Law and Ethics, and Medical Office Clinical Procedures.

AAMA AREAS OF COMPETENCE

This chapter, which discusses the female reproductive system, provides information or content within several areas listed in the Medical Assistant Role Delineation Study. These areas include: clinical, patient (client) care, general transdisciplinary, professionalism communication, legal concepts, and instruction.

AMT PATHS

This chapter, which discusses the female reproductive system, provides a path to AMT competency in general medical assisting knowledge, anatomy and physiology, medical terminology, and patient (client) education.

POINTS OF HIGHLIGHT

- The internal organs of the female reproductive system are found in the pelvic cavity.
- The uterus is a pear-shaped, hollow organ that expands to hold and nourish the growth and development of a baby.
- Menarche is the beginning of the first menstrual cycle in a woman at puberty.
- Puberty is the beginning of the reproductive years.
- Menopause is the end of a woman's reproductive years; it is a gradual process that is considered complete when the woman has not had a menstrual period for one full year.

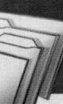

STUDENT PORTFOLIO ACTIVITY

Think about the career path you might take. What are your interests? Are there certain areas of medical assisting in which you would like advanced education? Can you see yourself in the future as an office manager? Do you prefer clinical medical assisting, or do you like a combination of administrative and clinical work? What are some of your short-term and long-term career goals? What steps do you need to take to reach these goals? Include these career objectives in your portfolio.

APPLYING YOUR SKILLS

As part of your clinical responsibilities, you obtain medical information from a teenaged girl about her menstrual cycles. What she tells you indicates that she does not understand what is happening to her body. How would you approach a discussion of this topic? What would you say to this client?

CRITICAL THINKING QUESTIONS

1. A woman in her first pregnancy confides in you that she is afraid she will not be able to breast-feed or nurse her baby because her breasts are too small. How do you respond? What would you tell her about the process of breastfeeding?

2. Identify the structures within the vulvar region. Why is good hygiene so important?

3. The vagina can be grouped with both the external and internal structures of the female reproductive system. How could you explain this?

4. Why are the ovaries also studied as part of the endocrine system?

5. What is the role of the ovaries in the development of females?

6. A young woman comes to the office for an appointment that will include her first pelvic examination. She appears anxious. How can you make this procedure less stressful for the client?

7. A client asks why it is necessary to use instruments for a pelvic examination. What would you explain about the instruments?

8. The doctor asks you, as a medical assistant, to provide information about puberty to a young client. What changes can the girl expect to occur in her body?

9. Describe the role of the uterus during pregnancy.

10. How do the ovaries function once a female has reached puberty?

11. Explain the relationship of ovulation to the menstrual cycle.

12. A client states that she does not perform breast self-examinations because she comes for a yearly visit to the gynecologist. How would you respond?

13. A woman in her fifties tells you that her menstrual periods are getting irregular. What is most likely happening to her reproductive system? Explain the process.

14. Go back to the beginning of this chapter and review the Anticipatory Statements. Reread each statement and then indicate whether it is true or false. If the statement is false, rewrite it to make it a true statement.

CLIENT TEACHING PLAN

Female Hygiene Practices

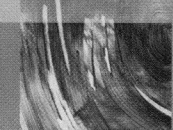

■ What Is to Be Taught:

- Female hygiene practices.

■ Objectives:

- Female client will practice hygiene activities that promote health.

■ Preparation Before Teaching:

- Review hygiene practices for females and the reasons and rationale for each.
- Get together handouts for use in teaching, and paper and pen for notes and written instructions.

■ Steps for the Medical Assistant:

1. Wash your hands.
2. Get supplies needed.
3. Introduce yourself to the client.
4. Explain what you are going to teach and why.
5. Inform the client that the goal of a healthy body can be helped by steps the client can take.
6. List steps that contribute to the working of a healthy female body.
   a. After using the toilet, wipe from front to back so as not to allow bacteria into the vagina.
   b. Do not use bubble bath.
   c. Do not douche unless ordered by the doctor.
   d. Wear cotton underpants or underpants that have a cotton crotch panel.
   e. Avoid tight underwear.
   f. Urinate and wash the genital area after intercourse.

■ Special Needs of the Client:

- Look at the client's chart to see if there is any factor that might interfere with the client's ability to follow these hygiene practices.

- Ask the client if there is anything you should know about her ability to follow these practices.

■ Evaluation:

- Client will be able to list female hygiene practices and the reasons for each.

■ Further Plans/Teaching:

- Provide the client with written instructions regarding these hygiene practices.
- Give the client printed pamphlets and the names of resources to contact for more information. Be sure to include telephone numbers, addresses, and Web sites.

■ Follow–up:

- At the next office visit, ask the client what steps she was able to follow and what problems she encountered. Do not ask a direct yes-or-no question that might make a client defensive, such as "Did you follow the steps that I taught you?"

Medical Assistant

Name: _____

Signature: _____

Date: _____

Client

Date: _____

Follow-up Date : _____

UNIT FOUR

Common System Disorders

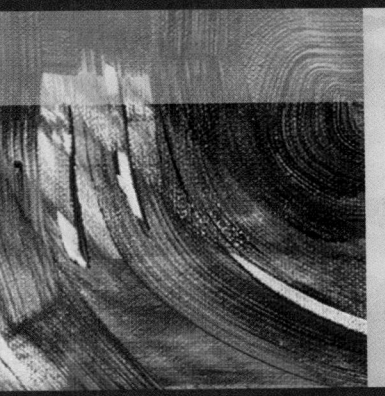

The chapters in the preceding unit discussed body systems and their organization and normal functioning. Now that you have learned the normal structure of each system and how each system should work, you can begin to look at what happens when something goes wrong in a system. When a system does not work well, the problem directly affects the other systems, which try to make up for the malfunctioning system and keep the body working.

This unit presents chapters that examine common disorders in each system. Each chapter contains three main topical areas:

1. Systemic disorders that may be seen by the medical assistant working in an ambulatory health care setting

2. Common tests and procedures to diagnose disorders of a system

3. The medical assistant's role in giving client-centered care to clients with specific disorders

While you are learning about common diagnostic tests and procedures, you may want to look at Unit Six, which examines specific diagnostic and laboratory tests in more detail. The medical assistant's role may be to prepare the client, teach the client, assist with or perform the tests, and/or give postprocedure care to the client.

At the end of the discussion about systemic disorders, you will be given a health care situation or client problem to solve by using what you have learned in the chapter and applying your critical thinking skills.

Throughout the unit, you will also find client teaching plans. As a medical assistant, you will find that giving competent care to clients includes teaching clients about their disorders.

C H A P T E R 20

Anticipatory Statements

People have different ideas about skin disorders and how to treat them. Read and think about the following statements based upon what you believe now. Decide whether you agree or disagree. Write the word **agree** after the statement if you think the statement is true. Write the word **disagree** after the statement if you think the statement is false. Read the chapter to find out if your current beliefs can be supported.

1. Skin cancer is a rare form of cancer.   _____

2. Unbroken, healthy skin is the best protection
   from infection.   _____

3. Athlete's foot is a fungal infection.   _____

4. Atopic dermatitis or eczema is the same as psoriasis.   _____

5. Herpes simplex is sometimes called a cold sore.   _____

Integumentary System Disorders

Learning Objectives

Upon completion of this chapter, the medical assistant student should be able to:

- List at least five skin lesions
- Tell the difference between atopic dermatitis and psoriasis
- Identify two common fungal infections
- Describe common treatments for bacterial infections of the skin
- Explain the process in acne vulgaris
- State ways to decrease the itching that is common in many skin conditions
- Describe the result of infection of hair follicles or sebaceous glands
- Develop a teaching plan for skin cancer prevention
- Teach another person steps to prevent skin cancer

Key Terms

atopic dermatitis Inflammation of skin caused by an allergic-type reaction.

basal cell carcinoma Common type of skin cancer.

bullae Blisters.

fissure Crack in the skin or mucous membrane.

lesion A specific difference in the appearance of the skin in a defined area.

malignant melanoma Serious cancer of the melanocytes in the skin and mucous membranes.

plaque A localized patch or area of skin.

psoriasis A chronic condition that causes dry, elevated, silvery lesions.

pustule Small, reddened, raised or elevated vesicle containing pus.

urticaria Hives.

vesicle Elevated area of skin containing liquid.

virus Smallest of the infectious organisms.

vitiligo Loss of pigment in patchy areas of the skin.

wheal Temporary swelling of an area of skin, such as hives or an intradermal injection.

■ INTRODUCTION

The skin is the largest organ; it covers and protects the entire body. Problems can occur in the skin itself, or the skin may manifest problems caused by a disorder in another body system. Sometimes the problem only affects the way the skin looks; in other cases, skin problems may be a sign of a very serious disorder. One of the functions of the integumentary system is communication (see Chapter 7). How the skin looks and feels communicates messages and an image to others. Companies manufacture and advertise many skin products to the public to help consumers create, enhance, or present a certain image via the skin.

When a client has an integumentary system disorder, the appearance of the skin may cause stress or worry for the client. The level of seriousness of the disorder does not necessarily match the client's level of concern. The medical assistant needs to be aware of how the client perceives the appearance of the skin. To find this out, the medical assistant needs to know the basic types of skin lesions, how they look, and what could cause them. An understanding of common disorders will aid the medical assistants in their role as care providers.

■ SKIN LESIONS

Lesions can occur anywhere on the skin. A *lesion* is a specific difference in the appearance of the skin in a defined area (Figure 20-1). Lesions can be primary, arising on their own, or *secondary,* which means they appear as a result of another lesion. The medical assistant should be able to recognize the differences between lesions. Some are common to several disorders; other, specific lesions occur only with certain disorders.

Recognition of common lesions helps in the diagnosis of skin disorders. Thick, flaky **plaques** are frequently seen in psoriasis. *Scales* are extremely dry patches of the upper layers of the skin. Scales are seen in **atopic dermatitis.** In many skin conditions where there is oozing of fluid, a crust will form, such as with impetigo and eczema. A *cyst* contains fluid or semisolid matter. If the cyst becomes infected, a **pustule** may form. During skin testing or tuberculosis (TB) testing, a **wheal** forms at the site. The temporary swelling of a wheal may be itchy and uncomfortable. An *ulcer* is a wearing away or opening of the skin, and may eventually destroy underlying tissue right down to and including the bone. Ulceration can often be prevented by relieving pressure and maintaining good circulation to all tissues of the body. Even after healing, ulcers usually leave a scar.

■ ACUTE DISORDERS

The skin reacts quickly to outside stimuli. The appearance of the skin can also indicate an underlying internal problem. Clients experience itching, pain, and discomfort with most acute skin conditions. Chronic skin disorders can flare up into acute situations. Medical assistants need to recognize that clients may be embarrassed about the appearance of their skin, in addition to experiencing discomfort from the problem.

Urticaria

The client who has **urticaria** has red, swollen, very itchy patches of skin. A common name for this condition is *hives.* The intense itching is a reaction that can last for 24 hours or more. This is an allergic-type reaction to an antigen such as food, medicine, or even heat or cold. The client with urticaria will be very uncomfortable and will be seeking relief from the itching.

■ CHRONIC DISORDERS

Several disorders can affect the skin over a lifetime. There is no cure, only treatment to keep these conditions from flaring up. Clients need a great deal of emotional support, as these conditions are long-term problems that can affect

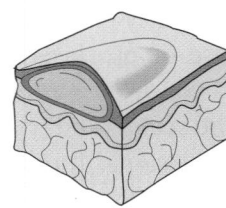

Bulla (large blister):
Same as a vesicle, but larger than 10 mm
Example:
Contact dermatitis, large second-degree burns, bulbous impetigo, pemphigus

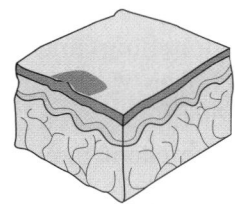

Macule:
Localized changes in skin color of less than 1 cm in diameter
Example:
Freckle

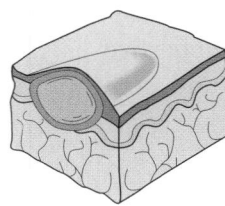

Nodules:
Solid and elevated; however, they extend deeper than papules into the dermis or subcutaneous tissues, more than 10 mm
Example:
Lipoma, erythema, cyst, wart

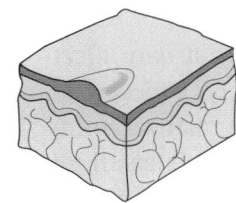

Papule:
Solid, elevated lesion less than 1 cm in diameter
Example:
Elevated nevi

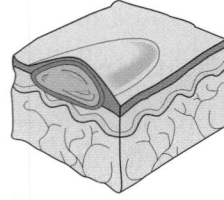

Pustule:
Vesicles or bullae that become filled with pus, usually described as less than 0.5 cm in diameter
Example:
Acne, impetigo, furuncles, carbuncles

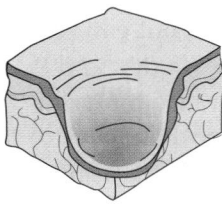

Ulcer:
A depressed lesion of the epidermis and upper papillary layer of the dermis
Example:
Stage 2 pressure ulcer

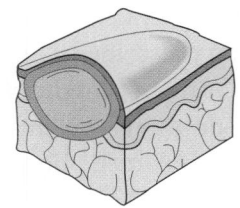

Tumor:
The same as a nodule, only larger than 2 cm

Example:
Benign epidermal tumor, basal cell carcinoma

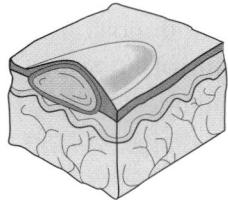

Vesicle (small blister):
Accumulation of fluid between the upper layers of the skin; elevated mass containing serous fluid; less than 10 mm
Example:
Herpes simplex, herpes zoster, chickenpox

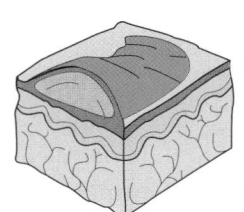

Wheal:
Localized edema in the epidermis causing irregular elevation that may be red or pale; may be itchy
Example:
Insect bite, hive, urticaria

FIGURE 20-1 Types of skin lesions.

every aspect of life. The client may often be uncomfortable (for example, from itching) and may be restricted in clothing choices if some materials irritate the skin. The client may even experience sleep disturbances. The client may also avoid social situations if the condition affects the face or hands.

Atopic Dermatitis

Atopic dermatitis is a condition that can affect only a part of the skin, or can be widespread over the entire body. It looks like a rash with reddened areas of scale that can ooze clear fluid and then crust over. Atopic dermatitis is not contagious. The area can become very itchy, and then the client may scratch, thus making the condition worse.

This condition may be acute, but can easily become chronic. The skin stays dry and is easily irritated. Scratching or continuous irritation over a long period of time can lead to thickened, tough-looking skin called *lichenified skin.* A client with this condition usually has a family history of allergies in some form. Atopic dermatitis is sometimes called by the general term *eczema.* Treatment consists of avoiding irritants, using only mild soaps and moisturizers, keeping allergies under control, applying topical medications, and (sometimes) taking oral medications.

Psoriasis

Psoriasis is a chronic skin disorder. The skin forms red patches with definite edges and thick silvery scales. The patches may be confined to a small area of the body, or can nearly cover the entire body surface. The cause of psoriasis is unknown. Treatment is aimed at lessening client discomfort, removing the scales, and trying to slow the growth of new lesions. Topical and oral medications are prescribed. Phototherapy with ultraviolet light may also be used to treat this condition. The medical assistant must teach the client how to use the prescribed treatments to keep the psoriasis under control. The medical assistant must be supportive as the client deals with treatment and body image issues.

Vitiligo

Vitiligo is the loss of melanocytes in specific areas of the skin, which causes loss of skin pigmentation in those areas. The face, hands, and genital areas are the most often affected. This condition can affect persons of all races, but is more pronounced in those with darker-pigmented skin. The skin looks patchy, with light areas surrounded by normal-looking, normally pigmented skin. Part of the treatment involves covering the patchy areas so that they match the rest of the skin. Topical and oral medications are often prescribed. One somewhat complicated treatment involves medications and specialized dressings; in this treatment, the dermis is destroyed in the hope that pigment will reappear after the dermis heals. The medical assistant should provide opportunities for clients to share their feelings about the loss of color. This condition can drastically affect a person's self-image.

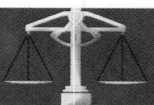

LEGAL/ETHICAL THOUGHTS

Try to understand how the client feels about the disorder. Show empathy. No matter how good their technical skills; if a client feels that health care providers do not care about the client as a person, the outcome will not be as good.

■ INFECTION

Unbroken, healthy skin is the best protection from infection. As the outermost portion of the body, the skin is constantly exposed to the many infectious organisms present in the environment. The person who has an itchy skin disorder with open, oozing lesions is at great risk of getting an infection, because of the nonintact skin. Infections can be fungal, bacterial, or viral.

Athlete's Foot

Athlete's foot is a fungal infection of the superficial skin layer, often affecting the toes. This is a contagious infection. **Bullae** (blisters), crusting, and scaling are seen. Treatment consists of topical application of antifungal medication. The medical assistant should instruct the client to keep the area clean and dry. Moisture and darkness encourage the growth and spread of fungal infections.

Ringworm

Ringworm is a highly contagious fungal infection. The affected area looks like a raised ring or circle. It often affects the face and scalp. It is treated with medication.

Acne Vulgaris

Acne vulgaris (often called *pimples* or *zits*) is very common in adolescents, but is also frequently seen in adults. Acne results when the oily sebum secreted by the skin becomes hard and plugs up a sebaceous gland opening. Leukocytes or white blood cells rush to the area, engulf bacteria trapped there, and then die, leading to pus formation. In a client with acne vulgaris, the medical assistant will observe pimples, cysts, blackheads, and sometimes scarring. Treatment includes topical medications and sometimes antibiotics.

Boils

The sebaceous glands or hair follicles may become infected, usually by Staphylococcus bacteria. A *boil* may become a furuncle or carbuncle when boils become joined or buried in the skin. A boil is tender, red, swollen, and very painful. Bacteria can enter the skin through cracks or **fissures.** Even dry, chafed skin with no obvious cuts or scrapes provides an opportunity for organisms to enter. Treatment is with medication; sometimes the boils are lanced open to drain.

Impetigo

Impetigo is a contagious infection. Little **vesicles** form, break open, and become crusted with a yellow scabby material. Impetigo is often seen in infants and children. It can also be seen in adults, particularly those who have other disorders that cause itching. When the person scratches or breaks open the skin, the lesion may become infected and spread the infection to other skin areas. Impetigo can also be spread to other family members. Care must be taken not to share the infected person's washcloths, towels, clothes, or bedding. Good handwashing, both before and after contact, is extremely important.

Viral Infections

Viral infections can affect the skin. They first appear as blisters. Herpes simplex, genital herpes, and herpes zoster (shingles) are the most common types. Herpes simplex is sometimes called a *cold sore* or *fever blister.* The blister is found around the mouth area. Oral contact often spreads the **virus** to another person. Genital herpes, the lesions of which are found on the genital area, can be spread through sexual contact. A woman who has an active outbreak of genital herpes during delivery can infect the baby. The doctor needs to be aware that the mother has genital herpes so that precautions can be taken to avoid transmission of the virus. Herpes zoster, or shingles, is a viral infection of the nerve endings, and presents as reddened areas of the skin. The affected area is itchy as well as painful. This is a serious viral infection in the elderly or frail client.

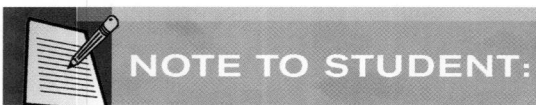

NOTE TO STUDENT:

Herpes infections can flare up (exacerbate) and then quiet down and go into remission. The client needs to be instructed about this process and what to do during a flareup.

Hemangioma

Hemangiomas are growths of dilated blood vessels (Figure 20-2). The area appears red. This primary, benign tumor can grow and then shrink. It is often present at birth. It is frequently found on the face and neck. People may call it a *strawberry birthmark* due to its appearance.

Skin Cancer

Skin cancer is a common type of cancer. Exposure to ultraviolet rays from sunlight or tanning booths increases the risk of skin cancer. The medical assistant must instruct clients about limiting exposure to sunlight and protecting the body by using sunscreen (Figure 20-3). The higher the number of the sunscreen product, the more protection it offers against harmful ultraviolet rays.

Three common types of skin cancer are basal cell carcinoma, squamous cell carcinoma, and malignant melanoma. **Basal cell carcinoma** occurs in the epidermis and may be limited to a specific area. This is the most common and least deadly type. It is often found on the face. Clients should be instructed to report to the doctor any small changes or discoloration on the skin. *Squamous cell carcinoma* is often found on the scalp and lower lip. This can spread to the lymph nodes, so it is critical that the cancer be found early and treated. **Malignant melanoma** spreads quickly to other areas of the body. This type of cancer often begins in the melanocytes, which give the skin its color. A new, dark area that may look like a mole should be checked by a doctor. Any change in an existing mole should be checked immediately. Surgery and chemotherapy are used to treat this potentially fatal cancer. The client will require a long period of follow-up.

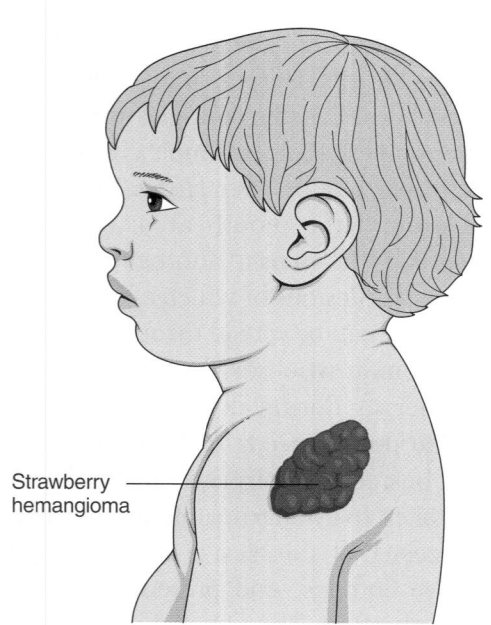

Strawberry hemangioma

FIGURE 20-2 Hemangioma.

 BRIDGE TO CAAHEP

This chapter, which discusses integumentary system disorders, provides information and content related to CAAHEP standards for Anatomy and Physiology, Common Pathology/Diseases, Diagnostic/Treatment Modalities, Medical Terminology, Medical Law and Ethics, Communication, Medical Assisting Clinical Procedures, and Professional Components.

 ABHES LINKS

This chapter, which discusses integumentary system disorders, links to ABHES course content for Anatomy and Physiology, Medical Terminology, Medical Law and Ethics, and Medical Office Clinical Procedures.

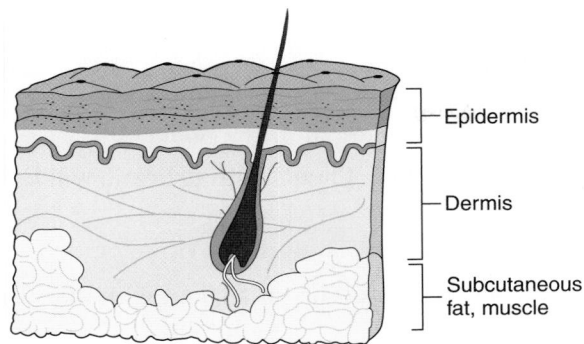
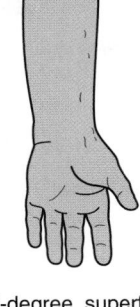

Skin red, dry

First-degree, superficial

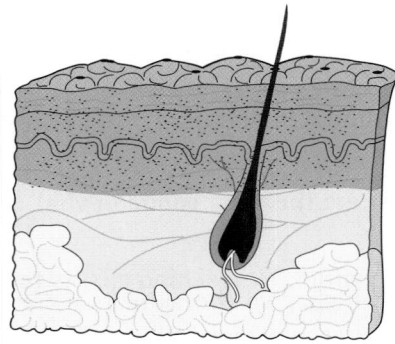
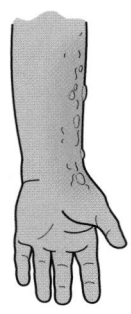

Blistered, skin moist, pink or red

Second-degree, partial thickness

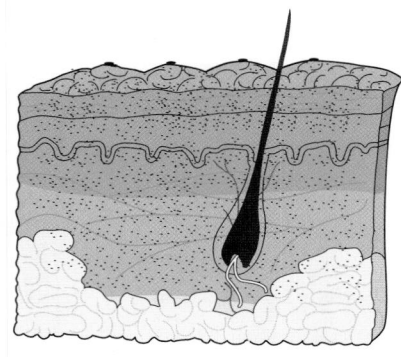
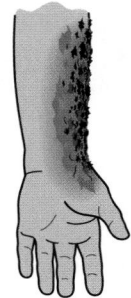

Charring, skin black, brown, red

Third-degree, full thickness

FIGURE 20-3 Sunburns are considered first-degree burns.

 AAMA AREAS OF COMPETENCE

This chapter, which discusses integumentary system disorders, provides information or content within several areas listed in the Medical Assistant Role Delineation Study. These areas include: clinical, patient (client) care, general transdisciplinary, communication skills, legal concepts, and instruction.

 AMT PATHS

This chapter, which discusses integumentary system disorders, provides a path to AMT competency in general medical assisting knowledge, anatomy and physiology, medical terminology, and patient (client) education.

POINTS OF HIGHLIGHT

- The skin, which covers and protects the body, is the largest organ of the body.
- Urticaria, commonly called hives, is a reaction to an antigen. Clients with urticaria will be uncomfortable and experience itching.
- Chronic skin disorders can affect the skin over a lifetime.
- Atopic dermatitis, sometimes referred to as eczema, usually occurs in a client with a family history of allergies.
- Scaly, well-defined patches are characteristic of psoriasis.
- Vitiligo can affect a client's self-image, as patches of skin lose their coloring pigment.
- Unbroken, healthy skin is the best protection against infection and many acute skin disorders.
- Athlete's foot and ringworm are two common, contagious fungal infections.
- Boils and impetigo are caused by bacterial infections.
- Herpes simplex, genital herpes, and herpes zoster (shingles) are the most common viral infections that affect the skin.
- The medical assistant plays a crucial role in skin cancer prevention by teaching clients to limit exposure to the sun and to use protection when in sunlight.

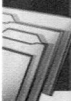

STUDENT PORTFOLIO ACTIVITY

Medical assisting is an allied health profession. Learn about the history of medical assisting. Why and how was it founded? What health care need did it fulfill? Talk with representatives from the medical assisting profession. Write a reflection about the role that medical assisting continues to play in today's health care environment. Place this in your portfolio and use it to help you discuss with potential employers the medical assistant's role as a health care team member.

APPLYING YOUR SKILLS

A client tells you that she is worried about getting skin cancer. The client says that she knows someone who died as a result of skin cancer. What steps can people take to lessen their chances of getting skin cancer? What should they do if they notice something different about the skin?

CRITICAL THINKING QUESTIONS

1. A client experiences severe itching as part of an integumentary system disorder such as atopic dermatitis. What steps could the client take to decrease the itching?

2. What is vitiligo? What happens to the client's skin? How might this affect the client's self-esteem?

3. What are some things that you, as a medical assistant, could teach a client about avoiding skin infections?

4. Psoriasis is a common chronic skin disorder. What are some treatment options for the client with psoriasis?

5. Why do clients need emotional support when they have chronic disorders of the skin? What effect can skin disorders have on social interactions?

6. A client is diagnosed with athlete's foot. What is this? What can the client do to avoid a recurrence?

7. What will a medical assistant observe in a client who has acne?

8. How is skin cancer related to the sun?

9. A parent brings in a child who is diagnosed with impetigo. Describe impetigo in your own words and discuss steps to keep it from spreading to other members of the family.

10. A client with a herpes infection asks you if he will be cured of herpes when he is finished with treatment. What do you know about the course of herpes over the course of a lifetime?

11. Go back to the beginning of this chapter and review the Anticipatory Statements. Reread each statement and then indicate whether it is true or false. If the statement is false, rewrite it to make it a true statement.

CLIENT TEACHING PLAN

Skin Self-Examination

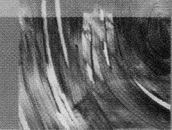

■ What Is to Be Taught:

- How to examine one's own skin surface.

■ Objectives:

- Client will be able to examine her own skin and look for anything different or unusual.

■ Preparation Before Teaching:

- Review information on the skin and its appearance. Get together items needed for teaching: a handheld mirror and a full-length mirror, and copies of a simple outline of the human body.

■ Steps for the Medical Assistant:

1. Wash your hands.
2. Get together supplies needed.
3. Introduce yourself to the client.
4. Explain what you are going to teach and why.
5. Explain to the client the purpose of examining the skin. Tell the client that by periodically examining her skin, the client can take part in keeping herself healthy. Problems will be found early and treatment started earlier. List what to look for.
6. Ask the client to hold the smaller mirror and look at her face, scalp, and neck. If the hair is long, pull it up off the client's neck and face to get a clear look. To view the back of the neck, the client should stand in front of the long mirror and adjust the handheld mirror as needed.
7. Instruct the client to remove her clothing from the waist up. Look at the front and back of the body. Lift the right arm and examine the right side; lift the left arm and examine the left side. Make sure the client looks in the mirror to see all areas of her back.
8. Tell the client to look at all areas of her hands and arms, including the palms of the hands, the elbows, and the underarms.
9. Instruct the client to put clothing back on her upper body.
10. Ask the client to remove the clothing from her lower body.
11. Have the client look at her abdomen, genital area, and the fronts of her legs.
12. Hand the small mirror to the client so she can examine the buttock area and the backs of her legs.
13. Tell the client to put clothing back on her lower body.
14. Ask the client to sit and look carefully at her feet, including between the toes.
15. Hand a simple outline drawing of the human body to the client.
16. Instruct the client to mark any findings on the outline. All moles should be marked on this (this chart is used for comparison, to find any changes when doing the next skin self-examination). Open or bleeding sores should be marked, as well as any itchy areas.
17. Ask the client if she has any questions or concerns.
18. Share the findings of the skin examination with the doctor.

■ Special Needs of the Client:

- Look at the client's chart to see if there are any factors that might interfere with the client's ability to perform skin self-examination or to follow the directions.
- Ask the client if there is anything you should know about that might affect her ability to perform the procedure.

■ Evaluation:

- Client will be able to perform the skin self-examination and complete the outline with the help of the medical assistant.

(Continues)

CLIENT TEACHING PLAN (Continued)

■ Further Plans/Teaching:

- Give the client written instructions to use as a guide when performing the skin self-examination at home.
- Instruct the client to call the doctor if she finds any change from what was found during this exam.
- Give the client a copy of the outline with the findings recorded. Also give her some blank outlines of the human body surface, to fill in as needed.
- Remind the client to bring the completed outline to the next office visit.

■ Follow-up:

- At the client's next visit, review the client's completed outline from her home exam(s).

Medical Assistant

Name: _____

Signature: _____

Date: _____

Client

Date: _____

Follow-up Date : _____

CHAPTER 21

Anticipatory Statements

People have varying ideas about skeletal system disorders. Read and think about the following statements based upon what you believe now. Decide whether you agree or disagree. Write the word **agree** after the statement if you think the statement is true. Write the word **disagree** after the statement if you think the statement is false. Read the chapter to find out if your current beliefs can be supported.

1. A client with scoliosis will appear to be standing crooked. _____

2. A strain is an injury to the bones. _____

3. Bone cancer is common in adults. _____

4. Arthritis is a normal part of aging. _____

5. A sprain may take as long as a broken bone to heal. _____

Skeletal System Disorders

Learning Objectives

Upon completion of this chapter, the medical assistant student should be able to:

- Identify major categories of skeletal system disorders
- List acute-onset disorders that are caused by injuries
- Explain arthritis
- State the difference between a strain and a sprain
- List at least four risk factors for osteoporosis
- Define dislocation
- Discuss the medical assistant's role in the treatment of clients who have skeletal system disorders
- Prepare a teaching plan to assist a client who has a skeletal system disorder

Key Terms

arthritis Inflammation of the joints.

bursa A space near the joints; holds synovial fluid to reduce friction between tendons, bones, and ligaments.

bursitis Inflammation of the bursa.

cancer Uncontrolled growth of abnormal cells, which can crowd out and damage healthy tissues.

dislocation Displacement of one or more bones at a joint.

ecchymosis Bruising; bleeding under the skin.

fracture To break; a break.

genetic Inherited.

inflammatory Describes the body's response to cell or tissue injury.

kyphosis Thoracic curvature of the spine; hunchback.

lordosis Lumbar curvature of the spine; swayback.

osteoporosis Loss of bone mass; puts a person at risk of fractures.

scoliosis Abnormal lateral curvature of the spine.

spinal fusion Surgical procedure in which selected vertebrae are joined together or fused.

sprain Injury to a joint.

strain Injury to a muscle or tendon caused by overuse.

■ INTRODUCTION

The medical assistant will work with many clients who have skeletal system disorders. These conditions affect movement and hamper the client's ability to move about freely and perform activities of daily living (ADLs). These disorders also affect a person's quality of life. Many conditions are painful, so the medical assistant needs to assess clients for pain and provide comfort measures. Some conditions are acute (sudden onset), such as fractured (broken) bones. Injuries such as sprains, strains, and dislocations occur as a result of injury to the skeleton and supporting structures. Disorders can develop gradually over time. Some are a result of aging and deterioration (wear and tear over time). Brief explanations of some common skeletal system disorders are given in the following sections. Causes, risk factors, and treatment options are included for further information on each disorder. The medical assistant's role may include assisting the doctor in the treatment of an acute injury, or teaching the client to care for an injury during the healing phase.

■ ACUTE CONDITIONS

Skeletal disorders can come on suddenly, as a result of injury or trauma. Four common problems are fractures, sprains, strains, and dislocations. These are often first seen in the emergency room of a hospital. After the initial assessment and treatment, the client is often seen at a physician's office for follow-up.

Fractures

Fractures can happen to anyone at any time. The three major signs of a fracture are pain, **ecchymosis** (bruising), and restricted motion or loss of motion. Fractures can be classified as *closed* (simple), *open* (compound), or *incomplete* (greenstick) (Figure 21-1). In a closed or simple fracture, the fractured bone has not protruded through the ligaments or the skin. Depending upon the site, a cast is usually applied to allow the bone to heal in alignment, prevent movement, and ease pain. In an open or compound fracture, the bone comes through the skin. A comminuted fracture is a fracture in which the bone has splintered. In addition to a cast, surgery is frequently needed to "pin" or set the bone in place. An incomplete or greenstick fracture occurs when a bone has bent and partially broken. This type of fracture is called "greenstick" because it is the kind of break seen when a green limb of a tree is broken. This type of fracture occurs most often in younger children.

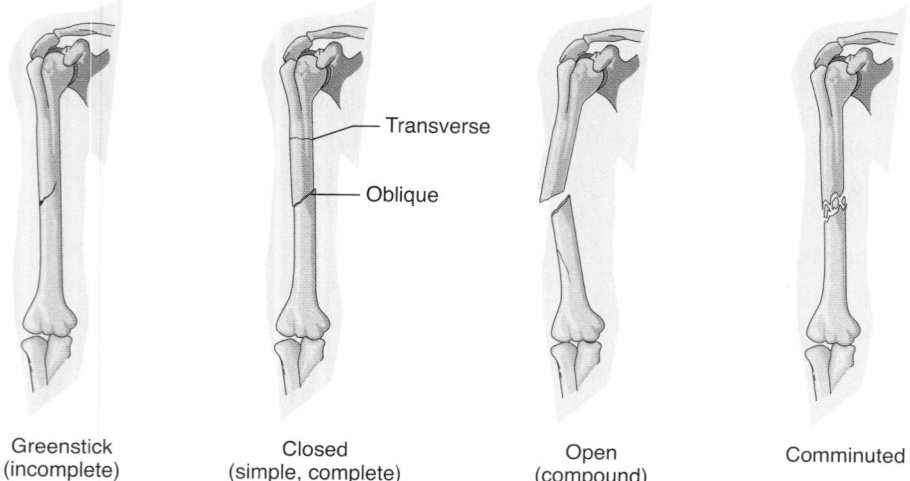

Greenstick (incomplete) Closed (simple, complete) Open (compound) Comminuted

FIGURE 21-1 Types of fractures.

Healing of a fracture can take from a few weeks to several months. The length of time depends on the type of fracture, the site of the broken bone in the body, and the health and condition of the client. Generally, younger, healthy individuals heal faster than elderly persons.

Sprains

A **sprain** is an injury to the ligaments. If the injury is severe enough, the ligament can be torn completely and can break off a piece of the bone (Figure 21-2). This is called a *sprain fracture.* The ankles and the back are two areas that are commonly sprained. The area near the sprain may feel warm and look discolored or swollen. The client experiences pain and often wonders whether the injured area is "broken." An examination by a physician and X-rays will help to determine if the injury is a broken bone or a sprain. Initial treatment includes application of ice to slow down swelling; if possible, the affected area should be elevated to decrease swelling and inflammation. The physician may also prescribe pain medication (analgesic) and anti-inflammatory medication. A sprain may take as long as a broken bone to heal. The medical assistant will need to be supportive and empathetic regarding the client's pain and interruption of his usual routine.

NOTE TO STUDENT:

Information about strains is included here because this type of injury must be distinguished from a broken bone or sprain. An injured client may at first appear to have any one of the three conditions.

Strains

A **strain** is an injury to the tendons or muscle from trauma or overuse. This type of injury often happens to a person who is not used to physical activity and suddenly decides to begin playing a sport or exercising strenuously without first getting into condition. If this happens, the medical assistant will need to offer support and encouragement to the client, who may become discouraged and give up trying to "get in shape." The medical assistant should explain the importance of warm-up exercises and not overdoing. It takes time for the benefits of exercise to occur and possible enjoyment of a sport affects willingness to continue exercising. The client should be encouraged to speak with the doctor before attempting any new strenuous physical activity.

Dislocations

A **dislocation** is the displacement of a bone from its usual position in a joint (Figure 21-3). There

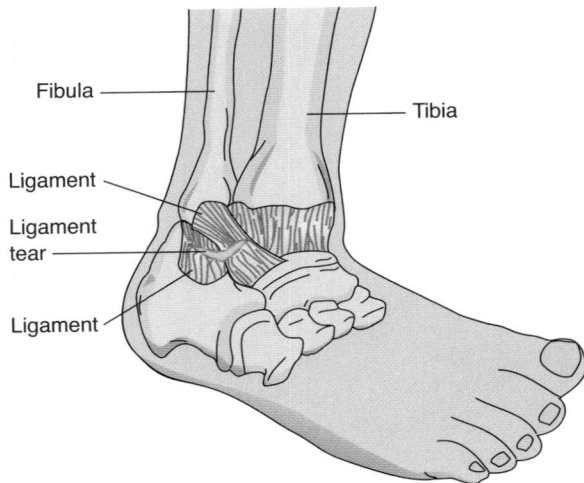

FIGURE 21-2 Sprained ankle.

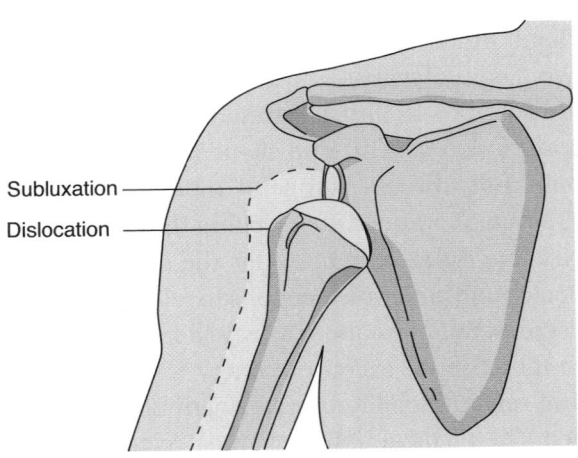

FIGURE 21-3 Dislocation.

are many classifications depending on the place where the dislocation occurs and the cause. Dislocations are often due to trauma. The treatment is reduction. To *reduce* a dislocation means to replace the bone in the correct position in the joint. Pain relief is almost immediate when reduction is complete.

■ CHRONIC DISORDERS

Many skeletal disorders are chronic, meaning that they are of long duration. Recovery may be slow. The client may experience chronic pain, long-term stiffness, and restrictions on some activities. The medical assistant will collect information, assist the doctor, and provide teaching. The role of the medical assistant is often mainly supportive, as it takes a long time for these conditions to heal or lessen and for the client to get better. The client is often uncomfortable, and the medical assistant should encourage clients to express their feelings.

Frozen Shoulder

Frozen shoulder is a disorder that often develops after an acute condition such as an injury or inflammation. The clavicle (collarbone), scapula (shoulder blade), and the humerus (upper arm bone) are all involved in the working of the shoulder joint. An injury to any of these areas can put a person at risk of developing frozen shoulder. Depending on the acute condition that initiates the problem, sometimes the shoulder is purposely immobilized; sometimes the client limits his own shoulder movement to avoid pain. Because of the inactivity, the shoulder loses its ability to stretch and move after contraction sets in. The client will complain of pain and stiffness. Range of motion is limited. Treatment is aimed at returning the client to his baseline range of motion for the shoulder. The doctor may order medications to relieve pain and decrease inflammation. This will help the client to take part in exercise therapy to help stretch and regain mobility or movement of the shoulder. The medical assistant must recognize that "unfreezing" the shoulder may take months. The

client needs to be encouraged to work steadily at the exercises. This is not a quick recovery.

Arthritis

Arthritis is an **inflammatory** disorder affecting the joints. There are many kinds of arthritis, but osteoarthritis is the type most likely to be seen by the medical assistant in an office (Figure 21-4). The inflammatory process causes swelling and stiffness in the joints. The person also experiences pain. The risk of acquiring arthritis increases with age, but this disorder is not a normal part of aging. Certain factors put an individual at risk for developing arthritis: in addition to aging, excess weight is a factor. Overuse of joints and strenuous activity, whether in a sport or during physical work, also affects the development of arthritis.

When obtaining a medical history and a social history from a client, the medical assistant should note risk factors. Does the client participate in sports that involve repetitive motion of joints? Tennis and golf are two examples. Does the client's work history consist of manual labor,

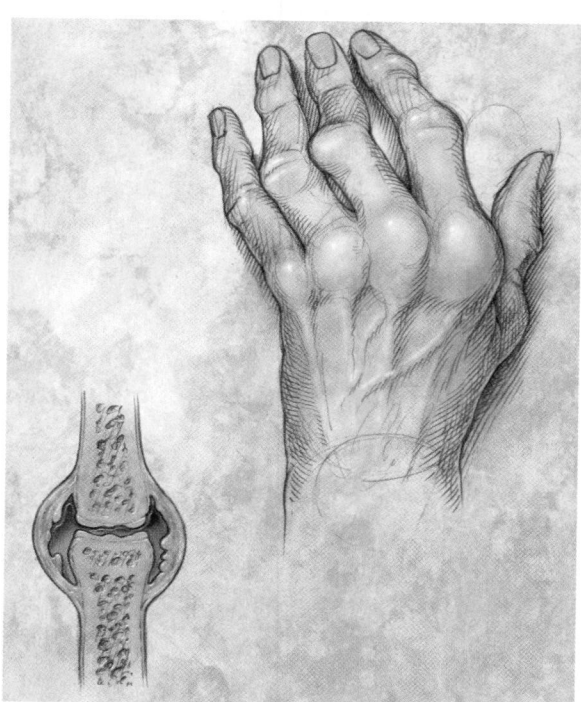

FIGURE 21-4 Arthritic hands. *(Courtesy of Getty Images)*

such as in manufacturing or construction work? Some clients may state that they have had to work hard all their lives and there is nothing they can do about it. The medical assistant needs to make the doctor aware of this so that the physician can prescribe an appropriate treatment.

The physician will prescribe a course of treatment aimed at symptom relief. Exercise is important, so the client may start with an exercise that is not stressful for the joints, such as swimming. Heat can provide relief. Rest is also important. If the client is obese, weight loss can decrease pain in the joints.

If all these treatments have been prescribed and followed, and the client has not gotten relief, surgery is a choice. If the joint affected with arthritis is a knee or hip, a knee or hip replacement may be performed.

The medical assistant needs to understand and work with the client who has arthritis. Arthritis is a long-term condition, and conservative treatment takes time to become effective. The medical assistant can help the client to pursue daily activities and treatments. For example, working, then resting to relieve fatigue, and then returning to work is better than doing an intense workout and resting for a long time.

Bursitis

Bursitis, which is common in the shoulder, knee, and elbow, is an inflammation of the **bursa** between the bony prominence and muscle. Tennis elbow and housemaid's knee are common layperson's terms describing this condition. When this condition first occurs (acute phase),

the client may experience pain or limitation of movement. The doctor may prescribe rest with little activity for the joints affected. Heat and pain medication are also used. If the condition does not improve, the client may be sent for physical therapy. The medical assistant needs to reinforce the prescribed treatment to help keep the client from developing chronic bursitis.

Bone Cancer

Cancer is the uncontrolled growth of abnormal cells; the cancerous cells, if not treated, will invade healthy tissue. Cancer that begins in the bone (primary bone tumor) is rare in adults. *Osteosarcoma,* which is a primary-site bone tumor, is seen mostly in children and teenagers, and only rarely in adults. Metastatic secondary bone tumors are more common in adults. Primary-site cancers can spread (*metastasize*) to the bone. Breast and prostate cancer, unless diagnosed and successfully treated, can easily spread to the bones and cause secondary bone cancer.

The medical assistant needs to follow the client's plan of care, which will be developed with input from everyone on the health care team. When giving physical care, the medical assistant must use clean, gentle techniques. The family should be given instructions on how to assist the client. The client and his family will also need emotional support. The medical assistant must use therapeutic communication in these situations and allow the client and family members the opportunity to share their feelings.

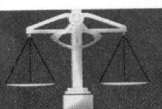

LEGAL/ETHICAL THOUGHTS

Clients who experience chronic pain are vulnerable to scams that promise cures and freedom from pain. Always be supportive of clients who have chronic pain. If they are able to share their frustrations and worries, they may be less susceptible to those who prey upon these individuals in order to obtain money fraudulently.

▇ SPINE CURVATURES

The spinal column (spine or backbone) is made up of 33 vertebrae: 7 cervical, 12 thoracic, 5 lumbar, 5 sacral, and 4 coccygeal. Various conditions can cause the spine to distort from the normal curve pattern (Figure 21-5). Three common conditions are kyphosis, lordosis, and scoliosis.

Kyphosis

In **kyphosis,** the normal postural curve is exaggerated (Figure 21-5A). The client appears to have a hunchback. The cause can be congenital (present at birth). Diseases such as syphilis and tuberculosis, as well as malignancy (cancer) or compression fractures, can also cause the condition. Sometimes the term *kyphosis* is applied to a spinal curvature with a backward convexity. This is usually caused by osteoarthritis, rheumatoid arthritis, or rickets.

Lordosis

Lordosis is a condition in which the lumbar spine (lower back) has a convexity in its anterior part (Figure 21-5B). The client appears to have a swayback. There can be a **genetic** cause, or disease can cause this curvature.

Scoliosis

Scoliosis is a lateral curvature of the spine (Figure 21-5C). In scoliosis, there are often two curves: a primary curve and another curve that compensates (makes up) for the primary abnormal curve. Scoliosis can be congenital, stemming from improper development of the vertebral bones. Various diseases can also cause scoliosis. Scoliosis can also be idiopathic (having no known cause).

The client with a scoliosis will appear to be standing crooked. The curve will be different depending on the location of the spinal deformity.

Routine scoliosis screenings are done at schools or in the pediatrician's office, to detect scoliosis at an early age. To do a basic screening, the medical assistant asks the child to bend at the waist, allowing the arms to hang down freely. The medical assistant stands behind the client and looks for symmetry of the back (same on both sides of the vertebrae). If the medical assistant sees a curve, he or she then uses a handheld ruler to measure the amount of curve. This number is noted and the doctor is informed.

Some types of scoliosis respond to the use of an orthopedic brace. In these cases, the client will need to wear the brace for a long period of time, up to several years. At each office visit, the medical assistant checks for any signs of skin irritation from the brace. It is necessary to teach the client about good skin care and make sure he follows the directions about use and care of the brace. Because the brace must be worn all the time, even when at school, work, home, or out with friends, the client may become self-conscious or embarrassed. Be a good listener and allow him to talk about these feelings.

Some scolioses are treated with surgery. A rod may be implanted in the back, or a **spinal fusion** may be performed to join the separate vertebrae together. The medical assistant will do preoperation teaching as directed by the physician. One long-term effect of a spinal fusion is a decrease in the amount of flexibility of the back. The amount of decrease in flexibility will be related to the number and location of the vertebrae to be fused.

▇ OSTEOPOROSIS

Osteoporosis is the loss of bone mass (Figure 21-6). This condition develops over time. In

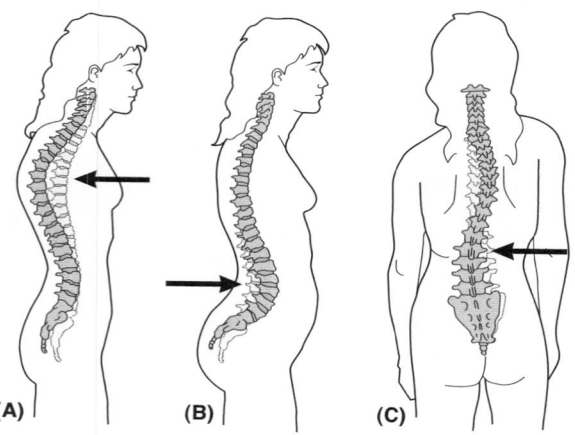

(A)   (B)   (C)

FIGURE 21–5 Abnormal curvatures of the spine.

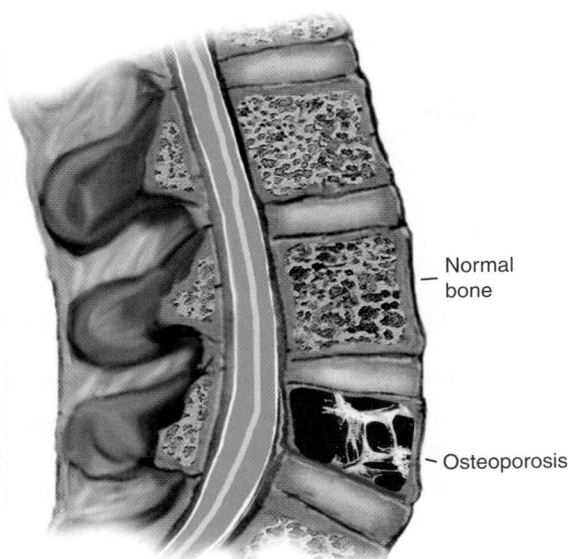

FIGURE 21-6 Normal and osteoporotic bone.

is painless and noninvasive. The medical assistant can reassure the client that no specific preparation is needed, other than to refrain from wearing clothing with metal clasps and fasteners. There are no precautions for the client after the completion of the test.

Certain factors increase a person's risk of developing osteoporosis. Some of these are nonmodifiable, meaning that they cannot be changed. The nonmodifiable risk factors are genetics, gender, race, body frame, and age of menopause. Inheriting a small-framed body increases a person's risk. Females are more likely than males to develop osteoporosis at an early age. Caucasian and Asian women are at increased risk. Experiencing menopause at an early age (before 45) also increases the risk.

Medication can increase bone loss. Phenytoin, used for seizure treatment, is one of these. Thyroid medication and the corticosteroids used in the treatment of many conditions also put a person at increased risk.

Endocrine disorders, such as Cushing's disease, hypertension, hyperparathyroidism, acromegaly, and hypogonadism, can contribute to bone loss. Smoking and excessive alcohol intake can start or increase the rate of osteoporosis.

Osteoporosis is a serious, debilitating disorder that causes pain, often leads to fractures, and may eventually cause loss of mobility because of multiple fractures. The medical

healthy bones, new bone is "laid down" as older bone is destroyed, in a process termed *bone remodeling*. In a person with osteoporosis, more bone is destroyed than is laid down. Osteoporosis is preceded by osteopenia. The client usually does not become aware of osteoporosis until after a fracture (Figure 21-7). Because there are no signs or symptoms of osteoporosis, it is important to prevent and/or treat the condition as soon as possible. It is important to have a bone density test done to verify a diagnosis of osteopenia or osteoporosis. A bone density test

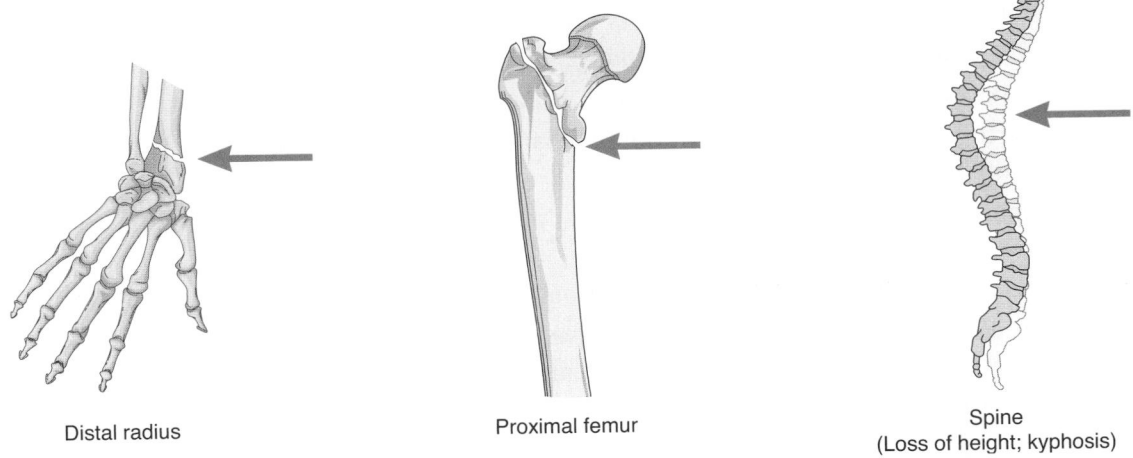

Distal radius   Proximal femur   Spine
(Loss of height; kyphosis)

FIGURE 21-7 Fractures due to osteoporosis.

assistant can teach clients to prevent or lessen this disorder through healthy lifestyle and appropriate activities. Diet should include sufficient amounts of calcium and vitamin D. Limiting caffeine is another positive step. Caffeine is found in coffee, tea, colas, and chocolate. Individuals need to do weight-bearing exercise frequently. Brisk walking is an excellent exercise for the skeletal system. For many health benefits, including decreased risk of osteoporosis, the medical assistant should give all possible help to a client who wishes to stop smoking.

 ## BRIDGE TO CAAHEP

This chapter, which discusses skeletal system disorders, provides information and content related to CAAHEP standards for Anatomy and Physiology, Common Pathology/Diseases, Diagnostic/Treatment Modalities, Medical Terminology, Medical Law and Ethics, Communication, Medical Assisting Clinical Procedures, and Professional Components.

 ## ABHES LINKS

This chapter, which discusses skeletal system disorders, links to ABHES course content for Anatomy and Physiology, Medical Terminology, Medical Law and Ethics, and Medical Office Clinical Procedures.

 ## AAMA AREAS OF COMPETENCE

This chapter, which discusses skeletal system disorders, provides information or content within several areas listed in the Medical Assistant Role Delineation Study. These areas include: clinical, fundamental principles, patient (client care), general transdisciplinary, professionalism, communication skills, legal concepts, and instruction.

 ## AMT PATHS

This chapter, which discusses skeletal system disorders, provides a path to AMT competency in general medical assisting knowledge, anatomy and physiology, medical terminology, and patient (client) education.

POINTS OF HIGHLIGHT

- Skeletal system disorders affect a client's ability to move about freely.
- Skeletal disorders can be acute or chronic.
- Acute skeletal disorders include fractures, sprains, strains, and dislocations.
- Osteoarthritis is an inflammatory disorder characterized by swelling, stiffness, and pain in the joints.
- Osteoporosis (loss of bone mass) is the most prevalent bone disorder; it leads to pain, fractures, and disability.
- Bone cancer often occurs when a cancer from another site spreads to the bone.
- The medical assistant needs to be supportive of clients who have skeletal system disorders, as these disorders are often accompanied by pain and frustrating mobility limitations.

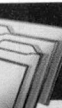

STUDENT PORTFOLIO ACTIVITY

Employers like to hire individuals who possess more than the minimum requirements for a job. For example, once you are competent in obtaining vital signs, find opportunities to take blood pressures. Medical assisting students might set up the clinical lab and offer free blood pressure readings to prospective students as they visit during your school's open house. Be sure to work with instructors who can verify your activity.

APPLYING YOUR SKILLS

Scoliosis is often detected during a routine checkup. What is scoliosis? What will you observe in the client who has it? What skills do you as a medical assistant need when working with a client who has a newly diagnosed scoliosis?

CRITICAL THINKING QUESTIONS

1. A client complains of itching under his leg cast. He tells you that his friend gave him a plastic backscratcher that he has been able to wedge under his cast to scratch. What would you tell him? What reasons would you give for not using it?

2. A client's bone density test report came back with a diagnosis of osteopenia. What can the client do to prevent further loss of bone?

3. A 65-year-old man has been diagnosed with osteoarthritis. What are some signs that you might observe in this client? What are some complaints that he might state when discussing his concerns about this disorder?

4. A client has a sprained ankle. He tells you that "it hurts a lot and it's not even broken." How would you explain sprains to him? What can you tell him about healing time?

5. A client's breast cancer has spread (metastasized) to the bone. What are some of the client's needs at this time?

6. Why is it important to check children for scoliosis?

7. You observe that a hunchback or kyphosis has developed in an older client. What are some causes of this condition?

8. You are working with a teenager and want to share ways for this client to build healthy bones and prevent osteoporosis later in life. What are some points to include in your discussion with this client?

9. Another health care worker does not understand why a client who has osteoarthritis complains about pain at every office visit. What would you explain to your fellow worker about chronic skeletal disorders and pain?

10. What are some ways to prevent acute bursitis from developing into chronic bursitis? How can the client's actions help in this prevention?

11. Go back to the beginning of this chapter and review the Anticipatory Statements. Reread each statement and then indicate whether it is true or false. If the statement is false, rewrite it to make it a true statement.

CLIENT TEACHING PLAN

Frozen Shoulder Exercises

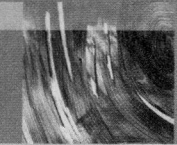

What Is to Be Taught:

- How to perform exercises for a frozen shoulder.

Objectives:

- Client will be able to do exercises to release a frozen shoulder and regain use of the joint.

Preparation Before Teaching:

- Review the anatomy of the shoulder and possible causes of a frozen shoulder, such as injury, fracture, or acute inflammation.
- Look up risk factors and who is most likely to have a frozen shoulder.
- Get together materials for teaching, such as a three-foot-long towel and paper and pen for written instructions.
- Make sure the area is free from distractions while you are teaching.

Steps for the Medical Assistant:

1. Wash your hands.
2. Gather needed supplies.
3. Introduce yourself to the client.
4. Explain what you are going to teach and why.
5. Explain to the client that immobility of the shoulder area, because of injury, illness, or surgery, can put a person at risk of a frozen shoulder.
6. A frozen shoulder can usually be unfrozen, although the client will have to work at it through exercise.
7. Inform the client that you will show him a series of exercises to help stretch the shoulder.
8. Tell the client that he should take a warm bath or shower to warm up the muscles before stretching.
9. Have the client sit. Using one arm, lift the other arm at the elbow (instruct client to use his unaffected or "good" arm to lift the affected arm) and bring it across the chest, using a little amount of pressure. Hold for 15 seconds. Tell

the client that he should repeat this 10 to 20 times once a day.

10. Have the client stand. With one arm, lift the injured arm and place it onto a ledge or shelf at about mid-chest height. Gently bend the knees, to stretch open the underarm area. Keep bending the knees slightly so as to not jerk the arm and cause pain. Slowly straighten up. Tell the client not to force this. (Remember, the client may also have arthritis in the knees.) This exercise should be repeated 10 to 20 times once each day.
11. Walk over to a wall. Have the client stand about three-quarters of an arm's length away. Ask the client to touch the wall with the fingertips of the affected arm at about waist height. Walk the fingers up the wall like a spider. Do this until level with the shoulder. Use the fingers, not the shoulder. Tell the client not to go that high if there is pain. Keep the elbow slightly flexed, and then slowly lower the arm. Tell the client that if the lowering portion of the exercise is uncomfortable, he can use the unaffected arm to assist.
12. Pick up the towel and hold it behind your back, using both hands. Hold the towel level and even. Demonstrate pulling the towel with one arm, which will in turn stretch the other arm. Remind the client to pull using the unaffected or "good" arm. Tell the client that he should repeat this exercise 10 to 20 times once each day.
13. Ask the client to perform these four exercises as you give prompts and encouragement.
14. Ask the client if he has any questions.
15. Hand the client written instruction with step-by-step directions for doing these exercises, and a list of the number of repetitions to be done each day.

Special Needs of the Client:

- Look at the client's chart to see if there are any factors that might interfere with the client's ability to remember and perform the exercises.

(Continues)

CLIENT TEACHING PLAN (Continued)

- Ask the client, before and after the teaching and demonstration, if there is anything you should know about that might affect his performance of these exercises.

Evaluation:

- Client is able to state the purpose of the stretching exercises.
- Client is able to demonstrate the four exercises with the steps in the correct order after observing your demonstration.

Further Plans/Teaching:

- Ask the client if he has any questions or needs any additional information.

Follow-up:

- Call the client at home in a few days. Ask the client if he has had any problems with the exercises.

- Encourage the client to continue with the stretching exercises at whatever level he can.
- At the next visit, ask the client to perform the exercises. Review any steps as necessary.

Medical Assistant

Name: _____

Signature: _____

Date: _____

Client

Date: _____

Follow-up Date : _____

Anticipatory Statements

People have different ideas about muscular system disorders. Read and think about the following statements based upon what you believe now. Decide whether you agree or disagree. Write the word **agree** after the statement if you think the statement is true. Write the word **disagree** after the statement if you think the statement is false. Read the chapter to find out if your current beliefs can be supported.

1. If muscles are not used, they can weaken and shrink. _____

2. People who are not well conditioned often injure themselves while attempting strenuous exercises or sports. _____

3. The disorder called "tennis elbow" is not related to use of the elbow. _____

4. Ice should never be used after an injury to the muscles. _____

5. When an organ pushes out through weak muscles, the condition is called a hernia. _____

Muscular System Disorders

Learning Objectives

Upon completion of this chapter, the medical assistant student should be able to:

■ Identify the medical assistant's role in caring for a client who has a muscular system disorder

■ Explain what happens to the client who has muscular dystrophy

■ Describe the appearance of a client who has myasthenia gravis

■ State the difference between a muscle strain and a muscle spasm

■ Describe sites where hernias commonly occur

■ Discuss the treatment of fibromyalgia

■ Discuss what happens to a client's muscles after a long period of inactivity or bedrest

Key Terms

atrophy Shrinking or decrease in size of tissue.

contracture Permanent shortening of tissue that causes a deformity.

fibromyalgia Painful musculoskeletal condition.

hernia Weakening of a muscular wall through which internal structures can protrude.

muscular dystrophy Inherited disorder characterized by progressive weakening of muscles.

myasthenia gravis Neuromuscular disorder with progressive weakening of voluntary muscles.

■ INTRODUCTION

Disorders of the muscular system can arise suddenly, as in the case of an injury; these are called *acute disorders.* They can also develop slowly over time; these are called *chronic disorders.* The medical assistant should be familiar with the more common disorders, as clients with these problems are often seen in the medical office. The medical assistant's role regarding these clients will vary depending on the disorder and the medical office policy.

■ ACUTE DISORDERS

With today's increased emphasis on exercise and sports exercise-related injuries are common complaints in the medical office setting. Some injuries are sustained by athletes, through a fall or accident, during the course of playing a sport. Many times, however, the muscle injury is due to stress or strain of a muscle that is not well conditioned or prepared for exercise.

Tendons are connective tissue that attaches muscle to bone. Tendons are often the site of injury. For instance, when someone takes up the popular exercise of jogging or running, she may develop "shin splints" if the tendons in the front of the shin are injured or overused. Injury is particularly likely if the person is not conditioned properly before starting the new exercise, or overdoes the amount when beginning.

Although the common name for another condition is *"tennis elbow,"* any activity can put a person at risk of this problem if it involves repetitive use of the elbow and forearm (Figure 22-1). Workers such as movers who are constantly lift-

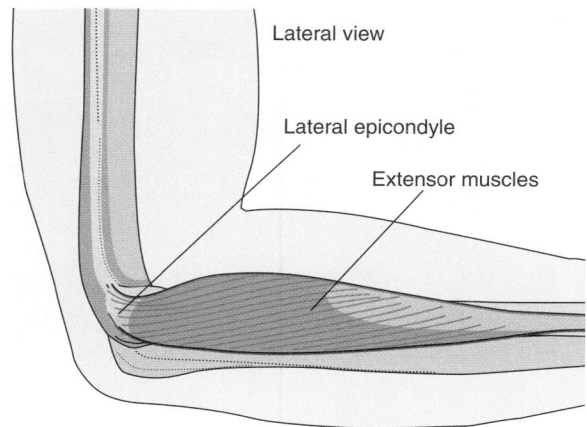

FIGURE 22-1 Tennis elbow.

ing, and carpenters who repeatedly hammer, are examples of people whose occupations put them at increased risk. The tendons and muscles at the elbow become irritated and then inflamed. The doctor may order pain medication, rest for the affected arm, and ice packs until healing takes place.

The tendons at the shoulder joint can also become inflamed from repetitive activity (Figure 22-2). Any activity that involves raising the arm overhead can affect the shoulder and put the client at risk. Tennis and baseball are two such activities. This type of injury can also occur from an accident, such as when an elderly person slips, falls, and tries to grab onto something to break the fall. The usual treatment is pain medication and physical therapy.

People may begin an intensive exercise plan or sport before getting into condition. They can overdo it and suffer muscle injuries, such as muscle stress or muscle spasm. A muscle strain can occur when a muscle is stressed

LEGAL/ETHICAL THOUGHTS

Clients often have misinformation or wrong ideas about diets, exercise, and weight loss. It is important that medical assistants always teach correct information about healthy eating, exercise, and weight loss. However, do not argue with clients. People are often reluctant to change their ideas, and arguing does not help.

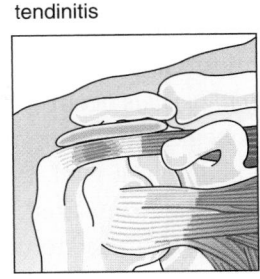

Overuse
tendinitis

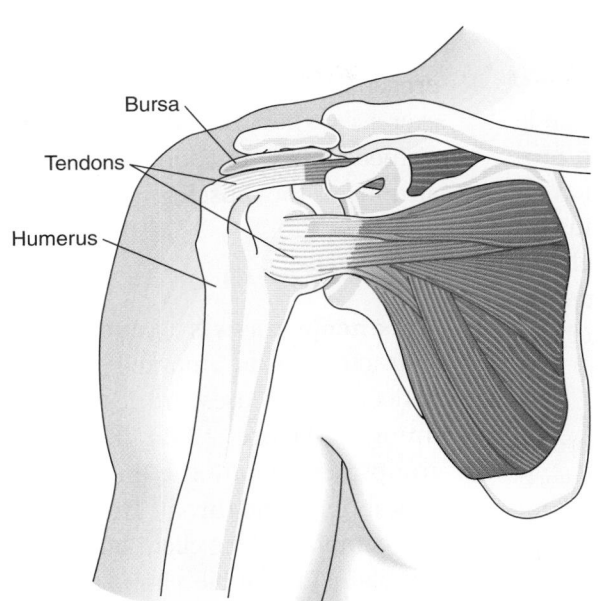

Bursa

Tendons

Humerus

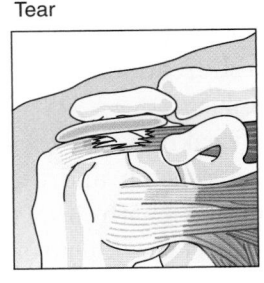

Tear

FIGURE 22–2 The shoulder in health (left) and with injuries (right).

or overused. Pain, swelling, and bleeding inside the muscle can result from overuse. Cramps or muscle spasms happen when a muscle is overused.

The medical assistant reinforces prescribed treatments for all acute muscular injuries. The medical assistant also allows the client an opportunity to express feelings. There is no quick fix for such injuries; the client must follow the treatment plan and allow time for the injury to heal.

■ CHRONIC MUSCLE PAIN

In addition to acute disorders, muscle pain can become a chronic problem. *Chronic pain* is defined as pain lasting longer than three months. Chronic muscle pain can become generalized; that is, involve more than one area.

Fibromyalgia

Fibromyalgia is a group of symptoms that includes muscle pain. Headaches, feelings of tiredness, aching, numbness, and tingling of muscles and joints are also often present. To help confirm the condition, the doctor will order

diagnostic tests to rule out other disorders. The diagnosis is frequently made only after all other problems that have similar symptoms are eliminated. In addition to pain medication, other treatments vary according to the needs of the client and the doctor's decision. The treatments are all based on healthy lifestyle behaviors. These include good sleep patterns, exercise, relaxation, and massage therapy. The medical assistant needs to be supportive of these clients, as chronic pain can interfere with a client's life.

■ CHRONIC DISORDERS

Clients who have chronic muscular disorders often have similar health problems. The muscles may weaken, atrophy, or become contracted due to lack of use, and mobility may be lost as a result of the chronic disorder.

Weakness

Muscles can become weak either through lack of use or from an underlying condition. Weak muscles can cause other conditions for which the client will seek help from the doctor. When muscles become so weak that internal structures cannot be supported and organs protrude, a **hernia** exists. Three common types of hernias are abdominal, inguinal, and hiatal.

Abdominal hernias occur when the abdominal muscles weaken and the organs protrude through the abdominal wall. If the organ protrudes through the groin area, it is termed an *inguinal hernia*. When the stomach extends up through the diaphragm muscle, it is called a *hiatal hernia*. Medical treatment is frequently prescribed for hiatal hernias, but surgery is often the best treatment for abdominal and inguinal hernias.

Muscle weakness can occur anywhere in the body. The skeleton and the muscles work together. A problem with either the bones or the muscles will affect the other. For example, weak muscles in the legs can injure the arches and cause flat feet. Eventually, the client will experience foot pain and may seek medical treatment to get relief from the pain.

Contractures

Immobility is a major risk factor for muscular problems. When muscles shrink and shorten, joints can become fixed in position, making the person unable to move that part of the body. This condition, called a **contracture,** is a very disabling problem. A stroke, fracture, or any pain or injury that hinders movement puts a client at risk. Treatment is aimed at restoring movement of the affected part before the contracture becomes permanent. Active range-of-motion (AROM), in which the client performs exercises on her own, and passive range-of-motion (PROM), in which another person puts the client's muscles through the exercises, are critical for a client with contractures.

Atrophy

When muscles are toned, they are always ready to be used. Good nutrition and exercise help keep the muscles ready for action. Prolonged bedrest, fractures, and stroke can cause the muscles to lose tone and thus lose the ability to

spring into action. Whatever the cause of the inactivity, when muscles are not used, they lose tone, shrink, and **atrophy.** Exercise is crucial to prevent this. If the client cannot perform AROM exercises, then PROM exercises must be performed for her, and done consistently to prevent atrophy of the muscles.

Myasthenia Gravis

Myasthenia gravis is a neuromuscular disorder characterized by marked fluctuations (very noticeable increases and decreases) in muscular strength (Figure 22-3). The affected muscle groups are usually the muscles governing the eyes, mouth, and throat. This is often the client's first complaint. The client often experiences and complains of double vision and/or drooping of the eyelids, or trouble with swallowing, chewing, and slurred speech, as well as nasal regurgitation. These symptoms are least noticeable in the morning, but as the day goes on the weakness

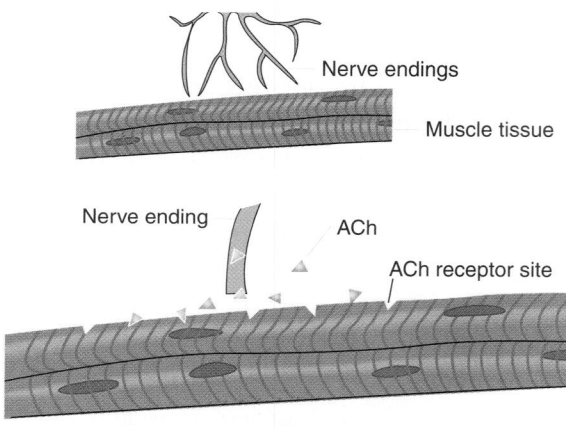

Normal (Magnified)

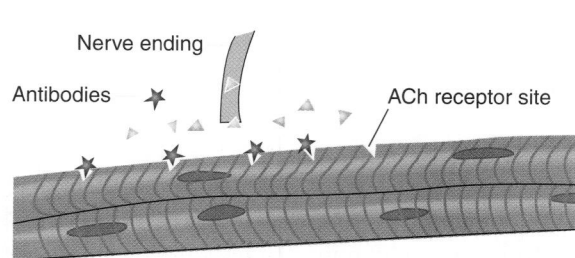

Myasthenia Gravis (Magnified)

FIGURE 22-3 Myasthenia gravis.

becomes worse. If the client rests for a while, the symptoms may improve, but only temporarily. As the disease progresses over months to years, the large muscle groups, especially of the neck and arms, will be affected. The client develops a characteristic drooping face or jaw appearance and often holds the chin up.

Myasthenia gravis often causes a pattern of greater proximal muscle involvement (muscles closer to the center of the body) as compared to weakness of the distal muscles (muscles farther away from the center of the body). This pattern of muscle weakness is often seen in Myasthenia Gravis. Less common types of myasthenia gravis include the neonatal type, called "floppy baby" syndrome; congenital types; and drug-induced types. Myasthenia gravis is an autoimmune disorder in which the body forms antibodies to the acetylcholine receptors in the postsynaptic region. This results in a defect of neuromuscular transmission, which causes the muscular weakness. Myasthenia gravis is also associated with other autoimmune diseases such as lupus and rheumatoid arthritis. The thymus, which is an organ of the immune system, is abnormal in more than 75% of these clients.

Myasthenia gravis clients frequently experience a marked worsening of weakness if they contract an infectious disease, develop certain thyroid disorders, or become pregnant. These clients' respiratory ability may change dramatically because of the weakness, even to the point of making respiratory support necessary. It is very important that clients who have myasthenia gravis be seen and treated quickly if they start to experience increased problems with respiration or swallowing.

A client can be tested in the office for suspected myasthenia gravis with the Tensilon test. Electromyographic studies can also detect the presence of myasthenia gravis. Testing the serum for acetylcholine receptor antibodies is yet another way to make this diagnosis. The client is treated with medication, and many times a thymectomy (surgical removal of the thymus) is done during the course of the disease.

Muscular Dystrophy

The various types of **muscular dystrophy** are all specific genetic disorders. The best-known type is Duchenne's, which is linked to an abnormal X chromosome. Initially, clients with muscular dystrophy are characterized by slow motor development. The client often has large calves and a waddling gait. The Gower's test is positive if the client needs to push himself up from the floor out of the prone position. He then "walks up" his legs until standing. Over time, the client develops a prominent lordosis (curvature of the back) when standing upright. Muscular dystrophy destroys the muscles, and as a result skeletal abnormalities develop as well. By the time clients are in their teens, most must use wheelchairs. The muscles of the chest wall are also weakened. The cause of death in many of these clients, which usually occurs in their teens or twenties, is respiratory illness. Physical therapy, splints, and braces are used to maintain the client's mobility for as long as possible, as well as to prevent skeletal deformities.

 BRIDGE TO CAAHEP

This chapter, which discusses muscular system disorders, provides information and content related to CAAHEP standards for Anatomy and Physiology, Medical Terminology, Medical Law and Ethics, Psychology, Communication, Medical Assisting Clinical Procedures, and Professional Components.

 ABHES LINKS

This chapter, which discusses muscular system disorders, links to ABHES course content for medical assisting for Anatomy and Physiology, Medical Terminology, Medical Law and Ethics, and Medical Office Clinical Procedures.

 AAMA AREAS OF COMPETENCE

This chapter, which discusses muscular system disorders, provides information or content within several areas listed in the Medical Assistant Role

POINTS OF HIGHLIGHT

- Overuse of muscles that are not toned and conditioned can cause muscle injury.
- Repetitive use of a set of muscles can result in a painful disorder of the affected joint.
- Myasthenia gravis is a neuromuscular disorder in which the client experiences drastic changes in muscle strength.
- Muscular dystrophy is a genetic disorder in which the muscles are progressively destroyed.
- Muscles that are not used will weaken, lose tone, and eventually atrophy.
- Fibromyalgia is a group of symptoms involving chronic pain.
- Hernias commonly occur in the hiatal, abdominal, and inguinal regions.
- When muscles shrink and shorten, joints can freeze so that the client cannot move the affected area. This is called a contracture.

Delineation Study. These areas include: clinical, fundamental principles, diagnostic orders, patient (client) care, general transdisciplinary, professionalism, communication skills, legal concepts, and instruction.

 AMT PATHS

This chapter, which discusses muscular system disorders, provides a path to AMT competency in general medical assisting knowledge, anatomy and physiology, medical terminology, and patient (client) education.

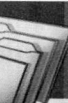 **STUDENT PORTFOLIO ACTIVITY**

Choose a disorder of interest to you. Think about an aspect of this disorder that you would include in client teaching. Using one of the sample client teaching plans as a blueprint, develop your own teaching plan. Put the completed teaching plan in your portfolio.

 APPLYING YOUR SKILLS

A client has sustained an injury to a muscle. Although the injury is healing in the expected time period, you observe that the client seems to hold the affected arm in a flexed or bent position. When asked to straighten the arm, she is very hesitant and is unable to extend or straighten the elbow. What is happening to the joint? What can be done to prevent this condition from becoming permanent?

CRITICAL THINKING QUESTIONS

1. An inactive individual decides to lose some weight and get in shape by taking up a sport such as tennis. Why is this individual now at a greater risk for a muscular injury?

2. What skills of a medical assistant can be applied to help a client who is being treated for fibromyalgia?

3. Describe some body-structure problems that can be caused by weak muscles.

4. Why is a client who has had a massive stroke at risk of contractures?

5. What happens to muscles that have lost much of their tone?

6. How can the problems identified in question 5 be prevented? Give specific examples to support your answer.

7. What might the client with myasthenia gravis observe about her symptoms throughout the day?

8. Why is important for a client with myasthenia gravis to contact the doctor immediately if she begins to experience problems with respiration and swallowing?

9. You work with a client who has fibromyalgia. What do you anticipate will be the client's major concerns?

10. Weakened muscles affect more than just the skeletal strength. Discuss other problems for which the client with weak muscles is at risk.

11. As a medical assistant, you have been asked to help a client's family perform PROM exercises on the client. How would you explain passive range of motion to the family?

12. What do you expect to see in a client with myasthenia gravis who has recently contracted an infection? What are some critical risks?

13. Many clients with chronic muscular disorders experience chronic pain. How can you, as a medical assistant, help these clients? What are your ideas?

14. You give care to many elderly clients at your place of employment. Why is it important for the client who is elderly to remain active? How does inactivity affect the muscular system?

15. A client does not seem to understand the meaning of hernia. How do you explain this in every-day language?

16. Another medical assistant asks you to explain why clients with muscular dystrophy often die in their teenage years. How would you describe this disease process to another health care provider?

17. Go back to the beginning of this chapter and review the Anticipatory Statements. Reread each state-ment and then indicate whether it is true or false. If the statement is false, rewrite it to make it a true statement.

CLIENT TEACHING PLAN

Passive Range-of-Motion (PROM) Exercises

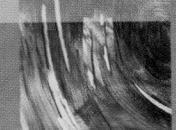

■ What Is to Be Taught:

• PROM exercises for the client's left hip and leg and right hip and leg.

■ Objectives:

• Caregiver will perform PROM exercises on the client's left hip and leg and right hip and leg.

■ Preparation Before Teaching:

• Review PROM exercises and the rationale or reasons for performing them. Make sure to put technical medical terms into words that the client and caregiver will understand.

■ Steps for the Medical Assistant:

1. Introduce yourself to the client.
2. Explain to the client and caregiver what you are going to teach and why.
3. Demonstrate handwashing to the caregiver.
4. Ask the caregiver to wash her hands.
5. Assist the client to a supine position on the examination table. Position yourself close to the table to ensure the client's safety.
6. Tell the client that you will be gentle, but if the movements cause pain or discomfort, the client should tell you and you will stop.
7. Instruct the caregiver also to watch for signs of pain, especially if the client has difficulty communicating.
8. Uncover only the left leg; maintain the client's privacy.
9. Support the left hip and leg.
10. Bend and then straighten the left hip and leg.
11. Repeat this three times.
12. Do not force the movement if you feel resistance in the muscles.
13. Straighten the left leg and bring the straight leg toward you. Then move the leg back to the center of the body.
14. Repeat this three times.

15. Do not force the movement if you feel resistance in the muscles.
16. Turn the left leg inward and then outward. This will rotate the left hip joint.
17. Repeat this three times.
18. Cover the client's left leg.
19. Ask the client and caregiver if they have any questions.
20. Uncover the client's right leg; maintain the client's privacy.
21. Show the caregiver how to support the right hip and leg.
22. Tell the caregiver to bend and then straighten the client's right hip and leg.
23. Instruct the caregiver to repeat this three times.
24. Inform the caregiver not to force the movement of the leg if she feels resistance in the muscles.
25. Tell the caregiver to straighten the right leg and bring the straight right leg toward herself; then have her move the leg back to the center of the client's body.
26. Repeat this three times.
27. Remind the caregiver not to force the movement if she feels resistance in the muscles.
28. Instruct the caregiver to turn the client's right leg inward and then outward. This will rotate the right hip joint.
29. Tell the caregiver to cover the right leg.
30. Ask the client how she feels.
31. Assist the client as needed.
32. Ask the client and caregiver if they have any questions.
33. Hand the client and/or caregiver written instructions.
34. Instruct the client and caregiver to call the office and speak with the doctor or medical assistant if any concerns or questions come up after they get home.

■ Special Needs of the Client:

• Look at the client's chart to see if there are any factors that might interfere with the caregiver's

(Continues)

CLIENT TEACHING PLAN (Continued)

performance of the exercises. (PROM exercises are being done because the client is unable to do them on her own; thus, there may be other factors or limitations to take into account.)

- Ask the client and caregiver, before and after the teaching and demonstration, if there is anything you should know that might affect their ability to perform these exercises.

Evaluation:

- Caregiver will be able to state the steps involved in the specific PROM exercises.
- Caregiver will be able to demonstrate the PROM to the client's hips and legs.

Further Plans/Teaching:

- Give written instructions to the client and caregiver to use as a reference at home.
- Give the client and caregiver the written telephone number and extension of the medical assistant to call if any questions arise while performing the exercises at home.

Follow-up:

- Call the client and caregiver within one week to see if they have any concerns or problems.
- At the follow-up visit, review the teaching plan for the range-of-motion exercises. Make any changes necessary to meet the client's health needs.

Medical Assistant

Name: _____

Signature: _____

Date: _____

Client

Date: _____

Follow-up Date : _____

CHAPTER 23

Anticipatory Statements

People have different ideas about the nervous system and sensory system disorders. Read and think about the following statements based upon what you believe now. Decide whether you agree or disagree. Write the word **agree** after the statement if you think the statement is true. Write the word **disagree** after the statement if you think the statement is false. Read the chapter to find out if your current beliefs can be supported.

1. All hearing loss can be corrected with a hearing aid.

   _____

2. A client who has Parkinson's disease may seem to lack any facial expressions.

   _____

3. High blood pressure is a risk factor for stroke.

   _____

4. Memory loss or dementia is always caused by Alzheimer's disease.

   _____

5. Almost half of all traumatic deaths in the United States are related to head injury.

   _____

Learning Objectives

Upon completion of this chapter, the medical assistant student should be able to:

- Recognize major disorders of the central nervous system
- Explain what is happening to the client with each of the major disorders
- Explain what is meant by dementia
- Describe what happens to a client who has a brain injury
- List types of common visual problems

Nervous System and Sensory System Disorders

- Identify two types of hearing loss
- Develop a teaching plan and put it into action

Key Terms

astigmatism Abnormal curve or shape of the cornea (lens of the eye); causes distorted or wavy vision.

bradykinesia Very slow movement.

cataract A clouding of the normally clear lens of the eye.

concussion Injury to the brain caused by trauma from outside of the head (for example, a blow to a boxer's head during a fight, or a soccer ball forcefully hitting a player's head).

dementia Steady decrease in mental ability that affects all parts of mental functioning. Dementia eventually impairs a person's ability to perform activities of daily living.

gait An individual's pattern of walking or ambulation.

hyperopia Farsightedness.

multiple sclerosis Progressive disorder in which the myelin sheath of the nerves is destroyed. Frequently begins in young adulthood.

myopia Nearsightedness.

otitis media Inflammation of the middle ear.

otosclerosis Condition that affects the bones in the ear and thus causes hearing loss.

Parkinson's disease Progressive neurological disorder characterized by muscle rigidity and tremors.

presbyopia Condition in which the lens of the eye loses the ability of accommodation; usually occurs as a person ages.

seizures Erratic, disorganized electrical impulses discharged within the brain. Seizures occur suddenly.

sensorineural Hearing loss caused by nerve damage to the inner ear or auditory nerve.

stroke Cerebral vascular accident; sometimes called a *brain attack.*

transient ischemic attack (TIA) Similar to a stroke, except that the symptoms resolve. A TIA may be a warning of a coming cerebral vascular accident (stroke).

■ INTRODUCTION

Nervous system disorders affect many people. A disorder can have a quick onset, as in the case of a head injury; or can develop gradually over time, as in the case of Parkinson's disease. The disorder can affect the central nervous system, the peripheral nervous system, or both. Sensory system disorders can be painful and acute, but more often develop slowly, with few warning signs. Sensory disorders can directly affect the sense organ, or a disorder in another body system can cause problems in the sensory system.

■ NERVOUS SYSTEM DISORDERS

There are many disorders that can affect the nervous system, and many have variations and subtypes. Many nervous system disorders can drastically change a client's life. The disorders discussed in this chapter are relatively common; the medical assistant may work with many clients who have at least one of these disorders. Therefore, it is important for the medical assistant to have a clear understanding of these disorders, what happens in the body of a client who has one of them, and an awareness of the causes of these disorders. Medical assistants must develop their therapeutic communication skills as they work with these clients and their families over a long period of time.

Parkinson's

Parkinson's disease is a degenerative disorder of the central nervous system. It results in *rigidity,* which is an increase in the tone of muscles. What the medical assistant will see is that the client has stiff movements (Figure 23-1). The **gait,** which is the way a person walks, is slow and shuffling. Along with the shuffling walk, the medical assistant may note a decrease in the normal arm swing that occurs while walking. Getting in and out of chairs is difficult; sometimes the client must make two or three tries to get up out of a chair. **Bradykinesia,** a decrease

in the pace or rate of movement, is another sign of Parkinson's. Because of the muscular stiffness, a client's face shows less expression, and at times will look very blank. There is a decrease in the eye blink, so that the client often appears to be staring. The medical assistant will also notice that the speech is slow and monotone, and often trails off toward the end of a sentence. Clients may also have increased saliva production that results in drooling.

Parkinson's disease often is accompanied by a *tremor* (a shaking movement), seen most often in the fingers and the feet. It is visible when the client is at rest and not moving, but it will either decrease or disappear when the client performs some voluntary action (for example, picking up a glass or using a pen). Early on in Parkinson's disease, the client will experience problems mostly on one side; however, as the disorder advances, both sides of the body will become involved. This is a progressive disease, which gradually becomes more limiting for the client. Mobility becomes impaired; help is needed for walking and also with dressing, because the ability to do fine movements and use the fingers becomes limited by the stiffness.

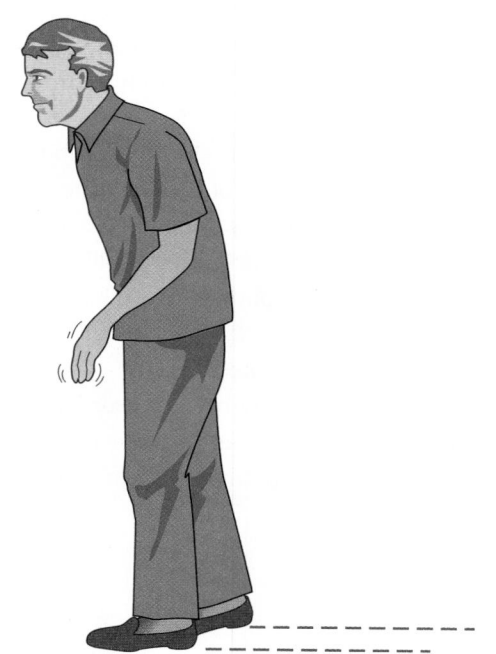

FIGURE 23-1 The effects of Parkinson's disease.

Seizures

Seizures are a disorder of the brain. There are many causes of seizures. For example, they can be caused by head injury, fever, brain tumors, or congenital metabolic conditions. In a large number of clients, though, the cause is never known. There are a number of different types of seizures, each of which looks different to the health care provider. There are two groups of seizures. The first group is generalized, meaning that the abnormal discharges in the brain that cause the seizures are generalized throughout the brain. The second group is partial (focal), in which the discharges are limited to a certain area of the brain. Both grand mal and petit mal seizures are generalized seizures.

A *grand mal seizure* has two phases. If the medical assistant is present when the seizure begins, he will usually hear a cry or a noise, at which time the client's arms and legs will suddenly go stiff and the client will lose consciousness. During this time the client may bite his tongue, foam at the mouth, become blue (cyanotic), and lose control of the bowels and/or bladder. This part of the seizure lasts one to three minutes. During the second phase, called the *clonic phase,* the medical assistant will see jerking movements of the client's body. This phase also lasts one to three minutes. Immediately afterward, the client will be unconscious, unresponsive, and limp. When the client wakes up, he will probably be confused, disoriented, and very tired; he will not remember having the seizure or what happened during it. Usually the client will go to sleep after a seizure. It often takes more than an hour for the client to return to his normal mental state. Even after sleeping for a while, the client may feel tired, and may have muscle soreness and headache. Clients can injure themselves while having a seizure, so they should be evaluated for injuries after the seizure is over. Possible injuries include cuts, head trauma, bruising, and even broken vertebrae or other fractures. Although seizures occur suddenly, many (but not all) clients experience an *aura,* which consists of certain feelings or sensations, immediately before a seizure.

Although there are many different types of auras, the client who experiences auras will have the same aura before most seizures.

The other type of generalized seizure that is commonly seen is the petit mal (absence) seizure. A petit mal seizure is a very short lapse of awareness, during which the client may stare, stop talking, or repeat movements. This can happen many times during the day, but the client is usually unaware of his loss of contact with the environment.

The other large category of seizures is *partial* or *focal seizures.* These seizures start in one part of the brain, often in the temporal lobe. The behaviors that the medical assistant sees depend on where in the brain the abnormal discharges occur. The most common type of partial seizure is the *complex-partial seizure.* The client does not usually fall to the ground, and there are no convulsive movements, as seen in the grand mal type. There can be abnormal, repetitive movements, or the client may experience abnormal sensations such as bad smells, sounds, vision changes, or emotional events, such as fear or anxiety.

Seizures are treated with medications. In some cases surgery is done on the brain to prevent further seizures. The medical assistant must be understanding and allow the client time to share his fears and anxieties. This is a chronic disorder to which the client will have to adjust in a daily routine. Some lifestyle changes may be necessary. Medication must be taken exactly as the doctor orders. If the client skips doses, his seizures could start again. Teaching in this area in particular will have to be reinforced. One of the greatest concerns for most clients is loss of independence, including restrictions on driving and working in certain types of occupations. The client should be encouraged to ask questions or share worries with the medical assistant and doctor.

Dementia

Dementia is a process that results in loss of the highest functions of the brain, including memory. The client who has dementia will also suffer a loss of personality and many of the skills needed for daily living. With the decline of these

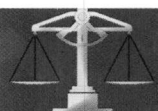

LEGAL/ETHICAL THOUGHTS

For an office visit, ask clients to bring a list of all the medications they are taking, or a bag containing their medication bottles. This includes nonprescription or over-the-counter (OTC) drugs, vitamins, and herbal supplements. This helps the health care professionals to monitor the client's health, as many client health complaints are the result of drug interactions.

functions, the client becomes dependent upon other people to provide many of his daily needs. Alzheimer's is one cause of dementia, but there are other causes as well. A major cause of dementia is vascular disease. Over a number of years, the decrease in the amount of oxygenated blood reaching to the brain causes a loss of neurons; the cumulative loss results in the deterioration of memory and personality. Other causes of dementia include thyroid diseases, certain types of anemia, certain infectious diseases, brain tumors, and alcohol or drug abuse.

In the beginning there is memory loss. The client forgets details regarding daily living and recent occurrences. This is known as *short-term memory*. The medical assistant will notice that the client's speech is less clear, and often the client will have difficulty naming objects. Clients with dementia may also lose their way in familiar surroundings. The client will progressively lose the ability to do daily tasks, such as get dressed properly, make a meal, or drive a car. The client may or may not be aware of these problems, but as the process continues the problems will accumulate and accelerate, such as a shuffling walk, a stiffening of the muscles, and a decrease in the amount and quality of speech. The client will become more withdrawn and able to do less and less. The client's personality may change markedly.

The medical assistant must be aware of these changes in the client and work with the client and the client's family members or caregiver. At each visit, the medical assistant should introduce himself and tell the client what will happen during the visit. The medical assistant needs to understand and remember that the client may not be able to understand or follow instructions.

Multiple Sclerosis

Multiple sclerosis is a neurologic disorder that affects mostly young adults. In multiple sclerosis, different areas of the brain and/or spinal cord do not work correctly, because of damage to the myelin sheath surrounding the nerves. This disrupts the transmission of nerve impulses and causes muscular problems. Many times, the client complains of something "not working right," such as being unable to see from one eye, numbness or tingling, or not being able to use one of his arms or legs. These problems can last from a few days to weeks; thereafter they may disappear and the client appears to return to normal or almost normal.

Common episodes involve the eye and vision. The client may have pain in the eye, blurred or double vision, or abnormal eye movements. There can be facial nerve weakness and/or pain. The arms or legs may feel numb, or have "pins and needles" tingling. Often the doctor orders an MRI study of the brain or spinal cord to confirm the diagnosis of multiple sclerosis. As the disorder continues, the client may lose control of bowel and bladder. His walk becomes more unsteady, and sometimes the client will need a wheelchair to maintain mobility.

Stroke

There are two major types of **stroke.** One type is *ischemic stroke,* which is caused by a decrease of blood flow to the brain (Figure 23-2). This can be caused by a *thrombosis,* that is, the closing-off of an artery to the brain; or by an *embolus,* a small clot that becomes stuck in an artery. Both

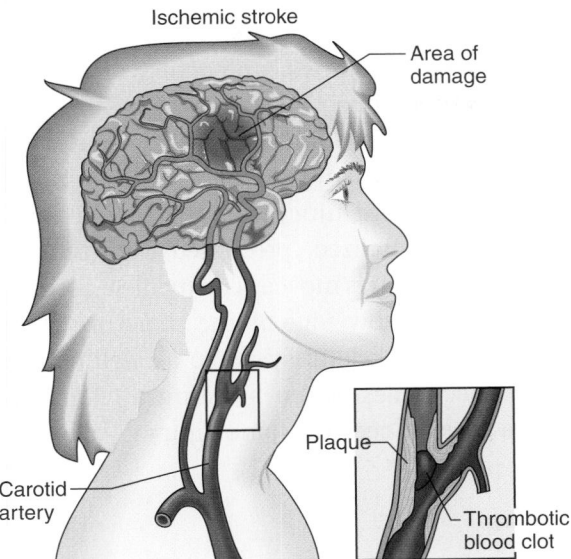

Ischemic stroke

Area of
damage

Plaque

Carotid
artery

Thrombotic
blood clot

FIGURE 23-2 A stroke is caused by the blockage of blood to the brain.

of these will result in a decrease or stoppage of blood flow to a part of the brain. With less blood and therefore less oxygen, the result will be changes in the brain itself, which may either result in complete destruction or partial damage of varying degrees of severity. What the medical assistant will see depends on what part of the client's brain has been affected. Ischemic stroke generally develops over a period of time.

Thromboses or clots in blood vessels are related to high cholesterol, high blood pressure, diabetes, smoking, advanced age, and certain types of blood disorders. An embolism, which is a clot that breaks off and gets stuck in a smaller artery, where it creates a blockage, generally can be caused by the same factors as thrombotic stroke. In addition, problems with the heart wall, heart valves, or blood vessels themselves can be sources of emboli. Irregularities of the heart rhythm (most often atrial fibrillation) can cause a stroke via embolism.

The other major type of stroke is called a *hemorrhagic stroke.* In a hemorrhagic stroke, the client gets a sudden, severe headache and may have loss of sensation, strength, and/or speech. Hemorrhagic stroke can be caused by a rupture of an *aneurysm,* a weakening in the wall of an artery. The client will have nausea and vomiting.

A hemorrhagic stroke that involves bleeding in the brain itself is often caused by high blood pressure, and generally occurs in older people.

With both major types of strokes, there can be warning signs. In thrombotic stroke, these are called **transient ischemic attacks (TIAs).** These mini-strokes may appear to be a stroke, but the symptoms go away within 10 minutes to 24 hours. It is estimated that one out of three stroke victims have at least one TIA before they have a major stroke. It is important for a health care provider to recognize a TIA and try to prevent a stroke thereafter. Treatment of the underlying causes of stroke, which is the third most common cause of death in the United States, can avoid a stroke. Irregularities of cardiac rhythm can be detected by the medical assistant and reported for evaluation. If they turn out to be due to atrial fibrillation, medication will be prescribed.

The medical assistant can work with clients to teach them ways to decrease their risk of stroke. Lowering cholesterol through diet and exercise can reduce the risk. Encourage clients who have diabetes to become active participants in their diabetic health care. Helping the client who is overweight to lose the weight and lower the blood pressure will aid in preventing stroke. Encourage the client who smokes to stop, or at least decrease, smoking. Smoking is a major risk factor for stroke.

NOTE TO STUDENT:

It is important for the medical assistant to recognize that getting medical care as soon as possible, to correctly diagnose and treat a stroke, is critical to the client's recovery. Time lost is brain lost. Teach clients to seek care quickly if they notice the signs of a stroke; early treatment greatly improves the chances of recovery. Teaching clients to check their own pulses and report irregularities to their health care providers may result in prevention of an embolic stroke.

■ INJURIES TO THE NERVOUS SYSTEM

Injuries to the nervous system are usually acute and happen suddenly. They frequently occur in young people who are in good health. Injuries to the nervous system can cause damage that is long term or permanent. The medical assistant needs to be patient and show empathy with clients and families, as the extent to which an injury will affect the person and his lifestyle may not be known for a while. A client faced with a nervous system injury may react with fear, anxieties, anger, withdrawal, and/or denial.

Head Injury

Almost half of all traumatic deaths in the United States are related to head injury. Head injuries can result from car accidents, falls, sport injuries, or accidents at work. They also can be caused by certain conditions and behaviors, such as alcohol or substance abuse.

Sometimes a person gets a head injury but does not get a skull fracture. However, just because a person does not get a skull fracture does not mean that the head injury is not serious. Bleeding within the skull may be immediate and heavy, or there can be a slow leakage of blood. If a client complains of certain signs and symptoms after a head injury, even if the injury occurred more than a week before and nothing happened then, the medical assistant must make sure that the doctor sees the client.

Concussion

A **concussion** is a brain injury. It may occur along with a very brief loss of consciousness, and usually the client has some memory loss about what happened right before or right after the injury. A concussion may be minor and cause few or no permanent problems. However, a concussion can also be so severe that the client dies. The medical assistant must take seriously any client report about a possible concussion.

Cervical Spine Injury

Cervical spine injuries can occur with or without head trauma. Falls, car accidents, and diving accidents, among other events, can cause spinal cord injuries (Figure 23-3). Whenever a spinal cord injury is suspected, the client's neck is immobilized (prevented from moving) before the client is moved. The medical assistant must apply knowledge of the structure of the nervous and skeletal systems, as well as good body mechanics, when assisting a client who has a possible cervical spine injury.

Headache

Headaches are a common problem. They can be a transient problem, easily treated with medications, or a sign of a serious, life-threatening condition. A client's headaches should be evaluated. Even though pain is a feature of headaches, a doctor can differentiate between different kinds of headache pain and what they signify.

■ SENSORY DISORDERS

Sensory disorders can directly affect the sense organs, and those organs alone. Often, however, a sensory disorder affects or is caused by a nervous system problem.

Chronic Eye Disorders

Disorders of the eye are often painless, with few symptoms noticeable to the client until the disorder has progressed far enough to cause damage.

Cataracts. A **cataract** is a clouding of the normally clear lens of the eye. It is seen most often in older persons, but may also occur in younger persons as a result of trauma, an endocrine disorder, or use of medications such as steroids. In the early stages, while the cataract is growing, the client may complain of being sensitive to bright light. This sensitivity is called *photophobia*.

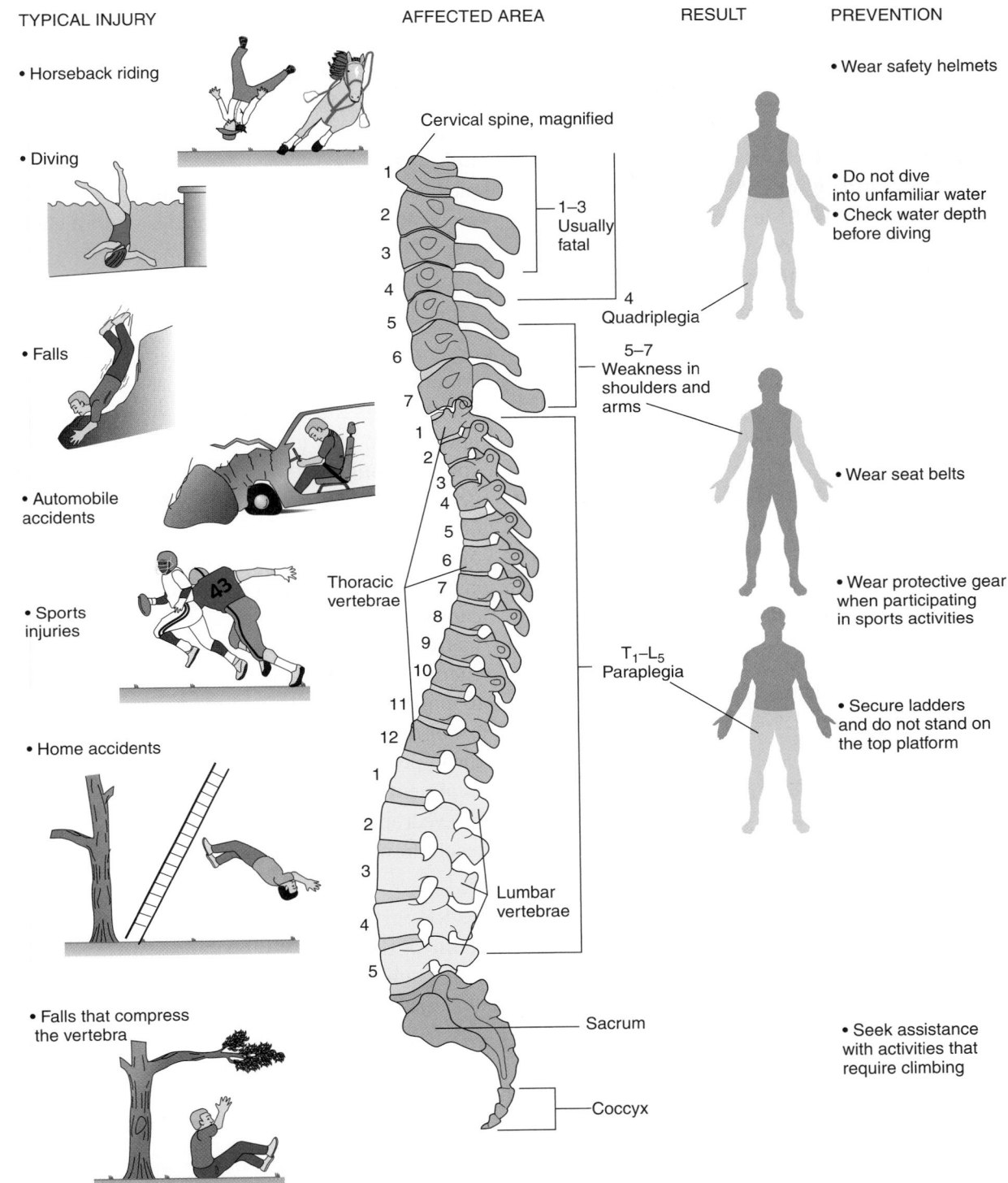

TYPICAL INJURY

- Horseback riding
- Diving
- Falls
- Automobile accidents
- Sports injuries
- Home accidents
- Falls that compress the vertebra

AFFECTED AREA

Cervical spine, magnified

1
2
3
4
5
6
7

1–3 Usually fatal

4 Quadriplegia

5–7 Weakness in shoulders and arms

Thoracic vertebrae

1
2
3
4
5
6
7
8
9
10
11
12

T_1–L_5 Paraplegia

Lumbar vertebrae

1
2
3
4
5

Sacrum

Coccyx

RESULT

PREVENTION

- Wear safety helmets
- Do not dive into unfamiliar water
- Check water depth before diving
- Wear seat belts
- Wear protective gear when participating in sports activities
- Secure ladders and do not stand on the top platform
- Seek assistance with activities that require climbing

FIGURE 23-3 Spinal cord injuries.

The person may not see as well at night, particularly while driving. Eventually the client will have severe difficulty in seeing at all. The medical assistant may notice a whitish coloration around the eye in a client who has severe cataracts.

The treatment for cataracts is removal by surgery (Figure 23-4). Surgery and the recovery time thereafter have become quicker and easier. Surgery to remove cataracts can be safely done even on very elderly clients. With the restoration of sight, the client can regain greater independence and the ability to carry out activities of daily living.

Macular Degeneration. *Macular degeneration* affects the retina or screen of the eye, causing a loss of pigment in the central part of the retina. Central vision is lost in the early stage of this disorder. The client will see a large black circle in the middle of whatever he looks at directly. Because the client can see only at the outer

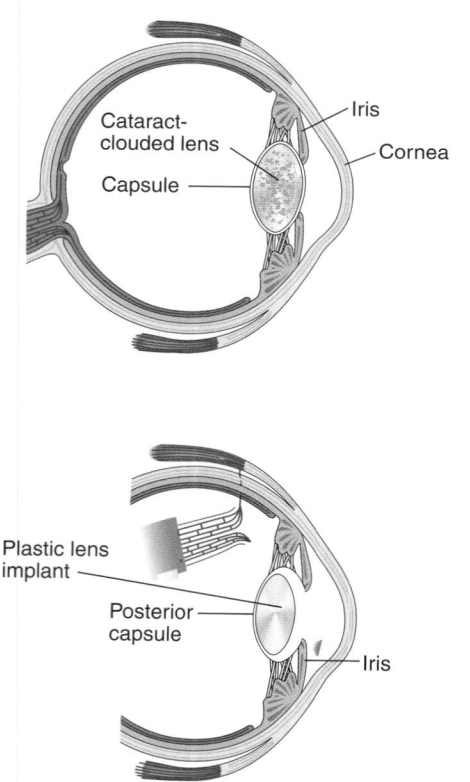

FIGURE 23-4 The cataract-clouded lens is replaced with a plastic lens implant.

edges, he will often try to see the complete image by turning the head and using peripheral vision. Eventually, macular degeneration will lead to permanent vision loss. Some factors may increase the risk, but the exact cause is unknown. The disorder is more common in people over the age of 50; so it is important for the medical assistant to check the vision of a client who is age 50 or over.

Glaucoma. *Glaucoma* is actually a group of disorders that have three characteristics in common. First, there is increased pressure in the eye, which then leads to a shrinking of the optic nerve and finally often blindness. Glaucoma, along with cataracts and macular degeneration, is one of the three leading causes of blindness in the United States. Glaucoma often goes undetected because there are few symptoms. Certain medications can significantly worsen glaucoma if the client already has it. The medical assistant should check all the client's medications if the client has glaucoma, to make sure that the medications do not worsen the disorder. The medical assistant needs to stress the importance of regular eye examinations. The treatment for glaucoma is medication in the form of eyedrops. The medical assistant will need to teach the client how to administer eyedrops.

Retinopathy. *Retinopathy* is a disorder of the retina of the eye. Common causes are hypertension (high blood pressure), atherosclerosis, and diabetes mellitus. Retinopathy can lead to blindness. The medical assistant should emphasize the importance of regular eye examinations, because retinopathy will not be apparent to either the client or the medical assistant.

Detached Retina. A *detached retina* occurs when the amount of fluid inside the eye decreases; the shrinkage of the tissues pulls on and causes a rip or tear in the retina, thereby detaching it. (Detachment may also be caused by trauma to the eye.) The detachment or tearing away starts at the outer edges first (Figure 23-5). Peripheral

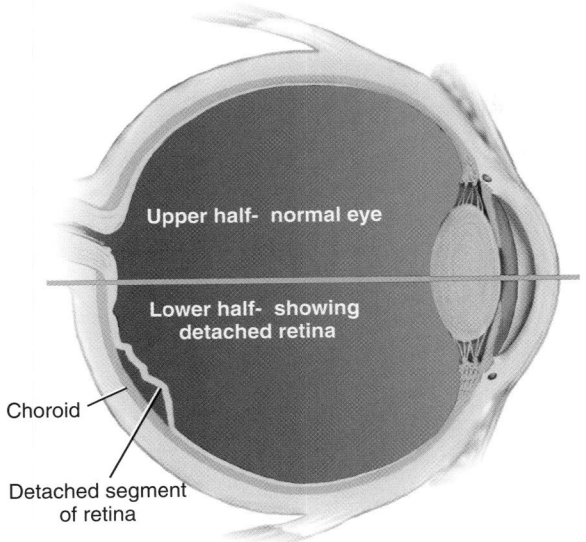

FIGURE 23-5 Detached retina.

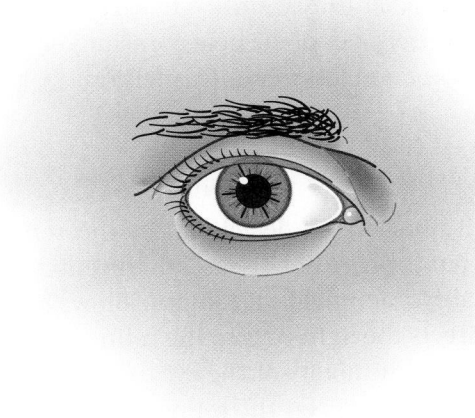

FIGURE 23-6 Conjunctivitis.

vision (vision at the outer edges of the visual field) is lost first; then vision loss progresses to the central vision. Treatments are available if a detachment is caught in the early stages, so it is very important to seek help when any vision problem is noticed.

Acute Disorders of the Eye. Acute disorders, caused by disease or trauma, can affect the organ of sight. Common problems include conjunctivitis, hordeolums, and corneal abrasions.

Conjunctivitis is an inflammation of the membranous lining of the eyelids and the exposed part of the eyeball. People may refer to conjunctivitis as "pinkeye," because the normally white area of the eye appears pink to red (Figure 23-6). The medical assistant must use strict aseptic methods, and teach these techniques to the client as well, as conjunctivitis is easily spread to the other eye and other people. Hand and face towels in the home must not be shared, even among family members. Medications in the form of eyedrops are usually ordered. The medical assistant will teach the client how to instill the drops in an aseptic manner.

Hordeolum is commonly called a *sty*. A sty is a small infected gland in the eyelid. The client's eyelid will look swollen, red, and tender

(Figure 23-7). The condition will end when the collected matter (pus, dead white blood cells, etc.) drains. Warm, moist compresses applied periodically to the eyelid for a few days usually help the condition. If not, the doctor can drain the sty.

The cornea of the eye can easily be scratched or abraded. This is called a *corneal abrasion.* A fingernail, a foreign particle, or any irritating substance in the eye can scratch the cornea. Dry eyes put a person at higher risk. This is a very painful acute disorder. The client will complain of pain in the eye, tearing, and sensitivity to light. A patch is placed over the

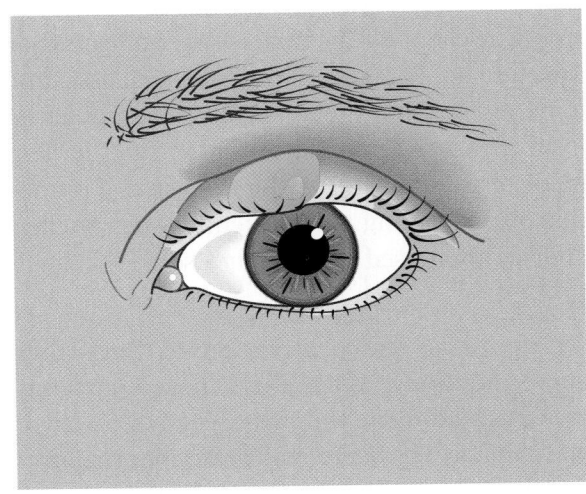

FIGURE 23-7 Sty.

affected eye after medicated drops are instilled. The eyes need to rest until the abrasion heals. Frequent episodes of corneal abrasions can lead to scarring and loss of contrast vision.

Visual Disorders

Visual disorders or defects affect the sense of sight, but they are not diseases or infections. The normal eye, acting like a camera, allows light in and directs the light rays to the retina or screen of the eye. The ability of the eye to bend parallel light rays to focus on the retina is called *refraction*. The shape of the eyeball or eye muscle ability may interfere with this process. These problems are called *errors of refraction*. Some common errors of refraction are myopia, hyperopia, and astigmatism (Figure 23-8).

Myopia. In **myopia,** or nearsightedness, the eyeball is too long and the focused light falls short of the retina, in front of the correct focus spot. The client will be unable to see objects that are far away. The medical assistant can test for this error of refraction by performing a visual acuity test; a Snellen chart is often used for this purpose.

Hyperopia. In **hyperopia,** or farsightedness, the eyeball is too short, and the light rays focus at a spot past the retina, behind the correct focus spot. The client will be unable to see objects that are close up. For example, the medical assistant may observe that a client holds a pamphlet or form at arm's length in order to read it. The medical assistant can test for this error of refraction by performing a visual acuity test; a Snellen chart is often used for this purpose.

Astigmatism. The cornea or lens of the eye may curve unevenly. With this uneven curving, called **astigmatism,** the client sees a distorted or wavy image. The doctor will prescribe eyeglasses or contact lenses to help correct for the waves or distortions.

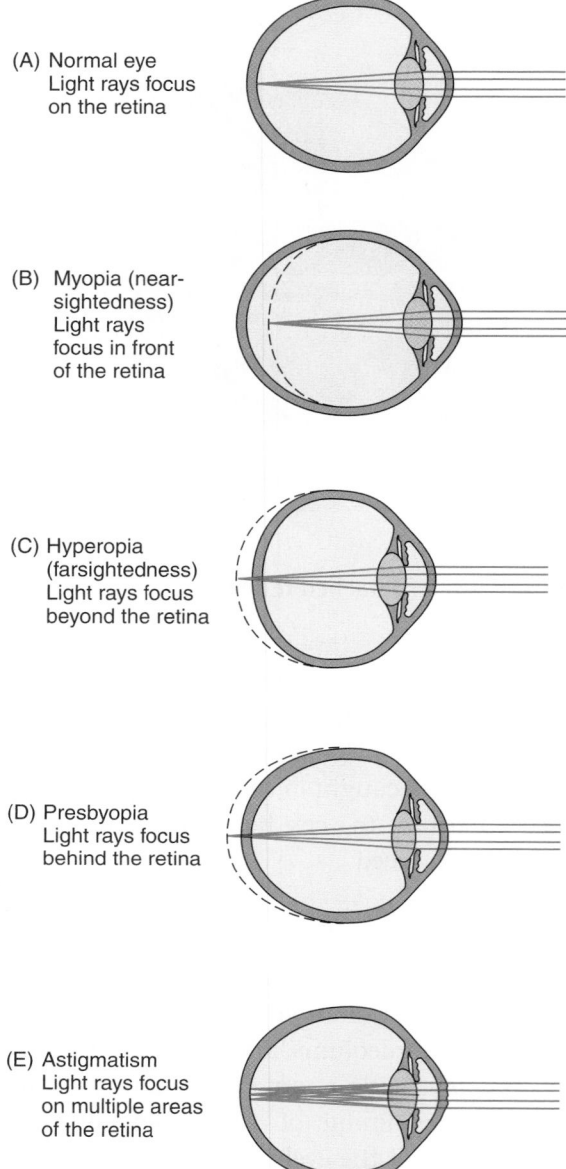

(A) Normal eye
Light rays focus
on the retina

(B) Myopia (near-
sightedness)
Light rays
focus in front
of the retina

(C) Hyperopia
(farsightedness)
Light rays focus
beyond the retina

(D) Presbyopia
Light rays focus
behind the retina

(E) Astigmatism
Light rays focus
on multiple areas
of the retina

FIGURE 23–8 Normal vision, nearsightedness, farsightedness, presbyopia, and astigmatism.

Presbyopia. **Presbyopia** is a visual disorder in which the lens of the eye loses elasticity. When this happens, the eye has difficulty changing focus quickly, as when focusing first on near objects and then objects farther away. The client who earlier did not have a visual problem may complain about not being able to focus quickly and clearly when looking at items close up. The medical assistant will observe this condition most often in clients who are over the age of 40.

Ear Disorders

Disorders of the ear can cause pain, loss of balance, and loss of the sense of hearing.

Otitis Media. An acute infectious disorder of the ear is **otitis media** (Figure 23-9). The middle ear becomes infected, causing pain and sometimes temporary hearing loss. The client with otitis media is often a child who has just had a cold or upper respiratory infection. Children are more susceptible to otitis media because of the structure and location of the middle ear and nasopharynx. Frequent, intense episodes of middle ear infection can lead to ear damage and permanent hearing loss. The doctor will prescribe antibiotics to cure the infection. The medical assistant must include in client teaching the importance of completing the entire course of antibiotics treatment, even if the pain goes away after only a few days.

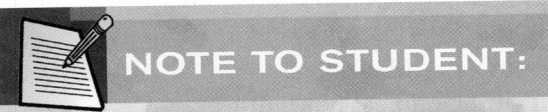

NOTE TO STUDENT:

Failure to take all of an antibiotic medication as directed can leave some bacteria alive. These bacteria can then become resistant to the drug, and the medication will not work the next time it is needed to combat an infection.

Hearing Loss

Several conditions can affect both the sense of hearing and the sense of balance, and may cause hearing loss. The tiny bones found in the ear, which normally vibrate or move to conduct sound waves, can become fixed and immoveable. This condition is **otosclerosis**, which means hardening of the ear. A possible treatment is surgery.

Ménière's disease is a condition involving the inner ear. During an acute attack, the client will experience ringing in the ear, extreme dizziness, and nausea and vomiting. Medication and bedrest are often prescribed. The medical assistant needs to listen with empathy to the client's fears, as the attacks come on suddenly and without warning.

The inability to hear, especially high-pitched sounds, can develop with aging. This condition is called *presbycusis.* The client or family members of the client may complain that the client is unable to hear certain things or some people's voices. The medical assistant should explain that as a person ages, it can become more difficult to hear the higher pitch of some voices. Hearing aids may help this difficulty.

Hearing Loss Groups. Hearing loss can be grouped into two major types: conductive hearing loss and **sensorineural** hearing loss. When the transmission of sound waves is hindered at any place, as the sound travels from the outside environment through all the parts of the ear to

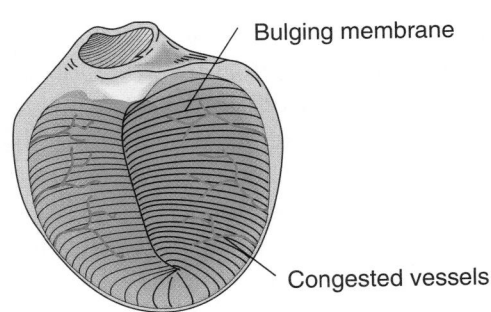

Malleus

Cone of light reflection

(A) Normal

Bulging membrane

Congested vessels

(B) Bulging tympanic membrane

FIGURE 23-9 Otitis media.

the auditory nerve, hearing is impaired. This is *conductive hearing loss*: the sound waves cannot be conducted or carried to their destination. An object put into the ear, such as a little piece of a toy in a child's ear, can cause a hearing loss. Growths in the ear canal may also be responsible for loss of hearing. A buildup of cerumen (earwax) can cause a conductive hearing loss, because the sound waves cannot travel through the thick wax. This is a temporary loss. The doctor will order an ear irrigation, which the medical assistant will perform. Hearing should then return to the level the client had before the buildup of cerumen.

Sometimes, even though the sound waves are conducted through the ear properly, the client still cannot hear. This *sensorineural hearing loss* can be caused by damage to the sensory auditory nerve (cranial nerve VIII). Heredity, disease, and age are all factors in hearing loss. Exposure to loud noises, such as noise exposure at work or while listening to loud music, can cause sensorineural hearing loss.

The medical assistant should look at the hearing-impaired client when speaking with him. Speak slowly and clearly. Do not talk loudly or exaggerate lip movements, as this will hinder the client's ability to understand what is said.

Smell

The sense of smell can be impaired by infections, inflammations, growths in, and structural problems of the nose. Inflammation of the lining of the nose, from irritants or allergens, can result in sneezing and a mucous discharge. The client may complain of these symptoms in addition to a feeling of fullness and difficulty breathing and smelling. Treatment is directed at treating the cause. Damage to the olfactory nerve, which is the first cranial nerve (cranial nerve I) can also cause loss of the ability to smell. Permanent loss of the sense of smell can occur after an especially severe cold or from certain types of head trauma, usually when there has been a skull fracture.

Taste

The effects of aging on the taste buds may impair the elderly person's ability to sense the different tastes in food. Damage to the facial nerve (cranial nerve VII) or the glossopharyngeal nerve (cranial nerve IX) can diminish a person's ability to taste. Certain prescribed medications may also cause a loss of taste.

 ## BRIDGE TO CAAHEP

This chapter, which discusses nervous and sensory system disorders, provides information and content related to CAAHEP standards for Anatomy and Physiology, Medical Terminology, Communication, Medical Assisting Clinical Procedures, and Professional Components.

 ## ABHES LINKS

This chapter, which discusses nervous and sensory system disorders, links to ABHES course content for Anatomy and Physiology, Medical Terminology, Medical Law and Ethics, and Medical Office Clinical Procedures.

 ## AAMA AREAS OF COMPETENCE

This chapter, which discusses nervous and sensory system disorders, provides information or content within several areas listed in the Medical Assistant Role Delineation Study. These areas include: clinical, fundamental principles, diagnostic orders, patient (client) care, general transdisciplinary, professionalism, communication skills, legal concepts, and instruction.

 ## AMT PATHS

This chapter, which discusses nervous and sensory system disorders, provides a path to AMT competency in general medical assisting knowledge, anatomy and physiology, medical terminology, and patient (client) education.

POINTS OF HIGHLIGHT

- Parkinson's disease is a degenerative disorder of the central nervous system.
- Seizures are abnormal electrical discharges in the brain; they can result from fever, head injury, brain trauma, or unknown causes.
- The most important action to take during a seizure is to protect the client from injury.
- Clients with dementia will lose memory and eventually their ability to perform activities of daily living.
- Vascular disorders are a major cause of dementia.
- A stroke is often called a brain attack. A stroke must be diagnosed and treated quickly if the client is to have a chance of recovery. Time lost is brain lost.
- Transient ischemic attacks are a warning sign of a coming stroke.
- Head injuries account for almost half of all traumatic deaths in the United States.
- A concussion is a bruising of the brain. Even a mild concussion can cause permanent problems for the client.
- Disorders of the sensory system can be caused by a disorder of the sense organ itself, or by disorders in other body systems that affect the senses.
- The medical assistant needs to stress the importance of regular eye examinations to detect and treat eye disorders early and prevent blindness.
- Cataracts are a clouding of the lens of the eye.
- Macular degeneration begins as a loss of central vision and progresses to a permanent loss of all vision.
- Glaucoma has few symptoms. The increased pressure in the eye leads to shrinking of the optic nerve and eventually blindness.
- Conjunctivitis, or "pinkeye," is an inflammation of the membranous lining of the eyelids and part of the eyeball. It is highly contagious, and strict aseptic methods must be practiced during treatment.
- Errors of refraction are not infections or diseases, but do affect the client's ability to see. Nearsightedness (myopia) and farsightedness (hyperopia) are examples of errors of refraction.
- Otitis media is a common infection of the middle ear, often seen in young children.
- Hearing impairment can be either conductive hearing loss or sensorineural hearing loss.
- The medical assistant should look at the hearing impaired client when speaking with him. Speak slowly and clearly. Do not talk loudly or exaggerate lip movements as this will hinder understanding by the client.

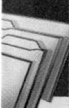

STUDENT PORTFOLIO ACTIVITY

Ethical dilemmas occur every day. You have probably discussed these concerns in your courses. Select an assignment in which you applied ethical decision-making steps to a client scenario. The assignment selected should illustrate your understanding of the steps involved in reaching a decision.

APPLYING YOUR SKILLS

A client who has Parkinson's disorder has been coming to the office for a long time. Gradually, over time, his symptoms have been worsening. How can you, as a medical assistant, help the client during the visit? What steps can you take to ensure the client's safety and comfort?

CRITICAL THINKING QUESTIONS

1. A client has been diagnosed with otitis media. The doctor has ordered antibiotics for the client and has asked you (the medical assistant) to teach the client about the medication. What are some key points that you would include on the teaching plan?

2. A client with early-stage dementia comes to the office with a family member. What are some changes that you expect to see as the dementia progresses?

3. After vision testing, a client is found to have myopia. The client asks you to explain what that means. What do you tell him?

4. A client who has diabetes mellitus and high blood pressure has not had an eye examination for several years. What would you tell this client about the need for regular eye exams? Why are eye exams important?

5. You will be teaching how to care for a family member during and after a seizure. Identify the key points that you will teach.

6. What are some difficulties that a child with petit mal seizures might encounter in school?

7. What are some behaviors that a client can practice to lessen the chance of sustaining a head injury?

8. An elderly client confides to you that he has not been to an "eye doctor" in years. What do you tell him about the importance of regular visits? What eye conditions can be prevented or treated successfully if detected early?

9. A parent complains that her child was sent home from school with "pinkeye" even though the child did not feel sick. What do you tell the parent about conjunctivitis? What are some ways to prevent its spread?

10. Go back to the beginning of this chapter and review the Anticipatory Statements. Reread each statement and then indicate whether it is true or false. If the statement is false, rewrite it to make it a true statement.

CLIENT TEACHING PLAN

Stroke Warning Signs

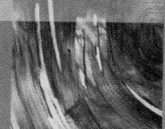

What Is to Be Taught:

- Warning signs of a stroke or cerebral vascular accident (CVA).

Objectives:

- Client will recognize symptoms that may be a warning of an impending stroke, and will understand how to respond to these symptoms.

Preparation Before Teaching:

- Review information about strokes, including risk factors and symptoms. Make sure to change technical medical terms into everyday language that the client will understand.
- Gather any pamphlets or printed materials available in the office. (Nonprofit associations may have printed information to supply to medical offices.)
- Have paper and a pen available for notes and written instructions.
- Make sure that the area is free from distractions while you are teaching.

Steps for the Medical Assistant:

1. Wash your hands.
2. Gather needed supplies.
3. Introduce yourself to the client.
4. Explain what you are going to teach and why.
5. Inform the client that stroke or cerebral vascular accident (also sometimes called a brain attack) is common and can have serious consequences. There are steps the client can take to lessen the chances of a stroke, and one of these is to recognize and respond to warning signs.
6. Show the client any pictures or printed material you have to help illustrate the following signs of stroke:
   a. Weakness or numbness of any part of the body, such as the arm, leg, or face, especially if it is only on one side of the body and happens all of a sudden

   b. Difficulty walking or keeping balance; uncoordination and/or dizziness that happens suddenly
   c. Trouble seeing, either in both eyes or in one eye
   d. Trouble speaking or understanding speech
   e. An unusual feeling of confusion
   f. Severe, painful headache for no apparent reason
7. Tell the client that if he notices one or more of these symptoms, do not ignore it or wait to see if it goes away. Call 9-1-1 immediately and get to the hospital right away.
8. Explain to the client that time lost is brain lost. Treatments may be available, but will be effective only if the problem is caught in time and acted upon immediately.
9. Teach the client to take his pulse and contact a heath care provider if he detects irregularities.
10. Ask the client if he has any questions or if anything is unclear.

Special Needs of the Client:

- Look at the client's chart to see if there are any factors that might interfere with the client's ability to recognize and respond to the warning signs of stroke.
- Ask the client, before and after teaching, if there is anything you should know that might affect his ability to follow these instructions.

Evaluation:

- Client will be able to list symptoms that may indicate an impending stroke or brain attack.
- Client can state what action to take if any of the warning signs occurs.

Further Plans/Teaching:

- Give the client a written listing of and instructions regarding warning signs of a stroke or brain attack.

(Continues)

CLIENT TEACHING PLAN (Continued)

■ **Follow-up:**

- Review the information at the client's next office visit and ask if he has any questions.

Medical Assistant

Name: _____

Signature: _____

Date: _____

Client

Date: _____

Follow-up Date : _____

Anticipatory Statements

People have different ideas about endocrine system disorders. Read and think about the following statements based upon what you believe now. Decide whether you agree or disagree. Write the word **agree** after the statement if you think the statement is true. Write the word **disagree** after the statement if you think the statement is false. Read the chapter to find out if your current beliefs can be supported.

1. Diabetes is also called "sugar." _____

2. An underactive thyroid is responsible for most obesity. _____

3. A person has no control over whether she develops diabetes. _____

4. Hormones help to determine how much a person grows. _____

Learning Objectives

Upon completion of this chapter, the medical assistant student should be able to:

■ Identify the medical assistant's role in client preparation for diagnostic tests of the endocrine system

■ Explain the effects of hypersecretion of the thyroid and parathyroid glands

■ Explain the mechanism and results of hyposecretion from the thyroid gland

■ State differences between type I diabetes and type II diabetes

■ Discuss the effects of hypersecretion of growth hormones

■ Discuss the effects of hyposecretion of growth hormones

Endocrine System Disorders

- ■ Discuss the effects of hypersecretion of adrenal cortical hormone
- ■ Develop a teaching plan for a client with diabetes mellitus
- ■ Teach another person how to use a home glucose monitoring unit to test blood glucose

Key Terms

acromegaly Condition in which the bones of the face, hands, and feet become larger as a result of overproduction of growth hormone during adulthood.

Addison's disease Disorder in which the adrenal glands do not make enough corticosteroids.

antidiuretic hormone (ADH) Released by the pituitary gland; tells the kidneys to conserve water.

cretinism Severe hypothyroidism in children; causes mental retardation and retardation of physical development.

Cushing's syndrome Disorder in which too much cortisol is made; a disease of the pituitary gland.

diabetes insipidus Lack or insufficient amount of antidiuretic hormone, which causes excess urination of dilute urine.

diabetes mellitus Chronic disorder affecting metabolism; associated with too little production of insulin or inability to use insulin (insulin resistance).

gestational diabetes Diabetes that occurs during pregnancy.

gigantism Overproduction of growth hormone during childhood.

glucose Used by the body as a source of energy.

goiter Enlargement of the thyroid gland.

Grave's disease Hyperthyroidism; condition in which the thyroid gland produces too much of the thyroid hormones.

myxedema Severe form of hypothyroidism in adults; caused by not enough thyroid hormones.

■ INTRODUCTION

The endocrine system helps to regulate bodily functions through the secretion of substances called *hormones*. The hormones travel through the circulatory system to various target destinations, and have far-reaching effects. A problem in any of the glands can affect the homeostasis (balance) of the entire body. Most endocrine disorders arise when the secretion of hormones is out of balance, resulting in either too much activity or too little activity.

■ PITUITARY DISORDERS

The pituitary gland secretes many different hormones and affects many bodily functions (Figure 24-1). Pituitary hypersecretion often takes the form of overproduction of growth

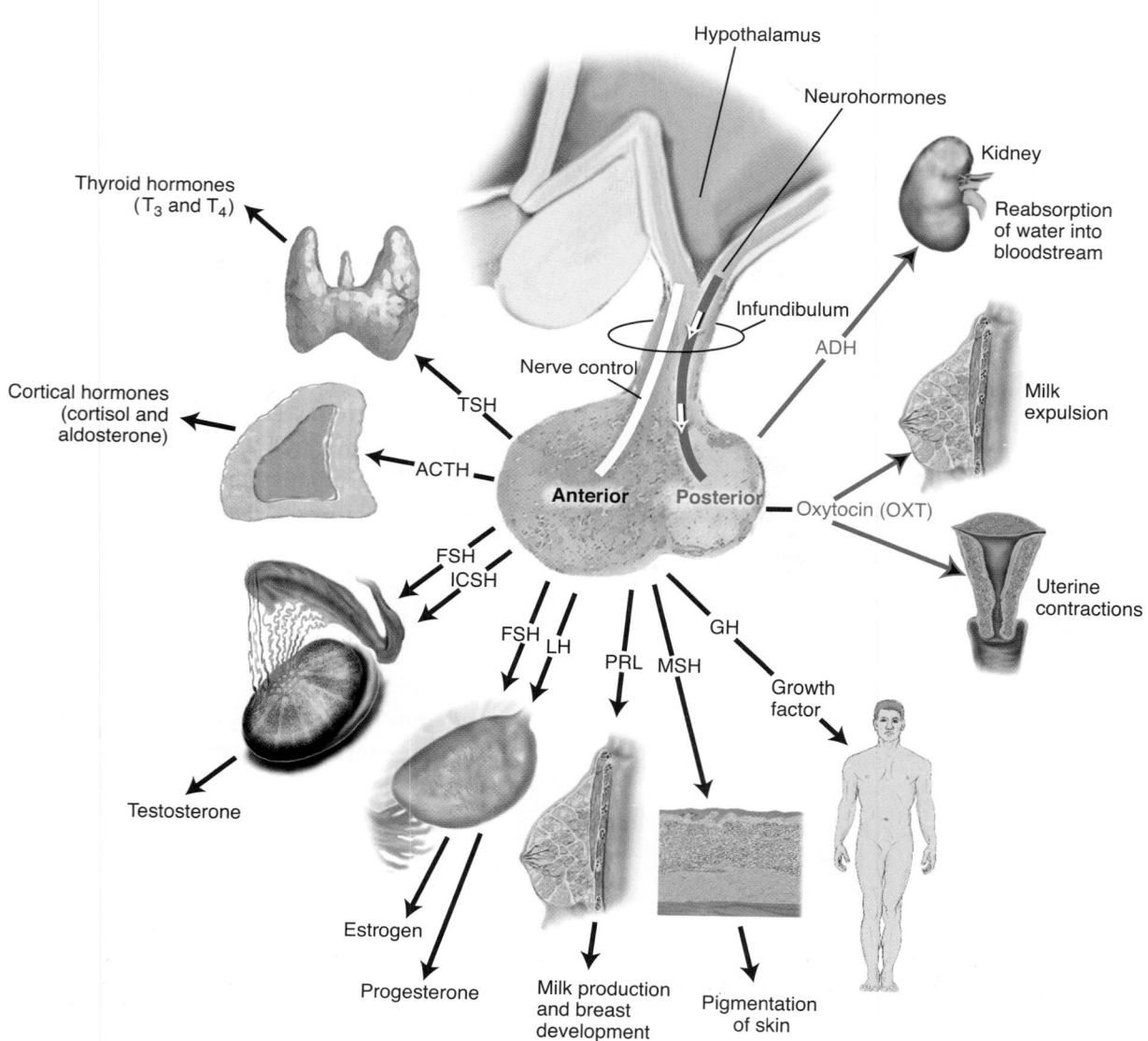

FIGURE 24-1 The pituitary gland affects many body functions.

hormone from the anterior pituitary and anti-diuretic hormone from the posterior pituitary.

With overproduction of growth hormone (GH), the medical assistant will observe different features in the client depending on whether the disorder occurs in childhood or adulthood. In children, overproduction of GH results in **gigantism.** Overall, the body tissue grows too much; the child can grow well above the normal range (up to eight feet tall). Although such a child is tall, this client does not have corresponding strength. Radiation therapy or surgery may be done to stop the growth process. The client will then need to take pituitary hormone replacement therapy.

If the overproduction of GH happens to an adult, **acromegaly** is the result. The adult does not grow taller; rather, the bones thicken, growing and enlarging horizontally. Although the clinical features (what can be observed) develop slowly, changes in the face and hands are the most prominent. The jaw becomes more pronounced, and the tongue thickens. The ears and nose become larger. The hands become thick and soft-feeling, with big fingers. Medication, therapeutic radiation, or surgery may be done to stop the process.

Whether the client is a child or an adult, the medical assistant needs to be supportive and understanding, as the changes in appearance caused by these conditions can dramatically affect the client's self-esteem.

If the posterior pituitary undersecretes, **diabetes insipidus** can occur. In this disorder, not enough **antidiuretic hormone (ADH)** is produced. The client will complain of extreme thirst (*polydipsia*). The client will also complain of having to urinate all the time; this excessive urine production is called *polyuria*. The client may void as much as 10 liters a day, compared to the average person who urinates about 1½ to 2 liters per day. The medical assistant may notice that a urine specimen looks like water, because the urine is so dilute. The specific gravity (relative weight) of the urine of such a client will be low, around 1.001 to 1.005 instead of the normal range of 1.005 to 1.030. In medical treatment of this disorder, the client will receive ADH preparations.

NOTE TO STUDENT:

Diabetes insipidus can also result from ingestion of lithium, which is used to treat manic-depressive, bipolar disorders and some behavioral problems. The client who takes this medication must be closely observed clinically and through frequent laboratory tests. Clients who take lithium may need assistance in self-monitoring for this potentially very serious side effect.

■ THYROID AND PARATHYROID DISORDERS

Thyroid disorders result from the overproduction or underproduction of thyroid hormones. The thyroid affects metabolism, pregnancy, hair production, texture of the skin, sleep, muscle function, memory, joints, voice, and weight. Undersecretion of the thyroid hormone is called *hypothyroidism* or **myxedema.** Clients with underactive thyroids or hypothyroidism will complain of weight gain, huskiness of voice, feeling extremely tired, poor memory, depression, menstrual difficulties, hair loss, and dryness of skin and eyes. People may blame an underactive thyroid for obesity, though this is not the major cause of obesity. Hypothyroidism can be caused by an autoimmune disorder such as Hashimoto's disease, a **goiter,** or an enlargement of the thyroid. In times past, goiter was caused by a lack of iodine, though this is rare today. A pregnant woman who has hypothyroidism can give birth to a baby who is thyroid deficient. This condition is called **cretinism,** which is characterized by severe cognitive impairment. A thyroid blood test on a newborn can detect this before any physical or developmental impairments appear. Such an infant will need thyroid replacement therapy over the course of a lifetime.

A client with hyperthyroidism will complain of *insomnia* (inability to sleep). She will describe feeling hot, jittery, and anxious. The medical assistant may observe that the client has bulging eyes and tremors or shakiness (Figure 24-2). Hyperthyroidism can be caused by thyroid nodules; occasionally thyroid nodules are malignant. **Graves' disease** is a form of hyperthyroidism.

Tests will be ordered to diagnose and help determine treatment. The medical assistant may obtain a blood sample and send the specimen to an outside laboratory for testing. An ultrasound of the thyroid may also be ordered. The medical assistant's role will be to prepare the client for the ultrasound and then to make sure that the report is received and the doctor is informed according to office policy.

The parathyroid gland produces parathormone, which is needed for calcium utilization, especially as it relates to the formation of bone. Tumors or growths that develop in the parathyroid gland can result in abnormal deposition or placement of calcium in the body.

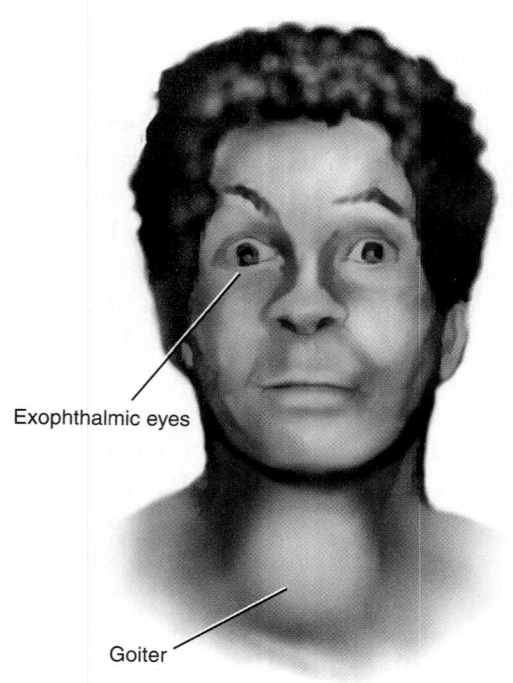

Exophthalmic eyes

Goiter

FIGURE 24-2 Hyperthyroidism.

ADRENAL GLAND DISORDERS

The adrenal gland produces adrenaline and corticosteroids. One disorder that can affect the adrenal glands is **Addison's disease,** a condition in which the cortex or outer layer of the adrenal gland does not make enough hormones. The medical assistant may observe that these clients look tanned or bronze; sometimes this skin coloration is mistaken for an ordinary tan. The medical assistant may also observe that the client's blood pressure is low. The client may complain of feeling very tired and not having enough energy for normal activities. The doctor will order laboratory tests to confirm the diagnosis. The medical assistant's role is to obtain a blood specimen, label it properly, and send it to the testing laboratory. The medical assistant also receives the laboratory report, informs the doctor that results are in, and files the report according to office policy. If the lab report is positive for Addison's, the medical assistant may note decreased sodium and blood **glucose** levels among electrolyte changes.

Overproduction of the glucocorticoid called *cortisol* can lead to a disorder called **Cushing's syndrome.** A growth on the pituitary gland or the adrenal cortex can cause this syndrome. The client will have a very round, "moon" face, and a "buffalo hump" or bump between the shoulder blades. The client will also appear to have thin arms and legs, as a result of muscle wasting. In addition to tumors, Cushing's syndrome can be caused by corticosteroid medications. Besides the clinical appearance, the doctor will order blood laboratory tests to confirm the diagnosis. The medical assistant should watch for bruising, edema, or swelling, all of which can occur with this disorder. The medical assistant must also watch closely for any signs of infection in these clients, as infection is often masked.

PANCREAS DISORDER

The most common metabolic disorder of the pancreas is called **diabetes mellitus.** In the past, nonmedical people have called this "sugar" diabetes. However, in diabetes mellitus, the body has difficulty metabolizing carbohydrates, proteins, and fats, because of a lack of the hormone insulin, underproduction of insulin, or ineffectiveness of insulin (insulin resistance). There are two major types of diabetes: Type I diabetes, or insulin-dependent diabetes (IDDM); and Type II diabetes, or noninsulin-dependent diabetes (NIDDM). These used to be called *juvenile diabetes* and *adult-onset diabetes*, respectively, but the new names better reflect the characteristics of the disorders.

In both types of diabetes, the most common clinical symptom of the disorder is hyperglycemia. Type I diabetes is thought to be an autoimmune disorder with a genetic component; there is a predisposition or tendency to develop it that runs in families. The onset is frequently sudden. In Type I diabetes, the problem is the lack of production or underproduction of insulin. A slower onset is characteristic of Type II diabetes, in which the problem seems to be an inability to use insulin effectively. Obesity is a major risk factor in this type of diabetes.

A third type of diabetes is **gestational diabetes.** This is usually discovered in a routine examination during pregnancy. The client may not have complaints or symptoms. This type is treated and managed as is diabetes mellitus. This type can disappear after delivery of the baby. However, the woman is at risk of developing Type II diabetes later on.

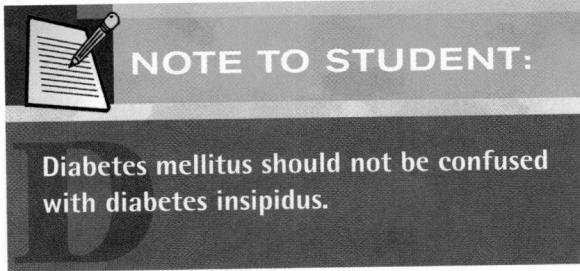

NOTE TO STUDENT:

Diabetes mellitus should not be confused with diabetes insipidus.

The doctor will order diagnostic tests to reach or confirm a clinical diagnosis of diabetes. The specific laboratory tests and the role of the medical assistant are discussed in Chapter 44.

The aim of treatment in all types of diabetes is to assist the client in living a healthy,

normal life. To accomplish this goal, the medical assistant works with the client in several major areas: medication and self-medication, physical activity, healthy eating, learning, and self-monitoring. Understanding how her actions and choices affect the course of the disorder, and following an individually designed plan, can help the client achieve a healthy lifestyle. Although the medical assistant will do much teaching and guidance, it is up to the client to assume the major role in her own care.

Both oral and injectable medications are used in the treatment of diabetes mellitus. Insulin pumps, that deliver constant, controllable amounts of insulin, have proven valuable for many individuals who have diabetes. These pumps provide better control over blood sugar levels and allow individuals to maintain healthier, active lifestyles with fewer of the long-term complications of diabetes.

Lack of understanding or not following prescribed health care decisions can put the client at great risk of developing complications. Cardiovascular problems, stroke, blindness, and kidney failure are major complications of long-term diabetes. Complications of diabetes are the largest cause of blindness and peripheral neuropathy in the United States. Because of problems with carbohydrate and fat metabolism, the client is at risk of heart attacks, strokes, and peripheral vascular disease. In turn, peripheral vascular disease results in poor circulation, which can cause death of tissue, especially in the feet and legs. In the past, this death of tissue, called *gangrene,* meant that many individuals eventually had to face amputation of toes, feet, and even legs. Harm to the kidneys from diabetes can lead to kidney failure and death.

 BRIDGE TO CAAHEP

This chapter, which discusses the endocrine system, provides information and content related to CAAHEP standards for Anatomy and Physiology, Medical Terminology, Medical Law and Ethics, Communication, Medical Assisting Clinical Procedures, and Professional Components.

POINTS OF HIGHLIGHT

- The endocrine system, through production and secretion of hormones, regulates many bodily functions.
- Overproduction or underproduction of any hormone can affect the homeostasis or balance in other areas.
- Overproduction of the growth hormone secreted by the anterior pituitary can cause major bodily changes. In a child, this results in gigantism; in an adult, it causes an overgrowth of bone and tissue called acromegaly.
- Underproduction of antidiuretic hormone from the posterior pituitary can result in diabetes insipidus.
- Diabetes insipidus and diabetes mellitus are not the same.
- Undersecretion by the thyroid gland is called hypothyroidism. This condition is characterized by feelings of extreme tiredness, weight gain, and loss of hair.
- Hyperthyroidism or overproduction by the thyroid gland will result in the client being anxious and overly active, with increased metabolism. The client's eyes will appear to bulge.
- Underproduction by the adrenal gland can result in Addison's disease. The client, who may appear to have a tan and look healthy, will complain of feeling tired, and the medical assistant will find that this client's blood pressure is low.
- The clinical signs of Cushing's syndrome are a round, "moon" face, thin arms and legs, and a "buffalo hump" between the shoulder blades.
- Diabetes mellitus is a serious metabolic disorder affecting a large number of Americans.
- The two major types of diabetes are type I (insulin-dependent diabetes or IDDM) and type II (noninsulin-dependent diabetes or NIDDM).
- Type I diabetes usually has a sudden onset, first occurs in childhood, and has a genetic component predisposing the client to the disorder.
- Obesity is a major risk factor for Type II diabetes.
- A client who has diabetes needs to take an active role in her own care if she is to lead a healthy, normal lifestyle.

ABHES LINKS

This chapter, which discusses the endocrine system, links to ABHES course content for Anatomy and Physiology, Medical Terminology, Medical Law and Ethics, and Medical Office Clinical Procedures.

AAMA AREAS OF COMPETENCE

This chapter, which discusses the endocrine system, provides information or content within several areas listed in the Medical Assistant Role Delineation Study. These areas include: clinical, fundamental principles of diagnostic orders, patient (client) care, general transdisciplinary, professionalism, communication skills, legal concepts, and instruction.

AMT PATHS

This chapter, which discusses the endocrine system, provides a path to AMT competency in general medical assisting knowledge, anatomy and physiology, medical terminology, and patient (client) education.

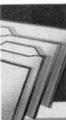

STUDENT PORTFOLIO ACTIVITY

Health care proxies and living wills are becoming more common, but many people still misunderstand what they are, or are confused about how they are used. Find out the legal issues involved with these documents. Write a brief summary that shows your awareness of these issues and the role of the medical assistant regarding these advance directives in a health care setting.

APPLYING YOUR SKILLS

A client comes to the office. She states that her hands seem to be getting bigger; she can tell because her rings do not fit anymore. She also tells you that her nose appears thicker than it used to be. You observe that the client's jaw is very prominent. The doctor orders laboratory tests of pituitary function. What could be happening with this client's pituitary gland? What condition seen in children is this related to?

APPLYING YOUR SKILLS

A client was recently diagnosed with diabetes mellitus. You know that the client needs to become an active participant in her own health care. In what ways can she become involved?

CRITICAL THINKING QUESTIONS

1. What are some points for the medical assistant to remember in working with clients who have diabetes mellitus?

2. What symptoms might you observe in a client with hyperthyroidism?

3. Identify some symptoms of hypothyroidism that a client might attribute to "getting older" or "too much stress" in life?

4. Describe what you, as a medical assistant, might observe when a client's body is overproducing cortisol?

5. What is the name of the syndrome in which there is overproduction of cortisol?

6. Uncontrolled diabetes mellitus can lead to complications. What is the client at risk of developing?

7. What is the difference between diabetes insipidus and diabetes mellitus?

8. The doctor diagnosed a client as having diabetes insipidus. The client questions how that can be, because she does not eat a lot of sugar and no one in her family has diabetes. This statement indicates that the client has misunderstood. What is the confusion?

9. How would you help the client in question 8 to understand her condition?

10. Explain how hypersecretion by the thyroid gland can affect a client. As a medical assistant, what would you observe in this client?

11. Steps should be taken to prevent complications from Cushing's disorder. What are some symptoms that the client needs to report to the doctor right away?

12. Identify steps that a client can take to decrease the risk of developing type II diabetes.

13. The doctor has ordered laboratory tests to detect diabetes in a pregnant client. What do you say to the client when she asks why blood has to be drawn?

14. Explain to a medical assistant student how the endocrine system regulates bodily function. What does she need to understand about "target" organs and overproduction or underproduction of hormones by the glands?

15. Go back to the beginning of this chapter and review the Anticipatory Statements. Reread each statement and then indicate whether it is true or false. If the statement is false, rewrite it to make it a true statement.

CLIENT TEACHING PLAN

Behaviors for Kidney Health in Diabetes

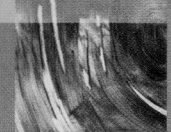

■ What Is to Be Taught:

- Behaviors to foster healthy kidneys in clients who have diabetes.

■ Objectives:

- Client who has diabetes will be able to identify steps to promote healthy kidneys.

■ Preparation Before Teaching:

- Review the long-term effects of diabetes on kidney function. Make sure that you put technical medical terms into everyday language that the client can easily understand.
- Look over actions that a person can take to promote kidney health.
- Get together teaching materials, such as diagrams or pictures of the kidneys, paper and pen for written instructions and notes, and any printed informational material about diabetes and the kidneys.
- Make sure that the area is free from distractions while you are teaching.

■ Steps for the Medical Assistant:

1. Wash your hands.
2. Gather needed supplies.
3. Introduce yourself to the client.
4. Explain what you are going to teach and why.
5. Tell the client that diabetes can have long-term effects on the kidneys and impair their ability to work efficiently. Inform the client that there are many steps she can take to promote kidney health. She can take an active part in her own health care in addition to testing for blood glucose levels and taking prescribed medications.
6. Show the client the pictures of the kidneys and urinary system. State in simple terms how the kidneys work. (The blood flows through the kidneys, and healthy kidneys filter the blood, retaining the nutrients the body needs and making urine to get rid of waste.) Certain factors can damage or destroy the kidney's ability to do these tasks. Uncontrolled diabetes is one such factor.
7. Tell the client that with knowledge of only a few facts, she can take steps to help the kidneys do their work. Tell her that:
   a. Uncontrolled blood sugar can damage the nephrons (working units of the kidneys). If the client tests her blood sugar with a home glucose (sugar) monitoring kit as directed, and follows through with the correct action based on the results as prescribed by the doctor, the kidneys can continue to do their work.
   b. There is no such thing as a "diabetic diet." Eating a well-balanced diet, with the right amount (portions) of carbohydrates, proteins, and fats to meet daily activity levels is the important idea. This will provide the vitamins, minerals, and energy needed. Eating less protein puts less strain on the kidneys.
   c. It is important to consume the right amount of calcium, which is critical for strong bones. Kidneys that are not working well will not adequately process or absorb the vitamin D in foods.
   d. Be careful with over-the-counter medications. Medicines such as aspirin, acetaminophens, ibuprofen, and naproxen can also damage the kidneys. Always check with the doctor about any over-the-counter medications.
8. Give written instructions and information about diabetes and kidney health for the client to use as a reference at home.

(Continues)

CLIENT TEACHING PLAN (Continued)

■ Special Needs of the Client:

- Check the client's chart to see if there are any factors that might interfere with the client's ability to understand and follow these steps.
- Ask the client, before and after the teaching, if there is anything you should know that might affect her ability to follow these steps.

■ Evaluation:

- Client is able to explain that diabetes is related to potential problems with the working of the kidneys.
- Client can state steps that she can take to help promote kidney health.

■ Further Plans/Teaching:

- Ask the client if she has any questions or needs any additional information.

■ Follow-up:

- At the next office visit, review the information on diabetes and kidney function with the client.
- Check the client's blood sugar readings and medication amounts.

Medical Assistant

Name: _____

Signature: _____

Date: _____

Client

Date: _____

Follow-up Date : _____

CHAPTER 25

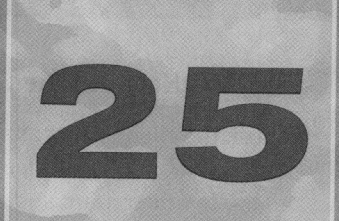

Anticipatory Statements

People have different ideas about cardiovascular system disorders. Read and think about the following statements based upon what you believe now. Decide whether you agree or disagree. Write the word **agree** after the statement if you think the statement is true. Write the word **disagree** after the statement if you think the statement is false. Read the chapter to find out if your current beliefs can be supported.

1. Cardiovascular disorders only happen to people who are very elderly.

   _____

2. The symptoms of a heart attack are the same for males and females.

   _____

3. Whether a person develops a heart disorder depends only on whether he has a family history of heart disorders.

   _____

4. Congestive heart failure usually develops slowly over time.

   _____

5. Smoking, inactive lifestyle, and obesity are risk factors for cardiovascular disease.

   _____

Learning Objectives

Upon completion of this chapter, the medical assistant student should be able to:

- Identify the medical assistant's role in client preparation for diagnostic tests of the cardiovascular system
- List three risk factors for a heart attack
- Explain how arteriosclerosis develops

Cardiovascular System Disorders

- Explain why hypertension is often called the "silent killer"
- Discuss the effects of angina pectoris
- State signs and symptoms of heart dysrhythmias
- Define endocarditis
- Develop a teaching plan for a client who has congestive heart failure
- Teach another person how to do activities of daily living after being treated for congestive heart failure

Key Terms

angina pectoris Condition in which the vessels to the heart are narrowed, causing pain upon physical activity or stress.

arteriosclerosis Coronary artery disorder in which the coronary arteries narrow and harden.

atherosclerosis Condition in which the walls of the arteries harden and collect fatty deposits.

cardiac dysrhythmia Irregular heart conduction cycle, rate, and rhythm.

congestive heart failure Inability of the heart to perform its work as a pump.

coronary heart disease Common term for any heart disorder.

hypertension High blood pressure.

inflammation Body's response to defend against invasion and to help heal injured tissue.

myocardial infarction Heart attack; complete blockage of one or more vessels to the heart.

phlebitis Inflammation of a vein.

rheumatic fever Occurs after a respiratory infection that was not healed successfully.

rheumatic heart disease Autoimmune disease in which, after an infection, the antibodies produced then attack and damage the heart, valves, and joints.

INTRODUCTION

Cardiovascular disorders are very common. Cardiovascular disease is the number-one cause of death in the United States. It is not just a disorder of the elderly client, nor of males; 50% of all women will die from **coronary heart diseases.** Heart disease kills more people than all the cancers combined, including breast and lung cancer. Prevention and early, effective treatment are essential. The medical assistant will need to understand the common disorders and the causes and risk factors for these diseases so that he can teach the client. Part of the medical assistant's responsibility will be to help care for clients with cardiac problems. The medical assistant will also teach clients about heart-healthy behaviors to prevent and avoid cardiac disorders. Client preparation for cardiac diagnostic tests is yet another responsibility of the medical assistant (these diagnostic tests are discussed in Chapter 43).

MYOCARDIAL INFARCTION

A **myocardial infarction** is commonly called a *heart attack* (Figure 25-1). Blood carries oxygen and nutrients to the heart. When the blood supply is cut off, for any reason, the heart is deprived of oxygen. The heart demands a constant supply of oxygen; even a short interruption will cause damage to the heart muscle and possibly death. Without oxygen, the heart muscle dies, and thus the heart can no longer keep the rest of the body supplied with essential oxygen and nutrients.

There are certain warnings signs of an impending heart attack that the client should learn to recognize. The classic signs are a crushing pain or heavy pressure in the chest. Sometimes the pain travels (radiates) down the arm. The client will begin to perspire or sweat. If the client experiences these symptoms, it is important to call 9-1-1 and the emergency medical services (EMS) squad. Women often do not experience the classic symptoms during a heart attack. Their feelings may be more vague. Instead of crushing chest pain, they may experience back pain near the scapula or shoulder blades. Other signs of heart attack in women include a feeling like indigestion, fatigue, and problems with sleep. If a woman experiences these symptoms, she should call 9-1-1 or EMS.

ANGINA PECTORIS

When the heart muscle does not receive enough oxygen and the proper amount of blood, the client will experience pain or pressure in the chest. This pain, called **angina pectoris,** occurs

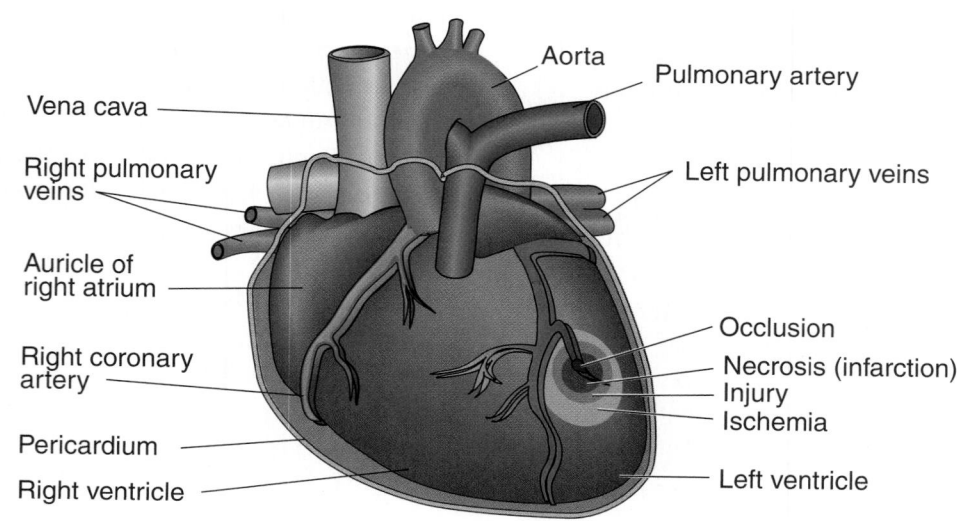

Vena cava

Right pulmonary veins

Auricle of right atrium

Right coronary artery

Pericardium

Right ventricle

Aorta

Pulmonary artery

Left pulmonary veins

Occlusion

Necrosis (infarction)

Injury

Ischemia

Left ventricle

FIGURE 25-1 Myocardial infarction.

when the blood vessels that supply the heart become clogged and thus decrease the flow of blood to the heart. The client often comes to the medical office complaining of chest pain after increased activity such as climbing the stairs, playing a sport, or doing heavy physical work; or after eating a heavy meal or being outside in the cold. When a person increases activity, the heart needs more oxygen and nutrients to keep up with the exertion. When it does not get an adequate amount, the client experiences pain. Treatment consists of pain medication and other medications such as nitroglycerin. In the acute stage, oxygen, pain medications, and aspirin or other clot-busting drugs may be given.

CARDIAC DYSRHYTHMIA

In addition to an adequate blood supply, the heart must maintain a regular rhythm to effectively meet the needs of the body. The conduction system of the heart sends electrical impulses to start and coordinate the beating of the heart and thus the blood flow. There should be an equal amount of time between each beat. If there is not, the heartbeat is *irregular.* Sometimes the initial impulse from the pacemaker fires too fast or does not allow completion of one heartbeat before it starts another. Sometimes there are extra impulses. The client may complain of "skipped" beats, or a feeling of palpitations or extra and fast beats. Any heart rhythm that is abnormal or out-of-order is called a **cardiac dysrhythmia.** Some are short-term and correct themselves. Others are life-threatening and require quick intervention.

The type and location of a dysrhythmia affect the seriousness of the condition. The doctor may order an electrocardiogram and a Holter monitor for the client (see Chapter 43). Treatment is aimed at identifying both the type and cause of the dysrhythmia. Medications may be prescribed. Often the client will have to avoid stimulants such as caffeine. Many clients who drink coffee and cola drinks consume more caffeine than they realize. The medical assistant will have to work with these clients to help them

adjust to the elimination of caffeine from the diet. The medical assistant will also teach the client to find and count the pulse, and the client will be asked to take the pulse whenever he feels that he has "skipped" beats or is feeling poorly.

INFLAMMATION OF THE HEART

Inflammation and infection can affect any part of the heart, including the muscle, valves, and pericardial sac. **Rheumatic fever** is an acute problem seen more in children than adults. This acute infection can lead to a chronic condition called **rheumatic heart disease.** Rheumatic fever can damage the heart valves; however, this problem usually does not become apparent until middle age. A new test for heart inflammation, which measures the amount of C-reactive protein, is administered when a client complains of chest pain. Additionally, doctors are using the test as a screening device or tool to detect heart disease.

Endocarditis

The membrane that lines the heart and its valves, the *endocardium,* can become infected. This infection is called *endocarditis.* When pathogenic microorganisms enter the bloodstream, they can travel to the heart valves. Upper respiratory infections and even dental work can introduce these pathogens. Once infected, the client will have a fever, loss of appetite, and loss of weight. This condition used to be fatal, and still can be today if it goes unrecognized and untreated. Currently, the condition is treated with antibiotics.

Pericarditis

The sac that surrounds the heart can become inflamed and infected. This inflammation is called *pericarditis.* The client will complain of pain in the chest upon movement; even the act of breathing can cause pain. The doctor will order medications to treat the infection and reduce the inflammation.

Phlebitis

A blood vessel inflammation is called **phlebitis.** This condition can occur in either a superficial or a deep vein. The affected vein may become red, swollen, and tender. At times, a clot (thrombus) can form as a reaction to the inflammation. This is called *thrombophlebitis.* If the clot forms in a deep vein, it is called a *deep vein thrombosis* or *DVT.* Certain factors can increase a client's risk of developing deep vein thrombosis. Obesity is one such factor. Inactivity, or remaining still for a long period of time, can also put the client at risk. Sitting on an airplane, or in a bus or car, for a long time without exercise or movement increases the risk of DVT. For some clients, doctors prescribe anticoagulants before surgery or prolonged bedrest. A very serious worsening of thrombophlebitis is the formation of an embolism, when a clot breaks loose. The embolus can travel through the blood vessels and eventually block a vessel leading to a vital organ.

Aneurysm

An *aneurysm* is a weakening of a blood vessel. The damaged vessel balloons out, thus making the vessel wall thinner and more fragile in that area. If the pressure of the blood flowing through the vessel becomes too great, the weakened, ballooned-out part can burst. If the aneurysm is found before it bursts, and is in a spot where it can be reached, surgery may be done to correct it. In many cases, however, the client is not aware of the aneurysm until it bursts. Keeping blood pressure down and vessels open will help to prevent stress on a weakened vessel. If a client's parent or sibling has or had an aneurysm, the client has an increased risk of having an aneurysm himself. If the medical assistant finds a history of aneurysm while taking a client's medical history, the doctor will screen for aneurysm and the possible need for repair.

ARTERIOSCLEROSIS

The blood vessels can become thickened; when that occurs, the vessels become less elastic, less spongy, and less able to contract. This is called **arteriosclerosis.** The most common form of arteriosclerosis is **atherosclerosis** (Figure 25-2), in which fatty deposits and calcium deposits line the blood vessels. These deposits make the *lumen* (passageway or interior diameter) of the vessels narrower, thus restricting the flow of blood. Certain factors put the person at risk for continued progression of arteriosclerosis. Family history and age are two factors, but there are other factors that a person can change to decrease the risk of worsening the condition. Smoking, inactive lifestyle, and obesity all put a person at risk. Diabetes, high cholesterol, and high blood pressure increase the risk. If the client, with the help of the medical assistant, works at reducing the risks, such as by eating low-fat foods and foods low in cholesterol and becoming more active, the risks will decrease. The client *must* stop smoking. Medications may also be prescribed. If a treatment plan is not developed, or the client does not take an active part in carrying out the plan, this can lead to serious consequences. If complete blockage of a vessel occurs, a stroke or heart attack may result.

HYPERTENSION

Hypertension, or high blood pressure, is defined as a systolic pressure above 140 mm Hg and a diastolic pressure of more than 90 mm Hg. Many people have high blood pressure and are not aware of it. The client feels no pain or other uncomfortable feeling. Often the client does not become aware of the problem until the hypertension has already done damage to body systems. Thus, it is critical that everyone be screened for high blood pressure. In most health care settings, the medical assistant will obtain and record the client's blood pressure reading. Free blood pressure clinics are sometimes set up in the community to screen for hypertension.

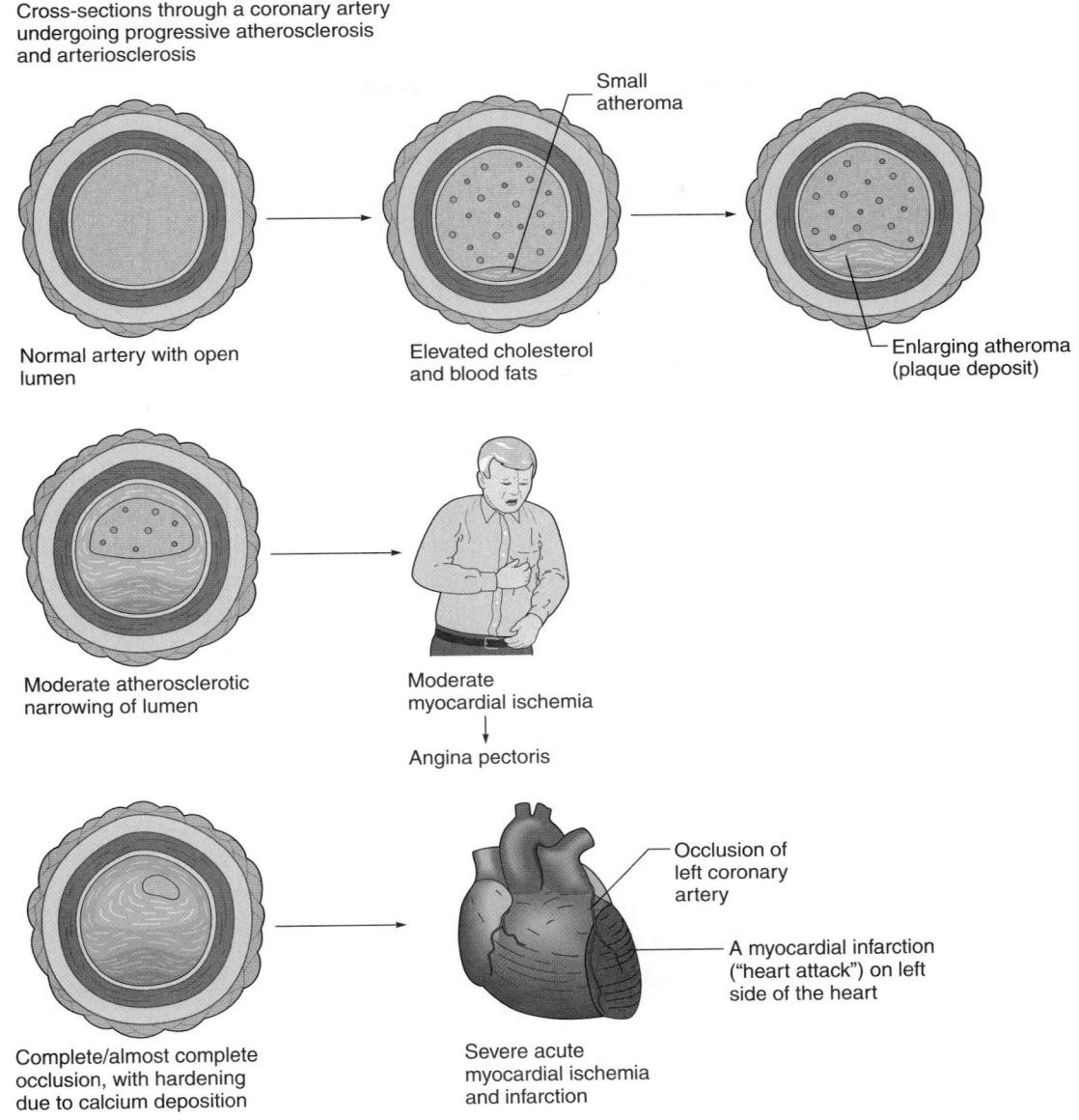

Cross-sections through a coronary artery undergoing progressive atherosclerosis and arteriosclerosis

Small atheroma

Normal artery with open lumen

Elevated cholesterol and blood fats

Enlarging atheroma (plaque deposit)

Moderate atherosclerotic narrowing of lumen

Moderate myocardial ischemia

Angina pectoris

Complete/almost complete occlusion, with hardening due to calcium deposition

Occlusion of left coronary artery

A myocardial infarction ("heart attack") on left side of the heart

Severe acute myocardial ischemia and infarction

FIGURE 25-2 Atherosclerosis.

Hypertension is often called the "silent killer" because there are no warning signs, and unfortunately sometimes a person learns about his hypertension only after a stroke. Healthful eating, including lowering the amount of sodium in the diet, is helpful. The client must increase physical activity. If the client is overweight, it is critical that he lose weight. In addition, the doctor may order medication. Clients may experience some side effects with these medications, and may declare that they felt better before they started to take the medication. The medical assistant needs to actively listen to the client and then work with him in changing to a healthier lifestyle.

Recently, the blood pressure guidelines have been expanded to include a prehypertension classification; once a client's blood pressure is 120/80, he is considered prehypertensive. At this stage, the medical assistant will review with the client the lifestyle changes needed to decrease the blood pressure, such as weight loss, decreased salt intake, and increased exercise.

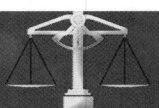

LEGAL/ETHICAL THOUGHTS

Clients who are sick or have chronic disorders are often angry or afraid. Sometimes, in trying to cope, clients express anger at or speak hurtfully to the health care provider. The medical assistant should remain calm and professional, and not take any angry words personally.

VALVULAR HEART DISORDER

When functioning properly, the valves of the heart allow blood to flow in one direction only. Correctly functioning valves open to allow blood to flow from the atria to the ventricles; the valves then close to prevent the blood from flowing backward. Any malfunctioning of the valves is grouped under the general term *valvular heart disorder.* If the valve does not close properly, it is *insufficient.* If the valve is too narrow, the blood cannot completely empty into the ventricles. When the valves do not work properly, a sound or *murmur* can be heard with a stethoscope.

Valvular heart disorder puts the client at risk of blood clots. These blood clots can become emboli, breaking off and traveling to vital organs. In addition, valvular heart disorder makes the heart work extra hard, eventually causing congestive heart failure. Clients who have damaged or abnormal heart valves, such as mitral valve prolapse, need to use prophylactic antibiotics before dental and certain surgical procedures to prevent endocarditis. The medical assistant must teach these clients the importance of taking antibiotics each time before having teeth cleaned and before certain other procedures.

CONGESTIVE HEART FAILURE

When the heart cannot perform its work any more, it becomes congested and fails as a pump. In the early stages of **congestive heart failure**, the client may have difficulty breathing when doing light exercise such as walking up stairs. Eventually, even less strenuous activities cause

shortness of breath and difficulty in breathing. The heart increases the number of beats in an attempt to circulate blood to all parts of the body. As a result, the client increases the number of breaths. If the right side of the heart fails, the liver and spleen become congested. If the left side fails, there is congestion and fluid buildup in the lungs. Fluid buildup in the lungs is called *pulmonary edema.*

Congestive heart failure occurs over time. It can come on slowly, so that the client is not aware of a problem until activities of daily living become difficult (Figure 25-3). The medical

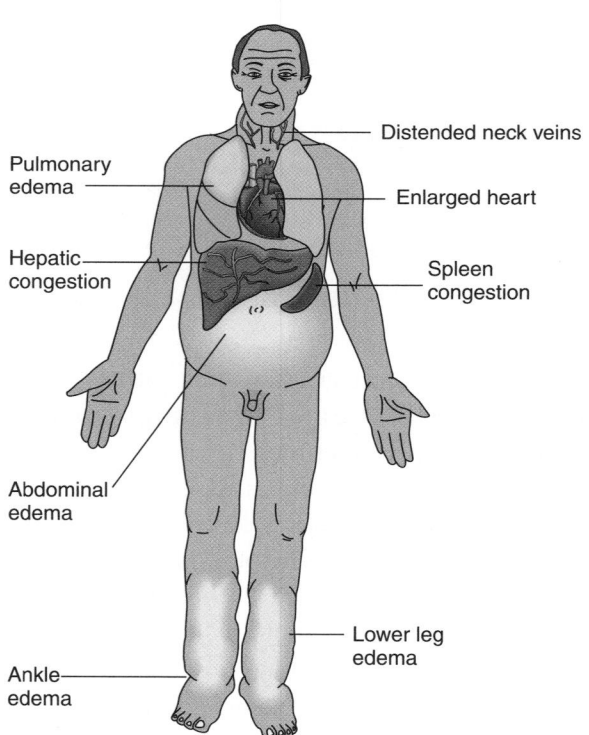

FIGURE 25-3 Symptoms of congestive heart failure.

assistant will work with the client on a daily plan to lessen the strain on the heart. Daily activities, such as eating, dressing, doing errands, and any work or social activities, are planned to use the heart most efficiently and allow rest periods.

Keeping the heart healthy by reducing the number of risk factors can help prevent many cardiovascular disorders. Increasing one's amount of exercise little by little will help. Eating a more healthful diet, and reading food labels to avoid foods high in fatty acids and sodium, will keep the blood vessels clear. Recognize stress and find ways to decrease or deal with it. Cardiovascular disorders require lifestyle changes to prevent more serious damage to the body.

 ## BRIDGE TO CAAHEP

This chapter, which discusses cardiovascular disorders, provides information and content related to CAAHEP standards for Anatomy and Physiology, Common Pathology/Diseases, Diagnostic/ Treatment Modalities, Medical Terminology, Medical Law and Ethics, Communication, Clinical Procedures and Professional Components.

 ## ABHES LINKS

This chapter, which discusses cardiovascular disorders, links to ABHES course content for Anatomy and Physiology, Medical Terminology, Medical Law and Ethics, and Medical Office Clinical Procedures.

POINTS OF HIGHLIGHT

- Cardiovascular disease is the leading cause of death in the United States.
- Decreasing the number of risk factors can help prevent many cardiovascular disorders.
- Signs and symptoms of a heart attack are not the same for males and females. Males may experience the classic symptoms of crushing pain in the chest, pain in the arm and/or jaw, and difficulty breathing. Symptoms in females are more subtle and vague, and may include back pain and fatigue.
- Individuals may have hypertension and not be aware of it. Hypertension may proceed silently and lead to a heart attack or stroke.
- Rheumatic fever can lead to a chronic problem called rheumatic heart disease.
- The client with angina often experiences chest pain after activity because not enough blood and oxygen are delivered to meet the additional needs of the heart during increased activity.
- Endocarditis is an infection of the endocardium that lines the heart and its valves.
- Any abnormal rhythm of the heart is called a cardiac dysrhythmia. Dysrhythmias can be mild and short-term or severe and life-threatening.
- The chances of developing chronic disorders such as arteriosclerosis can be lessened by not smoking, increasing physical activity, and maintaining ideal body weight through healthy eating and exercise.
- Medical assistants can support clients in understanding and following treatment plans prescribed by the doctor to keep blood pressure within the guidelines.
- Medical assistants can help clients who have congestive heart failure by working with them to schedule activities of daily living efficiently and lessen the strain on the heart.

AAMA AREAS OF COMPETENCE

This chapter, which discusses cardiovascular disorders, provides information or content within several areas listed in the Medical Assistant Role Delineation Study. These areas include: clinical, patient (client) care, general transdisciplinary, communication, legal concepts, and instruction.

 ## AMT PATHS

This chapter, which discusses cardiovascular disorders, provides a path to AMT competency in general medical assisting knowledge, anatomy and physiology, medical terminology, and patient (client) education.

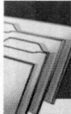 ### STUDENT PORTFOLIO ACTIVITY

Employers are looking for individuals who think creatively and take individual responsibility for their actions. Think about classroom or laboratory instructors you have worked with. Ask if an instructor would be willing to write a letter about you addressing these characteristics. Do not wait to do this until you are near graduation and looking for a job!

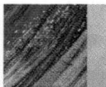 ### APPLYING YOUR SKILLS

Your clinical procedures instructor has stressed blood pressure competency through numerous practice sessions and attention to detail. Why is this skill so vital to you as a medical assistant? How do the client and doctor depend upon your skill in obtaining and recording the client's blood pressure?

CRITICAL THINKING QUESTIONS

1. Why is hypertension or high blood pressure called the silent killer?

2. The conduction system of the heart sends electrical impulses to regulate the heartbeat. What happens to the client, and what might the client feel or experience, if the conduction system becomes abnormal?

3. Identify risk factors for developing atherosclerosis. What can a client do to reduce the risk factors?

4. If a client feels crushing pain in the chest and is perspiring excessively, what should he do? What might be happening?

5. If a person was sick with rheumatic fever as a child, what condition might he develop during adulthood? How does this condition affect the heart?

6. A client has been told that she has a heart murmur. How do you explain this in everyday language?

7. Why is it important for women to understand risk factors for cardiovascular disorders?

8. In angina pectoris, why does physical activity increase the chance that the client will experience pain symptoms?

9. What is the relationship of dental work and endocarditis?

10. Deep vein thrombosis is a serious condition. What can put a client at risk of developing DVT?

11. Go back to the beginning of this chapter and review the Anticipatory Statements. Reread each statement and then indicate whether it is true or false. If the statement is false, rewrite it to make it a true statement.

CLIENT TEACHING PLAN

Reducing Risks of High Blood Pressure

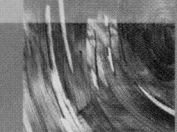

■ What Is to Be Taught:

- How to reduce the risks of high blood pressure.

■ Objectives:

- Client will understand the risks of high blood pressure and how to live a healthy life while coping with high blood pressure.

■ Preparation Before Teaching:

- Review the health risks associated with high blood pressure.
- Look over actions that a person can take and choices he can make to promote and follow a healthy lifestyle.
- Get together teaching materials, such as diagrams or pictures of how blood flows throughout the body and the effects on the various organs if the person has high blood pressure. Make sure you have paper and pens for written instructions and notes.
- Make sure the area is free from distractions while you are teaching.

■ Steps for the Medical Assistant:

1. Wash your hands.
2. Gather needed supplies.
3. Introduce yourself to the client.
4. Explain what you are going to teach and why.
5. Inform the client that high blood pressure can be harmful and even deadly. Tell him, however, that there are certain steps and actions he can take to lower his blood pressure and help reduce these risks.
6. Show the client pictures and diagrams of how the blood flows throughout the body and how high blood pressure can damage the normal rate and flow of the blood. Explain to the client what problems this can cause.
7. Tell the client that knowing the right steps to take in living a healthy lifestyle can reduce the risks of high blood pressure. These include:

a. Cutting down on salt and sodium in the diet by keeping the salt shaker away from the table. Always taste the food before considering adding any salt. If the client desires salt, use a lower-sodium product.

b Eat a heart-healthy diet that includes an adequate amount of fiber and vegetables.

c. Exercise is key to living a heart-healthy life. Changing little things can make a big difference. For instance, instead of taking the elevator, walk the stairs. If you work in a safe environment, park farther away and walk the extra distance.

d. Take prescribed medication as directed.

e. Call the doctor with any questions or concerns.

■ Special Needs of the Client:

- Check the client's chart for any factors that might interfere with the client's ability to follow through on all the steps discussed.
- Ask the client if there is anything you should know that might affect his ability to participate in any of these steps to help maintain a healthy blood pressure.

■ Evaluation:

- Client will be able to list steps to help reduce the risks of high blood pressure.
- Client states that he is willing to start incorporating these steps into his daily life.
- Client agrees to call the doctor if he has any questions or concerns regarding his blood pressure.

■ Further Plans/Teaching:

- At the next visit, review the information with the client.
- Ask the client what steps he was able to take and if he has had any problems incorporating these steps into his daily activities.

(Continues)

CLIENT TEACHING PLAN (Continued)

■ Follow-up:

- Call the client after one week and ask how he is feeling.
- Ask the client if he has been able to start taking the steps to maintain healthy blood pressure.
- Ask the client for details and if he has any problems or questions. Be nonjudgmental.

Medical Assistant

Name: _____

Signature: _____

Date: _____

Client

Date: _____

Follow-up Date : _____

Anticipatory Statements

People have different ideas about blood and hematologic system disorders. Read and think about the following statements based upon what you believe now. Decide whether you agree or disagree. Write the word **agree** after the statement if you think the statement is true. Write the word **disagree** after the statement if you think the statement is false. Read the chapter to find out if your current beliefs can be supported.

1. With hemophilia, a client's blood thickens and forms clots.

   _____

2. Iron-deficiency anemia is often seen in adult women and teenage girls.

   _____

3. Sickle cell anemia is found most frequently in Black people, of African origin or descent.

   _____

4. "Mono" or mononucleosis has symptoms similar to those of flu.

   _____

5. Leukemia is a disorder of the blood's clotting mechanisms.

   _____

Hematologic and Lymphatic System Disorders

Learning Objectives

Upon completion of this chapter, the medical assistant student should be able to:

- Identify the medical assistant's role in preparing clients for diagnostic tests of the hematologic and lymphatic systems
- State signs and symptoms of an acute stage of sickle cell disorder
- List clotting disorders of the hematologic system
- Compare Hodgkin's and non-Hodgkin's lymphoma
- Develop a teaching plan for a client with sickle cell disorder
- Teach another person how to recognize and react to the onset of a sickle cell crisis

Key Terms

anemia Condition in which too little oxygen is delivered to the cells, either because there are not enough red blood cells or because the cells lack hemoglobin.

hemophilia Genetic disorder found mostly in males; causes slow clotting of blood, which can lead to severe blood loss from even a minor cut.

Hodgkin's disease Malignant disorder with progressive enlargement of lymphoid tissue.

leukemia Condition in which bone marrow makes abnormal white blood cells that the body cannot use to fight off infections.

lymphedema Swelling caused by fluid that cannot flow easily through the lymphatic system.

mononucleosis Increase in the number of mononuclear lymphocytes (a type of white blood cell).

neutropenia Decrease in the number of neutrophils, a type of white blood cell.

polycythemia Too many erythrocytes or red blood cells.

sickle cell anemia Disorder in which red blood cells become sickle-shaped because of abnormal hemoglobin.

thrombocythemia Too many platelets in the blood.

thrombocytopenia Too few platelets in the blood.

■ INTRODUCTION

The blood carries oxygen and nutrients to the cells and carries away waste. Blood volume, infection fighting, and blood clotting are also part of the tasks of the hematologic system. The lymphatic system acts as a protector against infection and filters waste products and foreign substances from the blood. *Hematology* is that branch of medicine that studies the hematologic and lymphatic systems. *Hematologists* are medical doctors who practice in that specialty. Disorders of the hematologic and lymphatic systems can begin in the blood, or they can originate elsewhere in the body and be carried and spread to other systems by the blood and lymph.

■ DIAGNOSTIC TESTS

Laboratory tests to diagnose hematologic and lymphatic disorders consist of blood tests and biopsies. A complete blood count (CBC) with differential is the most common laboratory test. A CBC looks at red blood cells, white blood cells, and platelets. The differential part of the complete blood test examines in detail the number of cells. Tests will determine the oxygen-carrying ability of the red blood cells. Bleeding-time tests, such as prothrombin time (PT) and thromboplastin time (PTT), examine blood-clotting ability. Biopsies may be taken from the blood-forming organs or lymph nodes.

The medical assistant's role in diagnostic testing of the hematologic and lymphatic systems will vary according to the scope of practice, office policy, and regulatory laws. The medical assistant will prepare the client with any special instructions for the two tests. If properly taught and permitted by law and policy, the medical assistant may perform a venipuncture and obtain a blood sample. The sample is then labeled with all required information, processed, and sent to the laboratory that will perform the tests. When the lab report is returned to the office, the medical assistant

notifies the doctor and files the lab report according to office policy.

■ RED BLOOD CELL DISORDERS

The red blood cells work to bring oxygen to all parts of the body; they exchange oxygen for carbon dioxide, carry nutrients, and take away waste products. If the hematologic system is to work well, there must be the right amount of red blood cells. Too many or too few will upset the balance and create problems. Too many cells, especially red blood cells, is called **polycythemia.**

A different, and much more common, problem with red blood cells, is **anemia,** a condition in which there are fewer red blood cells and less hemoglobin, which is the oxygen-carrying part of the red blood cell. Anemia is not a separate disease or entity; rather, many disorders can cause anemia, usually by changing the oxygen-carrying capacity of the red blood cells. There are many types of anemias, which are named and grouped according to their cause. However, the client's symptoms are similar in all types of anemia. Medical assistants should be familiar with the symptoms common to all anemias and the major causes of anemia.

Iron-Deficiency Anemia

Iron-deficiency anemia is the most common type of anemia. It is seen most often in women, children, and the elderly. In iron-deficiency anemia, either not enough iron is absorbed or too much iron is excreted. This may be due to poor dietary habits or lack of iron-rich food. Teenage girls who have heavy menstrual flows may develop anemia, particularly if they do not eat iron-rich foods. During pregnancy, there is also a higher demand for iron. The elderly client often has dietary problems. Their diets may not supply enough iron because of tooth, chewing, or digestive problems. Mobility or financial problems may mean that they cannot obtain or afford the food for an adequate diet. Older adults may also not eat well because they are alone.

Folic Acid Anemia

Folic acid anemia is also related to dietary intake. Folic acid is necessary for the development of red blood cells. There is a critical demand for folic acid during pregnancy; deficiencies can cause birth defects such as neural tube defects. It is recommended that everyone include folic acid as part of a daily vitamin regimen. This will prevent folic acid anemia.

Hemorrhagic Anemia

Anemia can also result from acute or chronic hemorrhage. A sudden loss of a large amount of blood can decrease the volume of blood drastically and cause anemia. Treatment aims first to replace the volume and then to remedy the lack of oxygen. For example, if a large blood vessel is ruptured by a traumatic injury, the blood will first have to be replaced; then treatment will focus on the oxygen level.

Less easily recognized is anemia from chronic blood loss. It takes longer to cure this type of anemia because the blood is lost at a much slower pace. Gastrointestinal disorders, such as peptic ulcers, may cause chronic blood loss. Chronic hemorrhagic blood loss will eventually lead to iron-deficiency anemia. The doctor will need to identify the source of the bleeding and treat the cause. The medical assistant will instruct the client about eating a diet rich in iron. The doctor may also order iron supplements.

Pernicious Anemia

Pernicious anemia has a very specific cause. In a client with pernicious anemia, the stomach does not secrete the intrinsic factor necessary to absorb vitamin B12 from food. Vitamin B12 enables the body to use iron. This is a slow-onset disorder and is usually in advanced stages before the diagnosis is made. Taking vitamin B12 supplements orally will not help; the client will need vitamin B12 by injection. The medical assistant will need to work closely with this client, as these injections will be necessary for the rest of the client's life.

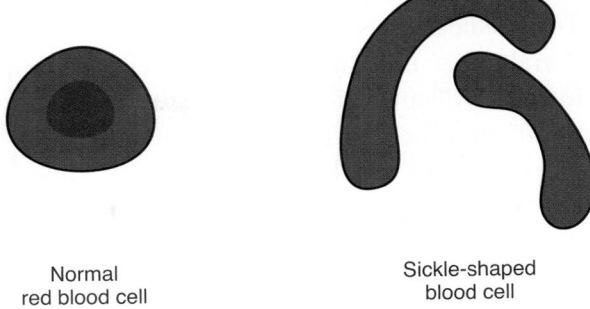

Normal red blood cell

Sickle-shaped blood cell

FIGURE 26-1 Normal red blood cells and sickle-shaped red blood cells.

Sickle Cell Anemia

Sickle cell anemia is a genetic, inherited disorder of the red blood cells (Figure 26-1). People of African, Mediterranean, or Southwest Asian origin or descent are most often affected by this disorder. Their red blood cells have a shorter life span. When there is less oxygen, the red blood cells become "sickled" or crescent-shaped. The cell shape hinders the transportation of oxygen. The cells become sticky and hard and clump together. When the cells clump, they do not circulate well and oxygen cannot get to vital organs. The client will then have symptoms of anemia. Clots called thrombi can break off the clumped red blood cells. Clots that break off and travel through the bloodstream are called *emboli*. Clients with emboli are at risk of strokes. During a sickle cell crisis, the client will have severe pain because the tissues lack oxygen.

■ WHITE BLOOD CELL DISORDERS

The white blood cells work to protect the body from invasion by foreign harmful organisms. They have a role in fighting off infections and providing immunity. Any disorder of the white blood cells will reduce a person's ability to stay healthy.

Neutropenia

Neutropenia is a decrease in the number of neutrophils. A person with a low number of neutrophils is at risk of acquiring an infection. The medical assistant will need to take additional measures to protect the client from infection. Clients who are having chemotherapy treatments for cancer cannot fight off infections, because the drugs that treat the cancer also destroy the neutrophils. **Leukemia** is a malignant disorder (cancer) of the white blood cells in which abnormal white blood cells grow and multiply rapidly, replacing normal white blood cells. Without normally functioning white blood cells, the client cannot fight off infection. Leukemia can be acute or chronic. In all types of leukemia, though, anemia is present. **Mononucleosis**, also called *mono*, is a disease that stimulates production of a high number of mononuclear lymphocytes, which are a type of white blood cell.

Infectious mononucleosis is caused by a virus spread through saliva. After entering the body, the virus then invades the lymph nodes. The client will complain of a sore throat, headache, chest pain, and other flu-like symptoms. Treatment includes pain relief medication; more importantly, lots of rest is required. The spleen can become enlarged in mononucleosis. If the spleen is enlarged, the client must not participate in sports or strenuous physical activity, to avoid the possibility of rupture (breaking open) of the spleen.

■ PLATELET DISORDERS

The ability of the blood to clot is crucially important to prevent continuous bleeding and death from injuries. Having too many or too few of the clot-forming cells called *thrombocytes* can cause problems.

Thrombocythemia

Thrombocythemia is an increase in the number of platelets. Blood vessels can be closed off because of the increase in the number of abnormal blood-clotting cells. The doctor may prescribe aspirin or other medication to prevent the formation of clots.

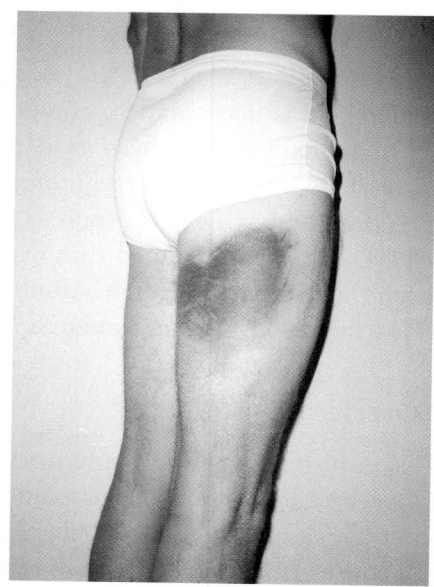

FIGURE 26-2 Hematoma.

Thrombocytopenia

Thrombocytopenia is a decrease in the number of platelets. In some cases, the cause is unknown, but thrombocytopenia is a known complication of cancer treatment. Treatments involve preventing or controlling excessive bleeding and hemorrhaging. The client may notice a bruise or *hematoma* (Figure 26-2), which is a collection of blood in a particular area. This can happen anywhere in the body. The medical assistant will teach the client steps to reduce the chance of excessive bleeding. For example, the client should use an electric razor for shaving. Extreme caution should be used when cutting toenails; it is best to have a podiatrist (foot doctor) cut and trim the nails. A soft toothbrush should be used to avoid bruising or cutting the gums around the teeth.

Hemophilia

Hemophilia is a disorder in which either there are too few blood-clotting proteins or those proteins do not exist (are not made in the body). This is a genetic disorder that affects males almost exclusively. Women are the carriers of the trait. The condition can range from mild to severe. Bruising and bleeding from even minor scratches or bumps can occur. The medical assistant will work with the client and his family concerning lifestyle changes to maintain the client's health and safety.

■ INFECTIOUS DISORDERS

Septicemia is an infection of the blood by pathogenic microorganisms. This is a systemic response. The client often has a fever and a fast pulse and respiration rate. Sepsis can result from a lung, abdomen, or urinary tract infection. A client with septicemia is acutely ill and must be treated in a hospital.

■ LYMPHATIC SYSTEM DISORDERS

The lymphatic system filters bacteria and waste products. Its job is to keep these from entering the general circulation. It is therefore closely interconnected with the hematologic system. Lymphatic disorders can be inflammatory, or they can result from disorders in other systems. **Lymphedema** is a swelling caused by fluid that cannot flow easily through the lymphatic system (Figure 26-3). Cancers that affect the lymphatic system, as well as some surgeries, can cause this condition. Lymphedema puts a client at high risk of infection. *Lymphadenitis* is caused by an infection. The lymph nodes become enlarged and are often referred to as "swollen glands."

In *lymphangitis*, the vessels that drain a body part become inflamed and can be identified by the red streaks along the vessels. The area will be hot, swollen, and painful. Lymphangitis is sometimes referred to as "blood poisoning."

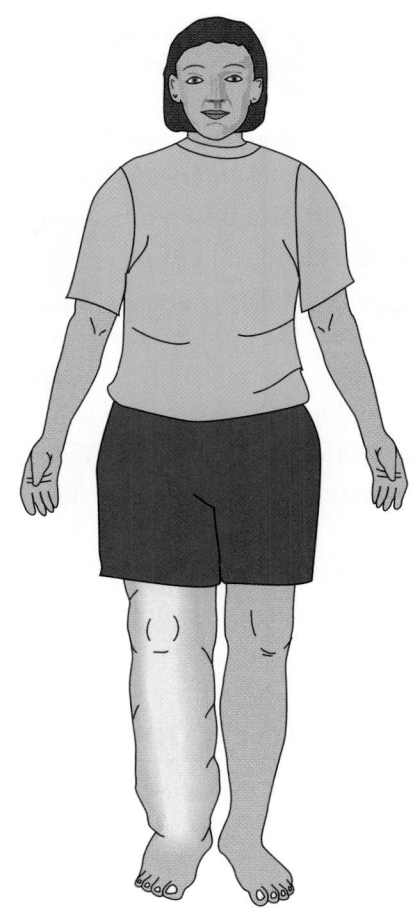

FIGURE 26-3 Lymphedema.

Lymphoma is a cancer affecting the lymphocytes. **Hodgkin's disease** is a type of cancer that affects the lymphatic system. Though the enlargement is painless, the client will have enlarged, swollen lymph nodes and other lymphoid tissue structures. Epstein-Barr virus (EBV) has been linked to the disorder. Non-Hodgkin's lymphoma is another type of lymphoma. Fever, extreme fatigue, and weight loss may be present in both types of lymphoma.

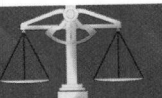

LEGAL/ETHICAL THOUGHTS

When working with terminally ill clients, do not offer false reassurance, such as "Everything will look better tomorrow," or shallow encouragement such as "Cheer up." False reassurance does not allow clients to express their feelings, and is a roadblock to communication.

POINTS OF HIGHLIGHT

- Hematology is the area of medicine that studies the hematologic and lymphatic systems and the disorders of these systems.
- A CBC with differential is the most common laboratory test to diagnose blood problems.
- Red blood cell disorders affect the cell's ability to use and carry oxygen.
- Iron-deficiency anemia, folic acid anemia, pernicious anemia, and sickle cell anemia all affect the red blood cells and their functioning.
- Sickle cell anemia is an inherited disorder in which red blood cells become sickle-shaped and unable to carry oxygen efficiently.
- White blood cell disorders affect the cell's ability to fight off infection.
- Platelet disorders affect the cell's ability to clot. Too many or too few clot-forming cells will cause problems.
- Lymphatic system disorders hinder bacteria and waste product filtration.
- Lymphoma is a cancer that affects the lymphatic system.

 ## BRIDGE TO CAAHEP

This chapter, which discusses hematologic and lymphatic system disorders, provides information and content related to CAAHEP standards for Anatomy and Physiology, Common Pathology/ Diseases, Diagnostic/Treatment Modalities, Medical Terminology, Medical Law and Ethics, Psychology Communication, Medical Assisting Clinical Procedures, and Professional Components.

 ## AAMA AREAS OF COMPETENCE

This chapter, which discusses hematologic and lymphatic system disorders, provides information or content within several areas listed in the Medical Assistant Role Delineation Study. These areas include: clinical, patient (client) care, fundamental principles, diagnostic orders, general transdisciplinary, professionalism, communication, legal concepts, and instruction.

 ## ABHES LINKS

This chapter, which discusses hematologic and lymphatic system disorders, links to ABHES course content for medical assisting for Anatomy and Physiology, Medical Terminology, Medical Law and Ethics, and Medical Office Clinical Procedures.

 ## AMT PATHS

This chapter, which discusses hematologic and lymphatic system disorders, provides a path to AMT competency in general medical assisting knowledge, anatomy and physiology, medical terminology, and patient (client) education.

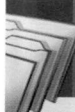 ### STUDENT PORTFOLIO ACTIVITY

Expand your computer skills. Do not rely solely on what you learned in the computer course. Ask for technical help from resource staff at the school. Seek out any short, specialized computer sessions offered through community education programs.

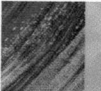 ### APPLYING YOUR SKILLS

A client has neutropenia as a result of chemotherapy treatment for cancer. Why is this client at risk of infection? As a medical assistant, what precautions would you share with the client and the family to protect the client from infection?

CRITICAL THINKING QUESTIONS

1. A client who has thrombocythemia has been prescribed aspirin. What is the purpose of the aspirin? What would you include in client teaching?

2. Why is it recommended that folic acid be part of everyone's daily vitamin intake? What can happen to a woman who is pregnant and does not have enough folic acid?

3. How does sickle cell disorder affect the shape of the red blood cell?

4. How does the change in the red blood cell affect the client? What symptoms will the client notice?

5. During an infection, a client may complain of "swollen glands." How do you explain this?

6. What are methods commonly used to diagnose hematologic and lymphatic disorders?

7. Describe the functions of the red blood cells. If there are too few circulating red blood cells, what symptoms might the client experience?

8. What age group is susceptible to iron-deficiency anemia? Why do you think this might be? What are some common behaviors in this high-risk age group?

9. Why does a client with sickle cell anemia crisis experience pain? What is happening inside the body?

10. How does a person develop hemophilia? What must be present for a person to acquire this disorder?

11. While you are completing the past medical history with a client, she states that several years ago she had "blood poisoning." What does this mean?

12. How can a person develop septicemia?

13. You are asked to teach a client who has thrombocytopenia. Describe safety steps for this client to incorporate into her activities of daily living.

14. Go back to the beginning of this chapter and review the Anticipatory Statements. Reread each statement and then indicate whether it is true or false. If the statement is false, rewrite it to make it a true statement.

CLIENT TEACHING PLAN

Foot Care for Clients with Blood Circulation Disorders

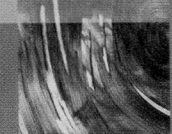

■ What Is to Be Taught:

- Foot care to promote health of feet.

■ Objectives:

- Client will be able to perform foot care to promote and keep healthy feet.

■ Preparation Before Teaching:

- Review blood circulation and its effect on feet.
- Review healthy practices for foot care.
- Get together teaching supplies: soap, water, towel, basin, paper and pen.

■ Steps for the Medical Assistant:

1. Wash your hands.
2. Gather supplies needed.
3. Introduce yourself to the client.
4. Explain what you are going to teach and why.
5. Tell the client that, when bathing, she should wash her feet carefully with soap and warm water. Pat feet dry with a soft towel. Demonstrate to the client how to wash and dry one foot. Then ask the client to wash and dry the other foot.
6. Ask the client to carefully look at all skin surfaces on her feet, including the soles or bottoms of the feet and in between toes. If she finds any cuts, sores, or cracks, tell her to inform the doctor.
7. Inform the client that light-colored cotton socks will help to circulate air and discourage the growth of fungus and bacteria.
8. Instruct the client never to go barefoot. This increases the risk of stubbing a toe or stepping on a sharp object, resulting in a cut or sore that will not heal.
9. Tell the client that toenails should be cut by a podiatrist (foot doctor). With poor circulation, increased age, and other problems, the toenails can become hard and thick, making them

difficult to cut. It is very easy for nail clippers to slip and cut the skin on the toes. The podiatrist has special instruments that greatly reduce the chances of accidental injury.

■ Special Needs of the Client:

- Look at the client's chart to see if there are any factors that might interfere with the client's ability to practice steps for healthy feet.
- Ask the client, before and after teaching, if there is anything you should know that might affect her ability to do proper foot care.

■ Evaluation:

- Client will be able to list the components of good foot care.
- Client will be able to wash, dry, and inspect her feet after observation of your demonstration.

■ Further Plans/Teaching:

- Review foot care information with the client at the next visit.

■ Follow-up:

- Check the client's feet at the next visit.
- Ask the client what steps she was able to follow and if she encountered any problems.

Medical Assistant

Name: _____

Signature: _____

Date: _____

Client

Date: _____

Follow-up Date : _____

CHAPTER 27

Anticipatory Statements

People have different ideas about immune system disorders. Read and think about the following statements based upon what you believe now. Decide whether you agree or disagree. Write the word **agree** after the statement if you think the statement is true. Write the word **disagree** after the statement if you think the statement is false. Read the chapter to find out if your current beliefs can be supported.

1. Only homosexual men are at risk of getting AIDS.   _____

2. Hives may result from an allergic response to
   inhaled substances.   _____

3. HIV and AIDS are the same.   _____

4. An extreme sensitivity to a substance can
   cause death.   _____

5. Hay fever happens only during certain seasons.   _____

Learning Objectives

Upon completion of this chapter, the medical assistant student should be able to:

- Identify the medical assistant's role in client preparation for diagnostic tests of the immune system
- Define *allergen*
- List at least five common substances that can cause an allergic reaction
- Explain the medical assistant's role with a client who is experiencing a severe allergic reaction
- Discuss the difference between an immune disorder and an autoimmune disorder

Immune System Disorders

- Explain what is meant by immunodeficiency
- Develop a teaching plan for a client who has an allergy to a food substance
- Teach another person how to stay healthy and to avoid allergy triggers

Key Terms

acquired immunodeficiency syndrome (AIDS) Disorder that causes the immune system to be suppressed; a serious, life-threatening disorder.

allergen A protein or substance that sets off an allergic response in a person.

autoimmune disorders Describes a response in which the body mistakes its own tissue as foreign and begins to attack itself.

contact dermatitis Inflammation of skin caused by coming into contact with an irritant.

hay fever Seasonally related form of allergic response. Sneezing, runny nose, and watery or itchy eyes are common symptoms.

human immunodeficiency virus (HIV) Viral infection that weakens a person's immune system.

hypersensitivity disorders Overly sensitive or reactive to a substance or stimulus.

immunodeficiency disorders Conditions in which the immune system does not respond, or responds insufficiently, to an invasion.

intradermal Within the dermis part of the skin.

patch test Test to determine a person's level of allergic response to common allergens. The test involves putting a small amount of substances on the skin and covering them with a dressing. After the dressing is removed, the response on the skin is noted.

rheumatoid arthritis Autoimmune disorder that attacks the joints.

systemic lupus erythematosus (SLE) Autoimmune disorder that can cause inflammation of one or more organs of the body.

■ INTRODUCTION

The immune system overall works as a defense system to protect the body against foreign invaders. With immune system disorders, the immune system may become overly alert and sensitive, or deficient and unable to put up a good fight. There are also immune disorders in which the system does not seem to recognize the enemy. In others, the immune system appears confused and treats some parts of the body as the enemy. With disorders in which the body is overly sensitive—the **hypersensitivity disorders**—the immune system creates an allergic inflammatory response. The "confusion" disorders, in which the immune system sees part of the person's own body as foreign, are the **autoimmune disorders.** Disorders in which the immune system is deficient or lacking in response are the **immunodeficiency** disorders.

■ HYPERSENSITIVITY/ ALLERGIC DISORDERS

In an allergic reaction, the immune system reacts to a normally harmless substance as if it were dangerous. The foreign protein, substance, or material that causes an allergic reaction is called an *antigen.* When a susceptible person comes into contact with the **allergen,** the body releases antibodies. One of the chemicals most commonly released is histamine. These chemicals begin a chain reaction of events throughout the body, including swelling and inflammation.

Allergens are grouped or classified according to how they enter the body, as they can enter the body through different routes. An individual can come into contact with an allergen through breathing, eating, ingesting, or touching it. Table 27-1 lists some common allergens and the possible means of contact.

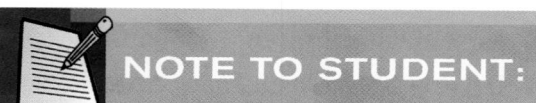

NOTE TO STUDENT:

Contacts made after the first exposure to an allergen can often result in a more serious reaction or response than previously experienced. The medical assistant must teach the client to be aware of this, take precautions, and not disregard an allergy as merely a minor annoyance.

TABLE 27-1 Common nonfood allergens.

ALLERGEN	COMPONENTS, CONTACT AREAS, AND WHEN ACTIVE
House dust	Mix of indoor allergens, including dust mites, animal dander, insect feces, and molds; year-round
Feathers	Protein found in down pillows, comforters, and upholstery; year-round
Dust mites	Found in mattresses, pillows, carpeting, furniture, and dusty environments; year-round
Cat dander	Protein from hair, skin, saliva, and urine of all cats; year-round
Dog dander	Protein from hair, skin, saliva, and urine of all dogs; year-round
Tree pollens	Outdoors; usually from April through May
Grass pollens	Outdoors; usually from May through late July
Ragweed pollen	Outdoors; usually from mid-August until after the first frost
Alternaria mold	Outdoor mold found on damp grass, leaves, and vegetation; from July through end of autumn
Molds	Can occur indoors or outdoors, in damp areas of home or on vegetation

Types of Allergic Responses

There seems to be an inherited tendency toward allergies; however, the type of allergic response or form that it takes may be different. Although it is commonly thought that children get allergies and then outgrow them, allergic responses can happen or begin at any age. Types of allergies are medically named by the reaction that occurs on the cellular level with immunoglobulins. The medical assistant may find it more helpful, though, to learn about the allergic responses based on what might be observed in a client.

Atopic/Skin. Allergic responses to allergens often include an atopic or skin response, no matter what the route of entry of the allergen. When exposed to an allergen, the skin often becomes red, itchy, and swollen. Small, red, swollen, itchy, circular areas called *urticaria* or *hives* may appear. It is important to find out what caused the reaction so that the client can avoid it in the future. The doctor may order medications such as antihistamines to reduce the itching. Epinephrine or steroids may also be ordered, depending upon the severity of the reaction.

Eczema or *atopic dermatitis* is often clinically seen as a chronic disorder. The client experiences itching on patches of skin that ooze and then crust over. Over a period of time, the skin can become thickened or *lichenified.* Treatment is aimed at finding the cause or trigger and then avoiding the substance. The doctor may order antihistamines and medicated creams, such as steroid preparations.

Direct contact with an allergen may result in **contact dermatitis.** Soaps, metals such as nickel in jewelry, latex gloves, and materials in clothing may cause this response. Identification of the cause is important. For example, if a client's hands are affected, latex gloves, soaps, hand lotions, or materials encountered in the client's work may be the reason. The medical assistant needs to work with the client to help find the cause.

Respiratory/Breathing. **Hay fever,** or *allergic rhinitis*, is caused by an inhaled allergen. The client will complain of sneezing, runny nose, scratchy throat, itching inside the mouth and ears, and itchy, watery eyes. Sometimes this is a seasonal problem; that is, it only happens at specific times of the year. This is particularly so if the allergen is a pollen.

An allergic response in a client may result in a condition known as *asthma.* In response to an allergen, the muscles of the bronchi go into spasm. There is swelling, mucus production, coughing, and wheezing. The client will complain of difficulty in breathing. The medical assistant will also observe wheezing, labored breathing, and the use of accessory muscles. The client will appear short of breath and may talk in short, choppy sentences. Asthma can be mild, but may be so severe that it progresses to respiratory failure and death.

Gastrointestinal. Food may cause a gastrointestinal or digestive system response. In addition to the other allergic responses listed previously, the client may experience nausea, vomiting, diarrhea, and abdominal pain.

Anaphylaxis

Anaphylaxis is a severe, systemic hypersensitivity to an antigen. This reaction occurs in clients who are extremely sensitive to an allergen. Anaphylaxis can begin almost immediately after contact with the allergen and, if not treated quickly and successfully, can result in death within minutes. Anaphylaxis is a medical emergency. The client will have difficulty breathing, may not be able to swallow the saliva, and may appear to be drooling. The client will be restless, irritable, and feel that the throat is swelling shut. The medical assistant may note that the client's face and hands swell, possibly within seconds of contact with the allergen. The client

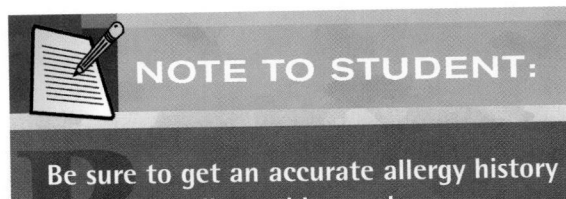

NOTE TO STUDENT: Be sure to get an accurate allergy history from every client; this may become critical in providing care.

will develop a rapid, thready pulse and then the blood pressure will drop sharply.

Peanuts are the most common food allergy that can lead to anaphylactic shock. Bee stings also are a common antigen that triggers anaphylaxis. Iodine, which is sometimes used as a contrast medium in X-ray procedures, can cause this reaction.

Treatment consists of giving the client epinephrine (0.1 to 0.5 mL injected subcutaneously), intravenous medications, steroids, vasopressors, and/or antihistamines.

■ DIAGNOSTIC TESTING

In addition to a carefully taken history and physical examination, certain tests may be conducted to identify allergens. Skin testing is frequently done. This can be in the form of a scratch test, an intradermal test, or a patch test. In a *scratch test*, an area on the arm or back is used. Scratches are made at numbered points, and one or two drops of an allergen are placed in each numbered scratch. If the client is allergic to a substance, a positive reaction is seen. A positive reaction is characterized by a *wheal*, a round, swollen area. An **intradermal** test involves injecting the allergen intradermally (under the skin). With a **patch test,** a patch or strip containing small amounts of allergens is placed on a client's back. It remains on the client for one to four days and is then inspected to see if there are any positive reactions to the substances.

The medical assistant's role in allergy diagnostic testing consists mainly of client preparation. The client may not take any allergy or antihistamine medication before the testing, or the reactions will not accurately reflect the true allergic response. The medication will dull or stop a positive response. The medical assistant must be sure to ask the client if he has taken any allergy or antihistamine medications. If he has, the test cannot be done and the client will have to reschedule. During the test, the medical assistant should remain close to the client and offer support. Clients may become very uncomfortable near injection needles.

Additionally, a RAST test can be performed. For this test, the medical assistant

performs a venipuncture and sends the blood sample to a specialized laboratory for testing.

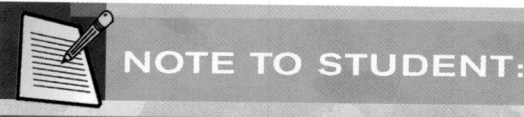

NOTE TO STUDENT:

The client must remain in the medical office for at least 30 minutes after allergy testing to be observed for a delayed allergic reaction.

■ AUTOIMMUNE DISORDERS

Sometimes the body's defense system becomes confused and does not seem to recognize enemies. Instead, it starts producing antibodies against the body's own cells. Any body tissue, organ, or system can be affected by this type of autoimmune response. The exact cause of these disorders is not known. There may be a family risk factor, and women have a greater risk than men of developing an autoimmune disorder. Chemical substances may trigger an inappropriate response, or immune cells that are not normal may act inappropriately.

Autoimmune disorders may affect only one organ, or involve several organs. The whole body can be affected, in which case the disorder is called *systemic*. An example of a systemic autoimmune disorder is **systemic lupus erythematosus (SLE),** which damages many organs and structures such as connective tissue, blood, the heart, the brain, and the kidneys. Laboratory tests will be ordered to check antibodies and affected organs. After the diagnosis is made, the doctor may order anti-inflammatory medications and steroids.

Rheumatoid arthritis affects the musculoskeletal system. The joints become inflamed and swollen (Figure 27-1A). Very commonly, the fingers deviate (point away) from the ulnar side of the wrist (Figure 27-1B). Nodules or bumps may appear at various joints (Figure 27-1C). This is a painful condition, but it is not the same as osteoarthritis. The main focus of treatment is relief of symptoms. The doctor may order pain

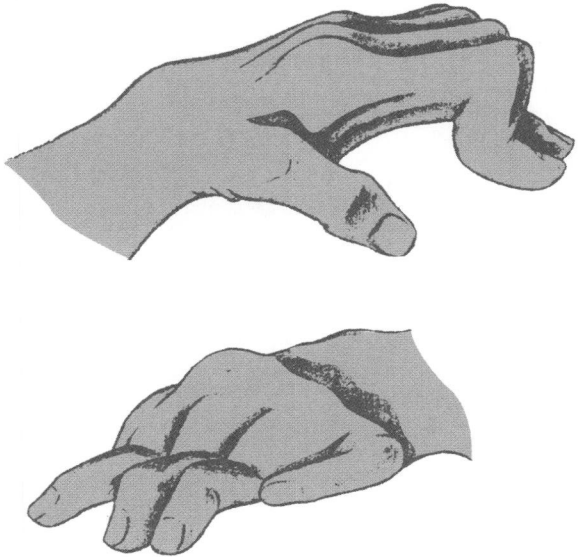

FIGURE 27–1A Joint changes from rheumatoid arthritis.

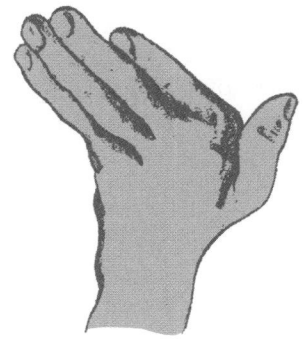

FIGURE 27–1B Ulnar deviation from rheumatoid arthritis.

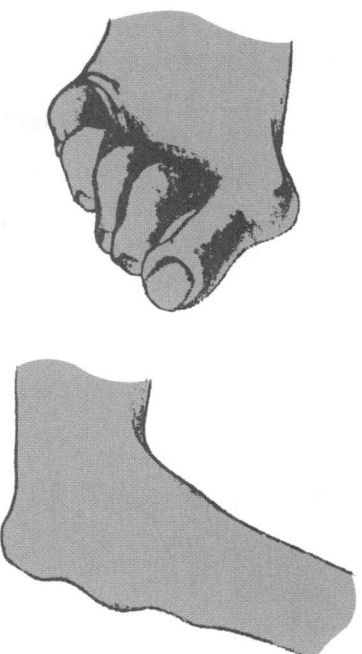

FIGURE 27–1C Rheumatoid nodules.

■ IMMUNODEFICIENCY

Acquired immunodeficiency syndrome (AIDS) is a group of clinical problems or symptoms in which the body's immune response is compromised and eventually destroyed. The body cannot fight off invaders and opportunistic infections. *Opportunistic infections* are caused by pathogens that take advantage of the person's weakened defense or immune system (Figure 27-2). In a healthy person, these infections would be mild, and easily taken care of, but they are devastating in a person who has a compromised immune system. In clients who have AIDS, 90% of all deaths are due to opportunistic infections.

Human immunodeficiency virus (HIV) is the virus that causes AIDS. This virus, which can remain dormant for years, affects the

medications, anti-inflammatory drugs, and sometimes therapeutic radiation.

Treatment of autoimmune disorders can be very difficult. The aim is to quiet down or suppress the immune system response, but to avoid so much suppression that the immune system cannot do its work of protection against invaders.

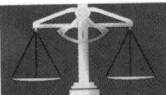

LEGAL/ETHICAL THOUGHTS

Be aware of your own feelings about HIV and AIDS and the people who are affected by this virus and disorder. Do not allow any negative feelings to affect your interactions with clients. Judgmental attitudes have no place in health care services.

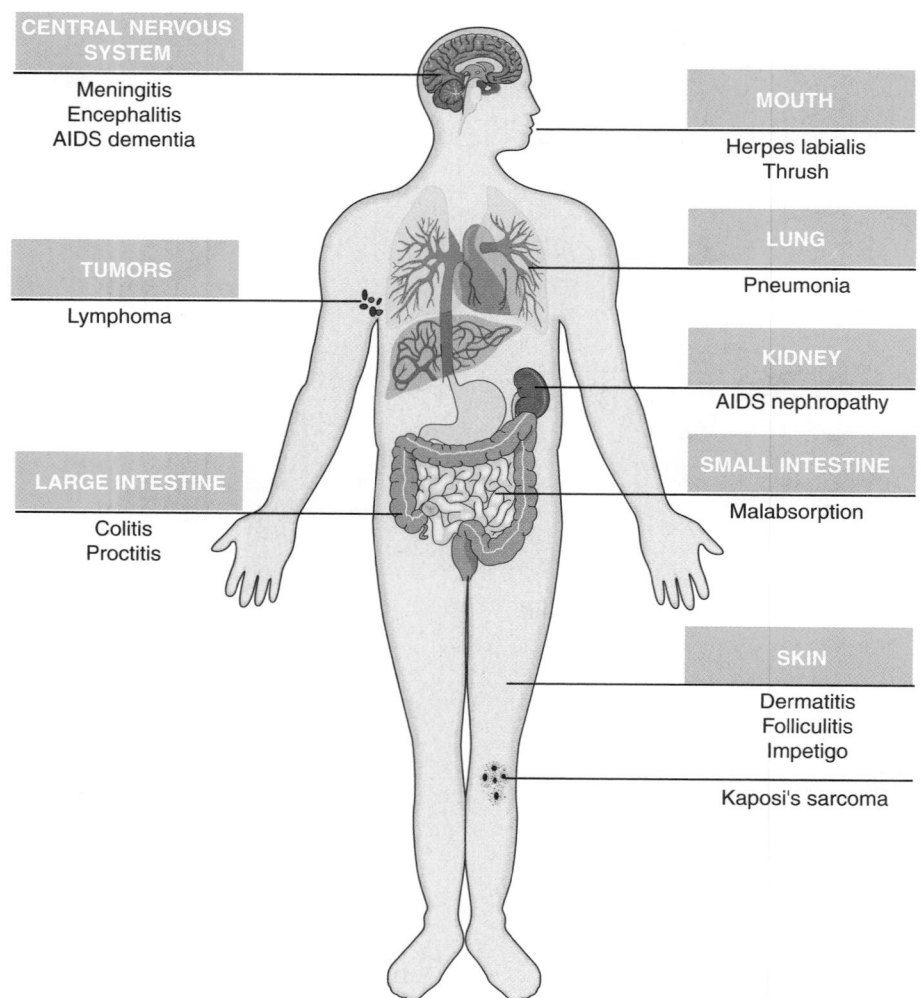

FIGURE 27-2 Pathologies connected with AIDS.

lymphocytes, which are essential to the working of the immune system.

The HIV virus can be transmitted through contact with blood, semen, or vaginal and cervical secretions contacted during intercourse. Since testing of donor blood was initiated, transmission of HIV through blood transfusions has occurred much less frequently. Sexual contact is the most common way of spreading the virus. People who abuse drugs, using dirty or shared needles to inject them intravenously, are at great risk of contracting the HIV virus. Once common among homosexual and bisexual men, the rate of infection has increased among women and children. Infants can be infected during perinatal transmission. HIV

can also be transmitted to an infant through breast milk from an infected mother.

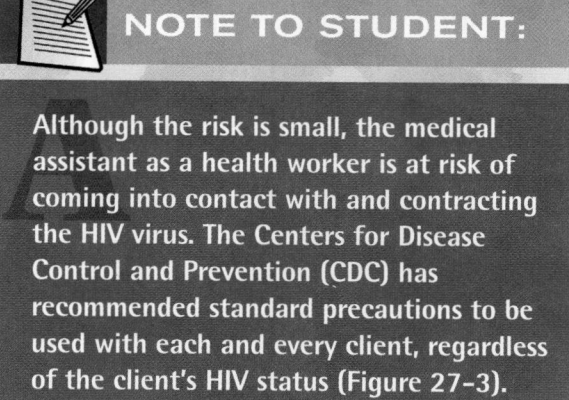

NOTE TO STUDENT:

Although the risk is small, the medical assistant as a health worker is at risk of coming into contact with and contracting the HIV virus. The Centers for Disease Control and Prevention (CDC) has recommended standard precautions to be used with each and every client, regardless of the client's HIV status (Figure 27-3).

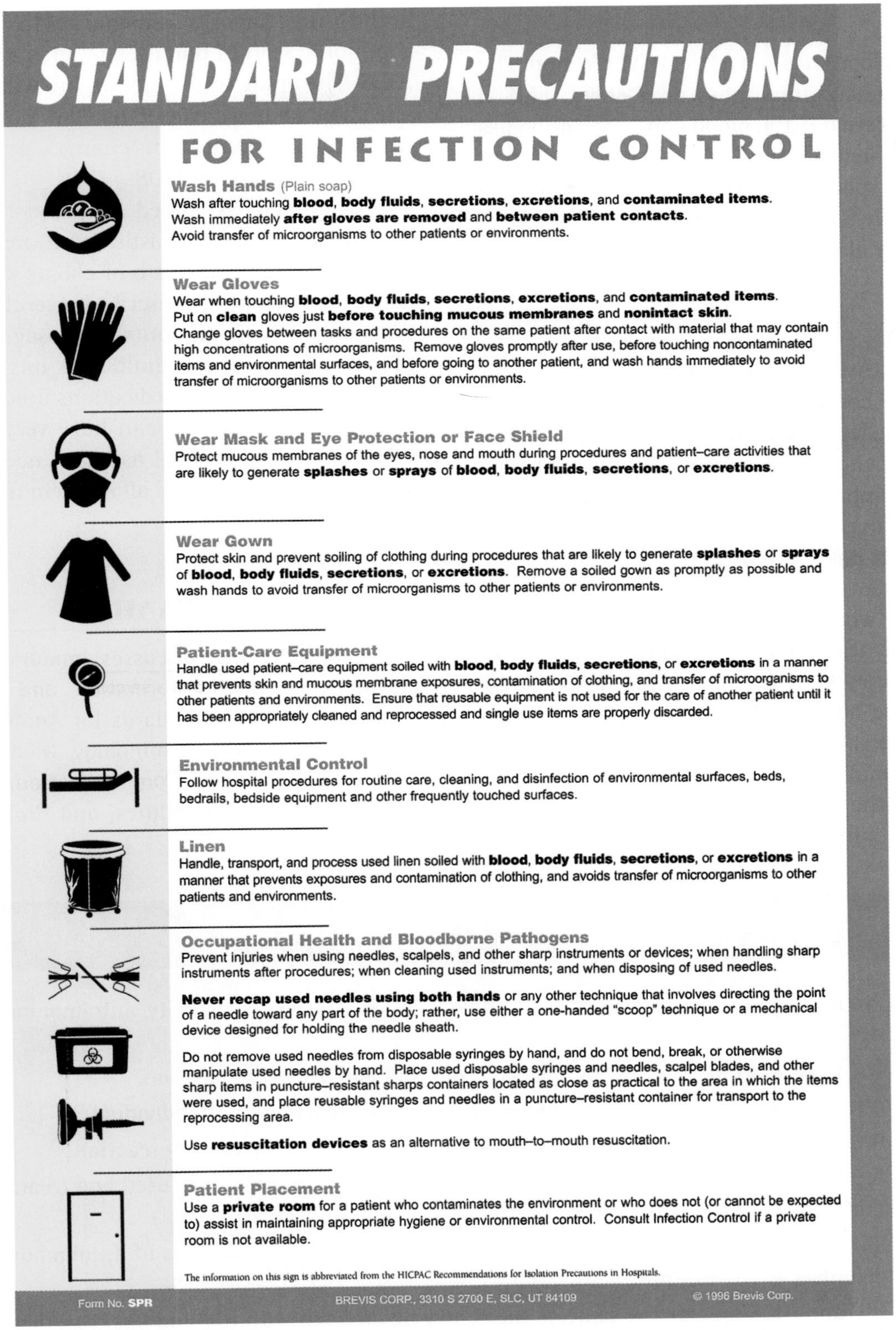

STANDARD PRECAUTIONS

FOR INFECTION CONTROL

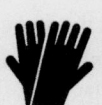
Wash Hands (Plain soap)
Wash after touching **blood**, **body fluids**, **secretions**, **excretions**, and **contaminated items**.
Wash immediately **after gloves are removed** and **between patient contacts**.
Avoid transfer of microorganisms to other patients or environments.

Wear Gloves
Wear when touching **blood**, **body fluids**, **secretions**, **excretions**, and **contaminated items**.
Put on **clean** gloves just **before touching mucous membranes** and **nonintact skin**.
Change gloves between tasks and procedures on the same patient after contact with material that may contain
high concentrations of microorganisms. Remove gloves promptly after use, before touching noncontaminated
items and environmental surfaces, and before going to another patient, and wash hands immediately to avoid
transfer of microorganisms to other patients or environments.

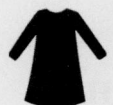
Wear Mask and Eye Protection or Face Shield
Protect mucous membranes of the eyes, nose and mouth during procedures and patient–care activities that
are likely to generate **splashes** or **sprays** of **blood**, **body fluids**, **secretions**, or **excretions**.

Wear Gown
Protect skin and prevent soiling of clothing during procedures that are likely to generate **splashes** or **sprays**
of **blood**, **body fluids**, **secretions**, or **excretions**. Remove a soiled gown as promptly as possible and
wash hands to avoid transfer of microorganisms to other patients or environments.

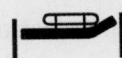
Patient-Care Equipment
Handle used patient–care equipment soiled with **blood**, **body fluids**, **secretions**, or **excretions** in a manner
that prevents skin and mucous membrane exposures, contamination of clothing, and transfer of microorganisms to
other patients and environments. Ensure that reusable equipment is not used for the care of another patient until it
has been appropriately cleaned and reprocessed and single use items are properly discarded.

Environmental Control
Follow hospital procedures for routine care, cleaning, and disinfection of environmental surfaces, beds,
bedrails, bedside equipment and other frequently touched surfaces.

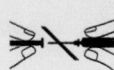
Linen
Handle, transport, and process used linen soiled with **blood**, **body fluids**, **secretions**, or **excretions** in a
manner that prevents exposures and contamination of clothing, and avoids transfer of microorganisms to other
patients and environments.

Occupational Health and Bloodborne Pathogens
Prevent injuries when using needles, scalpels, and other sharp instruments or devices; when handling sharp
instruments after procedures; when cleaning used instruments; and when disposing of used needles.

Never recap used needles using both hands or any other technique that involves directing the point
of a needle toward any part of the body; rather, use either a one-handed "scoop" technique or a mechanical
device designed for holding the needle sheath.

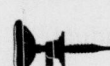
Do not remove used needles from disposable syringes by hand, and do not bend, break, or otherwise
manipulate used needles by hand. Place used disposable syringes and needles, scalpel blades, and other
sharp items in puncture–resistant sharps containers located as close as practical to the area in which the items
were used, and place reusable syringes and needles in a puncture–resistant container for transport to the
reprocessing area.

Use **resuscitation devices** as an alternative to mouth–to–mouth resuscitation.

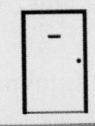
Patient Placement
Use a **private room** for a patient who contaminates the environment or who does not (or cannot be expected
to) assist in maintaining appropriate hygiene or environmental control. Consult Infection Control if a private
room is not available.

The information on this sign is abbreviated from the HICPAC Recommendations for Isolation Precautions in Hospitals.

Form No. **SPR**   BREVIS CORP., 3310 S 2700 E, SLC, UT 84109   © 1996 Brevis Corp.

FIGURE 27–3 Standard precautions should always be followed for infection and disease **control.** *(Courtesy of Brevis Corporation)*

Diagnostic Tests

Specific blood tests can detect HIV infection. The enzyme linked immunosorbent assay (ELISA) test can reveal if the blood contains antibodies to HIV proteins. If the ELISA test is positive, then the more specific Western Blot test, which looks specifically for HIV, is ordered. Biopsies and cultures may also be done.

Treatment

The client with an HIV infection may come to the office complaining of shortness of breath, coughing, fever, numbness and burning of feet, night sweats, loss of appetite, and weight loss. With a compromised and deficient immune system, lacking effective T lymphocytes, the client is at high risk for many infections and other body system disorders. These infections, which normally would not be able to establish themselves in the body, are called *opportunistic* because they take the opportunity available to attack the body in its weakened state. In the early stages, thrush (a fungal infection) and/or shingles may occur. Athlete's foot is common. Later on the client may contract *Pneumocystis carinii* pneumonia (PCP), which is an infection in the lungs. Kaposi's sarcoma, a skin cancer, is commonly seen in homosexual men who have AIDS. The brain, as a major organ, will eventually show changes caused by HIV. Many times dementia or mental-status changes are the presenting complaint of AIDS.

Treatment is aimed at preventing and treating early opportunistic infections, which frequently cause the death of clients who have AIDS. Clients may be prescribed several medications in varying amounts or dosages; often people refer to these multidrug mixtures as "drug cocktails." The medications used to treat AIDS are powerful and can have very serious side effects. The medical assistant needs to be supportive of clients and allow them to express their fears and concerns.

 BRIDGE TO CAAHEP

This chapter, which discusses immune system disorders, provides information and content related to CAAHEP standards for Anatomy and Physiology, Medical Terminology, Medical Law and Ethics, Psychology, Communication, Medical Assisting Clinical Procedures, and Professional Components.

POINTS OF HIGHLIGHT

- Problems with the immune system can be classified as hypersensitivity, autoimmune, or deficiency disorders.
- The first focus in treating allergies is to identify and avoid the allergen.
- Allergens are substances that can cause an allergic reaction in an individual.
- Anaphylaxis is a medical emergency resulting from a hypersensitivity reaction.
- Autoimmune disorders arise when the immune system becomes confused and treats the body's own cells as the enemy.
- Rheumatoid arthritis and systemic lupus erythematosus are examples of autoimmune disorders.
- HIV and AIDS are not the same. A client may be infected with HIV and not have developed AIDS.
- The medical assistant must follow standard precautions with each and every client—no exceptions.

ABHES LINKS

This chapter, which discusses immune system disorders, links to ABHES course content for Anatomy and Physiology, Medical Terminology, Medical Law and Ethics, and Medical Office Clinical Procedures.

AAMA AREAS OF COMPETENCE

This chapter, which discusses immune system disorders, provides information or content within several areas listed in the Medical Assistant Role Delineation Study. These areas include:

administrative, administrative procedures, clinical, fundamental principles, diagnostic orders, patient (client) care, general transdisciplinary, professionalism, communication skills, legal concepts, and instruction.

AMT PATHS

This chapter, which discusses immune system disorders, provides a path to AMT competency in general medical assisting knowledge, anatomy and physiology, medical terminology, and patient (client) education.

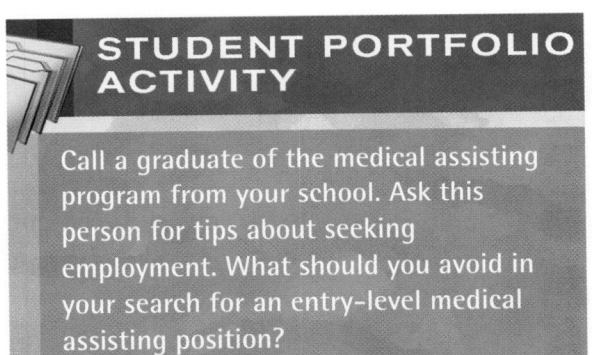

STUDENT PORTFOLIO ACTIVITY

Call a graduate of the medical assisting program from your school. Ask this person for tips about seeking employment. What should you avoid in your search for an entry-level medical assisting position?

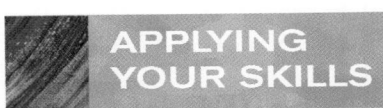

APPLYING YOUR SKILLS

A co-worker is about to perform a dressing change on a client. The co-worker asks you to check on the client's HIV status in case the client has AIDS. What should you do? What would be your response, and why?

CRITICAL THINKING QUESTIONS

1. A client who was recently diagnosed with an allergy to peanuts comes to the office for treatment of an allergic reaction. After treatment, the doctor asks you to speak with the client. The client tells you that he did not eat any peanuts and cannot imagine what happened. What is your response? Where do you begin as you try to identify the cause of the reaction? What are some possible ways that the client could have accidentally ingested peanuts?

2. Explain how HIV and AIDS are related.

3. A client has been diagnosed with an allergy to several substances. How would you explain allergy to this client? What happens in the client's body?

4. List some ways that a client can lessen the number of flare-ups of eczema or atopic dermatitis.

5. What should clients who might have anaphylactic reactions always carry with them? Why is this so important?

6. Allergy testing has been completed and the client gets up to leave the office. What do you tell the client, and why?

7. What is the treatment goal with autoimmune disorders?

8. Systemic lupus erythematosus is a systemic autoimmune disorder. What does it mean to call this disorder systemic?

9. A medical assistant student is confused about rheumatoid arthritis and osteoarthritis. What do you tell him about the similarities and the differences between the two disorders?

10. Why are opportunistic infections so harmful to clients who have AIDS? How is the client's immune system status involved?

11. What happens in the body as a person experiences anaphylaxis?

12. Select an autoimmune disorder and describe what it does to the immune system.

13. What are hives, and why do they happen?

14. Why are opportunistic infections such a serious concern in clients who have weakened immune systems?

15. Go back to the beginning of this chapter and review the Anticipatory Statements. Reread each statement and then indicate whether it is true or false. If the statement is false, rewrite it to make it a true statement.

CLIENT TEACHING PLAN

AIDS Prevention

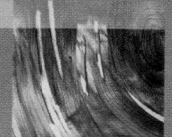

■ What Is to Be Taught:

• Methods to prevent AIDS.

■ Objectives:

• Client will be able to identify ways to decrease the risk of acquiring AIDS.

■ Preparation Before Teaching:

• Review information about HIV infection and AIDS. Make sure that you put technical medical terms into everyday language that the client can easily understand.
• Gather materials such as diagrams, and paper and pen for writing notes and instructions.
• Make sure that the area is free from distractions while you are teaching.

■ Steps for the Medical Assistant:

1. Wash your hands.
2. Get together supplies needed.
3. Introduce yourself to the client.
4. Explain what you are going to teach and why.
5. Tell the client that AIDS is the end stage of a continuum that starts with HIV exposure and infection. Heterosexual, bisexual, and homosexual individuals can all contract AIDS; the riskiest sexual behavior is unprotected receptive anal intercourse. HIV is transmitted in three ways: anal or vaginal intercourse, use of contaminated needles for injecting drugs, and through breast milk. Blood, semen, cervicovaginal secretions, and breast milk are the substances that can transmit the virus if they come from an infected person. HIV is not transmitted by insects, or sharing pencils, computers, and other dry objects.
6. Inform the client that understanding the disorder and having correct information about preventing and treating AIDS will help the client to participate in his own health care.

7. State simple guidelines for the client:
   a. HIV testing and counseling can help prevent transmission. Instruct the client to ask himself if he engages in any behaviors or attitudes that put him at risk. If he does, then he needs to decide when, how, or whether he will be tested.
   b. Safer sexual behaviors can help to decrease the risk. The most effective method is to abstain from sexual activities. A relationship that is mutually exclusive, with neither partner at risk of infection from injecting drugs and with no history of exposure to the HIV infection from previous sexual activities, decreases the risk of becoming infected.
   c. Never share any supplies that are used to inject drugs. The use of any illicit drugs, even if inhaled or swallowed, can put a client at risk of HIV infection. For example, drugs of abuse can lower the client's inhibitions so that he engages in other risky behaviors.
8. Give written instructions or printed informational materials to the client for use as a reference at home.
9. Provide the client with names and telephone numbers of agencies or other community resources if the client wants more information.

■ Special Needs of the Client:

• Check the client's chart for any factors that might interfere with the client's ability to understand and follow the safety guidelines.
• Ask the client, before and after teaching, if there is anything you should know that would affect his ability to follow the safety guidelines.

■ Evaluation:

• Client is able to explain how HIV is transmitted.
• Client is able to describe safety precautions to prevent the transmission of HIV.

(Continues)

CLIENT TEACHING PLAN (Continued)

■ Follow-up:

- At the next office visit, review the safety guidelines with the client.
- Ask the client if he has any questions or wants any additional information.

Medical Assistant

Name: _____

Signature: _____

Date: _____

Client

Date: _____

Follow-up Date : _____

Anticipatory Statements

People have different ideas about what can cause disorders of the respiratory system and how to treat those disorders. Read and think about the following statements based upon what you believe now. Decide whether you agree or disagree. Write the word **agree** after the statement if you think the statement is true. Write the word **disagree** after the statement if you think the statement is false. Read the chapter to find out if your current beliefs can be supported.

1. Pulmonary or lung function studies are commonly performed in the medical office. _____

2. Sore throats and colds can trigger asthma attacks. _____

3. Smoking is a risk factor for lung cancer. _____

4. Asthma and emphysema are the same. _____

5. Only a doctor can obtain a throat swab specimen for testing. _____

Respiratory System Disorders

Learning Objectives

Upon completion of this chapter, the medical assistant student should be able to:

- Identify the medical assistant's role in preparing clients for diagnostic tests of the respiratory system
- Explain what happens in the lungs of a client who has asthma
- Explain what happens in the lungs of a client who has emphysema
- List the signs and symptoms of an acute asthma attack
- State ways to help a client who has chronic breathing problems to prevent flare-ups
- Discuss ways to keep from getting a cold
- Identify common causes of lung cancer
- Develop a teaching plan for a client who has COPD
- Teach another person ways to improve breathing

Key Terms

acute coryza Respiratory viral infection; also called the common cold.

asthma Reactive airway disorder in which the tubes of the bronchial tree become narrowed; often caused by allergies or infection; client experiences difficulty in breathing during an acute episode.

atelectasis Collapsed lung.

emphysema Chronic pulmonary disorder in which the alveoli of the lungs are damaged; often connected to smoking.

influenza A respiratory infection that comes on suddenly; in frail individuals or those with chronic conditions, may be fatal. More commonly called the *flu*.

lung cancer Cancer that affects the lungs; very frequently connected to smoking.

pleurisy Inflammation of the pleura in the thoracic (chest) cavity.

pneumonia Inflammation or infection of the lungs.

pulmonary Refers to the lungs.

tuberculosis Infection of the lungs by the *myobacterium tuberculosis*.

■ INTRODUCTION

Clients who have problems related to breathing, ranging from a feeling of nasal stuffiness to extreme difficulty in just getting air in and out of the lungs, are commonly seen in the medical office. Therefore, the medical assistant must have a basic understanding of common respiratory disorders. Many of these disorders can be classified as either acute or chronic. Although all the disorders involve difficulty with breathing, clients will look different and their treatment will differ based on the cause of their problems.

■ ACUTE DISORDERS

Acute respiratory disorders are frequently the reason clients seek help from a primary health care provider. The occurrence of acute disorders caused by viruses will increase in frequency during the winter months in colder climates. Many disorders, especially those caused by viruses, are treated symptomatically; that is, only the symptoms are treated while the client's immune system deals with the actual infection. Medical assistants have an opportunity to teach clients to prevent and control the spread of acute respiratory disorders.

The doctor may order tests to determine specifically what is causing a client's acute respiratory disorder. A throat culture may be ordered. The medical assistant will swab the client's throat and place the swab in a sterile container, label the specimen, and send it to a laboratory (see Procedure 40-3). The lab will test and culture the specimen to isolate any bacteria. The doctor will then decide if medications such as antibiotics are necessary to treat the acute respiratory disorder.

Acute Coryza

Acute coryza is the common cold. This respiratory inflammation is caused by a virus. The client will complain of a running nose, sneezing, scratchy throat, and a cough. On average, a person gets a common cold about once a year; smokers often get colds more frequently. An infected person is contagious before any signs or symptoms are noticeable. The cold virus is spread through droplets from coughing or sneezing. It is also spread by direct contact with the mucous secretions. For example, a person who sneezes or coughs and does not wash her hands and then shakes hands with another person will spread the cold virus. People who live, work, play, or go to school in close contact with many others can easily spread the virus from one to another.

Frequent handwashing is the most effective way to keep from spreading or getting a cold. The treatment of acute coryza is supportive. Rest, warm fluids, and medications to relieve the symptoms are prescribed. Clients who have an underlying chronic illness, such as asthma or any cardiac condition, need to protect themselves from colds and call their doctors as soon as they notice any symptoms.

Influenza

Influenza is a respiratory disorder caused by a virus. Influenza is not the same as a cold. The client with influenza will have a mucous discharge and fever, will feel achy all over, and will be extremely tired. The "flu" can be a very serious illness, especially for a very young child, an elderly person, or someone who has an underlying chronic problem. Keeping oneself healthy is the best protection—and that includes good handwashing. The elderly and those with a chronic condition should get vaccinated against the flu (a flu shot) before the beginning of the flu season. This immunization offers protection from whatever particular flu strain has been determined to be most prevalent that year.

Pneumonia

Pneumonia is an infection of the lungs caused by a bacterial organism or virus (Figure 28-1). Pneumonia is a serious condition that can lead to death, especially if the client has an underlying chronic condition. A pneumonia vaccine can protect a person; it is recommended for older adults and those with a chronic condition. The client who has pneumonia will complain of

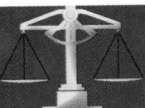

LEGAL/ETHICAL THOUGHTS

If a client seems to be acutely ill, infectious, or contagious, do not allow the client to remain in the reception or waiting area. Inform the doctor and follow the doctor's instructions and office policy.

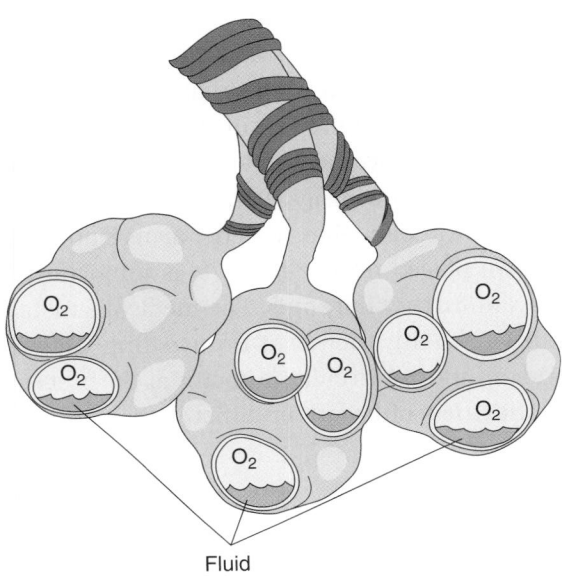

FIGURE 28-1 Pneumonia: fluid filling alveolar sacs.

shortness of breath, cough, and a fever. She may experience chest pain and chills. In addition to any medication the doctor prescribes, the treatment plan should include techniques for improvement of breathing. Coughing and deep breathing exercises will help the client get rid of the thick mucous secretions in the lungs. The client can become very tired from these exercises, especially if she is frail. Clear liquids will keep the client hydrated and help to loosen the secretions.

Tuberculosis

Tuberculosis is a contagious infection that is caused by the mycobacterium *tuberculosis*. It mainly attacks the lungs, although other systems can be the target. Transmission is commonly through respiratory droplets from

sneezing or coughing. The medical assistant is at risk of contracting tuberculosis through casual contact with infected clients.

After declining for several decades, the incidence of tuberculosis began to climb. Among other factors, this increase is linked to the increasing number of individuals with AIDS and immigrants from countries where tuberculosis is common. These groups of people, along with substance abusers and those who live in crowded, close conditions such as institutionalized settings, are of great risk of contracting tuberculosis.

Months of treatment with prescribed medications is necessary. Multidrug-resistant tuberculosis is also on the rise. This form is more difficult to treat successfully.

Pleurisy

The *pleurae* are membranes that line the lungs and the diaphragm; these membranes reduce friction during breathing. If the pleurae become inflamed, the client will feel pain when breathing in and out. This condition is called **pleurisy.** The client should rest in a sitting position with the back supported. Because breathing is painful, the client may breathe shallowly, which puts her at risk of a collapsed lung. Deep breathing and coughing are encouraged to prevent collapsed lungs. Medication to relieve the pain will also make it easier for the client to take deep breaths.

Atelectasis

Atelectasis is a collapsed lung. A person who hypoventilates (takes shallow breaths) is at risk of developing this condition. For example, a person who has pleurisy, and takes shallow breaths because of the pain, is at high risk of atelectasis. Coughing, deep breathing, adequate fluid intake, and humidified air will help to prevent a collapsed lung.

■ CHRONIC DISORDERS

Chronic respiratory disorders make a person's breathing more difficult; this in turn can affect a person's ability to perform everyday tasks. Medical assistants need to understand how chronic disorders affect the breathing process. A key point in treating any chronic respiratory disorder is to prevent flare-ups. Medical assistants will teach clients ways to breathe easier and promote respiratory health.

Asthma

Asthma is a reactive airway disorder (Figure 28-2). The airways become swollen and inflamed. There is increased mucus production. The passageway through which air comes in and goes out becomes narrowed. The client with a flare-up of asthma will have difficulty in getting air out. As the client exhales, the air traveling through the narrowed, uneven passageways makes a wheezing sound. The client will have difficulty breathing, and in an acute flare-up will use the diaphragm and accessory muscles to try to assist in moving air. She may show retraction of the muscles near the clavicle or collarbone. The client may not even be able to speak in complete sentences. Asthma can be triggered by allergens, such as pollen or dust, infections, stress, or even cold air. Treatment is aimed at discovering the trigger and then avoiding or removing it.

Medications that relieve bronchospasm and open the airways will be ordered. It is important for the client to get an adequate amount of fluids and rest. The medical assistant can instruct the client in ways to ease breathing and get rest. Sitting at the side of the bed, with arms resting on an overbed table, will help the client to breathe more easily. At home, the client can sit at the kitchen table, with her arms leaning on pillows placed on the table. It is important to prevent further flare-ups. The medical assistant can work with the client on avoiding triggers, and remind her to call the doctor at the first sign of shortness of breath or difficulty breathing.

Emphysema

Emphysema is a chronic **pulmonary** disorder. Gases are exchanged in the alveoli of the lung (Figure 28-3). In emphysema, the alveoli lose their elasticity and gases become trapped. This is a chronic, progressive disorder. Smoking is a major risk factor for developing emphysema. The client will have difficulty breathing and a chronic cough. As the disease advances, the

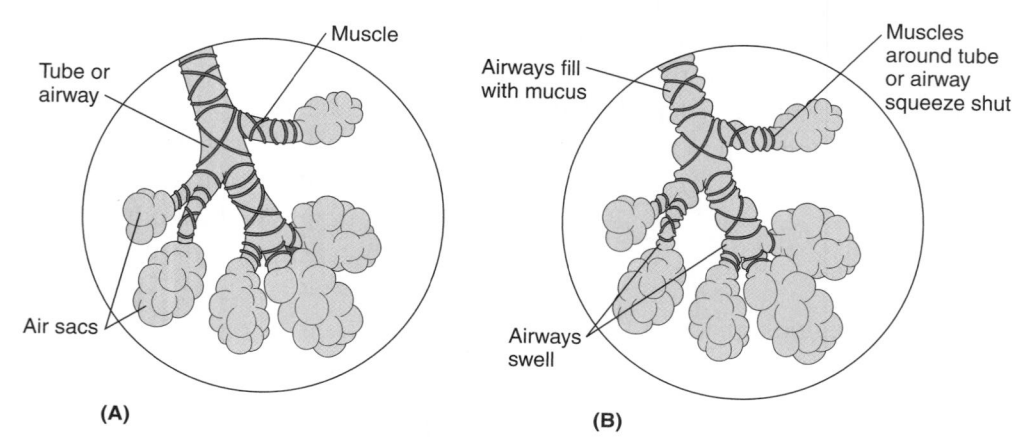

FIGURE 28-2 (A) Before an asthma attack, the airways are open. (B) During an attack, the airways fill with mucus, tightening the muscles.

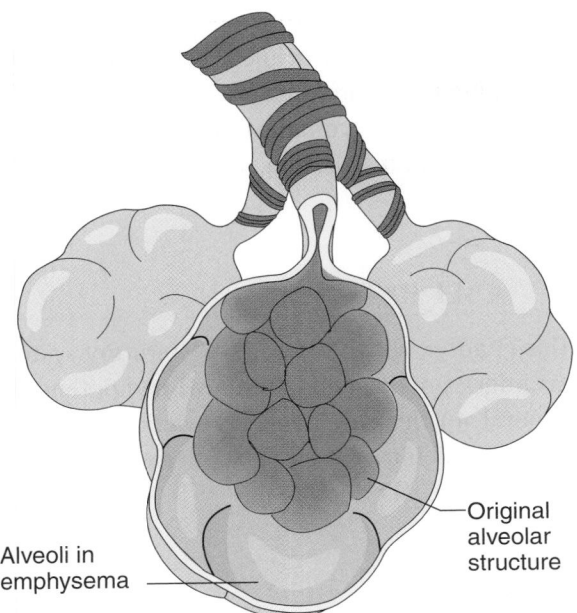

Alveoli in emphysema

Original alveolar structure

FIGURE 28-3 Changes in the alveoli with emphysema.

client will have to make lifestyle changes to be able to perform activities of daily living.

Pulmonary function tests are performed to aid in the diagnosis of many respiratory disorders. The results can also be used to track the progress of clients who have respiratory disorders and their responses to medications and treatments.

■ LUNG CANCER

Lung cancer can be prevented in many cases, but is difficult to cure. It is a very serious, deadly type of cancer. The majority of lung cancers—about 97%—can be traced or related to smoking. Health education that teaches young people not to start smoking could significantly decrease the number of cases. Those who already smoke can decrease their chances of getting cancer, even if they have smoked for years, just by stopping.

 BRIDGE TO CAAHEP

This chapter, which discusses respiratory system disorders, provides information and content related to CAAHEP standards for Anatomy and Physiology, Medical Terminology, Communication, Medical Assisting Clinical Procedures, and Professional Components.

POINTS OF HIGHLIGHT

- Handwashing is the best protection against spreading the cold virus.
- Influenza can be a life-threatening condition, especially for the very young, the very old, and those who have a chronic respiratory or cardiac disorder.
- The ability to perform daily tasks often decreases in those who have respiratory disorders, because of the difficulty in breathing.
- Asthma is a reactive airway disorder often triggered by allergens, infections, stress, or cold air.
- Emphysema is a chronic, progressive pulmonary disorder.
- Smoking is the major risk factor for lung cancer.
- The medical assistant can instruct the client on ways to ease breathing and get needed rest.
- The goal of client teaching in respiratory disorders is to increase the client's ability to breathe and avoid flare-ups of respiratory problems, thus helping the client to continue with daily activities.

ABHES LINKS

This chapter, which discusses respiratory system disorders, links to ABHES course content for Anatomy and Physiology, Medical Terminology, Medical Law and Ethics, and Medical Office Clinical Procedures.

AAMA AREAS OF COMPETENCE

This chapter, which discusses respiratory system disorders, provides information or content within several areas listed in the Medical Assistant Role Delineation Study. These areas include:

administrative, administrative procedures, clinical, fundamental principles, diagnostic orders, patient (client) care, general (transdisciplinary) professionalism, communication skills, legal concepts, and instruction.

AMT PATHS

This chapter, which discusses respiratory system disorders, provides a path to AMT competency in general medical assisting knowledge, anatomy and physiology, medical terminology, and patient (client) education.

STUDENT PORTFOLIO ACTIVITY

With your peers, plan a study group in preparation for a national certification examination. Brainstorm how the group should be organized. When, where, and how frequently should the group meet?

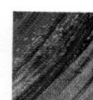

APPLYING YOUR SKILLS

A client who has been diagnosed with a cold (coryza) is upset because the doctor did not prescribe an antibiotic. As a medical assistant, what would you tell her about the usefulness of antibiotics against the common cold? What are some steps that might help the client to feel better (symptom relief)?

CRITICAL THINKING QUESTIONS

1. The primary care office where you are employed has just received a supply of influenza vaccine. Which clients are most in need of the protection this vaccine offers? Why are they at greater risk of getting seriously ill with influenza?

2. In addition to taking prescribed medication, what steps can the client who has pneumonia take to help herself get better?

3. Asthma and emphysema are disorders that affect the respiratory system. How are these disorders alike? What are major differences between them?

4. Explain the difference between influenza (the flu) and coryza (a cold).

5. How can a person protect herself from becoming ill with the flu?

6. Why are coughing and deep breathing helpful in many respiratory disorders?

7. Smoking is a major risk factor for many respiratory disorders. Select two and describe their connection to smoking.

8. The client with pleurisy takes shallow breaths. Shallow breathing places this client at increased risk of serious problems. Discuss these potential problems.

9. It is important to prevent flare-ups of asthma. As a medical assistant, what would you include in a client teaching plan on this subject?

10. A client with chronic breathing difficulties comes to the office. As part of the exam, you know that the client will need to sit and then lie supine (on her back). How can you make the client more comfortable in these positions?

11. What do you tell a client is the single best way to prevent the spread of colds or the flu?

12. Another health care provider does not understand the difference between asthma and emphysema. What explanation would you give her?

13. Carrying out activities of daily living is often difficult for the client who has a chronic respiratory disorder. What are some practical ways for such a client to organize her day?

14. What factors put elderly individuals at risk of pneumonia and acute respiratory disorders?

15. Go back to the beginning of this chapter and review the Anticipatory Statements. Reread each statement and then indicate whether it is true or false. If the statement is false, rewrite it to make it a true statement.

CLIENT TEACHING PLAN

Taking an Oral Temperature Using a Disposable Thermometer

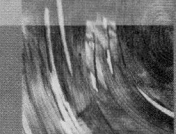

■ What Is to Be Taught:

- How to take and read an oral temperature using a disposable thermometer.

■ Objectives:

- Client will be able to take, read, and report her temperature using a disposable thermometer.

■ Preparation Before Teaching:

- Review the procedure for taking, reading, and reporting an oral temperature using a disposable thermometer.
- Get together teaching supplies, including a disposable oral thermometer, a watch with a second hand, and paper and pen.
- Make sure the area is free from distractions while you are teaching.

■ Steps for the Medical Assistant:

1. Wash your hands.
2. Gather supplies needed.
3. Introduce yourself to the client.
4. Explain what you are going to teach and why.
5. Show the client how to wash her hands. Discuss the importance of handwashing to prevent the spread of bacteria and other germs. (The client will not be wearing gloves at home.)
6. Open the box and show a disposable oral thermometer to the client.
7. Point out the dots and explain what they mean.
8. Ask the client to open her mouth.
9. Instruct the client to place the thermometer under her tongue toward the back.(The numbers on the thermometer can be facing up or down.)
10. Tell the client to keep her tongue down and to leave the thermometer there for one full minute (60 seconds).
11. Hand the client the watch with the second hand and ask him her start counting when the second hand gets to the 12.
12. Remove the thermometer from the client's mouth after one full minute.
13. Tell the client to wait a few seconds before reading the temperature, to let the color on the dots lock in.
14. Instruct the client to read and write down the number at the last colored dot. Check the dots to verify that the client read correctly. Inform the client not to pay attention to any skipped dots.
15. Tell the client to throw the disposable thermometer into the wastebasket.
16. Ask the client to wash her hands.
17. Give written instructions to the client. Be sure to include the office telephone number and the hours to call.

■ Special Needs of the Client:

- Check the client's chart for any factors that might interfere with the client's ability to take, read, and report her temperature.
- Ask the client, before and after the demonstration, if there is anything you should know that might affect her ability to perform this procedure.

■ Evaluation:

- Client is able to list the steps for obtaining an oral temperature.
- Client is able to demonstrate the steps after she has done it with your assistance.
- Client is able to call the office and accurately report the oral temperature reading.

■ Further Plans/Teaching:

- Ask the client if she has any questions or needs any additional information.

■ Follow-up:

- Call the client at home at the end of the next day if the client has not called the office.
- At the next office visit, review the steps as needed.

(Continues)

CLIENT TEACHING PLAN (Continued)

Medical Assistant

Name: _____

Signature: _____

Date: _____

Client

Date: _____

Follow-up Date : _____

Anticipatory Statements

People have different ideas about digestive system disorders. Read and think about the following statements based upon what you believe now. Decide whether you agree or disagree. Write the word **agree** after the statement if you think the statement is true. Write the word **disagree** after the statement if you think the statement is false. Read the chapter to find out if your current beliefs can be supported.

1. Straining while having a bowel movement can be very harmful. _____

2. Diarrhea is a common disorder with no serious effects on the body. _____

3. Stress is the major cause of stomach ulcers. _____

4. Irritable bowel syndrome causes increased activity of the intestines. _____

5. Hepatitis is easily cured. _____

Digestive System Disorders

Learning Objectives

Upon completion of this chapter, the medical assistant student should be able to:

- Identify the medical assistant's role in preparing clients for diagnostic tests of the digestive system
- Explain the differences between diverticulosis and diverticulitis
- State what is meant by GERD
- List the causes of hepatitis
- Explain the differences between Crohn's and ulcerative colitis
- Develop a teaching plan for a client who has chronic constipation

Key Terms

appendicitis Inflammation of the appendix.

cirrhosis Liver disorder that damages the cells of the liver.

constipation Condition in which the feces are hard, dry, and difficult or painful to pass.

Crohn's Inflammatory bowel disorder affecting all layers of the digestive tract. Can occur at any point along the tract.

diarrhea Passing of loose or liquid feces or waste material.

diverticulitis Inflammation of diverticula (sacs or pouches in the intestine).

diverticulosis Formation of sacs or pouches in the intestine; does not cause any symptoms.

flatulence Excessive gas in the digestive tract.

gallbladder Organ that stores bile made in the liver; found under the right lobe of the liver.

gastroenteritis An inflammation of the stomach and intestine.

hepatitis Inflammation or infection of the liver.

intestinal obstruction Blockage in the intestines that interferes with movement of the contents through the intestine.

irritable bowel syndrome (IBS) Motility disorder of the colon that sometimes causes diarrhea and other times causes constipation.

pancreatitis Inflammation of the pancreas.

ulcerative colitis Inflammatory bowel disorder affecting only the lining of the digestive tract. Usually affects the large intestine.

■ INTRODUCTION

Disorders of the digestive system are commonly seen in the medical office. Several diagnostic tests are available to identify digestive system disorders. Gastrointestinal studies and colonoscopies are commonly done (see Chapter 45). Disorders of the digestive system can be caused by the actual structure of the organs. They may also be due to what and how much a person eats and his corresponding lifestyle. Disorders in other systems can also affect the digestive system. Clients who have digestive disorders are often uncomfortable and experience difficulties with activities of daily living, especially eating, which is not only necessary for survival but also has social and environmental consequences. The medical assistant needs to understand the basic disorders and how they affect the many aspects of a client's life.

■ DIARRHEA

Diarrhea affects almost everyone at some time. It can last for only one bowel movement, or it can persist, leading to dehydration and a need for hospitalization. In underdeveloped countries, it is a leading cause of death in young children. *Diarrhea* is loose, unformed stool. The severity of the problem will depend on the amount of stool passed, the frequency of defecation, the client's age, and his general health. A young child will become sicker faster because of the percentage of water in the body and the size of the child. An elderly person or someone who has an underlying condition will also be affected more severely than an otherwise healthy young adult.

The medical assistant must ask the client how many times there have been loose stools and how long (hours, days) this condition has lasted. Did the client take any over-the-counter medications, or any herbs or other preparations, to try to stop the diarrhea? Clients often try quite a few different remedies before giving up and calling the doctor. Has the client been able to drink any fluids? Sometimes acute diarrhea is combined with nausea and vomiting and the client is not able to keep anything down.

The treatment of diarrhea is aimed at finding the cause and replacing the fluid that has been lost. Knowing whether the diarrhea is a more chronic problem, or if the client's condition has alternated between diarrhea and constipation, will help the doctor to find the cause and develop appropriate treatments.

NOTE TO STUDENT:

A person need not have a specific number of loose bowel movements before diarrhea is diagnosed. "Normal" varies from person to person. More important than the number and times is a change in bowel habits for the individual client. Changes in number of times defecation occurs, and changes in the shape, consistency, and/or color of feces, should be reported to the doctor.

■ CONSTIPATION

Constipation is a decrease in the number of times that stool is passed (compared to normal for the client). Often it is difficult for the client to pass the stool, and the stool that is passed is hard and dry.

There are many causes of constipation, and some are easier to correct than others. First, lack of fiber or bulk in the diet can lead to constipation. Second, an adequate amount of water is needed each day to avoid constipation. Third, changes in normal eating habits can put a person at risk. Fourth, lack of activity, such as sitting for long periods of time, will hinder bowel movements. Fifth, some vitamins and minerals, such as iron preparations, are very constipating. Finally, some prescription medications can cause constipation as a side effect.

NOTE TO STUDENT:

Constipation can be a symptom of an underlying disorder.

Clients can become very uncomfortable when they are constipated. Over-the-counter medications to correct constipation are heavily advertised. Clients may begin to use *laxatives*, substances that help to loosen and aid the passage of stools. Clients can become physically dependent on laxatives: Depending on the way the laxative works, the body may not keep moving the stool through the intestine without the help of the laxative. When the client abruptly stops using the product, constipation occurs or reoccurs. Laxatives can be helpful in the treatment of occasional constipation, but they should be used as directed for temporary relief.

The cause of the constipation must be identified. Treatment is based on the underlying cause. In addition to laxatives, sometimes a client benefits from the use of a stool softener. A stool softener helps the stool to pass more easily out of the rectum, without straining or pain.

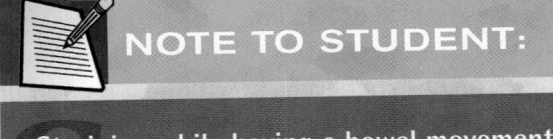

NOTE TO STUDENT:

Straining while having a bowel movement can be very harmful. It raises the blood pressure and could cause a cardiovascular event.

The medical assistant can help the client to promote good bowel habits. The client should drink plenty of water each day, eat meals at regular intervals, allow time each day to have a bowel movement, and eat a diet high in fiber, fruits, and vegetables.

■ GASTROESOPHAGEAL REFLUX DISORDER

When the sphincter of the esophagus leading into the stomach relaxes, or does not close properly, the contents of the stomach back up into the esophagus. In addition to food, gastric secretions also back up. The client will complain of chest pain or "heartburn." (A client's complaint of heartburn must be clearly distinguished from cardiac pain.) In addition to medication, the medical assistant can teach the client some steps to help control gastroesophageal reflux disorder (GERD). Eating small meals and remaining upright for at least two hours afterward will alleviate many of the problems. Clients should avoid foods that seem to make the discomfort worse. Drinking enough fluids, maintaining normal weight, and increasing exercise also seem to improve the condition.

■ ULCERS

Ulcers are lesions, sores, or open areas. They can appear on the skin or any mucous area of the body, including those that line the digestive tract. The ulcer is named by the location of the open area (Figure 29-1). For example, the very common duodenal ulcer appears in the duodenum, which is the first part of the small intestine. Although stress can aggravate a gastrointestinal ulcer, often a bacterial infection is responsible for the lesion. Antibiotics, antacids, and prescription medications are ordered.

■ GASTROENTERITIS

Gastroenteritis is an inflammation of the stomach and intestine. It can be caused by an allergic reaction to food, or by food that has "gone bad"

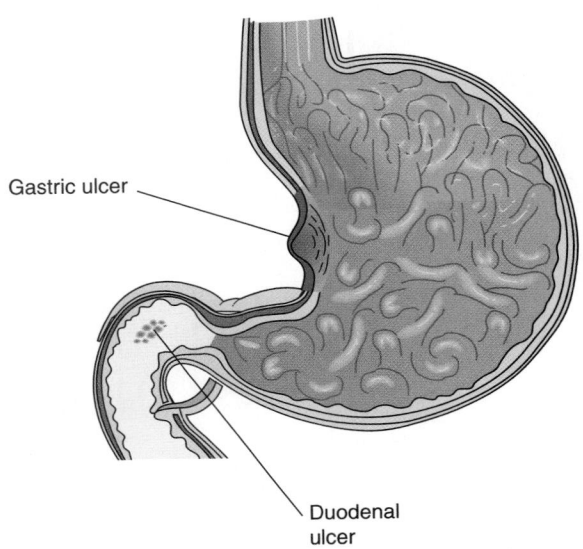

Gastric ulcer

Duodenal ulcer

FIGURE 29-1 Gastrointestinal ulcers.

(is spoiled). It is also caused by microorganisms. Gastroenteritis may come on suddenly. The client will have nausea and vomiting, abdominal pain, and diarrhea. Medication to treat the diarrhea and nausea may be ordered. Good handwashing technique is very important to avoid getting gastroenteritis. Proper precautions must be taken when preparing and handling food, and uneaten food should be refrigerated quickly to avoid growth of harmful pathogens.

■ DIVERTICULOSIS AND DIVERTICULITIS

Diverticulosis is a condition in which little pouches or sacs form on the walls of the intestine (Figure 29-2). Diverticulosis is common in older adults and often causes no symptoms. If the sacs become inflamed, the condition is called **diverticulitis.** During the acute stage, the client will lose his appetite, and have pain and fever. Pain medication and medication to relieve the spasms, as well as antibiotics and stool softeners, are the usual treatment. The client should rest during the acute stage to avoid additional strain on the intestine. The client will need to be instructed to inspect the stool for consistency and the presence of mucus and/or blood.

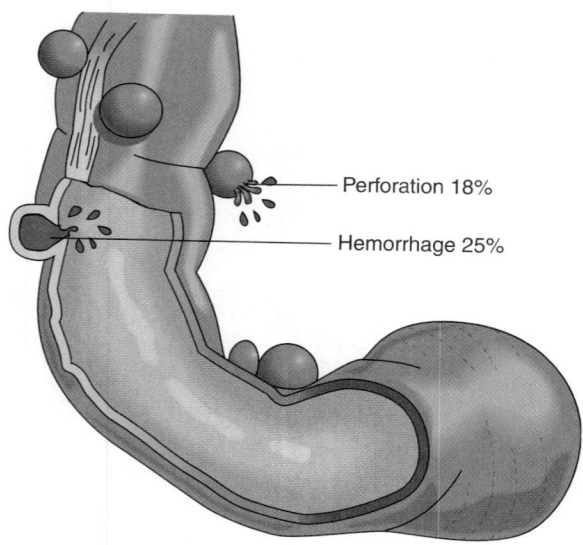

FIGURE 29-2 Diverticulosis.

Perforation 18%

Hemorrhage 25%

If chronic diverticulitis develops, the bowel walls thicken, leading to narrowing, strictures, and possibly obstruction. The medical assistant will need to provide teaching regarding nutrition and diet. The client must drink enough fluid (two to three liters per day); the diet must include fiber and roughage in the form of vegetables and fruit. However, the client must avoid seeds in vegetables or fruits. Seeds can get stuck in the diverticuli (pouches) and lead to further inflammation.

■ INTESTINAL OBSTRUCTION (COLON BLOCKAGE)

Intestinal obstruction is commonly called a *bowel obstruction.* Peristalsis (wavelike movements of the muscles) move the digestive contents along the gastrointestinal tract. In a bowel obstruction, neither gas nor fluid can move through the intestine (Figure 29-3). The contents get stopped or blocked at some point along the way. The client's symptoms will depend on where the obstruction is, how large a section of the intestine is involved, and how complete the obstruction is. The abdomen will be distended (stick out more than usual). The client may also have nausea, vomiting, and cramps. The client will not have an appetite and will feel constipated.

The treatment for intestinal obstruction depends on the site of the obstruction. Tubes may be inserted to straighten out the kinks and twists in the intestine. Suction may be used to empty the intestine. Sometimes surgery must be done to correct the problem.

■ INFLAMMATORY BOWEL DISEASE (IBD)

The digestive tract can become inflamed, red, and swollen. Two major types of inflammatory bowel diseases are **Crohn's** and **ulcerative colitis.**

Crohn's affects all layers of the digestive tract. Although frequently seen in the small intestine, it can happen at any point along the entire digestive tract from the mouth to the

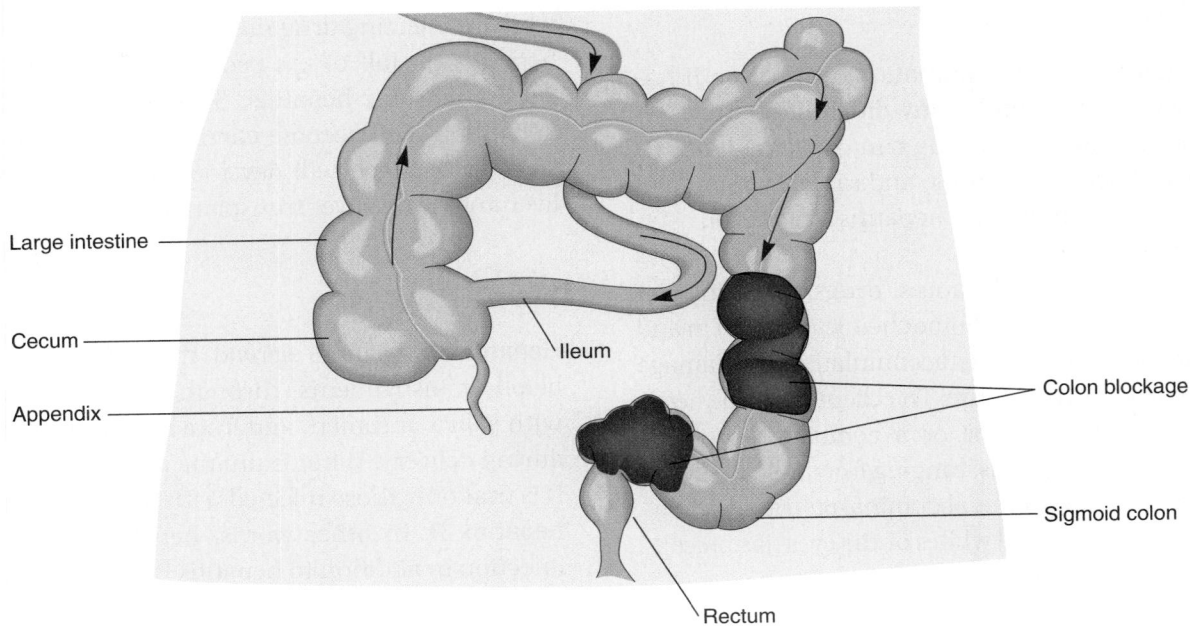

Large intestine

Cecum

Appendix

Ileum

Colon blockage

Sigmoid colon

Rectum

FIGURE 29-3 Intestinal obstruction.

anus. It may affect one area of the digestive tract, skip a section, and then affect another area. This chronic disorder has both flare-ups and quiet times. The client will experience abdominal pain, diarrhea and often rectal bleeding, fever, and weight loss. Complications include blockage, fistulas (sores or ulcers that develop into tracts), and malnutrition (most absorption of nutrients takes place in the small intestine). Treatment includes long-term medications and possible surgery. The medical assistant needs to be supportive as this chronic disorder can affect many aspects of a client's life.

Ulcerative colitis affects the lining of the digestive tract. It occurs most frequently in the large intestine. The client will experience many loose stools per day, bowel urgency, straining with bowel movements, incomplete bowel movement feeling, and blood with and pus in the feces. Treatment includes long-term medication and surgery may be needed. Surgery may "cure" ulcerative colitis if the diseased section can be completely removed. The medical assistant will need to help the client adapt to the disorder and its effects on the client's activities.

■ IRRITABLE BOWEL SYNDROME

Irritable bowel syndrome (IBS) is known by several different names. It can be called *spastic* or *irritable colon* or *spastic* or *mucous colitis*. It is the most common disorder causing increased activity of the intestines. The client will complain of **flatulence** (gas) and bouts of diarrhea followed by bouts of constipation. Nausea and abdominal pain are common. Other disorders must be ruled out before a diagnosis is made.

The client who has this disorder may become very upset. Because the client might have the urge to have a bowel movement frequently and at inconvenient times, the client will always want to know where the nearest bathroom is. He may avoid social situations or traveling. The medical assistant can help the client to control and adapt to this disorder. The medical assistant will need to help the client examine his lifestyle and changes that can be made to that lifestyle. Regular mealtimes, with a high fiber diet, might help. Medications to quiet the bowels, as well as antispasmodics, can also be effective.

■ HEPATITIS

Hepatitis is an inflammation of the liver. It has several causes and many different subtypes. A virus, a toxin, or a drug can cause hepatitis. It can be acute or chronic and range from mild to life-threatening. Viral hepatitis is classified as A, B, C, D, or E.

Chemical substances, drugs, or toxins can also cause hepatitis. Some chemicals collect in and damage the tissue; this accumulation and damage can lead to liver failure. The client who has hepatitis will show some or a combination of the following symptoms, ranging from mild to severe: fever, loss of appetite, abdominal pain, and yellowing of the skin and whites of the eyes (jaundice).

Hepatitis A

Hepatitis A is the most common type. Often the client experiences only mild symptoms and the diagnosis is missed. Most frequently hepatitis A is transmitted through the oral–fecal route. Crowded living conditions are a primary risk factor. Hepatitis A can be prevented by vaccination, and does not lead to chronic hepatitis.

Hepatitis B

Hepatitis B used to be called *serum hepatitis.* Hepatitis B is spread through infected blood or instruments, through sexual contact with saliva or semen, and from mother to baby during delivery. Those who share needles, sexually active homosexual individuals, and babies of HBV carriers are at risk.

Health care providers, including medical assistants, are at great risk of contracting hepatitis B virus (HBV) and should strictly observe standard precautions. The Centers for Disease Control and Prevention (CDC) recommends vaccination for health care providers, including medical assistants.

Hepatitis C

Those who received blood transfusions before laboratories began screening blood, and those who are injecting drug users are at great risk of hepatitis C. Half of the people with hepatitis C develop chronic hepatitis; 50% of people with hepatitis C will become carriers for the rest of their lives. Some will develop cirrhosis of the liver and need a liver transplant later in life.

Hepatitis D

Hepatitis D virus is spread through infected blood or instruments, through sexual contact with saliva or semen, and from mother to baby during delivery. What is unique about hepatitis D is that only those infected with hepatitis B get hepatitis D. In other words, hepatitis D is an infection in addition to hepatitis B.

Hepatitis E

Hepatitis E is rare in the United States. However, those who travel to countries where it is prevalent, such as Mexico, India, and Pakistan, should take precautions to avoid contracting the disease.

■ CIRRHOSIS OF THE LIVER

Cirrhosis of the liver is a chronic degenerative disorder (Figure 29-4). The tissue of the liver becomes scarred and cannot function properly. The liver cannot detoxify (make harmless) toxins or harmful chemicals in the body. Viral hepatitis and alcoholism are the two most common causes of cirrhosis.

In the beginning, the client's symptoms may be vague. Severe cirrhosis will have many symptoms. Varicose veins appear in the esophagus and abdomen due to the increased fluid pressure. These distended veins can burst open and cause massive bleeding (hemorrhages). The spleen becomes enlarged. The liver is not able to play its role in blood clotting, so the client may have internal bleeding in the abdomen, signaled by blood in the stool and/or vomit. The ankles and feet swell with retained fluid (edema). Because the protein necessary for fluid balance, which is made in the liver, is not

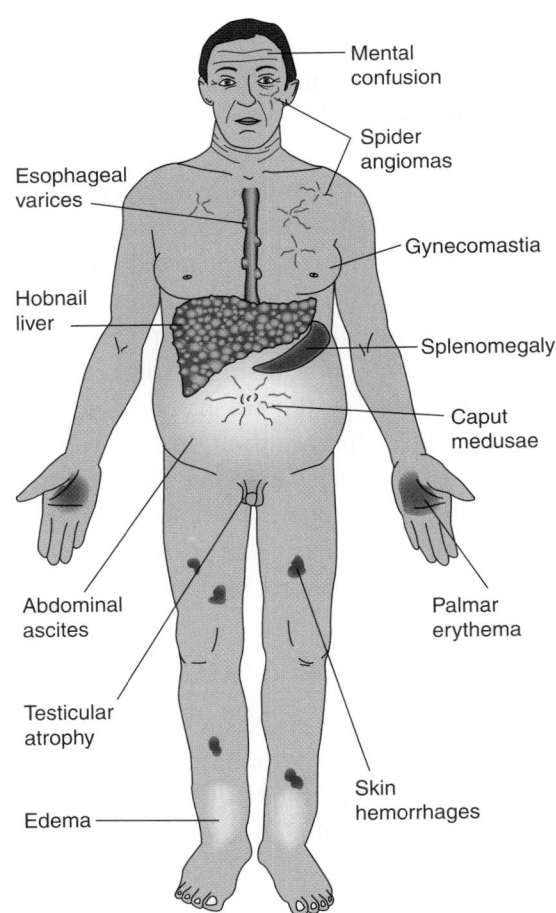

Mental confusion

Spider angiomas

Esophageal varices

Gynecomastia

Hobnail liver

Splenomegaly

Caput medusae

Abdominal ascites

Palmar erythema

Testicular atrophy

Skin hemorrhages

Edema

FIGURE 29-4 Complications of cirrhosis of the liver.

available, fluids seep into the tissues and stay there. Fluid also builds up in the abdomen; this is called *ascites.* The enlarged abdomen will cause pressure on the diaphragm and rib muscles and eventually make it difficult for the client to breathe. Because the liver cannot get rid of waste products, nitrogen builds in the blood and eventually affects the brain. The client may become confused and go into a semi-conscious state. Hallucinations may result, with shaking of the body called *delirium tremens.* Eventually, this condition leads to coma and death.

The doctor may try to drain off some of the fluid to try to make the client more comfortable and relieve some of the pressure. The only curative treatment, however, is a liver transplant.

■ GALLSTONES

Gallstones are solid accumulations of minerals in the **gallbladder.** Formation of gallstones is called *cholelithiasis.* The client will not have any symptoms until the stones block a duct or passageway. When that occurs, the client may experience nausea, vomiting, and pain in the right upper part of the abdomen, especially after eating foods containing fats. Gallstones vary in size and shape. Several factors increase a person's risk of getting gallstones: age over 40, overweight, and being female are all risk factors. Ultrasound and cholecystography are done to make the diagnosis cholecystectomy (surgical removal of the gallbladder). Lithotripsy (breaking up of stones) may be done with extracorporeal shock waves (ESWL).

Cholecystitis

Cholecystitis is an inflammation of the gallbladder, usually caused by gallstones. With this condition, many of the symptoms of gallstones become worse, especially the pain after eating. This is because the inflamed gallbladder is trying to send out bile. The treatment is surgery to remove the gallbladder. The surgery is called *cholecystectomy.*

■ APPENDICITIS

Appendicitis is an inflammation of the appendix (Figure 29-5). The appendix becomes obstructed and causes pain. The infecting bacteria reproduce and accumulate, and if the buildup causes too much pressure, the appendix can burst, releasing bacteria into the entire surrounding area and spreading the infection throughout the peritoneal cavity. The treatment is surgery to remove the appendix, called an *appendectomy.*

■ PANCREATITIS

Pancreatitis is an inflammation of the pancreas. There are several causes, although severe pancreatitis is usually related to alcoholism. The client may not have any symptoms

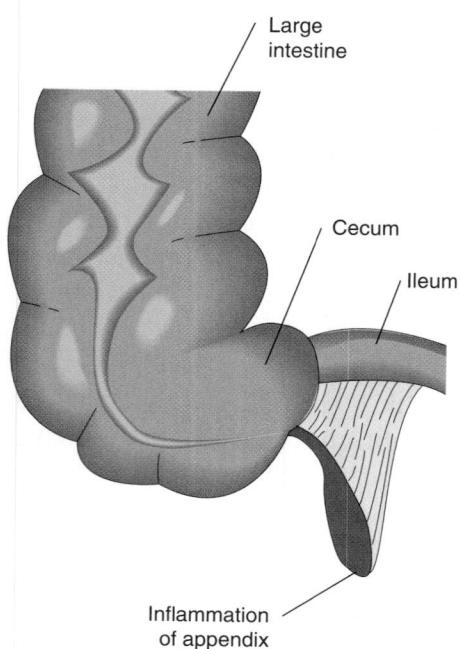

FIGURE 29-5 Appendicitis.

until the disease is advanced. If gallstones have caused the problem, they are removed. Otherwise, the treatment is supportive only.

■ CANCER

Cancer can occur anywhere in the organs and structures of the digestive system. The causes, symptoms, and treatments will depend on where the cancer is and how far advanced it is. For example, treatment of colon cancer is highly effective if the cancer is detected early. Stool samples should be obtained during the yearly physical examination to look for occult blood. Periodic colonoscopy (using an instrument to view the inside of the colon) can find *polyps*, small growths that are thought to develop into cancer. On the other extreme, the client with pancreatic cancer often will have no symptoms until late in the disease. The current treatments for pancreatic cancer are not very successful.

 BRIDGE TO CAAHEP

This chapter, which discusses digestive system disorders, provides information and content related to CAAHEP standards for Anatomy and Physiology, Medical Terminology, Psychology,

POINTS OF HIGHLIGHT

- Diarrhea is a common medical problem, which affects young children and older adults most severely.
- Laxatives should be used only for the occasional relief of constipation; frequent use can lead to dependence.
- The medical assistant can teach clients ways to promote bowel health.
- The duodenum is a very common site for gastrointestinal ulcers.
- Diverticulosis, which is the formation of little pouches on the intestinal wall, is increasingly common as a person ages. When the pouches become inflamed, the condition is called diverticulitis.
- Clients with chronic diverticulitis must take precautions in selecting foods that will not aggravate the condition.
- Irritable bowel syndrome can have a major effect on a client's lifestyle and social activities.
- There are many causes and subtypes of hepatitis, which is an inflammation of the liver. The disorder can be acute or chronic and the symptoms range from mild to life-threatening.
- Cancer can occur anywhere in the organs and structures of the digestive system.
- Dietary habits can greatly affect a client's digestive health.

Communication, Medical Assisting Clinical Procedures, and Professional Components.

ABHES LINKS

This chapter, which discusses digestive system disorders, links to ABHES course content for Anatomy and Physiology, Medical Terminology, Medical Law and Ethics, and Medical Office Clinical Procedures.

AAMA AREAS OF COMPETENCE

This chapter, which discusses digestive system disorders, provides information or content within several areas listed in the Medical Assistant Role Delineation Study. These areas include: administrative, administrative procedures, clinical, fundamental principles, diagnostic orders, patient (client) care, general transdisciplinary, professionalism, communication skills, legal concepts, and instruction.

AMT PATHS

This chapter, which discusses digestive system disorders, provides a path to AMT competency in general medical assisting knowledge, anatomy and physiology, medical terminology, and patient (client) education.

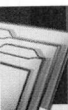

STUDENT PORTFOLIO ACTIVITY

Make an appointment with a staff member in the career center at your school. Ask for advice on the correct procedure for obtaining reference letters. How many should be character references? How many should be professional references? Does the career center keep graduate résumés or employment folders on file?

APPLYING YOUR SKILLS

After you weigh a client, you notice that he has lost several pounds since his last visit. When asked about his appetite, he tells you that his wife died a few months ago and that he just has not been hungry. How would you approach this client? What questions would you ask, and what else do you need to know? Who else should you involve to help this client?

CRITICAL THINKING QUESTIONS

1. You ask a client about bowel habits, and he tells you that everything is fine. He takes a laxative every day to have a bowel movement. What are the implications of excessive use of laxatives on bowel health?

2. Why does diarrhea affect young children more severely than adults?

3. When the sphincter muscles of the esophagus do not work well, what happens to the digestive process? What will the client experience?

4. What role does food play in gastroenteritis?

5. The client has a chief complaint of diarrhea. The severity of the problem depends upon what factors?

6. What questions would you ask the client from question 5?

7. How is a stool softener different from a laxative?

8. After examination and testing, the doctor has diagnosed a client with GERD. In addition to medication, how can the client help himself?

9. A client who has diverticulosis questions the need to avoid seeds from fruits and vegetables. What would you explain about the disorder and seeds?

10. What is the connection between lifestyle and irritable bowel syndrome?

11. A client's lab report indicates that he has hepatitis B. What does this place him at greater risk of developing, and why?

12. Explain the implications for a client who has cirrhosis of the liver. What are some of the major bodily effects from a diseased liver?

13. As a medical assistant, you understand that there are healthy practices to avoid conditions that might lead to cancer in the digestive tract. Discuss these steps.

14. Go back to the beginning of this chapter and review the Anticipatory Statements. Reread each statement and then indicate whether it is true or false. If the statement is false, rewrite it to make it a true statement.

CLIENT TEACHING PLAN

Preparation for Colonoscopy

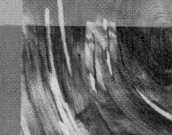

■ What Is to Be Taught:

- Client preparation before undergoing a colonoscopy examination.

■ Objectives:

- Client will understand the purpose and take the necessary steps before undergoing a colonoscopy.

■ Preparation Before Teaching:

- Review the colonoscopy procedure and any special office policies or procedures for colonoscopy.
- Get together colonoscopy prep kit, which contains laxatives, suppositories, magnesium citrate, disposable enema, and gloves.
- Get either samples or pictures of what is allowed on a clear liquid diet.
- Get paper and pen for any special written instructions.
- Check the client's chart thoroughly in case the doctor ordered something different from the standard preparation.

■ Steps for the Medical Assistant:

1. Wash your hands.
2. Gather supplies needed.
3. Introduce yourself to the client.
4. Explain what you are going to teach and why. Stress the need for the preparation steps and the importance of following the instructions to help ensure accurate test results.
5. Review any vitamins the client is taking. Make sure to find out if any iron is included. If they contain iron, the client must stop taking the vitamins three to four days before the procedure.
6. Review the client's medications. If he takes aspirin regularly, tell the client to stop taking it one week before the procedure. List common products that contain aspirin.

7. Inform the client what is included in the clear liquid diet that he must follow for two days. Show pictures and/or write down what may be eaten.
8. Instruct the client how to take magnesium citrate, which is a strong cathartic. Suggest ways to make it easier, such as with ice.
9. Show the client a sample suppository and how to unwrap it. Remind the client that it is made to melt at body temperature, so he should not leave it unwrapped in his hand for long before inserting it into the rectum.
10. Show the client the sample enema and how to use it.
11. Tell that client that he will need to use the bathroom frequently during the preparation steps, so he should schedule activities to take this into account.
12. Inform the client that he may experience gas pains for a few hours after the procedure.
13. Remind the client to drink plenty of fluids after the procedure.
14. Tell the client that if any blood appears in the stool afterward, he should call the doctor immediately.
15. If he has any questions or concerns during the preparation steps or after the colonoscopy, the client should call the doctor.

■ Special Needs of the Client:

- Look at the client's chart to see if there are any factors that might interfere with the client's ability to follow through with the preparation steps.
- Ask the client, before and after teaching, if there is anything you should know that might affect his ability to follow through with these instructions.

■ Evaluation:

- Client will be able to list the steps and explain what is included in preparation for a colonoscopy.

(Continues)

CLIENT TEACHING PLAN (Continued)

■ Further Plans/Teaching:

- At the next visit, review the client's experience. A review allows you to answer any remaining questions and also helps you discover if any part of the instruction was unclear; this will be useful in adjusting your teaching for future clients.

■ Follow-up:

- Call the client during the preparation time to check if the client is able to follow the steps or has any questions.

Medical Asssistant

Name: _____

Signature: _____

Date: _____

Client

Date: _____

Follow-up Date : _____

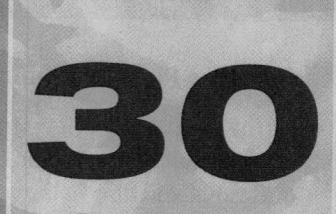

CHAPTER 30

Anticipatory Statements

People have different ideas about urinary system disorders. Read and think about the following statements based upon what you believe now. Decide whether you agree or disagree. Write the word **agree** after the statement if you think the statement is true. Write the word **disagree** after the statement if you think the statement is false. Read the chapter to find out if your current beliefs can be supported.

1. Urinary incontinence is a normal part of aging.

   _____

2. A urinary tract infection can turn into a recurrent, chronic disorder.

   _____

3. Sometimes clients are able to pass kidney stones out through the urethra.

   _____

4. In urinary retention, the bladder does not completely empty.

   _____

5. A client who has kidney failure should drink a lot of water.

   _____

Urinary System Disorders

Learning Objectives

Upon completion of this chapter, the medical assistant student should be able to:

- Identify acute infectious disorders of the urinary system
- Explain what is meant by an "ascending infection"
- Recognize the signs and symptoms of a urinary tract infection
- Describe how the structure of the female urinary system puts women at greater risk of developing urinary tract infections
- Explain what a kidney stone is
- List noninfectious disorders of the urinary system
- Identify the medical assistant's role in preparing clients for diagnostic tests of the urinary system
- Develop a teaching plan for a client who has chronic urinary tract infections
- Teach another person steps to prevent repeat urinary tract infections

Key Terms

cystitis Inflammation of the bladder.

glomerulonephritis Inflammation of the glomeruli; can harm the nephrons. This can be an acute or a chronic condition.

glomerulus The filtering unit of the kidney.

neurogenic Due to the nerves or nervous system.

polycystic Many cysts (in the kidneys).

pyelitis Inflammation of the cavities of the kidneys.

pyelonephritis Bacterial infection of the kidney; can be acute or chronic.

urethritis Inflammation of the urethra; most common in males.

■ INTRODUCTION

Disorders of the urinary system are frequently seen in the primary care office, as well as in urology and pediatric offices. The medical assistant needs to be familiar with the major disorders so that she can provide safe, competent care to clients. Learning about the acute inflammatory and infectious disorders, and how they can lead to or be related to other disorders, may help the medical assistant in understanding urinary disorders. Other noninfectious disorders, such as polycystic kidney disease, kidney stones, and kidney failure, are also discussed. Urinary disorders can affect anyone at any age. An understanding of the common disorders will enable the medical assistant to work with clients in a caring, knowledgeable way.

■ URINARY DISORDERS

An infection in any part of the urinary system can easily spread to the other structures. Prevention of infection is important. Any infection must be treated early and effectively to prevent it from spreading to the other structures or becoming a recurrent infection. The medical assistant teaches clients about the prescribed treatments. Follow-up and prevention should also be part of the teaching plan.

Clients may feel uncomfortable discussing problems with the urinary system. The urinary system, especially in males, is often identified with the reproductive system and sexuality. There may be cultural taboos in discussing these subjects and body parts with anyone. The medical assistant must be sensitive to the client's needs and approach the client in a calm, professional manner. The medical assistant should allow the client to express any concerns. Clients often have misinformation, and the office visit can be an excellent teaching opportunity through which the medical assistant helps the client. The medical assistant may also act as a liaison or advocate and inform the doctor about client concerns or misinformation.

Cystitis

A common infection of the urinary system is in the lower urinary tract (Figure 30-1). An inflammation of the urinary bladder is called **cystitis** (Figure 30-2). A client who is experiencing a bladder infection will complain of frequency, urgency, and pain upon urination. *Frequency* refers to the number of times a person has to urinate. Urgency refers to the feeling or need to void immediately. During urination, the client may experience pain or an itching, burning sensation.

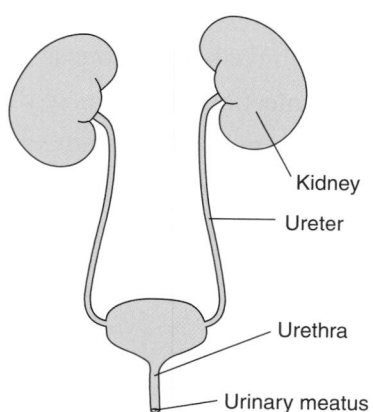

FIGURE 30–1 Infection of the entire urinary tract.

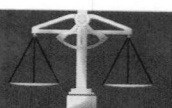

LEGAL/ETHICAL THOUGHTS

Remember that the client you are caring for is an individual. Treat each client with dignity and respect. It is the ethical way to act, as well as demonstrating legally responsible behavior.

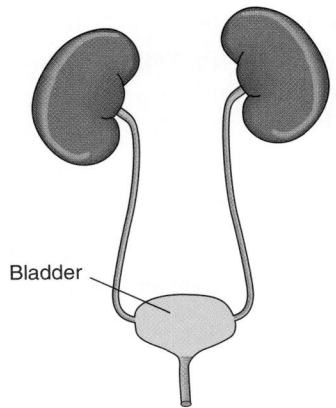

FIGURE 30-2 Cystitis.

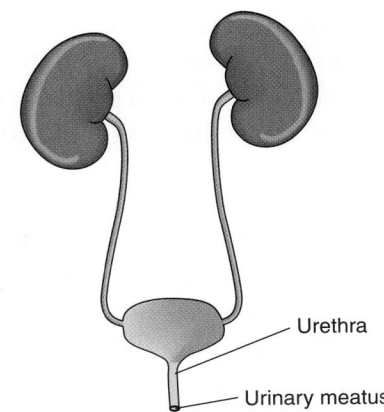

FIGURE 30-3 Urethritis.

The medical assistant will help the client obtain a urine specimen, which the medical assistant will test for a possible infection. A urine sample is always obtained for cultures and sensitivity (C & S) before a client is prescribed antibiotics. If there is an infection, the doctor will order an antibiotic medication. It is important that the client complete the ordered medication even though the symptoms may disappear before the last dose. If the client does not complete the course of treatment as prescribed, some bacteria may remain and become *resistant*, that is, not be killed by the antibiotic. If this happens, the medicine will not cure the infection and will not work on future infections. The medical assistant needs to reinforce the importance of follow-up. Additionally, after the course of treatment has been completed, the client needs to call the doctor at the first sign of any recurrence of symptoms, such as frequency, urgency, or pain upon urination.

An acute infection can become a chronic disorder, with the client having frequent recurring episodes of urinary tract infection. The infection can also travel to other structures in the urinary system, usually in an ascending order that begins in the urethra and travels up until it reaches and infects the kidneys. This is much more common in females than males. The female urethra is shorter and lies closer to the rectum. The short length and position allow easier entry of bacteria into the urethra. Secretions from the vagina may carry bacteria, which

can travel to and enter the urethral area. Sexual intercourse may cause irritation of the urethra and bladder and lead to possible infection.

Urethritis

Urethritis is an inflammation of the urethra. It can result from cystitis, as part of an ascending infection (Figure 30-3). However, it can also be a symptom of gonorrhea, herpes genitalis, or chlamydia.

Urinary Incontinence

Urinary incontinence is the inability to control the flow of urine. There are many causes of incontinence. *Stress incontinence* happens when a person laughs, coughs, sneezes, runs, or jumps. Women are more prone to this type of incontinence. There are treatment options for stress incontinence. A **neurogenic** bladder can also be the reason for incontinence. Neurogenic bladder develops when the nerves associated with control of urination are damaged. Accidents and spinal cord injuries account for some cases of neurogenic incontinence. A herniated disk can interfere with urination. A stroke or cerebrovascular accident, depending upon the type, can cause this problem. Diabetes mellitus, dementia, and Parkinson's disease can also leave a person with incontinence.

Urinary incontinence is a common problem. It is not a natural part of aging, although many elderly people do experience this. Incontinence is caused by one of the factors listed earlier, and these are common problems in older adults. Clients may be hesitant to mention any problem with incontinence, often because of embarrassment. Even if there is only leaking of urine, the client will be concerned about odor and may avoid social gatherings. It is up to the medical assistant to ask clients about this problem. The doctor will order different treatment options depending on the cause. Most treatments involve bladder retraining or other programs. The medical assistant needs to understand the possible causes and be willing to help the client and possibly her family with long-term solutions.

Urinary Retention

A second common urinary problem with varying causes is *urinary retention.* With retention, the bladder does not empty completely. The urine that remains in the bladder can lead to urinary tract infections. Normally, a person feels the urge to void when the bladder reaches a certain fullness. With retention, the person does not feel the urge to void until it is quite full. This can be a result of holding the urine for long periods of time. People do this for many reasons: A child may not want to use the bathroom at school, and will hold the urine until she is able to use the toilet at home, or a toddler may not want to stop playing to go to the bathroom. A person may need assistance to walk to the bathroom and help getting on and off the toilet. She may be hesitant to call for assistance, a caregiver might be available only at certain times, or the client may not want to be a "bother" to others.

An individual with a spinal cord injury may not feel the urge to void because of the nerve damage. This person needs to have a schedule of times for voiding. If left unrelieved for a long time, life-threatening problems could arise.

The doctor will diagnose the problem and cause of urinary retention and prescribe a treatment plan. The medical assistant will work with the client by teaching ways to improve urinary health and behaviors.

■ KIDNEY DISORDERS

Many disorders can affect the kidneys. Some of the most common disorders are discussed in this section.

Pyelitis

Pyelitis is an inflammation of the pelvis of the kidney (Figure 30-4). The renal pelvis is the area of the kidney that funnels or narrows to connect to the ureters. As a result of its position, it can easily succumb to an ascending infection. Quick and effective treatment is necessary to prevent infection of the rest of the kidney and **pyelonephritis.**

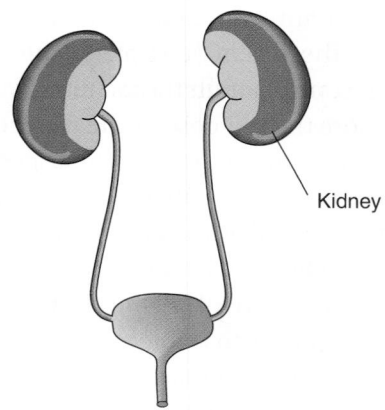

Kidney

FIGURE 30-4 Pyelitis.

Pyelonephritis

In pyelonephritis, the kidneys become inflamed from an infection (Figure 30-5). Pockets of pus form and then burst in the kidneys. Antibiotics are used to cure this condition. Incomplete treatment or repeated infection can turn this acute problem into a chronic condition.

Glomerulonephritis

Glomerulonephritis is the most common disorder of the kidneys. It affects the filtering unit,

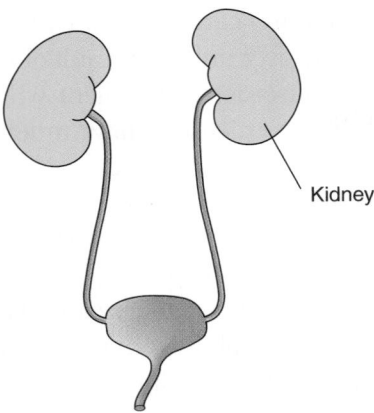

FIGURE 30-5 Pyelonephritis.

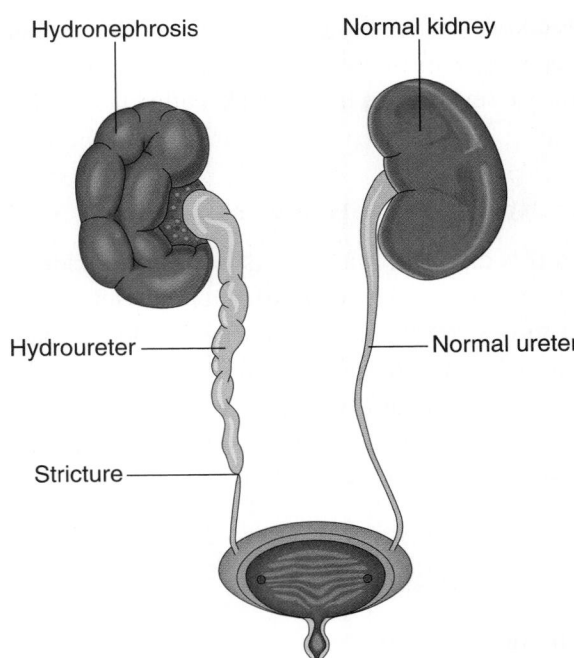

FIGURE 30-6 Hydronephrosis.

the **glomerulus,** of the kidney. A client will complain of back pain, not feeling hungry, and a general feeling of tiredness. The client will have a fever, and the medical assistant may notice that the client's eyelids and ankles are edematous (swollen with retained fluids). The medical assistant will see this most frequently in children and young adults. This usually occurs about one month after the client has recovered from a "strep throat" infection. It can also follow scarlet fever or rheumatic fever. The doctor will order medication to decrease the client's high temperature and will sometimes order antibiotics. Salt, proteins, and fluids may be restricted until healing takes place. Glomerulonephritis can become a chronic condition.

Hydronephrosis

When the kidney becomes blocked, trapped urine can collect in the kidney. This is called *hydronephrosis* (Figure 30-6). Infections, kidney stones, an enlarged prostate, and other conditions can cause such a blockage. The kidney must be unblocked to avoid permanent damage to the organ.

Kidney Stones

The formations commonly called *kidney stones* are actually renal calculi (Figure 30-7). Often the stones are made up of calcium deposits,

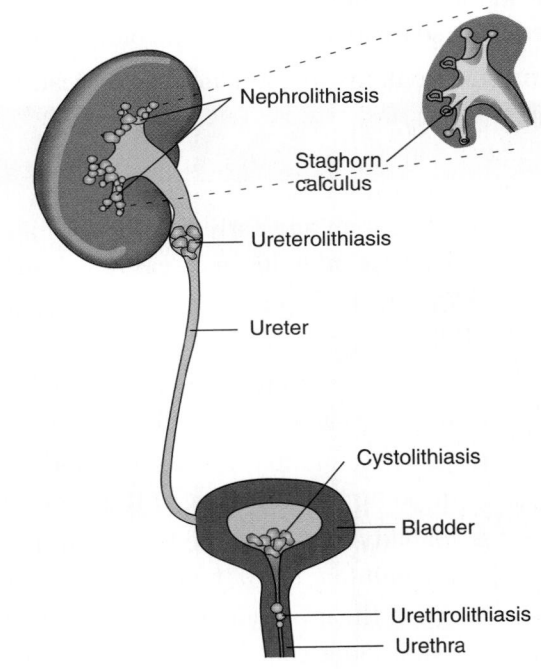

FIGURE 30-7 Types and locations of kidney stones.

although other substances may be included as well. These stones can become positioned, or grow so big, that they interfere with the kidney function. Some small stones will pass out through the urethra with the urine. Others can become stuck along the way. If the stones become stuck in the ureters, the client will experience severe pain in the back, called *flank pain.*

Polycystic Disorder

In this disorder, many cysts form in the kidney, giving it its name: **polycystic** kidney disease. The cysts destroy tissue and enlarge the kidney, leading to renal failure. There is no cure. The medical assistant will help most by offering emotional support, as this is a slow-progressing disease that destroys the kidneys.

Renal Failure

The nephrons are the functioning units of the kidneys. When too many of the nephrons are hurt or injured, the kidneys cannot function. The kidneys cannot filter waste products out of the blood, so toxins build up in the blood. Renal or kidney failure can come on suddenly, or develop slowly over time as a result of other urinary system disorders. The client will have to limit salt intake, measure how much fluid is taken in and how much is excreted (intake and output or I&O), and take medicine as prescribed. Eventually, the client may have to undergo dialysis or a kidney transplant.

When a person's kidneys cannot clean the blood of wastes, a dialysis machine must take over the work of the kidneys. Frequently the client must undergo the dialysis treatment two to three times a week. A common method involves inserting a needle and tube into the client's blood vessel. The client's blood travels through the tube to the dialysis machine, where it is filtered, and then the cleansed blood is returned to the client. The medical assistant will need to offer much support to the client who is undergoing dialysis. This is a long-term treatment, and the client will need to visit the health care facility frequently and indefinitely.

POINTS OF HIGHLIGHT

- Prevention and early treatment of an infection anywhere in the urinary system is critical because infections can easily spread to the other structures in the urinary system.
- Cystitis is an inflammation or infection of the urinary bladder; it can become a chronic disorder.
- Women are more prone to cystitis than men because the female urethra is shorter and bacteria can easily travel the short distance to the urinary bladder.
- An inflammation of the urethra, called urethritis, can result from an ascending (traveling or going up) infection, or it can be a symptom of a sexually transmitted disease.
- Inability to control the flow of urine from the body is called urinary incontinence (involuntary loss). It is not a normal part of aging.
- When the urinary bladder is not emptied completely, urine remains in the bladder. This condition is called urinary retention.
- Glomerulonephritis is the most common disorder of the kidney.
- Renal calculi or kidney stones can cause severe pain.
- Kidney or renal failure results when the nephrons are destroyed and are unable to do their work of filtering wastes and toxins out of the blood. Renal failure can happen suddenly or develop slowly over time.
- Clients of all ages can be affected by urinary disorders.

BRIDGE TO CAAHEP

This chapter, which discusses urinary system disorders, provides information and content related to CAAHEP standards for Anatomy and Physiology, Medical Terminology, Communication, Medical Assisting Clinical Procedures, and Professional Components.

ABHES LINKS

This chapter, which discusses urinary system disorders, links to ABHES course content for Anatomy and Physiology, Medical Terminology, Medical Law and Ethics, and Medical Office Clinical Procedures.

AAMA AREAS OF COMPETENCE

This chapter, which discusses urinary system disorders, provides information or content within several areas listed in the Medical Assistant Role Delineation Study. These areas include: clinical, fundamental principles, patient (client) care, general transdisciplinary, professionalism, communication skills, legal concepts, and instruction.

AMT PATHS

This chapter, which discusses urinary system disorders, provides a path to AMT competency in general medical assisting knowledge, anatomy and physiology, medical terminology, and patient (client) education.

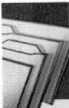
STUDENT PORTFOLIO ACTIVITY

Read professional journals. If possible, subscribe to a journal. Many journals offer reduced student rates. If not, be sure to check out the school library. Select an article that interests you. Read it and then write a thoughtful reflection on the article. Medical assistants need to keep up with current thinking in the health care field. Employers look for individuals who will grow with their profession to meet and lead changes in health care.

APPLYING YOUR SKILLS

Culture often plays a role in determining what topics a person talks about with others and with whom she discusses matters that are considered private. Think of your own cultural group. Are there any cultural reasons why clients from your culture might be hesitant to discuss problems of the urinary system?

CRITICAL THINKING QUESTIONS

1. A client has been diagnosed with a urinary tract infection. Why is it so important for the infection to be diagnosed and treated early and successfully? What complications can happen if the infection is not completely cleared?

2. A client calls complaining of frequency, urgency, and pain when she urinates. What is one of the first steps you should take? Why?

3. Why is cystitis seen more often in females than in males?

4. Why might a client who has kidney stones experience severe flank pain?

5. A client has inflammation of the urethra (urethritis). What other conditions might also be present?

6. What is meant by an ascending infection? Give an example.

7. A client with pyelonephritis does not finish the whole course of an antibiotic treatment. What can happen to this acute condition?

8. What disorders often occur before a client develops glomerulonephritis?

9. Explain what happens when renal calculi develop. What symptoms might a client experience as a result of this process?

10. What happens to the urinary system in renal failure? How will the client's life change?

11. Explain why a client might not ask or tell you about urinary incontinence. As a medical assistant, how do you approach this topic with a client? What do you explain about urinary incontinence?

12. How can dialysis help a client whose kidneys have failed?

13. Go back to the beginning of this chapter and review the Anticipatory Statements. Reread each statement and then indicate whether it is true or false. If the statement is false, rewrite it to make it a true statement.

CLIENT TEACHING PLAN

Prevention of Repeat Urinary Tract Infections

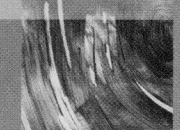

What Is to Be Taught:

- How to reduce the risk of a repeat urinary tract infection.

Objectives:

- Client will be able to list steps to take to prevent a repeat or recurrent urinary tract infection.

Preparation Before Teaching:

- Review the organization and working of the urinary system.
- Review potential complications of a urinary tract infection.
- Remember to put technical medical terms into simple, everyday language that the client can easily understand.
- Look over steps to promote urinary health.
- Get together teaching materials, such as pictures of the structures of the urinary system, paper and pen for written instructions, and any pertinent printed health information.
- Make sure that the area is free from distractions while you are teaching.

Steps for the Medical Assistant:

1. Wash your hands.
2. Gather supplies needed.
3. Introduce yourself to the client.
4. Explain what you are going to teach and why.
5. Describe in simple terms how the urinary system works and what happens when an infection occurs.
6. Show the client the pictures of the urinary structures while describing the system.
7. Tell the client, in a positive manner, that she can take steps to decrease her chances of getting another infection.
8. Inform the client of the risk factors for an urinary tract infection, such as:

   a. age (as a person ages, there is a greater chance of carrying bacteria in the urine).
   b. less acidic urine.
   c. greater chance of uterine or bladder prolapse and pelvic muscle weakening in women and enlarged prostate gland in men (all these can put a person at risk of infection).
   d. inadequate intake of water.
   e. unhealthy bladder practices.
   f. inactivity.

9. Instruct the client that the most important step she can take at this time is to complete the course of treatment prescribed by the doctor. Tell her that if the medication is not taken as directed, the bacteria will not be completely destroyed; they will grow again and the infection will return. If she has any difficulty with the prescribed treatment, she should immediately call the doctor's office.
10. Inform the client that drinking an adequate amount of water helps to keep the urine dilute and rinse out waste products and bacteria.
11. Suggest that the client regularly urinate and not try to go for long periods without urinating.
12. Maintain a reasonable level of physical activity. Prolonged sitting or bedrest predisposes a client to infections.
13. Restrict sugar intake; sugar encourages the growth of bacteria.
14. Take showers instead of baths if there are no factors that would make showers risky for the client.
15. Inform the client of the signs and symptoms of a urinary tract infection. Be sure to provide this information in writing as well. The signs and symptoms that the client should be aware of are: having to urinate more frequently, feelings of urgency or having to get to the bathroom in a hurry, getting up at night to urinate, incontinence (an "accident"). Pain is usually a symptom.

(Continues)

CLIENT TEACHING PLAN (Continued)

16. Instruct the client that if she notices any of these symptoms, or if she thinks that she feels the same as when she had this present infection, she should call the doctor's office.

■ Special Needs of the Client:

- Review the client's chart to see if there are any factors that might interfere with the client's ability to carry out this plan to prevent repeat urinary tract infections.
- Ask the client, before and after the teaching, if there is anything you should know that might affect her ability to take these steps.

■ Evaluation:

- Client is able to list signs and symptoms of a urinary tract infection.
- Client can list the steps she can take to prevent repeat urinary tract infections.

■ Further Plans/Teaching:

- Give the client a specimen container (sterile container). If she notices any signs or symptoms and calls the doctor, she may be asked to obtain a sample of urine and bring it to the office or diagnostic laboratory for testing.
- Ask the client if she has any questions or wants any additional information.

■ Follow-up:

- Call the client at home at the end of one week to see if she has been able to take any of these steps.
- Ask the client if she would like to review any of the information.
- Encourage the client to practice as many of the steps as she can.

Medical Assistant

Name: _____

Signature: _____

Date: _____

Client

Date: _____

Follow-up Date : _____

Anticipatory Statements

People have different ideas about how the male reproductive system works and what is or is not normal. Read and think about the following statements based upon what you believe now. Decide whether you agree or disagree. Write the word **agree** after the statement if you think the statement is true. Write the word **disagree** after the statement if you think the statement is false. Read the chapter to find out if your current beliefs can be supported.

1. The prostate gland enlarges as a male ages.   _____

2. Testicular cancer is never seen in a young male.   _____

3. Sexually transmitted diseases are easily cured and have no long-term effects.   _____

4. As a man ages, it is important that he continue to go for yearly checkups to detect possible prostate problems.   _____

5. Difficulty in urinating may be a sign of a problem with the prostate.   _____

Male Reproductive System Disorders

Learning Objectives

Upon completion of this chapter, the medical assistant student should be able to:

- Identify the medical assistant's role in preparing clients for diagnostic tests of the male reproductive system
- List signs and symptoms of benign prostatic hyperplasia
- State risk factors for cancer of the prostate
- Explain what is meant by sexually transmitted disease
- Define epididymitis, orchitis, and prostatitis
- Develop a teaching plan for a client to recognize abnormal signs in the male reproductive system

Key Terms

benign prostatic hyperplasia (BPH)
Nonmalignant enlargement of the prostate gland.

chancre Painless sore, often on the genitals, cervix, or anus.

epididymis The structure in which sperm cells mature.

genital herpes Sexually transmitted disease that is highly contagious.

genital wart Sexually transmitted condition; frequently reappears after initial treatment.

gonorrhea Common sexually transmitted disease; often seen in teenagers and young adults.

orchitis Inflammation of the testis.

prostate cancer An abnormal, harmful growth of the prostate gland.

tertiary Third order or stage; medical care available only in large health care centers.

testicular cancer Cancer of the testes; most commonly seen in young men.

■ INTRODUCTION

The male reproductive system is closely related to the male urinary system. There is no separate physician specialist for male reproductive disorders. Urologists who treat urinary tract conditions also treat male reproductive disorders.

■ DIAGNOSTIC TESTS

Common diagnostic tests use blood, urine and sperm specimens, biopsies, and ultrasound. Blood specimens are obtained and tested to determine the level of testosterone, the major male hormone, if the client is experiencing *erectile dysfunction* (sexual dysfunction or impotence). Another blood test checks the level of a protein—prostate specific antigen or PSA—in the prostate. The blood sample for this test is obtained before physical examination, because the PSA levels can be affected by palpation of the prostate tissue. The level of PSA will be high if benign prostate hyperplasia (BPH) or prostate cancer is present. It will also be high when the prostate is inflamed (*prostatitis*). Men over the age of 50 should have the PSA test done on a yearly basis.

A rectal examination should be performed by the doctor during the general physical exam of a male client, or whenever the client has symptoms. Doppler ultrasound examination can be done on tissue from the prostate. A small sample can be obtained either through the rectum or the urethra.

In the male, a doughnut-shaped gland called the *prostate* is found just below the urinary bladder. Secretions from the prostate get mixed into the semen, which helps sperm to move around. During *ejaculation,* which is the forceful expulsion of semen, the prostate muscle contracts to force the semen out through the urethra. As a male ages, his prostate gland continues to enlarge. Because the prostate encircles the urethra, it can constrict the urethra when it grows. This enlargement of the prostate is a common condition called **benign prostatic hyperplasia (BPH)** (Figure 31-1). Uncomfort-

able symptoms will prompt the male client to seek medical help. The client cannot completely empty his bladder, and so must urinate often, including several times during the night. It may be difficult to start or continue the urine stream. The doctor will perform a digital rectal examination and order diagnostic laboratory tests to make sure of the diagnosis and rule out cancer. Early treatment may consist of prescription medicine, but often the treatment eventually includes surgery.

■ PROSTATE CANCER

Prostate cancer is a common cancer in men; its incidence increases with the man's age. The highest incidence occurs in men in their 70s. In the early stages of the cancer, there are few symptoms. The symptoms seem to be associated with the urinary system and are similar to those seen in BPH. In addition, the client may experience urgency (the need to urinate quickly after first feeling the urge to void). The client may have blood in the urine (*hematuria*) and pain upon voiding (*dysuria*). The treatment for prostate cancer depends upon the client's health and age and the stage of the cancer. The medical assistant needs to be supportive of the client and his family when the diagnosis is prostate cancer.

Testicular cancer is most common in young men aged 20 through the mid-30s. Symptoms are few, and so by the time it is detected, the cancer has often spread to other areas (*metastasized*). Depending upon the kind of cancer, the treatment is surgery. In addition to young age, risk factors include Caucasian race, history of mother using oral contraceptives or diethylstilbestrol (DES) during pregnancy, marriage later in life, or sexual inactivity. Because there are so few symptoms, it is important to find the lumps that signal cancer early. The medical assistant should instruct the male client on the steps for performing a testicular self-examination (TSE) (Figure 31-2). Men should examine their own testes each month starting at the age of puberty.

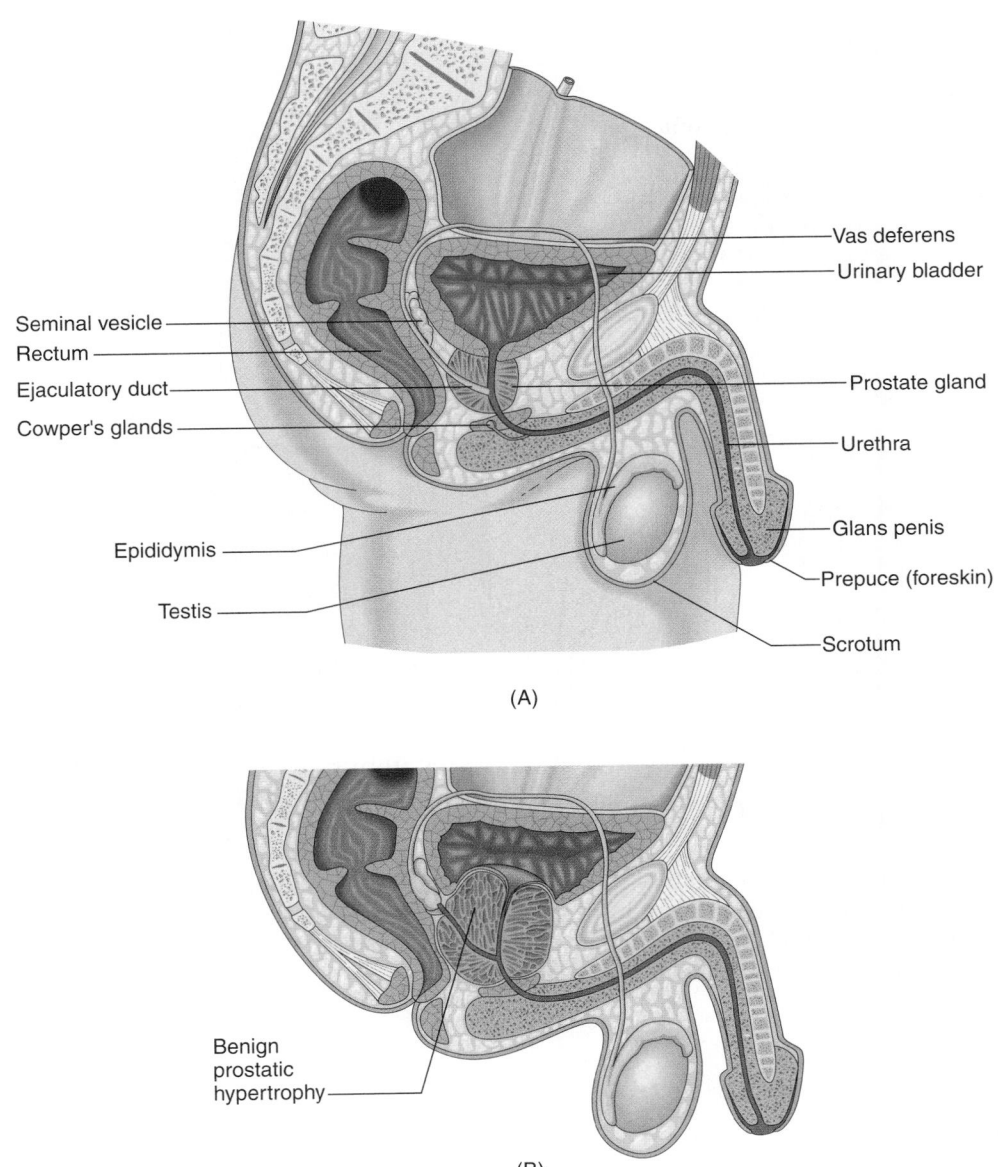

Seminal vesicle
Rectum
Ejaculatory duct
Cowper's glands

Epididymis

Testis

Vas deferens
Urinary bladder

Prostate gland

Urethra

Glans penis

Prepuce (foreskin)

Scrotum

(A)

Benign
prostatic
hypertrophy

(B)

FIGURE 31–1 (A) Normal prostate. (B) Enlarged prostate.

■ INFLAMMATION OR INFECTIONS OF THE MALE REPRODUCTIVE SYSTEM

Inflammation or infection can affect the tissue and organs of the male reproductive system. *Epididymitis* is an inflammation of the **epididymis,** a very small organ attached to the testes. Sperm mature in the epididymis. Several different organisms can cause this inflammation. The client will complain of pain and may

have difficulty walking. Medication, ice packs, and scrotal support are usually ordered.

The testes can also become inflamed. This condition is called **orchitis.** Orchitis can occur after mumps, other infection, or injury. The client will complain of pain and swelling of the scrotum.

Prostatitis is an inflammation of the prostate gland. The condition can be acute or chronic. Acute prostatitis may result from a urinary tract infection that spreads upward

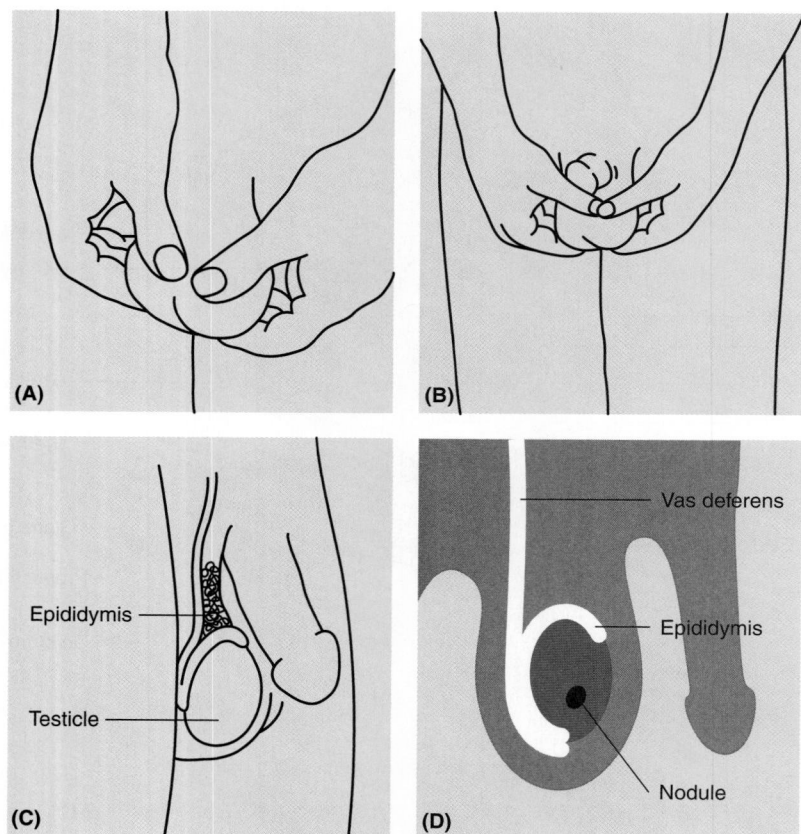

FIGURE 31–2 Testicular self-examination should be performed once a month, after a warm bath or shower. **(A)** Stand in front of a mirror and inspect the scrotum. Look for swelling. **(B)** Examine each testicle, using both hands. Roll each testicle between your thumbs and fingers. **(C)** Feel for the epididymis. **(D)** If you find a lump, contact your doctor right away.

(ascending urinary tract infection). Chronic prostatitis can occur if acute prostatitis was not completely cured. If acute prostatitis does not completely resolve with medical treatment, the condition can recur and become chronic.

■ SEXUALLY TRANSMITTED DISEASES

Sexually transmitted diseases (STDs) are a group of diseases that are spread through intimate or sexual contact. Blood, semen, and vaginal secretion, as well as infected skin and sores, are the sources that can spread the disease when another person comes into contact with them.

Contact with an infected person usually happens during oral, anal, or vaginal sexual activity. The causative agent may be the same, but the effects differ in males and females. People can prevent or avoid STDs by not having intimate contact with infected persons, persons whose sexual history is not known, or multiple sexual partners; having more than one partner increases the risk of contracting an infection. Condoms help to lessen the spread of these diseases. Treatment includes treating the client's sexual partners as well as the infected client. If the partners are not treated, the infection could be passed back and forth or given to new or different partners.

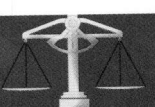

LEGAL/ETHICAL THOUGHTS

Cultural beliefs and family background may affect the client's comfort level when discussing sexual concerns, and may also govern with whom a client will discuss these matters. Be sensitive and professional.

Genital Herpes

Genital herpes is caused by a virus and is extremely contagious. Herpes simplex virus type I causes cold sores around the mouth. It is closely related to the herpes simplex II virus that causes genital herpes. Oral or anal sex and vaginal intercourse all spread the virus. Additionally, hands that touch an infected area and then touch mucous membranes can spread either virus. In a male, blisters may appear on the inner thigh, scrotum, shaft of the penis, or the glans penis (Figure 31-3). The blisters are very painful. This disease is not curable, though medications are available to lessen the severity and frequency of outbreaks.

Genital Warts

Genital warts are caused by a virus. In the male, warts are found along the penile shaft, on the head of the penis, or around the anus. The warts may be single or grouped together. Size will vary. The warts are chemically or surgically removed.

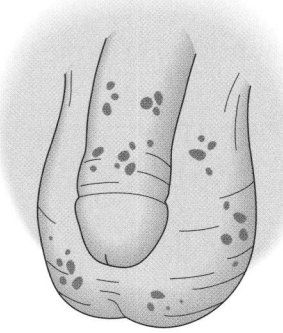

FIGURE 31-3 Genital herpes.

Gonorrhea

Gonorrhea is a common sexually transmitted disease, also known as the "clap." The male client may come to the office complaining of thick, colored discharge from the penis, as well as frequency and pain upon urination. Antibiotics are used to treat gonorrhea. Treatment is critical because if left untreated, systemic infection can occur and can be fatal. Additionally, if untreated, the male could develop arthritis as a result of the STD. Sterility is also common with untreated gonorrhea.

Syphilis

Syphilis is a sexually transmitted disease that quickly turns into a systemic disorder. If caught early, it is easily treated. Antibiotics are used to cure syphilis. If the infection is not halted, the client will progress through three stages. In the primary stage, the client will usually see a **chancre** on the head of the penis (Figure 31-4). The chancre is highly contagious, but will eventually disappear even without treatment. The client may believe that he is cured, but the disorder is actually progressing. Anywhere up to one year later, the client will enter the secondary stage, in which a highly contagious rash appears anywhere on the body. The rash may be misdiagnosed at this stage. A diagnosis is based upon a blood specimen. The third stage, **tertiary** syphilis, can affect many organs outside of the reproductive system. The brain and nervous system are frequently involved. Syphilis can also be spread to an infant; in this instance it is called *congenital syphilis*.

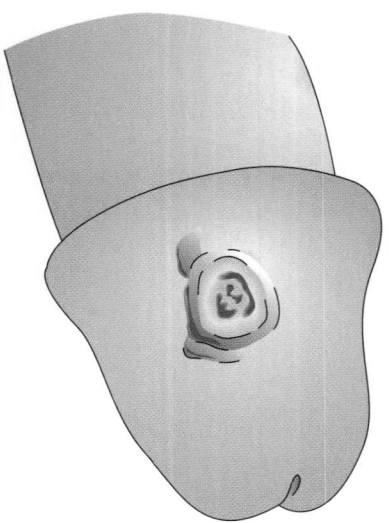

FIGURE 31-4 Syphilis chancre.

BRIDGE TO CAAHEP

This chapter, which discusses male reproductive system disorders, provides information and content related to CAAHEP standards for Anatomy and Physiology, Medical Terminology, Medical Law and Ethics, Communication, Medical Assisting Clinical Procedures, and Professional Components.

ABHES LINKS

This chapter, which discusses male reproductive system disorders, links to ABHES course content for Anatomy and Physiology, Medical Terminology, Medical Law and Ethics, and Medical Office Clinical Procedures.

AAMA AREAS OF COMPETENCE

This chapter, which discusses male reproductive system disorders, provides information or content within several areas listed in the Medical Assistant Role Delineation Study. These areas include: clinical, fundamental principles, diagnostic orders, patient (client) care, general transdisciplinary, professionalism, communication skills, legal concepts, and instruction.

POINTS OF HIGHLIGHT

- The male reproductive system and the urinary system are closely related.
- Prostate specific antigen, usually called PSA, is a protein produced by the tissue in the prostate gland. The PSA test, which uses a blood sample to look for elevated levels of the protein, is used for detection of cancer and to monitor treatment of cancer.
- As the male ages, the prostate gland continues to enlarge. This prostatic enlargement is called benign prostatic hyperplasia or BPH.
- Prostate cancer is a common cancer in men. The incidence rate increases with age; the highest incidence is in males in their 70s.
- Testicular cancer is most common in young men.
- Men should perform a testicular self-examination monthly, beginning at the time of puberty.
- Inflammation or infection of the tissues or organs in the male reproductive system must be diagnosed and treated effectively. If they are not, these acute problems can become chronic disorders.
- Epididymitis, orchitis, and prostatitis all involve inflammation of the tissues and organs in the male reproductive system.
- Sexually transmitted diseases include genital herpes, genital warts, syphilis, and gonorrhea. STDs are spread through sexual contact.

AMT PATHS

This chapter, which discusses male reproductive system disorders, provides a path to AMT competency in general medical assisting knowledge, anatomy and physiology, medical terminology, and patient (client) education.

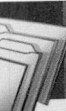 ### STUDENT PORTFOLIO ACTIVITY

The medical assistant is a multiskilled professional. Employers are more or less familiar with the many roles of the medical assistant. However, to make this idea easier for others to visualize (and for yourself, especially in preparation for job interviews), draw a diagram that looks like a spider. Medical assisting is written in the center of the page, as the "spider's" body, with lines extending out to the sides like the spider's legs. On each of the "legs," write one or two words to describe each of the functions or skills of a medical assistant.

 ### APPLYING YOUR SKILLS

The doctor has ordered a PSA blood test for a client. The client states that he does not have any problems, and asks why he needs to have his blood taken. As a medical assistant, what would you tell him about the PSA test and preventive health care?

CRITICAL THINKING QUESTIONS

1. A 60-year-old male comes to the office complaining that he has to get up frequently at night to urinate and that he has trouble starting the stream of urine. The doctor then performs an examination of the prostate. What relationship does the prostate have to the urinary system?

2. Explain how the male urinary system is related to the reproductive system.

3. If a man has problematic symptoms in his reproductive system, with what medical specialist might he make an appointment?

4. What should a male client know about testicular cancer?

5. What steps can a man take to decrease the chance of testicular cancer not being detected until it has spread?

6. Testosterone is the major male hormone, the effects of which are first seen at puberty. What can happen if the testosterone levels are too low? How will the doctor check this?

7. A client asks why he needs to do a testicular self-examination when he is only 25 years old. What do you explain?

8. Why are mumps in an adult male very serious? What are some possible complications?

9. What symptoms might a client with epididymitis experience?

10. If a client does not complete a course of antibiotic treatment, what can develop from acute prostatitis?

11. The doctor asks you to do health teaching with a young male client about sexually transmitted diseases. What do you say? How do you approach this client?

12. Identify symptoms that are associated with gonorrhea. What are potential complications if this STD is left untreated?

13. Go back to the beginning of this chapter and review the Anticipatory Statements. Reread each statement and then indicate whether it is true or false. If the statement is false, rewrite it to make it a true statement.

CLIENT TEACHING PLAN

Recognition of Abnormal Signs in the Male Reproductive System

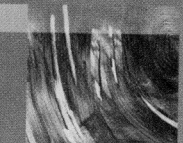

What Is to Be Taught:

- Recognition of symptoms that may indicate a problem with the male reproductive system and that should be reported to the doctor.

Objectives:

- Client will be able to identify symptoms that may indicate a problem with the male reproductive system.
- Client is aware that these symptoms should be reported.

Preparation Before Teaching:

- Review information about the structure and functioning of the male reproductive system, including common disorders. Remember to put technical medical terms into simple, everyday language that the client can easily understand.
- Get pictures of the male reproductive system, if possible, to assist in your teaching.
- Get together teaching materials, such as paper and pen for note taking and written instructions, and any printed educational materials available in your office.
- Make sure the area is free from distractions while you are teaching.

Steps for the Medical Assistant:

1. Wash your hands.
2. Gather supplies needed.
3. Introduce yourself to the client.
4. Explain what you are going to teach and why.
5. Tell the client that by understanding some facts about the male reproductive system, he can take an active role in preventive health care.
6. Explain that the male urinary system is closely related to the reproductive system and that a healthy urinary system will also help in achieving a healthy reproductive system.
7. Review both systems using diagrams and pictures.

8. Tell the client that the following are possible symptoms of a problem with the male reproductive system:
   a. The need to urinate frequently and/or urgently. Explain that this means that he feels he has to urinate more often than usual, and has to void right away, without waiting.
   b. The involuntary loss of urine (incontinence).
   c. Pain during urination.
   d. An increase in size or swelling of any reproductive structures. (The client should be aware of his organs and what is normal for him; refer to testicular self-examination.)
   e. Pain in any of the reproductive or urinary structures.
   f. Sexual dysfunction.
9. Instruct the client that if he has any of these signs or symptoms, or if something just doesn't seem right, he should contact his doctor.
10. Emphasize to the client that some male reproductive disorders have no symptoms until the disorder is far advanced. Some disorders can be detected only through an examination by a doctor or through laboratory tests. Even if the client has no symptoms, he should see his doctor regularly to help maintain optimal health.
11. Hand the client written information to use as a reference at home.

Special Needs of the Client:

- Look at the client's chart to see if there is any factor that might interfere with the client's ability to understand and follow these instructions.
- Ask the client, before and after teaching, if there is anything you should know about his ability to understand and use this information.

Evaluation:

- Client will list the symptoms that he should be aware of.

(Continues)

CLIENT TEACHING PLAN (Continued)

- Client is able to state that he will call the doctor if he becomes aware of any of these symptoms.

■ Further Plans/Teaching:

- Provide written information about the structure and functioning of the male urinary system and the male reproductive system, including signs and symptoms to watch for.

■ Follow-up:

- At the next office visit, review with the client the signs and symptoms to recognize.

Medical Assistant

Name: _____

Signature: _____

Date: _____

Client

Date: _____

Follow-up Date : _____

Anticipatory Statements

People have different ideas about the female reproductive system, how it works, and what can go wrong with the system. Read and think about the following statements based upon what you believe now. Decide whether you agree or disagree. Write the word **agree** after the statement if you think the statement is true. Write the word **disagree** after the statement if you think the statement is false. Read the chapter to find out if your current beliefs can be supported.

1. After menopause, women should continue to do monthly breast self-examinations. _____

2. The risk of breast cancer in women decreases with age. _____

3. Repeated episodes of sexually transmitted diseases can hurt a female's ability to conceive and give birth to children. _____

4. After menopause, a woman does not need to have a Pap test. _____

5. Lack of estrogen may cause vaginal secretions to lessen and the skin around the vagina to become dry and fragile. _____

Female Reproductive System Disorders

Learning Objectives

Upon completion of this chapter, the medical assistant student should be able to:

■ Identify the medical assistant's role in preparing a client for diagnostic tests of the female reproductive system

■ List the signs and symptoms of toxic shock syndrome

■ Explain premenstrual syndrome

■ Describe pelvic inflammatory disease

■ List ways to ease the discomforts of menopause

■ State risk factors for development of breast cancer

■ Explain the menstrual cycle

■ Develop a teaching plan to teach a client healthy feminine hygiene practices

Key Terms

cystocele Condition in which the bladder protrudes into the vagina.

dysmenorrhea Moderate or intense pain during the menstrual blood flow.

endometriosis Tissue that looks like the endometrium but is located outside of the uterus.

menopause End of a female's menstrual cycles and reproductive years.

menorrhagia Excessive bleeding during the menstrual flow.

metrorrhagia Bleeding between menstrual flow periods.

pelvic inflammatory disease (PID) Infection of the pelvic organs.

premenstrual syndrome (PMS) Symptoms that occur in some women about one week before the menstrual flow; may include bloating, breast tenderness, irritability, weight gain, and headaches.

prolapsed uterus Uterus that protrudes downward.

rectocele Condition in which the rectum protrudes into the vagina.

■ INTRODUCTION

The female reproductive system is a complex system that changes with a woman over time. Some changes can be normal; others are signs of a disorder. The study of the female reproductive system structure, function, and disorders is called *gynecology*. A *gynecologist* is a doctor who works in this area of medicine.

■ DIAGNOSTIC TESTS

The medical assistant takes part in preparing clients for and assisting the doctor with diagnostic tests of the female reproductive system. The medical assistant provides emotional support during many of these procedures.

Pelvic Examination

Commonly called a gyn exam (pronounced *gee-why-en*), a pelvic examination involves examining a woman's external genitalia and internal structures. Beginning after puberty, every woman should have an annual pelvic examination, which includes a Pap smear (Papanicolaou test) every one to three years to detect cervical cancer. The frequency of the Pap test depends upon several factors.

To prepare the client, the medical assistant asks the client to go into the bathroom and empty her bladder. Often a urine specimen is needed, so the medical assistant should check the doctor's orders in advance. The client takes off all her clothing and puts on a gown. (Whether the gown opens in the front or the back is decided by the doctor.) The client then sits on the examination table until the doctor comes in to perform the exam.

The instruments and supplies needed for a gynecological examination should be assembled beforehand, according to office policy and the doctor's preference. When the doctor comes in to perform the examination, the medical assistant remains in the room and gives emotional support to the client, in addition to assisting the doctor. When the doctor completes the examination, the medical assistant helps the client to get her feet out of the stirrups and sit up out of the lithotomy position. Tell the client to remain seated on the edge of the table for a minute before standing up, to avoid dizziness and fainting. This is especially important with elderly clients whose blood pressure and circulation may take longer to return to normal after a position change. A pregnant client may also need assistance, as the center of gravity and balance changes with pregnancy.

Breast Examination

A breast examination by the doctor should be part of the annual gynecological examination. This is in addition to the monthly breast self-exams performed by the client. The first part of the exam should be done with the client sitting on the exam table. The second portion of the breast examination is then done with the client lying down. The medical assistant should remain in the room to ease any client concerns. The client's privacy must be guarded at all times.

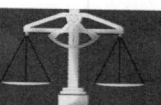

LEGAL/ETHICAL THOUGHTS

Although medical assistants are used to seeing the undressed body when caring for clients, clients must be draped to expose only what is necessary for the procedure. This is done out of respect for the client and deference to the client's desire for modesty.

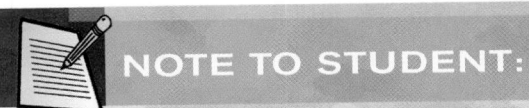

NOTE TO STUDENT:

The medical assistant must always be considerate of and aware of the client's feelings. Age and cultural differences will affect the client's ease and comfort with testing and gynecological procedures.

■ MENSTRUAL CYCLE CONCERNS

Many factors can affect the menstrual cycle. Hormones can change the frequency and amount of bleeding. Stress, birth control medications, and birth control devices can also affect the menstrual cycle. The medical assistant must be able to recognize common disorders of the menstrual cycle.

Amenorrhea

Amenorrhea is the absence of menses or bleeding. A female does not bleed before the start of puberty or after menopause. If a female still has amenorrhea (has not begun her menstrual cycles) by the age of 15, the doctor may order tests to find out why. A problem with hormone secretion or levels may be the cause. **Menopause** marks the end of the menstrual cycles and a woman's reproductive years. A client who experiences bleeding after menopause should talk to the doctor to discover the cause; bleeding is not normal at this point. A woman also experiences amenorrhea during pregnancy, but the menstrual cycle should resume after the birth of the baby. A female who has anorexia nervosa or high levels of stress for an extended period of time will experience changes in the levels of hormones, resulting in amenorrhea. Athletes with very low body fat content, such as marathon runners, may also experience amenorrhea for some time.

Irregular menstrual cycles may affect women throughout the years of reproductive capability. When a girl first reaches puberty, the menstrual cycles may be irregular, meaning that the time between monthly blood flows is not equal. For example, the monthly menstrual blood flow may come every 28 days for a few months, then extend to 31 or 32 days, then go back to 28 days. The flow of blood may be heavy or scant. If the irregularity lasts for a long time or is very irregular, tests can be ordered to discover the cause. The medical assistant should instruct each female client to keep a calendar of her cycles, marking the start day and end day and noting whether the flow was heavy or light.

Dysmenorrhea

Dysmenorrhea means painful or difficult menstrual periods. It is very common for women to experience pain or cramping during the days of the menstrual flow. Some women experience quite a lot of cramping for the first day or two. Others feel discomfort throughout all the days of the blood flow. Eating a healthful diet and exercising regularly seems to lessen the severity of cramping. Resting, drinking warm liquids, and taking over-the-counter (OTC) medications as directed may also relieve the pain. If menstrual pain keeps a woman from carrying out her daily activities, she needs to discuss this with the doctor. People experience pain differently, and pain during menstruation is no exception. The medical assistant should ask the client to keep a diary noting the amount of pain and what remedies helped to ease that pain. It is helpful if the client brings the diary with her on follow-up visits.

Menorrhagia

Menorrhagia is heavier-than-normal bleeding during the menstrual flow. In some cases menorrhagia can lead to anemia, because of the excessive blood loss. There are various reasons for and causes of this condition. The medical assistant should teach the client to recognize what is normal for her. The client should be aware of how many days the flow usually lasts, and how heavy the flow is. The client can figure out the amount of blood flowing by noting how many changes of tampons or pads are needed in a 24-hour period. The absorbency number of the pad or tampon should also be noted. Any concerns about heavy bleeding should be brought to the doctor's attention.

Metrorrhagia

When a woman bleeds between the menstrual periods, she has a condition called **metrorrhagia.** This is not normal; the client needs to seek medical help to discover the cause and correct the problem.

Toxic Shock Syndrome

Although *toxic shock syndrome* (TSS) is not a disorder of the menstrual cycle, it is related to the use of tampons during menstruation. A bacterial toxin causes the problem. The menstrual blood remains in the tampon inside the warm, dark body cavity, providing an excellent environment for bacterial growth. The client who develops TSS will have a fever, nausea, and vomiting, and may feel dizzy. If not diagnosed and treated, the symptoms could worsen and the client could die.

The number of TSS cases overall has decreased, as manufactures have made tampons less absorbent and included material that hinders the growth of bacteria. The medical assistant should teach the client ways to prevent toxic shock syndrome. The client must wash her hands thoroughly when inserting or changing a tampon. Tampons should be changed frequently and not pushed to the limit of their absorbency. If the client cannot remove a tampon, she must seek medical help quickly. Because pads are situated outside the body, TSS does not occur in women who use sanitary napkins.

Premenstrual Syndrome

Premenstrual syndrome or **PMS** is common. The symptoms begin one to two weeks before the menstrual flow and end with the beginning of the menstrual flow. People commonly think of PMS only as moodiness and irritably. However, these are only two symptoms of many possible with this disorder: The client may also retain fluid, gain weight, and have abdominal distention and backaches. Headaches are another frequent symptom.

Menopause

Menopause is the end of menstruation in a woman's life and the end of her reproductive years. As the woman ages, her body stops secreting the hormones estrogen and progesterone. The woman no longer ovulates or has menstrual periods. This is a normal part of life, not an illness or disorder. However, many women experience discomfort and health concerns at this time.

The most common symptom associated with menopause is hot flashes. A woman may suddenly begin to perspire, feel her heart racing, and experience tiredness, in addition to feeling extremely overheated. Most hot flashes subside quickly, but they may occur frequently. Women may feel embarrassed when this happens in front of others, and the problem may even disturb her sleep at night. (Other sleep disturbances due to menopause may also occur.) Women can feel differently about menopause. A woman's attitude toward what is happening to her body, and what menopause means to her lifestyle and aging process, can directly affect her health.

Vaginal Dryness

Vaginal dryness is another common symptom of menopause. This may cause a woman to experience pain with sexual intercourse. The dryness may even cause discomfort during exercise such as running or walking.

■ INFLAMMATORY DISORDERS

Vaginitis is an inflammation of the vagina. The inflammation can be caused by a yeast infection. Low estrogen levels during menopause cause a loss of moisture and secretions in the vagina. This loss can lead to extreme dryness and susceptibility to irritation and inflammation. Treatment of the condition will depend on the cause.

Pelvic Inflammatory Disease

Pelvic inflammatory disease (PID) is a serious infection of the ovaries, oviducts, uterus, and pelvic cavity. The client will come to the office complaining of lower abdominal pain and nausea and vomiting. The client will have a fever and a foul-smelling vaginal discharge. It is critical that the infection be identified and treated properly, because this acute infection can develop into a chronic infection. Chronic infection can in turn lead to sterility; that is, an inability to become pregnant and have children. Sterility is caused by scar tissue that forms in the fallopian tubes after infection.

Endometriosis

Endometriosis is a condition in which endometrial tissue is found outside of the uterus. It may be located on any of the organs in the abdominal or pelvic cavity. This happens more frequently in women who have never given birth. The client will complain of pain or pelvic pressure and dysmenorrhea. Pregnancy often relieves this condition. Medications may also decrease the symptoms. Extreme and chronic cases of endometriosis may require surgical intervention. The medical assistant will need to provide much emotional support to a woman who is experiencing this disorder.

Ovarian Cyst

Ovarian cysts are growths or tumors in an ovary (Figure 32-1). These cysts, which are fluid-filled sacs, enlarge and can often be felt during an examination. Sometimes there are no symptoms connected with the cyst. However, in some cases the client experiences pain and a change in the amount of menstrual blood flow (heavier or lighter). Ovarian cysts are usually removed surgically.

Fibroid tumors are also called *uterine tumors* (Figure 32-2). Ovarian hormones stimulate the growth of these tumors, which tend to occur after the woman reaches the age of 30. The client may experience heaviness in the pelvic area, abnormal bleeding, or excessive bleeding during

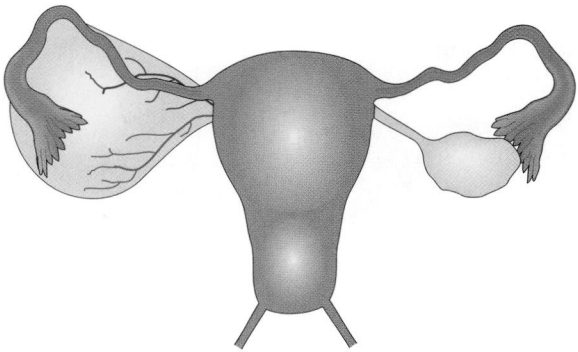

FIGURE 32-1 Ovarian cyst.

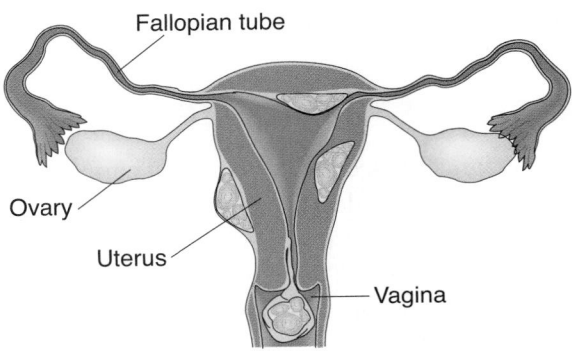

FIGURE 32-2 Fibroid tumors.

the menstrual flow. Depending on their location, these tumors may cause infertility or excessive bleeding at the time of delivery of a child.

■ DISORDERS OF ORGAN STRUCTURE

The pelvic muscles support the internal female reproductive organs. If anything affects the ability of the muscles to give support, the internal structures may be displaced and sag (move downward in the body). Cystocele, rectocele, and prolapsed uterus are three conditions that can result. A **cystocele** occurs when the urinary bladder sags downward into the vagina. A **rectocele** occurs when the rectum moves downward into the vagina. A **prolapsed uterus** has descended into the vagina (Figure 32-3). A client who has a prolapsed uterus often has a cystocele and a rectocele at the same time (Figure 32-4). Causes can include multiple pregnancies, perineal tearing during childbirth, and weakening of the muscles with aging.

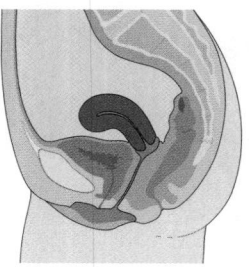 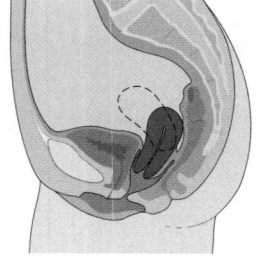 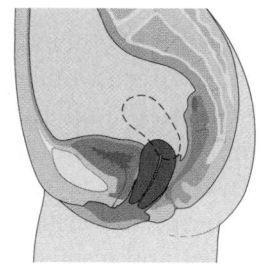 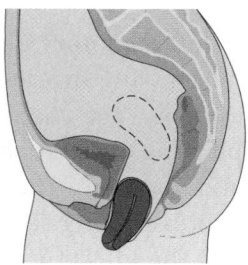

Normal uterus   First-degree prolapse   Second-degree prolapse   Third-degree prolapse

FIGURE 32–3 Prolapse of the uterus.

Depending on the severity of the condition, medical or surgical treatment will be needed.

■ BREAST CANCER

Breast cancer is second only to lung cancer as a cause of cancer deaths in women. However, early detection and treatment can lead to a very positive outcome. The risk of breast cancer increases with age, and certain other factors also put a woman at greater risk. A woman who has never had children, or who has given birth after the age of 35, is at increased risk. Starting the menstrual cycles (*menarche*) before the age of 11, or entering menopause after the age of 50, are also risk factors for breast cancer. A family history of breast cancer increases a woman's risk. Long-term use of oral contraceptives has been associated with breast cancer.

Some risk factors cannot be changed; others can be modified to decrease or eliminate the risk. Obesity and a diet high in fats and protein

have been associated with breast cancer. The medical assistant needs to work with female clients to encourage healthful eating and to help them increase the level of physical activity or exercise in their lives.

Breast cancer risk increases with age; the highest incidence is in women in their 70s. The medical assistant needs to explain and reinforce the importance of breast self-examinations, mammograms, and clinical examinations by the doctor even after menopause. Some women feel that it is not necessary to have gynecologic examinations and breast examinations after menopause, but the risk of cancer does not disappear because a woman can no longer have children.

Breast cancer develops quietly, in a subtle manner. This is one reason that a thorough breast self-examination should be done monthly. The medical assistant should teach the client what to look for during the examination. There are signs and symptoms that the woman needs to be aware of and follow up on if found.

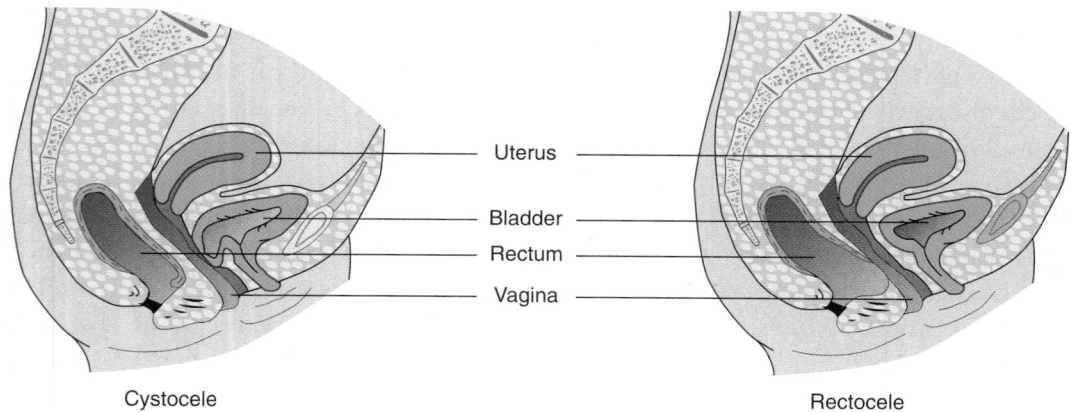

Uterus
Bladder
Rectum
Vagina

Cystocele   Rectocele

FIGURE 32–4 Cystocele and rectocele.

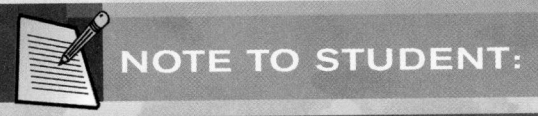

PROCEDURE

32-1

Breast Examination Assistance

Student Competency Objective: The medical assistant student will assist the doctor to do a breast examination on a female client.

Items Needed: Gown, drapes, paper and pen for notes and any instructions

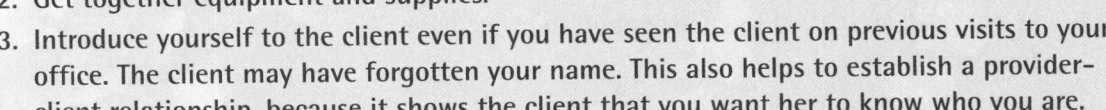

NOTE TO STUDENT:

The breast examination is usually done first at the annual visit to the gynecologist. It is followed by the pelvic examination.

Steps:

1. Wash hands
2. Get together equipment and supplies.
3. Introduce yourself to the client even if you have seen the client on previous visits to your office. The client may have forgotten your name. This also helps to establish a provider-client relationship, because it shows the client that you want her to know who you are.
4. Identify the client. Ask the client to state her name to establish that this is the right client, and then compare the name given to the name on the chart. Never enter a room and call out a client's name to determine if this person is the correct client. The client may not have heard you clearly and may just nod, smile, or answer yes. Clients almost never question if the medical assistant professional has the right client. It is up to the medical assistant to identify the right client before performing any procedure.
5. Tell the client, in everyday language, what you are going to do.
6. Ask if the client has any questions. If she does, give short and simple answers. Sometimes clients will start (and continue) talking because they are nervous about the procedure.
7. Ask the client to remove her clothing from the waist up.
8. Ask the client to put on the gown with the opening in front.
9. Help the client with buttons, zippers and undressing as needed.
10. Ask the client to sit at the end of the examination table.
11. When the doctor has completed examining the breasts with the client sitting, position the client supine on the table.
12. Drape the client as needed.
13. When the examination is finished, help the client into a sitting position.
14. Ask the client if she has any questions. The medical assistant should teach or review the steps for breast self-examination with the client.
15. Ask the client to dress and help her as needed.
16. Record the procedure in the client's medical record.

Charting Example:

9/12/20xx   1:45 P.M.   Assisted doctor with breast examination of client in sitting and supine positions. Reviewed breast self-examination steps with client.

Susan M. Smith, S.M.A.

Susan M. Smith, S.M.A. (printed name)

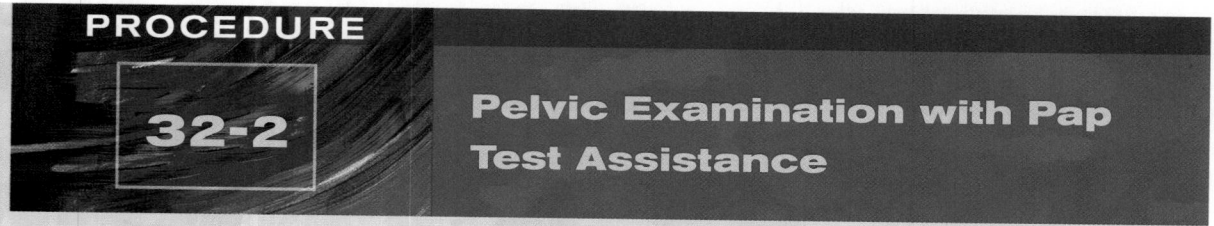

PROCEDURE 32-2 — Pelvic Examination with Pap Test Assistance

Student Competency Objective: The medical assistant student will assist the doctor with a pelvic examination, including a Pap test.

Items Needed: Gown, drape, water-soluble lubricant, vaginal speculum (correct size), gloves, exam light, cleansing wipes, uterine sponge forceps, cervical spatula, lab slips, labels, fixative

Steps:

1. Set up the examination room according to office policy.
2. Wash your hands.
3. Get together equipment and supplies.
4. Introduce yourself to the client even if you have seen the client on previous visits to your office. The client may have forgotten your name. This also helps to establish a provider-client relationship, because it shows the client that you want her to know who you are.
5. Identify the client. Ask the client to state her name to establish that this is the right client, and then compare the name given to the name on the chart. Never enter a room and call out a client's name to determine if this person is the correct client. The client may not have heard you clearly and may just nod, smile, or answer yes. Clients almost never question if the medical assistant professional has the right client. It is up to the medical assistant to identify the right client before performing any procedure.
6. Tell the client, in everyday language, what you are going to do.
7. Ask if the client has any questions. If she does, give short and simple answers. Sometimes clients will start (and continue) talking because they are nervous about the procedure.
8. Ask the client to empty her bladder and collect a urine specimen if needed (remember to check unless a urine sample is routinely collected at all visits).
9. Hand the client a drape and instruct her to remove all clothing from the waist down.
10. Assist the client to sit at the end of the examination table.
11. Adjust the drape on the client.
12. Talk with the client to reassure her.
13. When the doctor is ready, position the client in the lithotomy position, with her buttocks at edge of the table and her feet in the stirrups.
14. Pass instruments to the doctor in the correct order.
15. Help with the Pap smear by covering the slide with fixative and labeling the slide.
16. Tell the client when the doctor is going to take out the speculum and do a manual exam.
17. Hold the basin for the used speculum.
18. Squeeze water-soluble lubricant on the doctor's gloved fingers.
19. Instruct client to breathe deeply and slowly; this will relax the muscles.
20. Take the client's feet out of the stirrups when the doctor is finished.

(Continues)

PROCEDURE 32-2 (Continued)

21. Assist the client to a sitting position.
22. Give the client wipes to remove any excess lubricant; assist as needed.
23. Ask the client if she has any questions.
24. Help the client to get off the examination table, and assist with dressing as needed.
25. Complete processing for transportation of specimen to the lab.
26. Clean, disinfect, or discard equipment and supplies as required.
27. Clean the exam room.
28. Remove your gloves.
29. Wash your hands.
30. Record the procedure in the client's medical record.

Charting Example:
After a routine pelvic examination with Pap test, you would record the following:

9/12/20xx   1:45 P.M.   Assisted doctor with pelvic examination. Pap smear obtained and sent to lab.

Susan M. Smith, S.M.A.

Susan M. Smith, S.M.A.(printed name)

POINTS OF HIGHLIGHT

- Gynecology is the study of female reproductive system structures, functions, and disorders.
- From the onset of puberty, every woman should have a yearly pelvic examination.
- A woman should do a breast self-examination every month.
- It is very common for a woman to experience dysmenorrhea or pain during the menstrual flow.
- Toxic shock syndrome has been related to the use of tampons. Washing hands and changing tampons frequently can decrease the risk of TSS.
- The symptoms of premenstrual syndrome can begin one to two weeks before the menstrual flow.
- Menopause is the end of menstruation, and marks the end of the reproductive years for a woman. It is a normal part of life, not an illness.
- Pelvic inflammatory disease is a serious infection and can lead to sterility.
- Monthly breast self-examinations and periodic mammograms can help detect breast cancer.

BRIDGE TO CAAHEP

This chapter concerning the female reproductive system disorders provides information or content related to CAAHEP Standards for Anatomy and Physiology, Medical Law and Ethics, Medical Terminology, Communication, Medical Assisting Clinical Procedures, and Professional Components.

ABHES LINKS

This chapter, which discusses female reproductive system disorders, links to ABHES course content for Anatomy and Physiology, Medical Terminology, Medical Law and Ethics, and Medical Office Clinical Procedures.

AAMA AREAS OF COMPETENCE

This chapter, which discusses female reproductive system disorders, provides information or content within several areas listed in the Medical Assistant Role Delineation Study. These areas include: clinical, fundamental principles, diagnostic orders, patient (client) care, general transdisciplinary, professionalism, communication skills, legal concepts, and instruction.

AMT PATHS

This chapter, which discusses female reproductive system disorders, provides a path to AMT competency for general medical assisting knowledge, anatomy and physiology, medical terminology, and patient (client) education.

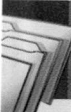

STUDENT PORTFOLIO ACTIVITY

Review the competencies of an entry-level medical assistant. Choose one area and think of an activity that would illustrate an understanding of and competency in the particular skill. Be creative as you decide how to document this competency.

APPLYING YOUR SKILLS

A woman who is past menopause states that she cannot remember when to do breast self-examinations now that she does not have menstrual periods. She explains that she used to coordinate the timing of the monthly exams with her cycles. She continues by saying that it probably does not matter, because only younger women get breast cancer. In your role as a medical assistant, what would you tell her about risk factors for breast cancer? What suggestions can you make to help her remember to do the exams?

CRITICAL THINKING QUESTIONS

1. A woman in her 60s tells you that she is glad she does not have to go through pelvic examinations now that she is past menopause. As a medical assistant, what would you tell her about preventive health measures?

2. It is important to be aware of normal, age-related changes in the body. Describe two normal, age-related changes in the female reproductive system.

3. What are some ways that a woman can reduce or lessen the severity of dysmenorrhea?

4. Why should a woman be aware of the amount of blood flood she normally experiences during her menstrual period? What should she do if she has concerns?

5. How can a woman determine the amount of blood flow?

6. What is the relationship of tampons to toxic shock syndrome?

7. A young woman tells you that she has severe pain and cramping during her menstrual flow. What can be done to ease these symptoms?

8. Describe some factors that can affect the menstrual cycle.

9. Anorexia nervosa involves more than disordered eating behaviors. What relationship does anorexia nervosa have to the female reproductive system?

10. The doctor asks you to do health teaching about sexually transmitted diseases for a young female client. What key points do you include? How do you approach this young woman?

11. Pelvic inflammatory disease (PID) can become a chronic disorder. What are some of the potential complications for a woman who has PID?

12. After childbirth, what can a woman do to decrease the chance of developing a prolapsed uterus later in life?

13. If a client has a prolapsed uterus, what other conditions might you expect to observe?

14. Go back to the beginning of this chapter and review the Anticipatory Statements. Reread each statement and then indicate whether it is true or false. If the statement is false, rewrite it to make it a true statement.

CLIENT TEACHING PLAN

Breast Self-Examination

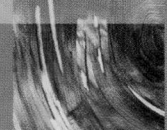

■ What Is to Be Taught:

• Breast self-examination.

■ Objective:

• Client will examine her own breasts on a monthly basis.

■ Preparation Before Teaching:

• Review the steps for breast self-examination, including information regarding reasons for performing self-exams.
• Set up a breast exam teaching model and mirrors.

■ Steps for the Medical Assistant:

1. Wash your hands.
2. Gather supplies needed.
3. Introduce yourself to the client.
4. Explain what you are going to teach and why.
5. Tell the client that examining her own breasts is important to maintain breast health and find any problems early. Tell the client that this is how she can take part in her own health care.
6. Inform the client that a breast self-exam should be done in three positions: standing in front of a mirror, lying down, and in the shower.
7. Using the teaching model, show the client the order of steps for a breast self-examination and what to look for. (A teaching model has different sizes and kinds of lumps so that the client can become familiar with how lumps feel.)
8. Ask the client to take off her clothing from the waist up. Provide privacy.
9. Ask the client to stand in front of the mirror with her arms at her sides and do the following:
   a. Look to see if breasts are similar in size, while looking for any swelling.
   b. Look to see if breast skin has any dimpling, like an orange peel.
   c. Look at the nipples to see if there is any discharge from or turning-in of the nipple.
10. Repeat steps 1, 2, and 3 with the client's arms raised straight up, and then again with hands on the hips and chest muscles contracted.
11. Ask the client to lie on the examination table with a towel under her right shoulder and her right arm under her head.
12. Tell the client to place the pads of the fingers on her left hand at the top of the right breast. Gently move the finger pads in circular movements around the breast. Instruct the client not to lift her left hand off the breast while moving, or she may miss a part of the breast tissue.
13. Instruct the client to gently squeeze the nipple between index finger and thumb.
14. Ask the client to move the towel under her left shoulder and put her left arm under her head. Tell the client to place the pads of the fingers on her right hand at the top of the left breast and repeat the steps done on the right breast.
15. Remind the client to repeat these steps while in a warm bath or shower. The skin will feel soft and somewhat slippery, and it might help her fingers to move over the breast tissue more easily.
16. Tell the client to dress; give assistance as needed.
17. Ask the client if she has any questions or wants any steps repeated or more fully explained.

■ Special Needs of the Client:

• Look at the client's chart to see if there is any factor, such as arthritis or poor vision, that might interfere with the client's ability to follow the steps and do a breast self-examination.
• Ask the client if there is any thing you should know that might affect her ability to perform this procedure.

■ Evaluation:

• Client will be able to find lumps in a breast examination teaching model.

(Continues)

CLIENT TEACHING PLAN (Continued)

- Client will name the positions used when doing a breast self-exam.
- Client will state the steps for doing a breast self-exam, in order.

■ Further Plans/Teaching:

- Give the client written instructions to help her remember the steps while doing the exam at home.
- Tell the client that if she notices anything, such as a lump, discharge, or dimpling, to call the medical office and speak with the doctor right away.

■ Follow-up:

- At the client's next visit, review the steps for doing a breast self-exam with the client.
- Ask the client if she had any problems while performing the breast self-examination.

Medical Assistant

Name: _____

Signature: _____

Date: _____

Client

Date: _____

Follow-up Date : _____

UNIT FIVE

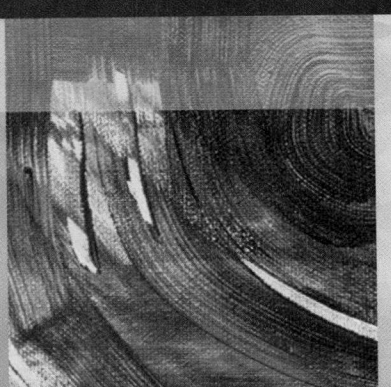

Specialty Topics in Clinical Medical Assisting

The medical assistant has a varied role working with different groups of clients and in different situations. The clinical competencies learned are adapted to the individual client and some skills may be specific to certain situations. Working with special populations and in specialty areas is the focus of this unit.

At the end of the discussion about each special population or specialty area, you will be given a health care or client care problem to solve, using what you have learned in the chapter and applying your critical thinking skills.

Throughout the Specialty areas unit, you will find client teaching plans. This unit deals with specific situations and the sample teaching plans focus on and expand upon those specialties. These plans can be used or changed to meet the unique health situations that you will see. In the future, you will find that you will work with the groups of clients, and their needs are discussed in these chapters in the many varied health care settings.

Anticipatory Statements

People have different ideas about clients with special needs. Read and think about the following statements based upon what you believe now. Decide whether you agree or disagree. Write the word **agree** after the statement if you think the statement is true. Write the word **disagree** after the statement if you think the statement is false. Read the chapter to find out if your current beliefs can be supported.

1. Medical offices must be accessible to the disabled and handicapped.

    _____

2. When speaking with a client who has hearing loss, talk very loudly.

    _____

3. When working with a client who has a cognitive impairment, talk only to the caregiver, because the client will not understand or remember what you said.

    _____

4. A client who has hearing loss should be given written instructions.

    _____

5. A client who cannot speak may still be able to understand what others are saying.

    _____

The Client with Special Needs

Learning Objectives

Upon completion of this chapter, the medical assistant student should be able to:

- List the causes of visual impairments
- List the causes of hearing impairments
- Explain the medical assistant's role in working with a client who has special needs
- Discuss ways to accommodate a client who has a visual impairment
- Discuss ways to accommodate a client who has a hearing impairment
- Discuss ways to accommodate a client who has a mobility impairment
- Discuss ways to accommodate a client who has a cognitive impairment
- Demonstrate a caring attitude toward all clients

Key Terms

caregiver A person who helps another with activities of daily living on a regular basis.

cognitive Intellectual ability and functioning.

hearing impairment Loss of part or all of the ability to hear.

impairment Loss of the use or function of part or all of a body system; may also include an abnormality of a structure.

nonverbal sign Communication by means other than the spoken word.

special needs General term describing clients who need either a procedure or service done somewhat differently to achieve the same results as with a client who does not have any impairment.

speech impairment Loss of part or all of the ability to communicate effectively with others through verbalizing.

visual impairment Loss of part or all of the ability to see.

■ INTRODUCTION

The medical assistant student learns many skills throughout the program, and is taught how to perform these skills competently with clients. The student may wonder why it is necessary to learn about clients with **special needs**. What, exactly, are special needs? Isn't the procedure for obtaining a blood pressure reading the same for everyone? Doesn't every client have to follow the same steps to prepare for a colonoscopy? This chapter introduces students to clients with special needs, including the types of special needs commonly encountered and the effect of various impairments on the client. Finally, it explores ways in which the medical assistant can understand the needs of and provide quality care to individuals with special needs.

■ PHYSICAL DISABILITIES

Many factors can cause an **impairment** and lead to a physical disability. Physical disabilities are often grouped according to the function affected. Five common groupings are:

- visual impairment
- hearing impairment
- speech impairment
- mobility impairment
- cognitive impairment (problems with thinking and judgment)

■ SIGHT IMPAIRMENT

Sight or **visual impairment** can be partial or complete; a person may be partially or completely blind. Visual difficulties can be caused by many things, including genetic disorders, injury or trauma to the eye, and metabolic conditions such as diabetes mellitus. Blindness often develops slowly over time, with little pain or discomfort. By the time a person is aware of symptoms, damage may be severe or irreversible. Macular degeneration, in which a person loses central vision, gradually progresses to total blindness. It is a leading cause of blindness among older adults.

Communicating with the Client Who Has a Visual Impairment

Clients who have visual impairments can still receive the same treatment and instructions as those who have sight; the difference is just a matter of how those instructions are communicated. As with any special-needs clients, the correct communication method is key to success. The medical assistant must know and understand which types and forms of communication will work best for a particular client.

Clients who have visual impairments will not be able to learn from the medical assistant through visual explanations or illustrations. Before you give verbal explanations, first check to make sure the client's hearing is adequate. Do not simply ask yes-or-no questions; rather, ask specific questions that require a more in-depth answer. Once it is determined that the client can in fact hear and respond to the medical assistant's questions, communication will be much easier. While explaining instructions to this client, it is critical for the medical assistant to take time to make sure the client comprehends the instructions given. For example, the medical assistant needs to instruct the client how to take

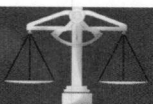

LEGAL/ETHICAL THOUGHTS

Clients who have disabilities can look to the Americans with Disabilities Act (ADA) to identify their rights under the law. The medical assistant should review this law and keep the ADA Web site address handy in the office.

a medication. Simply showing the client the medicine or medicine package will not work. Even handing the client the medicine will not work. The medical assistant must help the client learn to identify the differences between medications, and be sure the client understands the distinctions.

People who have visual impairments rely on their other senses to "see." Therefore, the senses of touch and hearing are very important. For example, the medical assistant might use various objects in teaching the client how to bandage a cut. Allow the client to feel the bandage and other objects so that he gets an idea and mental picture of what the object is like and can locate the bandage when needed. Also, ask the client to practice wrapping the bandage. Watch carefully to make sure the client fully understands how to perform the task.

It is critical for the medical assistant to remember that having a visual impairment does *not* mean the client is mentally incapable or incompetent. Good communication between client and medical assistant depends both on how the information is transmitted and also the manner in which information is given. It is never acceptable for the medical assistant to talk to a client in a condescending tone, whether or not he has a visual impairment. A medical assistant who treats the visually impaired client as though he cannot understand, just because he has a visual impairment, or speaks loudly to the client even though his hearing is fine, needlessly complicates the situation. This client has every right to feel alienated, offended, hurt, and even insulted by such behavior from a health care provider.

Good communication is impossible if clients do not feel that they can trust the medical assistant to give them the best possible care. If the medical assistant treats clients poorly or insensitively, they may not feel comfortable with that medical assistant and therefore be less cooperative. This can lead to dissatisfaction and eventually result in a poor outcome for the client. Even if a visually impaired client brings someone to assist, the medical assistant should not simply explain the instructions to this other person. The medical assistant needs to talk directly to the client; the client needs to know and comprehend the instructions because the client's health and well-being are at stake. Care should always be client-centered.

■ HEARING IMPAIRMENT

Clients who have visual impairments use their hearing and other senses to learn. Similarly, clients who have **hearing impairments** need to take in information in ways other than through sound. If the client who is hearing impaired still has his vision, visual teaching can be used. For example, the medical assistant can use diagrams and posters to explain a newly diagnosed condition or how a part of the body works. Written and pictorial materials work well for these purposes.

The medical assistant should continuously check to make sure that the client understands the instructions or information being taught. One way to check is to have writing materials available, so that the client can write down any questions or comments he has during the teaching session or meeting.

A client's hearing impairment may not be complete; he may still be able to hear some sounds. Use this capability if possible. For example, while showing a diagram, read the words aloud. When answering written questions, verbally answer the questions as well. Some clients who have hearing impairments can read lips, which makes communication easier.

The medical assistant should also be aware of **nonverbal signs** of communication, such as head-nodding or leaning forward. Facial expressions are a good indicator of whether the client understands the instructions being given. If the client has a wrinkled brow or a frown, the medical assistant should stop and ask the client if he would like anything repeated or reviewed. Also, if the client does not seem to be paying attention, is not focused on the diagram or teaching materials, or is not displaying any nonverbal signs of understanding, again stop and ask if he has any questions.

Even if the client says that he does not need to have information repeated, the medical assistant may feel that the client does not really understand. In this case, the medical assistant should not simply repeat the instructions, because the client has just told the medical assistant there is no need to do so. Instead, the medical assistant can ask the client questions to make sure that he really did comprehend what was being taught. If the client cannot answer the medical assistant's questions, the medical assistant can suggest going over the instructions again, emphasizing how important they are for the client's own health and well-being that he completely understand what is being explained.

Just as with clients who have visual impairments, the medical assistant should never treat a hearing-impaired client with disrespect or impatience. The medical assistant should never display frustration if it takes extra time to explain the instructions, or if the client does not understand and requires further details.

■ SPEECH IMPAIRMENT

We humans most commonly use speech (talking) to communicate with each other. The development of speech and language is a critical task that is closely watched by parents and pediatricians as a child grows. Early intervention with problems can help. For clients who do not have the ability to speak, or who have lost the ability because of a stroke, brain trauma, degenerative disorder, or other injury, communication can be difficult and frustrating. Society in general focuses on talking and often ignores those who cannot. Methods to help the nonverbal client—the client with a **speech impairment**—will vary depending on whether the inability to speak is congenital or traumatic, when the client lost or failed to gain the ability. The medical assistant needs to develop ways to communicate effectively and accurately with these clients while performing clinical procedures and skills during the office visit.

Clients with visual and/or hearing impairments are usually able to communicate verbally with the medical assistant. However, when a client does not possess this ability, the medical assistant must take a different approach to converse with and get information to the client.

Many younger clients can use sign language to speak. Many older clients, however, do not know sign language, because few education programs were available when they were children. The medical assistant should find out from the client whether he wishes to use sign language.

If the client is unable to communicate using sign language, nonverbal clues can work just as well to signal what the client is thinking. As with hearing-impaired clients, watch the nonverbal client's face for indications of whether he understands the information you are giving him. Any sign of confusion or disinterest from the client should be addressed by the medical assistant in a polite and patient manner. In working with any client, especially those with special needs, it is essential to exercise patience. It may take longer to give instructions, but that does not mean that it is impossible for instructions to be given and understood. The special need simply means that the medical assistant must take a different route to help the client.

Clients who have speech impairments can also benefit from having paper and writing material available during a meeting, so that they may write down any comments or questions. The medical assistant should periodically check to see if the client has written anything. If he has not, the medical assistant should pause to make sure the client understands and ask if he needs more explanation of anything that has been discussed.

■ MOBILITY IMPAIRMENT

Mobility impairment means more than not being able to walk. Such impairment can restrict a person's independence even to the point of interfering with performance of activities of daily living (ADLs). Mobility involves the smooth working together of the nervous, skeletal, and muscular systems. A breakdown in any of these systems will affect walking. For example, neuromuscular disorders, multiple sclerosis, muscular dystrophy, strokes (CVAs), and Parkinson's disease all affect mobility. Muscles that are weakened from disuse, atrophy, or inactivity imposed by other chronic conditions can make a person frail and unable to ambulate independently.

The medical assistant may encounter clients who have extensive mobility impairment. The most appropriate way to make sure that the client with mobility impairment receives the best possible care is to make sure that he has assistance and access. To ensure this, the medical assistant should frequently offer assistance to the client; for example, the client may need help getting on and off the examining table. Also, the client may need assistance changing into a gown before an examination. The medical assistant should remember never to lean toward or grab onto such a client, because he is often not stable and may fall.

Exam rooms should be accessible by wheelchair, if the client uses one. There should be enough space for the client to pass through the door and get in and out of the room. In addition, the medical assistant should make sure there are no objects in the way that the client could trip over if using a walker or other assistive device.

Any client may need to undergo several tests, not all of which will be administered in the same room. To best accommodate the client with mobility impairment, set up the tests so that the client has to travel as little as possible, and can do so in a systematic way. For instance, schedule appointments so that the mobility-impaired client does not have to go from one end of a building to the other, retracing his steps. Though it can be accomplished, moving takes more of an effort for these clients, compared to clients who have no mobility impairments. Therefore, it is only courteous and practical to have this client travel as little as possible; certainly, he will feel more comfortable when his limitations are respected.

■ COGNITIVE IMPAIRMENT

Cognitive impairment can result from trauma at birth, infections, certain diseases, or injury to the developing brain, such as trauma from being shaken or other child abuse. Strokes or temporary interruptions in the flow of oxygen-rich blood to the brain can cause cognitive impairment. Alzheimer's and neurologic disorders can also impair cognitive ability. Thinking, reasoning, judgment, and decision making may all be affected by a cognitive impairment. The amount of impairment ranges from mild to severe. Cognitive impairment can mean only that the client has a little trouble remembering some events, or it can mean that he is completely dependent on a **caregiver** to perform ADLs.

Communicating with the Cognitively Impaired Client

Whatever the cause of the impairment, the medical assistant still needs to communicate with clients who are cognitively impaired. Such a client will probably not be able to understand complicated instructions, so the medical assistant must give explanations in terms the client can understand. Explanations and procedures should be expressed in simpler terms that maintain respect for the dignity of the person. The medical assistant must remember that the adult client is not a child; no matter how cognitively impaired the client may be, he can still understand that he is being talked down to.

Many clients who are cognitively impaired will have caregivers with them. Although it is important to make sure the caretaker understands the various instructions, the medical assistant still needs to work with the client directly. Despite the fact that these clients are cognitively impaired, they are the ones who most need to understand the health information. Procedures to be performed on any client must be explained to the client beforehand. The medical assistant should make sure that the client understands what is going to take place before it happens.

As with all clients, the medical assistant needs to treat the client who has cognitive impairment with respect and dignity. Clients with impairments of any sort deserve the same respect given to a client who does not have any special needs.

Pain and Cognitive Impairment

When obtaining and recording the vital signs of a client who has a cognitive impairment, the medical assistant must be sure to gain the client's cooperation through clear, simple statements, a caring attitude, and patience. Measuring pain in a client who has a cognitive impairment is difficult. There are many myths regarding pain in this group of clients: some people believe that cognitively impaired clients are less sensitive to pain, or that they are not aware of it. It was often thought that if a client did not verbally communicate feelings of pain, then he must not be having pain. However, cognitively impaired clients who can communicate in the usual ways still complain of unpleasant, painful sensations; thus, we know that such clients can and do feel pain. Health care providers and caregivers should look for nonverbal and behavioral signs of pain. Does the client have an unhappy facial expression? Is he frowning or grimacing? Does the client guard or protect a body part, such as holding a painful arm close to the body? A reliable sign of unrelieved pain is restless or agitated behavior. Is the client unable to relax? Does he seem to be in constant motion? In the past, clients exhibiting this sort of behavior were often given sedating medications, when what they really needed was pain relief. The medical assistant should note any such findings and report these observations to the doctor.

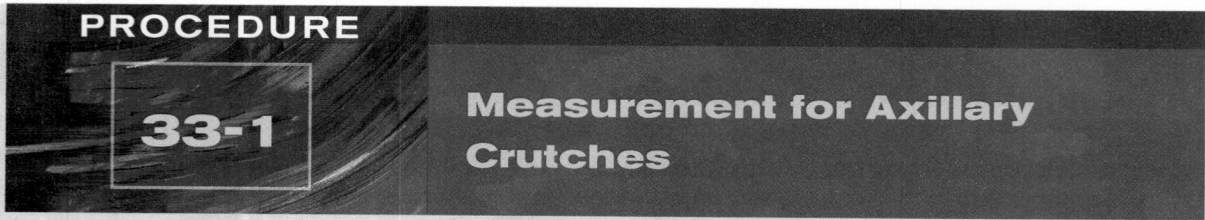

PROCEDURE

33-1

Measurement for Axillary Crutches

Student Competency Objective: The medical assistant student will measure a client for axillary crutches.

Items Needed: Axillary crutches, pads for axilla and hand rests, measuring tape, shoes client will be using for ambulation, paper and pen

Steps:

1. Wash your hands.
2. Gather equipment and supplies.
3. Introduce yourself to the client even if you have seen the client on previous visits to your office. The client may have forgotten your name. This also helps to establish a provider-client relationship, because it shows the client that you want him to know who you are.
4. Identify the client. Ask the client to state his name to establish that this is the right client, and then compare the name given to the name on the chart. Never enter a room and call out a client's name to determine if this person is the correct client. The client may not have heard you clearly and may just nod, smile, or answer yes. Clients almost never question if the medical assistant professional has the right client. It is up to the medical assistant to identify the right client before performing any procedure.
5. Tell the client, in everyday language, what you are going to do.
6. Ask if the client has any questions. If he does, give short and simple answers. Sometimes clients will start (and continue) talking because they are nervous about the procedure.

(Continues)

PROCEDURE 33-1 (Continued)

7. Ask the client to stand straight. Assist the client as needed for support. (Remember that the client who needs crutches may not be stable when standing.)

8. Place the tips of the crutches 2 inches in front of the client and 4 to 6 inches to the side of the client (Figure 33-1A). This is the tripod position, the starting point for all crutch walking gaits.

9. Adjust the length of the crutches by removing the bolts and wing nuts and sliding the central support up or down at the bottom until the shoulder rests or axillary bars are two finger's breadth below the client's axilla. Replace the bolts and wing nuts and fasten them securely (Figure 33-1B).

NOTE TO STUDENT:

Clients should never use another person's crutches unless the crutches are first brought in for adjustment. Ill-fitting crutches can harm the client. If the shoulder or axilla rests come up too high into the underarm, the client can suffer nerve damage.

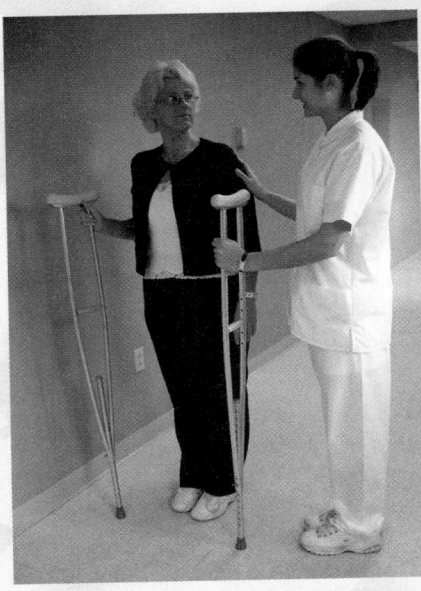

FIGURE 33-1A Assist the client to stand straight, and begin to measure for axillary crutches by placing the tips of the crutches 2 inches in front of the client and 4 to 6 inches to the side of the client.

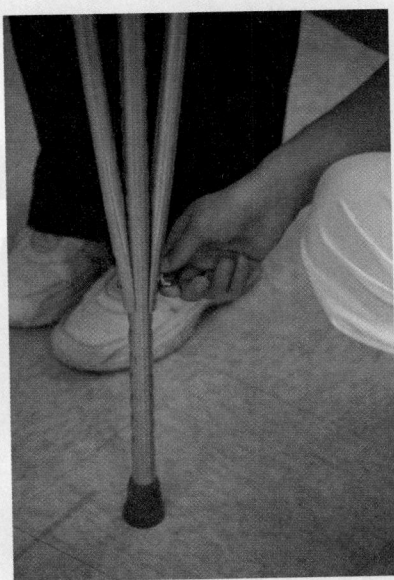

FIGURE 33-1B Adjust the length of the crutches by removing the bolts and wing nuts and sliding the central support up or down at the bottom. Replace and securely tighten the bolts and wing nuts.

(Continues)

PROCEDURE 33-1 (Continued)

10. Ask the client to stand with the crutches supporting the client's weight.

11. Move the handgrips to a level so that the client's elbows are flexed at a 30-degree angle (Figure 33-1C). This is done by removing the bolts and wing nuts and moving the handgrip bar up or down until the correct angle is achieved. Put the bolts and wing nuts back in and tighten them securely.

12. Make sure that the shoulder rests or axilla bars and handgrips are sufficiently padded for the client's comfort (hard or poorly padded bars and grips can cause skin irritation).

13. Check the fit of the crutches. You should be able to slip two fingers between the client's underarm and the top of the crutch (Figure 33-1D).

14. Give instructions as ordered. Be sure to tell the client to avoid getting the tips of the crutches wet. Wet tips can slip and cause the client to lose his balance and fall.

15. Ask the client if he has any questions or concerns.

16. Wash your hands.

17. Record the procedure in the client's chart.

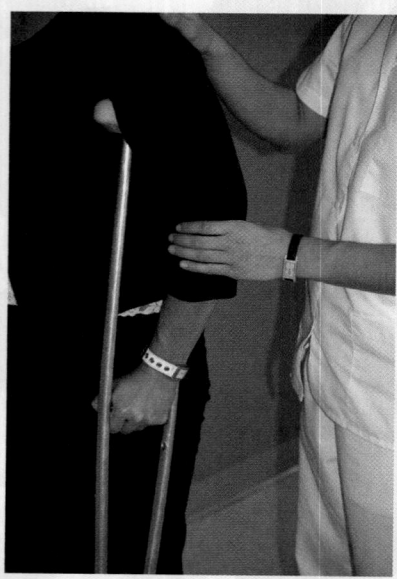

FIGURE 33-1C Ask the client to stand and use the crutches for support. Move the handgrips to a level where the client's elbows are flexed at a 30-degree angle when the hands are in position on the handgrips.

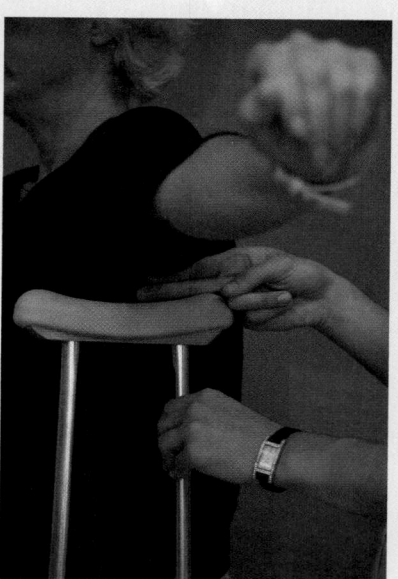

FIGURE 33-1D Test the fit of the crutches. There should be about two fingers' width between the client's underarms and the top of the crutch.

Charting Example:

10/16/20xx   8:30 A.M.   Client measured and fitted for axillary crutches. Elbows flexed to 30 degrees. Reviewed safety issues and gave client written instructions.

Edward John, S.M.A.

Edward John, S.M.A. (printed name)

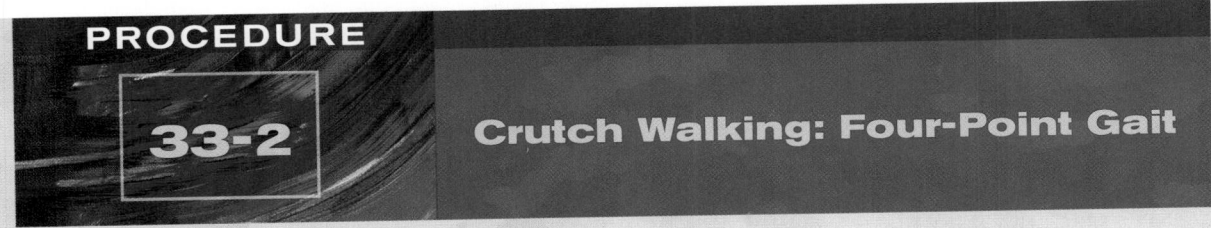

PROCEDURE

33-2

Crutch Walking: Four-Point Gait

Student Competency Objective: The medical assistant student will demonstrate the four-point gait for crutch walking.

Items Needed: Properly measured and fitted axillary crutches, comfortable shoes for walking

Steps:

1. Wash your hands.
2. Gather equipment and supplies.
3. Introduce yourself to the client even if you have seen the client on previous visits to your office. The client may have forgotten your name. This also helps to establish a provider-client relationship, because it shows the client that you want him to know who you are.
4. Identify the client. Ask the client to state his name to establish that this is the right client, and then compare the name given to the name on the chart. Never enter a room and call out a client's name to determine if this person is the correct client. The client may not have heard you clearly and may just nod, smile, or answer yes. Clients almost never question if the medical assistant professional has the right client. It is up to the medical assistant to identify the right client before performing any procedure.
5. Tell the client, in everyday language, what you are going to do.
6. Ask if the client has any questions. If he does, give short and simple answers. Sometimes clients will start (and continue) talking because they are nervous about the procedure.
7. Stand straight with crutches in tripod position (tips of crutches 2 inches in front and 4 to 6 inches to the side) (Figure 33-2A).

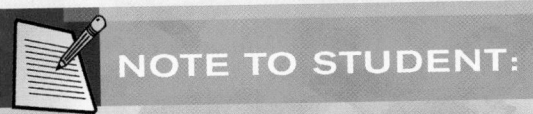

NOTE TO STUDENT:

Because three points of support are used in the four-point gait, this is a stable (though slow) gait. Clients who have problems of weakness, coordination, or balance may benefit from using this gait.

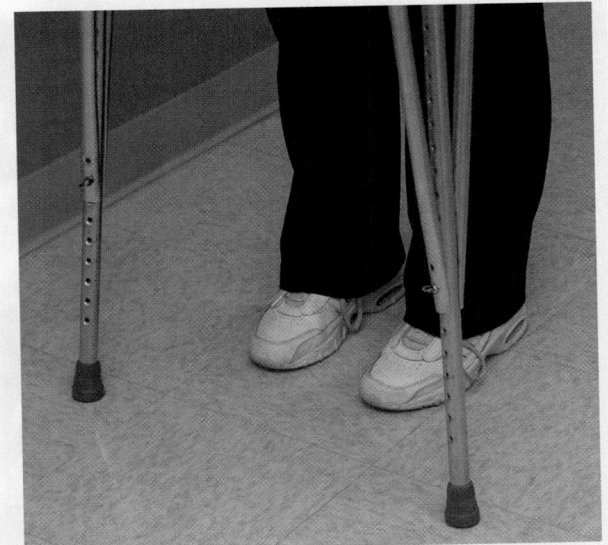

FIGURE 33-2A The medical assistant demonstrates walking with a four-point gait. Stand up straight in tripod position (with the crutch 2 inches in front and 4-6 inches to the side) before beginning to walk.

(Continues)

PROCEDURE 33-2 (Continued)

8. Move the right crutch forward about 6 inches (Figure 33–2B).
9. Move the left foot forward to just slightly ahead of the left crutch (Figure 33–2C).
10. Move the left crutch forward (Figure 33–2D).
11. Move the right foot forward to just slightly ahead of the right crutch (Figure 33–2E).
12. Move the right crutch forward and repeat the steps.

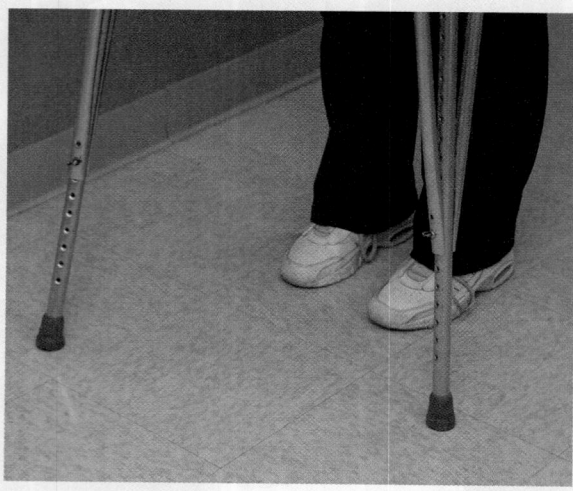

FIGURE 33–2B Move the right crutch 6 inches to the front.

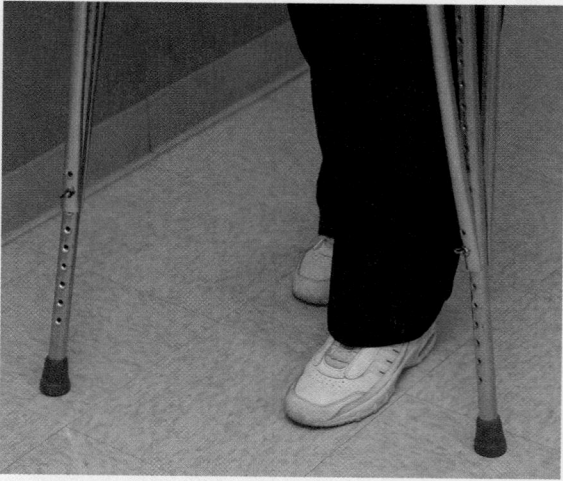

FIGURE 33–2C Move the left foot even with or slightly ahead of the left crutch.

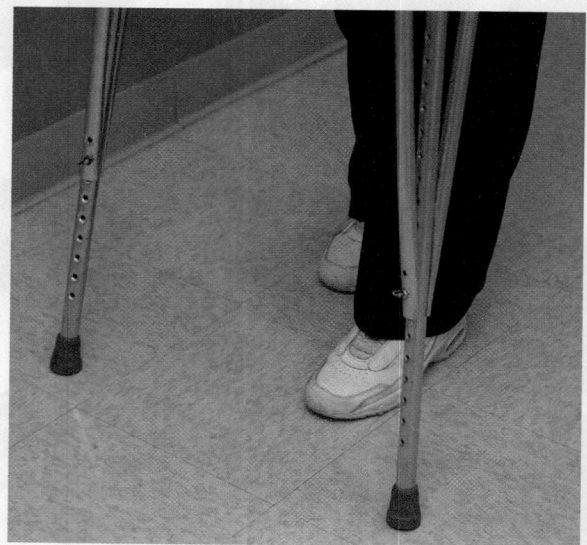

FIGURE 33–2D Bring the left crutch 6 inches to the front.

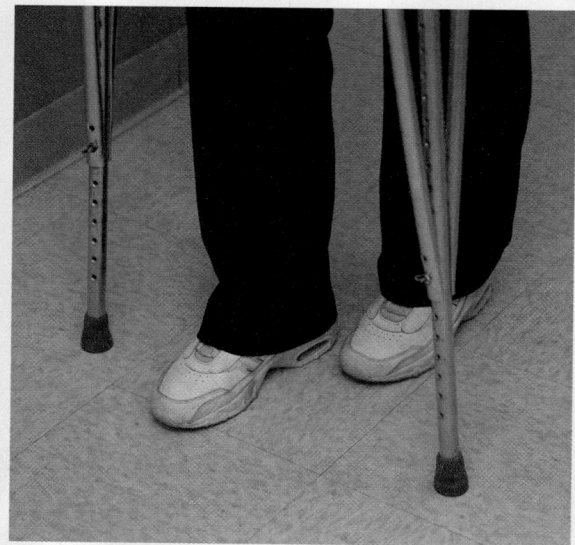

FIGURE 33–2E Move the right foot forward to just slightly ahead of the right crutch, then repeat the steps.

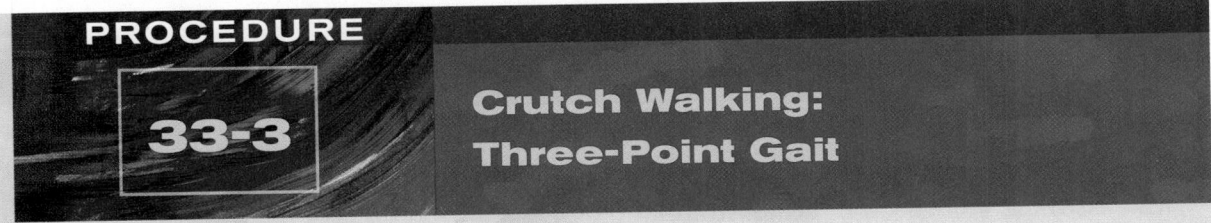

PROCEDURE

33-3

Crutch Walking: Three-Point Gait

Student Competency Objective: The medical assistant student will demonstrate the three-point gait for crutch walking.

Items Needed: Properly measured and fitted axillary crutches, comfortable shoes for walking

Steps:

1. Wash your hands.
2. Gather equipment and supplies.
3. Introduce yourself to the client even if you have seen the client on previous visits to your office. The client may have forgotten your name. This also helps to establish a provider-client relationship, because it shows the client that you want him to know who you are.
4. Identify the client. Ask the client to state his name to establish that this is the right client, and then compare the name given to the name on the chart. Never enter a room and call out a client's name to determine if this person is the correct client. The client may not have heard you clearly and may just nod, smile, or answer yes. Clients almost never question if the medical assistant professional has the right client. It is up to the medical assistant to identify the right client before performing any procedure.
5. Tell the client, in everyday language, what you are going to do.
6. Ask if the client has any questions. If he does, give short and simple answers. Sometimes clients will start (and continue) talking because they are nervous about the procedure.
7. Stand straight with the crutches in tripod position (tips of crutches 2 inches in front and 4 to 6 inches to the side).
8. Move both crutches and the affected leg forward (the affected leg can be held off the floor).
9. Balance weight on both crutches while moving the unaffected leg forward (Figure 33-3).
10. Move both crutches and the affected leg forward and repeat the steps.

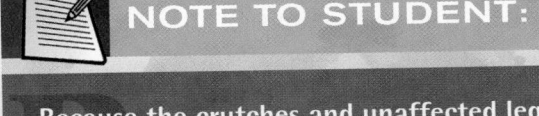

NOTE TO STUDENT:

Because the crutches and unaffected leg bear the weight in three-point crutch walking, the client must have sufficient arm strength and muscular coordination.

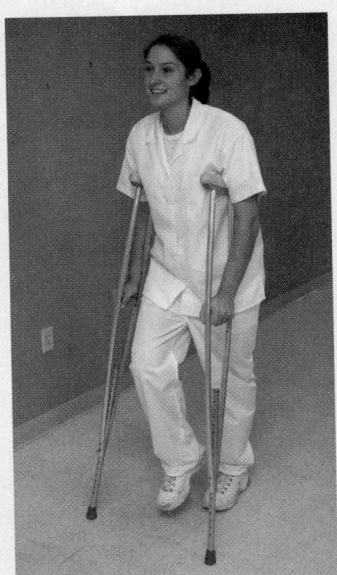

FIGURE 33-3 The medical assistant demonstrates walking with a three-point gait. Standing straight with crutches in the tripod position, move both crutches and the affected leg forward.

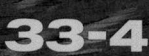

PROCEDURE

33-4

Crutch Walking: Two-Point Gait

Student Competency Objective: The medical assistant student will demonstrate the two-point gait for crutch walking.

Items Needed: Properly measured and fitted axillary crutches, comfortable shoes for walking

Steps:

1. Wash your hands.
2. Gather equipment and supplies.
3. Introduce yourself to the client even if you have seen the client on previous visits to your office. The client may have forgotten your name. This also helps to establish a provider-client relationship, because it shows the client that you want him to know who you are.
4. Identify the client. Ask the client to state his name to establish that this is the right client, and then compare the name given to the name on the chart. Never enter a room and call out a client's name to determine if this person is the correct client. The client may not have heard you clearly and may just nod, smile, or answer yes. Clients almost never question if the medical assistant professional has the right client. It is up to the medical assistant to identify the right client before performing any procedure.
5. Tell the client, in everyday language, what you are going to do.
6. Ask if the client has any questions. If he does, give short and simple answers. Sometimes clients will start (and continue) talking because they are nervous about the procedure.
7. Stand straight with crutches in tripod position (tips of crutches 2 inches in front and 4 to 6 inches to the side).
8. At the same time, move the left crutch and the right foot forward (Figure 33-4A).
9. Move the right crutch and the left foot forward together (Figure 33-4B).
10. Repeat the steps.

NOTE TO STUDENT:

In the two-point gait, only two points support the body. Therefore, the client must have muscular coordination and be allowed to bear some weight on the affected leg. This is faster than the basic four-point gait.

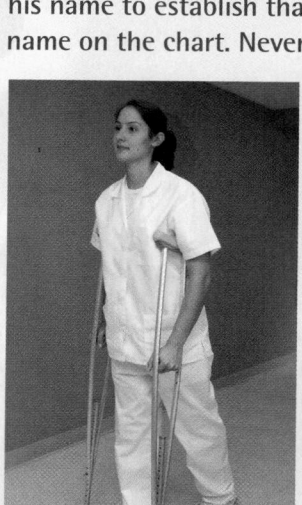

FIGURE 33-4A The medical assistant demonstrates walking with a two-point gait. Standing straight with crutches in the tripod position, move the left crutch and right foot forward at the same time.

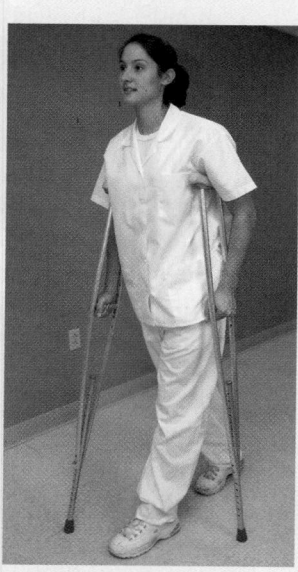

FIGURE 33-4B Move the right crutch and left foot forward at the same time.

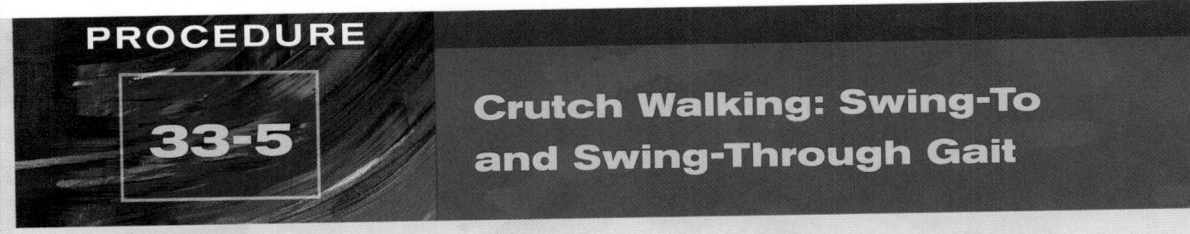

PROCEDURE

33-5

Crutch Walking: Swing-To and Swing-Through Gait

Student Competency Objective: The medical assistant student will demonstrate the swing-to and swing-through gait for crutch walking.

Items Needed: Properly measured and fitted axillary crutches, comfortable shoes for walking

NOTE TO STUDENT:

The swing-to gait is often taught before the swing-through gait.

Steps:

Swing-to:

1. Wash your hands.

2. Gather equipment and supplies.

3. Introduce yourself to the client even if you have seen the client on previous visits to your office. The client may have forgotten your name. This also helps to establish a provider-client relationship, because it shows the client that you want him to know who you are.

4. Identify the client. Ask the client to state his name to establish that this is the right client, and then compare the name given to the name on the chart. Never enter a room and call out a client's name to determine if this person is the correct client. The client may not have heard you clearly and may just nod, smile, or answer yes. Clients almost never question if the medical assistant professional has the right client. It is up to the medical assistant to identify the right client before performing any procedure.

5. Tell the client, in everyday language, what you are going to do.

6. Ask if the client has any questions. If he does, give short and simple answers. Sometimes clients will start (and continue) talking because they are nervous about the procedure.

7. Stand straight with crutches in tripod position (tips of crutches 2 inches to the front and 4 to 6 inches to the side).

8. Move both crutches forward.

9. Bear the weight on the hands.

10. Swing body to bring both feet to the level of the crutches (Figure 33-5A).

11. Repeat the steps.

Steps:

Swing-through:

7. Stand straight with crutches in tripod position (tips of crutches 2 inches to the front and 4 to 6 inches to the side).

8. Move both crutches forward.

9. Bear the weight on the hands.

(Continues)

PROCEDURE 33-5 (Continued)

10. Swing body to bring both feet through to a spot ahead of the crutches (Figure 33–5B).
11. Repeat the steps.

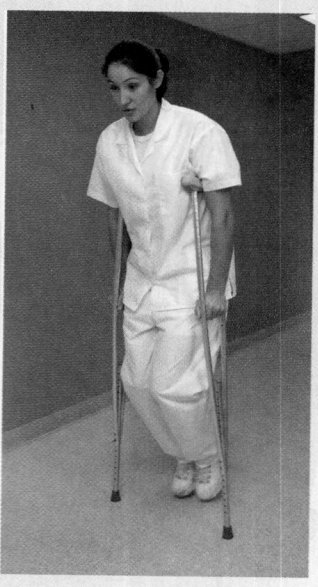

FIGURE 33–5A Standing straight with crutches in the tripod position, and bearing the weight on the hands, swing the body even with the crutches.

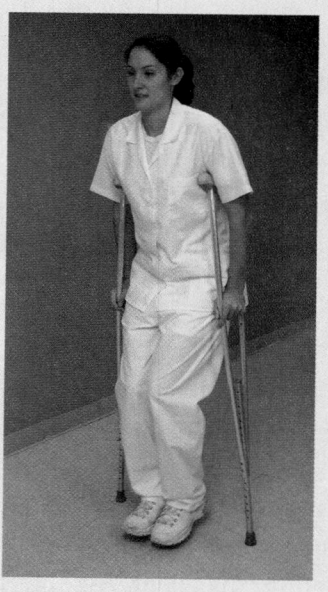

FIGURE 33–5B Standing straight with crutches in the tripod position, move both crutches forward. Then, bearing the weight on the hands, swing the body ahead of the crutches.

PROCEDURE

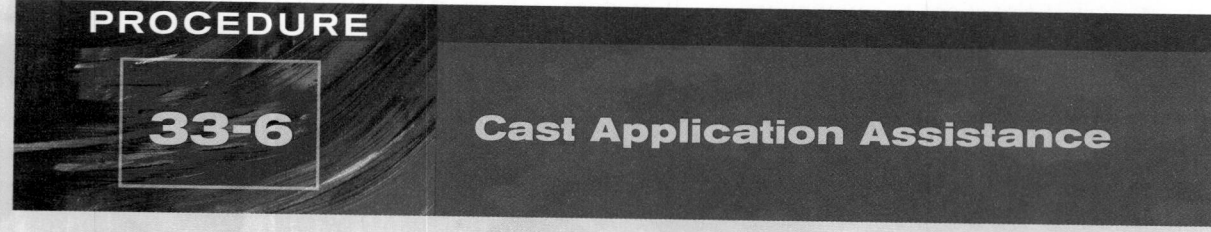

33-6   Cast Application Assistance

Student Competency Objective: The medical assistant student will demonstrate assistance in the application of a cast.

Items Needed: Casting material, soft stockinette, tubular or circular material, padding, bucket, room-temperature water, plaster cast knife, gloves (for both the medical assistant and the doctor), paper and pen

Steps:

1. Wash your hands.
2. Get together equipment and supplies.

(Continues)

PROCEDURE 33-6 (Continued)

3. Introduce yourself to the client even if you have seen the client on previous visits to your office. The client may have forgotten your name. This also helps to establish a provider–client relationship, because it shows the client that you want him to know who you are.

4. Identify the client. Ask the client to state his name to establish that this is the right client, and then compare the name given to the name on the chart. Never enter a room and call out a client's name to determine if this person is the correct client. The client may not have heard you clearly and may just nod, smile, or answer yes. Clients almost never question if the medical assistant professional has the right client. It is up to the medical assistant to identify the right client before performing any procedure.

5. Tell the client, in everyday language, what you are going to do.

6. Ask if the client has any questions. If he does, give short and simple answers. Sometimes clients will start (and continue) talking because they are nervous about the procedure.

7. The doctor performs many steps before the medical assistant has a role in cast application. The doctor inspects the area and places the stockinette and padding on the site.

8. Fill the bucket with room-temperature water.

9. Wait for the doctor's instructions; then put on gloves and place the casting material in the water bucket.

10. Wait for bubbles to stop rising from the water.

11. Take the roll out and gently squeeze it (do not wring).

12. Hand the roll to the doctor, who will wrap the limb.

13. Place the knife in the doctor's hand when wrapping is complete.

14. Wipe away any loose pieces of cast material from the client's skin with a warm, damp cloth.

15. Help the client to dress as necessary. Make sure not to cover the cast while it is still wet. Do not apply pressure or handle the cast with your fingertips; this can cause indentations and pressure points.

16. Teach cast care to the client, making sure to include any special instructions from the doctor.

17. Ask the client if he has any questions.

18. Clean, disinfect, or discard supplies and equipment according to regulations and office policy.

19. Wash your hands.

20. Record the procedure in the client's chart.

Charting Example:

7/16/20xx   4:00 P.M.   Assisted Dr. Simpson with short arm cast application to client's right arm. Good circulation noted in right extremity. Cast care information with written instructions given to client. Client verbalized understanding. Follow-up appointment scheduled.

James Olsen, S.M.A.

James Olsen, S.M.A. (printed name)

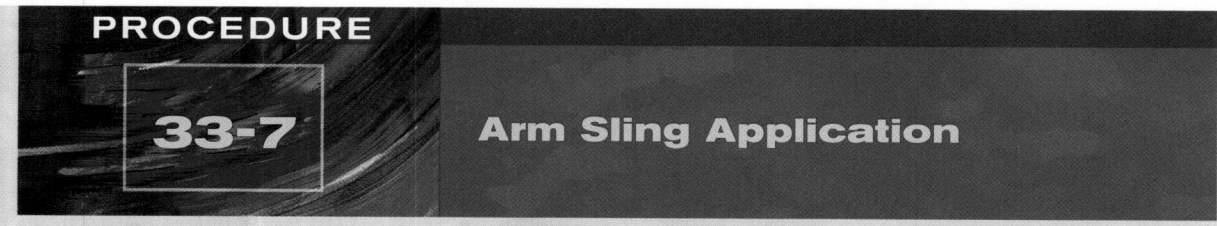

PROCEDURE

33-7

Arm Sling Application

Student Competency Objective: The medical assistant student will apply an arm sling.

Items Needed: Commercial arm sling, paper and pen

Steps:

1. Wash your hands.
2. Gather equipment and supplies.
3. Introduce yourself to the client even if you have seen the client on previous visits to your office. The client may have forgotten your name. This also helps to establish a provider-client relationship, because it shows the client that you want him to know who you are.
4. Identify the client. Ask the client to state his name to establish that this is the right client, and then compare the name given to the name on the chart. Never enter a room and call out a client's name to determine if this person is the correct client. The client may not have heard you clearly and may just nod, smile, or answer yes. Clients almost never question if the medical assistant professional has the right client. It is up to the medical assistant to identify the right client before performing any procedure.
5. Tell the client, in everyday language, what you are going to do.
6. Ask if the client has any questions. If he does, give short and simple answers. Sometimes clients will start (and continue) talking because they are nervous about the procedure.
7. Ask the client to sit.
8. Place the affected arm across the client's chest with the thumb pointing up (Figure 33-6A).
9. Gently place the arm in the sling so that the client's elbow fits snugly into the corner of the sling (Figure 33-6B).
10. Take the strap attached to the sling and bring it around the back of the client's neck. Pull it through the metal hoops.
11. Carefully pull on the strap until the sling is at a right angle to the body. The elbow of the affected arm should be flexed and the wrist slightly raised, to help circulation and prevent swelling (Figure 33-6C).
12. Check the position of elbow and wrist.
13. Ask the client if he is comfortable. Check neck area and apply padding if needed to ease pressure.
14. Give the client information and written instructions as ordered by the doctor.
15. Ask the client if he has any questions.
16. Wash your hands.
17. Record the procedure in the client's medical chart.

(Continues)

PROCEDURE 33-7 (Continued)

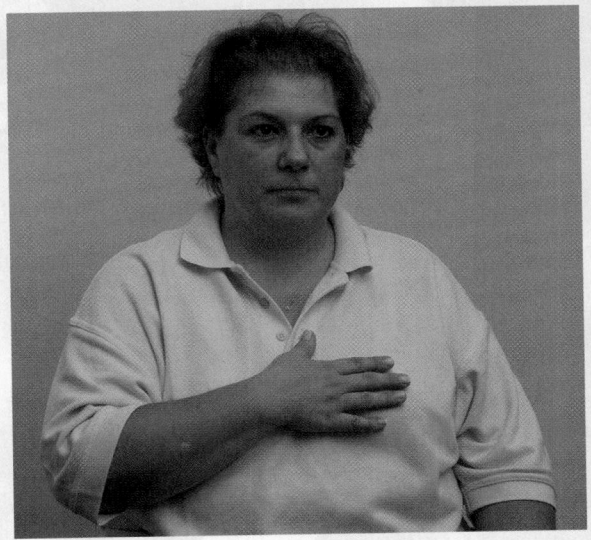

FIGURE 33-6A With the client sitting, place the affected arm across the client's chest with the thumb pointing upward.

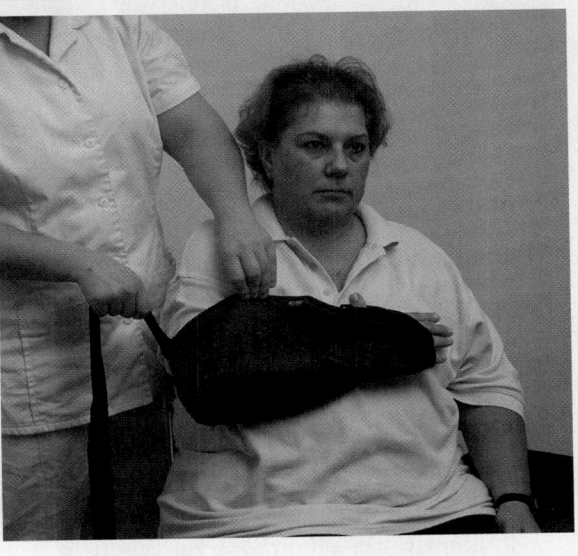

FIGURE 33-6B Place the client's arm in the sling, ensuring that the client's elbow fits snugly into the corner of the sling.

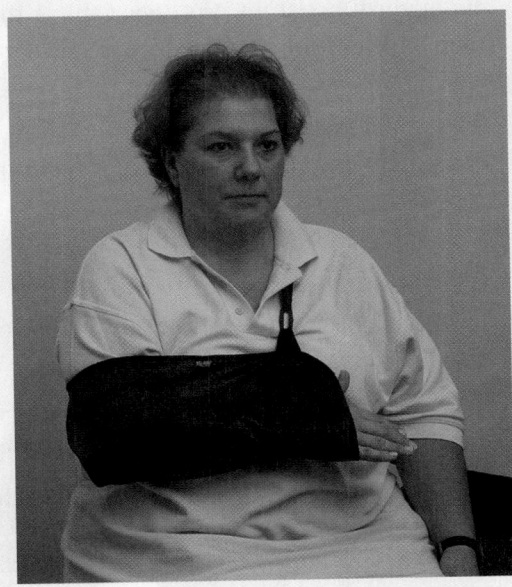

FIGURE 33-6C Bring the strap of the sling around the back of the client's neck and adjust the strap until the sling is at a right angle to the client's body.

Charting Example:

2/27/20xx   11:00 A.M.   Commercial arm sling applied to client's left arm. Circulation is good in extremity. Padding added to sling strap around neck. Information and written instructions given for commercial sling. Client verbalized understanding.

Mary Ann O'Grady, S.M.A.

Mary Ann O'Grady, S.M.A. (printed name)

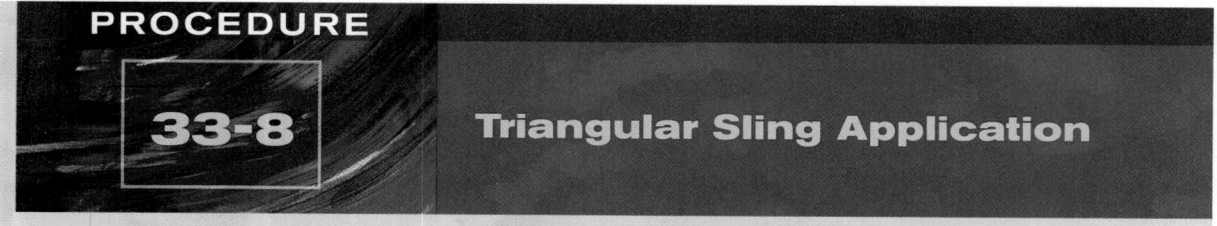

PROCEDURE

33-8

Triangular Sling Application

Student Competency Objective: The medical assistant student will apply a triangular arm sling.

Items Needed: Triangular sling, pins, paper, pen

Steps:

1. Wash your hands.

2. Gather equipment and supplies.

3. Introduce yourself to the client even if you have seen the client on previous visits to your office. The client may have forgotten your name. This also helps to establish a provider–client relationship, because it shows the client that you want him to know who you are.

4. Identify the client. Ask the client to state her name to establish that this is the right client, and then compare the name given to the name on the chart. Never enter a room and call out a client's name to determine if this person is the correct client. The client may not have heard you clearly and may just nod, smile, or answer yes. Clients almost never question if the medical assistant professional has the right client. It is up to the medical assistant to identify the right client before performing any procedure.

5. Tell the client, in everyday language, what you are going to do.

6. Ask if the client has any questions. If he does, give short and simple answers. Sometimes clients will start (and continue) talking because they are nervous about the procedure.

7. Ask the client to sit.

8. Bend the client's elbow with the hand at a little less than 90 degrees. (The fingers should be higher than the elbow to prevent swelling.)

9. Place one corner of the triangular cloth over the unaffected shoulder.

10. Extend the cloth down the client's chest.

11. Slide the cloth under the affected arm (Figure 33-7A).

12. Make sure that the middle point of the cloth is at the elbow.

13. Take the lowest point of the triangular cloth over the affected arm, with the point ending at the side of the neck.

14. Tie or pin the sling points at the side of the neck. Never tie a sling at the back of the neck, because the knot will cause pain and pressure (Figure 33-7B).

15. Take the loose folds of material at the elbow, fold them neatly, and fasten them with a pin (Figure 33-7C).

16. Give the client information and written instructions as ordered by the doctor.

17. Ask the client if he has any questions.

18. Wash your hands.

19. Record the procedure in the client's medical chart.

(Continues)

PROCEDURE 33-8 (Continued)

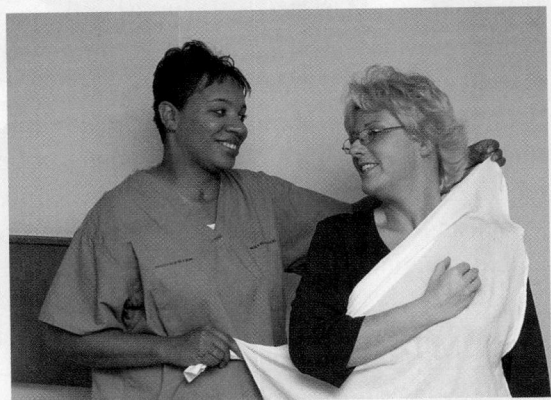

FIGURE 33-7A Bend the elbow of the affected arm a little less than 90 degrees. Place one corner of the cloth over the unaffected shoulder. Extend the cloth over the front of the client and slide it underneath the affected arm, making sure that the middle point of the cloth is at the elbow.

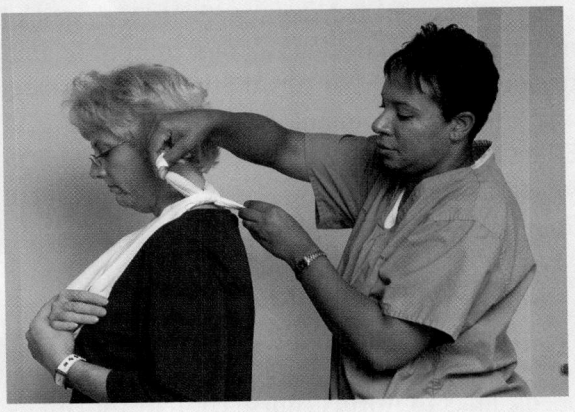

FIGURE 33-7B Take the lowest point of the cloth and move it over the affected arm to the side of the neck, tying or pinning the sling points.

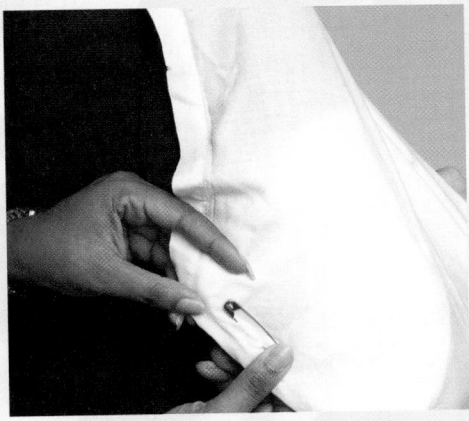

FIGURE 33-7C Take the loose folds of material at the elbow; fold and fasten them.

Charting Example:

4/1/20xx   2:30 P.M.   Triangular sling applied to client's right arm. Circulation is good with finger movement. Information and written instructions for arm sling given. Client verbalized understanding.

Tiffany Fitzgerald, S.M.A.

Tiffany Fitzgerald, S.M.A. (printed name)

BRIDGE TO CAAHEP

This chapter, which discusses clients with special needs, provides information and content related to CAAHEP standards for Anatomy and Physiology, Medical Terminology, Medical Law and Ethics, Psychology, Communication, Medical Assisting Clinical Procedures, and Professional Components.

 ## ABHES LINKS

This chapter, which discusses clients with special needs, links to ABHES course content for Orientation, Anatomy and Physiology, Medical Terminology, Medical Law and Ethics, Psychology of Human Relations, Medical Office Clinical Procedures, and Career Development.

 ## AAMA AREAS OF COMPETENCE

This chapter, which discusses clients with special needs, provides information or content within several areas listed in the Medical Assistant Role Delineation Study. These areas include: clinical, fundamental principles, diagnostic orders, patient (client) care, general transdisciplinary, professionalism, communication skills, legal concepts, and instruction.

 ## AMT PATHS

This chapter, which discusses clients with special needs, provides a path to AMT competency in general medical assisting knowledge, anatomy and physiology, medical terminology, medical law, medical ethics, human relations, and patient (client) education. It also links to clinical medical assisting, vital signs, physical examinations, and therapeutic modalities.

POINTS OF HIGHLIGHT

- Many factors can cause impairment and lead to a disability.
- Disabilities can be grouped according to the function impaired: sight, hearing, speech, mobility, and cognition.
- Clients with cognitive impairments need to be given clear directions beforehand so that they can understand and prepare for the procedure.
- The client is the focus of care and the medical assistant must direct teaching and care to the client.
- Clients who have special needs have a right to the same quality of care and respect given to any other client.
- Medical assistants must find ways to communicate with and meet the special needs of clients while giving competent, empathetic care.

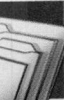

STUDENT PORTFOLIO ACTIVITY

Understanding the needs of clients who require care to be delivered in a different or special way is important to the medical assistant who works in a clinical setting. Service learning is one way to achieve this goal. Think about the special needs discussed in this chapter. Choose one that you want to learn more about. Visit a center that delivers services to clients with this need. Volunteer to help by donating your time and skills. While giving of your time, you will learn much. This volunteer time will help you become more aware of the needs of all clients. This will help you in your work as a medical assistant no matter in what type of health care setting you choose to work in. Keep track of your hours and ask a staff person from the site to evaluate you and document your service learning experience.

APPLYING YOUR SKILLS

You call a client from the waiting room to come back to the examination rooms. You notice that he needs to use a walker. How will this affect the examination? What additional steps do you need to take to prepare this client for the examination, care for him during the procedure, and assist him after the doctor is finished with the examination?

CRITICAL THINKING QUESTIONS

1. A client with a partial hearing loss seems confused about the instructions regarding preparation for laboratory testing that the doctor has just finished giving him. What are some possible reasons for this apparent confusion? What actions could you take to help this client?

2. You note on a client's chart that he is cognitively impaired. What do you need to know to provide quality care to this client?

3. A client is nonverbal. What are some possible ways to gain information from this client? As a medical assistant, what skills do you need?

4. A client has severe visual impairment. What do you need to remember in preparing this client for an examination by the doctor?

5. Blindness or severe visual impairment in the elderly is a major problem in the United States. However, blindness is not a natural part of aging. What are some ways to prevent blindness?

6. A caregiver comes to the office with a client who is cognitively impaired. The caregiver tries to talk and answers all your questions, while ignoring the client. Her back is to the client. How do you respond?

7. What precautions are needed to maintain the dignity of clients with special needs?

8. What are some clues that a client does not understand the points you are trying to make?

9. Accessibility of an office to the disabled is not only an ethical issue, but also a legal issue. Explain what this statement means.

10. Go back to the beginning of this chapter and review the Anticipatory Statements. Reread each statement and then indicate whether it is true or false. If the statement is false, rewrite it to make it a true statement.

Electroencephalogram Preparation

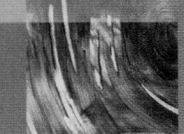

■ What Is to Be Taught:

- Client preparation for an electroencephalogram (EEG) diagnostic test.

■ Objectives:

- Client will be able to understand and follow the steps necessary before an electroencephalogram diagnostic test.

■ Preparation Before Teaching:

- Review the reasons for an EEG test.
- Review client preparation steps as well as the procedure itself.
- Assemble supplies for teaching, including paper and pen.
- Make sure that the area is free from distractions while you are teaching.

■ Steps for the Medical Assistant:

1. Wash your hands.
2. Gather supplies needed.
3. Introduce yourself to the client.
4. Explain what you are going to teach and why.
5. Inform the client that he will need to prepare for the test one day in advance. Tell him that following the steps will help to ensure an accurate test, which in turn will aid the doctor in diagnosing and treating the client's problem.
6. Instruct the client to wash his hair the night before the test. The hair must be free of dirt and oils.
7. Tell the client not to put on any hair gel, mousse, or sprays. These products interfere with the electrodes used for the EEG.
8. Ask the client not to eat or drink anything containing caffeine. This includes coffee, tea, many colas, soft drinks, and chocolate.
9. Instruct the client that he must stay up the night before the test and not sleep or take any naps.
10. Inform the client not to drive to the test site and that he needs to have someone bring him to the site.
11. Tell the client what to expect during the EEG test. This will help to gain the client's cooperation and allay any fears he might have. (Clients may worry about having electrodes attached to the head.)
12. Ask the client if he has any questions or concerns.

■ Special Needs of the Client:

- Check the client's chart to see if there are any factors that might interfere with the client's ability to follow the preparation steps.
- Ask the client if there is anything you should know that might affect the procedure or his ability to carry out the preparation steps.

■ Evaluation:

- Client is able to state the steps he needs to take the night before the test and the reasons for the steps.

■ Further Plans/Teaching:

- Ask the client if he has any questions or if he needs any more information about the EEG diagnostic test.

■ Follow-up:

- Call the client at home one or two days before the scheduled test. Review the steps with the client and ask if he has any questions or concerns you could help with.

Medical Assistant

Name: _____

Signature: _____

Date: _____

Client

Date: _____

Follow-up Date : _____

CHAPTER 34

Anticipatory Statements

People have different ideas about what it means to get old and what are normal health concerns in the elderly. Read and think about the following statements based upon what you believe now. Decide whether you agree or disagree. Write the word **agree** after the statement if you think the statement is true. Write the word **disagree** after the statement if you think the statement is false. Read the chapter to find out if your current beliefs can be supported.

1. Loss of memory is a normal part of aging. _____

2. As a person ages, the skin becomes thinner and drier and more easily bruised. _____

3. Many people who are elderly take several medications each day. _____

4. Medications and treatments are the same for the client who is elderly as for the client who is young. _____

5. The client who is elderly should take an active part in her own health care. _____

The Geriatric Client

Learning Objectives

Upon completion of this chapter, the medical assistant student should be able to:

- Identify the medical assistant's role in caring for the older client
- List physical changes in the older client that may affect the action and effectiveness of a prescribed medicine
- Explain how inactivity can lead to serious health problems
- Discuss ways in which the medical assistant can promote self-care in the older client
- List common eating problems in the older client
- Develop a teaching plan to assist a client who is elderly

Key Terms

absorption The taking up of a substance, such as medication, into or within the body.

comorbidity Two or more separate disorders or health problems that are occurring at the same time.

distribution Sending out to specific sites or places within the body.

excretion Getting rid of or moving a solid substance out of the body.

geriatrics Field of medicine related to aging and the older client.

mobility Ability to move and change place and direction.

sensorineural hearing loss Hearing loss due to nerve damage.

■ INTRODUCTION

Older Americans are the fastest growing segment of the U.S. population. The aging process puts the elderly person at increased risk of certain health problems. Disorders are not a natural part of aging, although many disorders are seen more often in the older person. Many of the clients with whom medical assistants work are elderly. This chapter introduces factors associated with aging that the medical assistant needs to understand in order to give competent and caring service to an elderly client. The absorption, distribution, and metabolism of medications in the body as a person ages is discussed. Sensory changes that can affect the client's quality of life and health care are discussed in relation to the medical assistant's role.

■ THE CLIENT WHO IS ELDERLY

Gerontology is the study of the older person. **Geriatrics** is the branch of medicine that works with the older client. The majority of clients seen in the adult care medical office are older individuals. Client-centered care is important throughout the life span. The elderly client is just as important as an infant client.

As a person gets older, the body and its responses slow down. An older person's reflexes might be slower, but the ability to respond is still present. Loss of the ability to think, remember, or solve problems is not a normal part of getting older. An older person who displays these limitations has a health problem, not an aging problem. The mind and body still work to sustain and promote life. However, when faced with trauma, other injuries, infection, or other sickness, the older body may not be able to correct the problem.

Chronic medical disorders that affect young people affect old people as well. For example, cardiovascular disorders affect children as well as adults. What differs is the treatment and the client's ability to tolerate or follow through with the treatment. This can happen for several reasons. The older person may have to manage other chronic conditions at the same time. This is called **comorbidity.** A person's ability to perform tasks as part of the treatment plan may also decrease. As people age, certain changes put them at risk of developing problems and inhibit their ability to respond successfully to treatment.

■ MEDICATION AND THE OLDER CLIENT

In addition to all the facts and safety precautions regarding medication that apply to everyone, there are some special concerns with the geriatric client. Major issues regarding older clients and medicine include:

- Physical changes in the body that affect the drug
- Use of over-the-counter (OTC) medicines
- Sensory changes that can affect the client's compliance with instructions for medication use

The older client may have several health problems at once, and may be taking prescribed medication to treat each condition. It is not uncommon for an older person to take 10 different medications every day. In addition, the client may also buy and take OTC medications to self-treat other problems; some of these other concerns may even be caused by the prescribed medications.

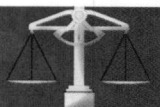

LEGAL/ETHICAL THOUGHTS

As a medical assistant, you may think that you are helping the older client by sharing her health care information with her spouse or adult children. Stop! The client must give permission before any health information is disclosed, even to relatives.

Medications in the Body

For a prescribed medicine to be successful (effective), it must go through four stages in the body (Figure 34-1): (1) **absorption,** (2) **distribution,** (3) metabolism, and (4) **excretion.** As the medicine travels to its destination, a breakdown at any of these stages will directly influence the effectiveness of the drug and client outcome.

Absorption. To work as intended, a medicine must be absorbed into the body. For example, when a client swallows a pill, the pill must be changed into a form in which it can reach the bloodstream and be carried to the cells. In this stage, several factors can affect the speed with which a medicine is absorbed and thus can begin to act. Gastric juices and other enzymes that help to break down pills decrease as the person ages. Also, the gastrointestinal tract of an older person slows down, meaning that a pill takes longer to get through this part of the path. This slowing down (slowed intestinal motility), along with the common problem of constipation, will directly affect the medicine's ability to work. Conversely, if motility is increased (such as if a client has diarrhea), the pill will not stay in the gastrointestinal tract long enough to be absorbed properly.

Distribution. Once a medication has been absorbed, it must be *distributed,* or sent to the right places in the body. Muscle mass decreases with age and is replaced with fat or adipose tissue, so drugs that are soluble in fat stay longer in these tissues. Fat-soluble vitamins, heparin, and many sleep medications will stay in fatty tissues for a long time, and thus will be active for longer. Also, if the blood circulation is slow or the client is dehydrated, medicines may take a long time to get to their intended destination.

Metabolism. As the body ages, metabolism slows down. This means that a pill, for example, is not changed from its active form into an inactive form as quickly on its way to leaving the body. The medicine remains in the body, and remains active, for a much longer time than it does in a younger person.

Excretion. Excretion is the part of the process that gets rid of waste. In an older person, the kidneys and respiratory system that help rid the body of waste slow down and are less efficient. Because they are not excreted quickly enough, drugs can build up to poisonous levels in the older person's body. This kind of overdose is a result of all the changes in the functioning of body systems: The medicine does not reach its destination in the amount or time it should; it may remain active in fat tissue for longer than intended; and it does not leave the body when it should. The medical assistant must observe older clients for side effects of medication and for symptoms of toxicity.

Over-the-Counter Medications

The use of OTC medication in any age group can be a concern for the medical assistant. With the client who is elderly, it is an even greater concern. As discussed earlier, bodily changes that occur with age can have a dramatic effect on prescribed medicines. This applies also to OTC medications.

OTC medicine is a big industry. Products include medications for pain, diarrhea, constipation, headaches, heartburn, arthritis, sleep disturbances, itching, and other skin problems, among many others. OTC medication is advertised directly to consumers through newspapers, magazines, radio, T.V., and lectures. People are often influenced to buy based on these sale pitches. Vitamins are also drugs, even though

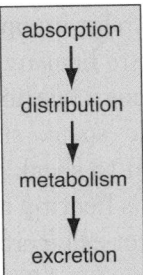

FIGURE 34-1 Medicine must pass through four stages (absorption, distribution, metabolism, and excretion) to work successfully.

clients may not intend to use them as medication. Sometimes clients take large doses of vitamins to treat some disorders; this is often done without any advice or input from the health care provider. It is helpful if the client brings in a written list of *everything* she is taking: all medications, vitamins, herbs, supplements, and so on. Sometimes clients even bring their prescription bottles and OTC medication bottles into the medical office.

At each office visit, the client needs to review all of her medicines, including OTC products and vitamins, with the medical assistant. It is not enough for the medical assistant to ask if there have been any changes or new medicines since the last visit. The client may not remember exactly when an OTC medication was added, or may not consider vitamins to be a new medicine.

■ SENSORY CHANGES IN THE ELDERLY

The senses help people interact with the outside world and be aware of the inside world. Sensory changes linked with getting older can have a dramatic effect on a client's ability to perform daily activities. The changes can also affect a person's ability to carry out treatment plans or participate in healthy behaviors. The medical assistant needs to be aware of these changes and how they can affect the client's care. Through observation and talking with the client, the medical assistant can promote ways for the client to maintain self-care ability and independence.

Sight

Age-related changes occur in the sense of sight. Disorders of the eye and other systems can affect vision. Whatever the cause, poor vision in the elderly can have dramatic effects. The medical assistant should observe clients while they are in the office. Is the client able to read the form that must be completed? Do clients have difficulty seeing as they walk from the waiting room to the examination room? Trouble with vision can affect the client's ability to follow written

directions. The client may not be able to read the small print on a prescription bottle, or handwritten instructions (or even printed directions) that the medical assistant gives her. If the client's sight is very poor, it might even be hard for her to find small pills. It might be helpful for the medical assistant to write a little larger and read the instructions to the client. The pharmacist should be asked to print larger prescription labels for an older client who has poor vision.

Older people usually see some colors better than others. It becomes harder to tell the difference between blue and green, although the distinction between red and yellow often remains the same. Knowing this, the medical assistant can suggest to the client that reds and yellows might be more enjoyable to look at and easier to work with. Reds and yellows in clothing can make garments easier to button and unbutton or to zip and unzip. Bright colors in hallways and at the edges of stairs will help alert the older client.

Hearing

As a person ages, higher-pitched sounds become more difficult to hear. Hearing loss may result from exposure to loud noise, either at work or over the course of a lifetime. **Sensorineural hearing loss** is common. Whatever the cause, the client may not be able to trust her hearing, although she may not recognize that she has a hearing impairment. For example, the client may not hear, or may misinterpret, what is said while the medical assistant or doctor is giving instructions or explanations. Some people just nod or say yes even if they have not clearly heard or understood what was said. The medical assistant needs to watch for inappropriate responses that may be a clue to hearing problems.

If the client has a hearing loss, the medical assistant needs to speak slowly and clearly. There is no reason to speak loudly; it does not improve the client's hearing and it may confuse some people. Do not exaggerate lip movements, as this will make it more difficult for the client to lip-read. It is important for the medical assistant to be positioned face to face with the client when speaking with her. Do not turn your back, look down, or write in the chart while speaking to the client. Written instructions should be provided in addition to oral directions.

Taste

The sense of taste affects eating and thus directly affects nutrition. With aging, the taste buds change, becoming dull and less sensitive to small differences in flavor (Figure 34-2). The client may complain that food is bland and needs spices. A client may lose her appetite when food is bland and unattractive. In contrast, the taste of sweetness may be heightened with age. The client may be surprised by a desire for sweets, especially if she did not have a "sweet tooth" in youth.

Smell

The sense of smell, which is closely related to taste, also seems to lessen as a person ages. Inability to smell may contribute to an older person's lack of appetite. It is also a safety concern, if the older client cannot smell gas or other odors

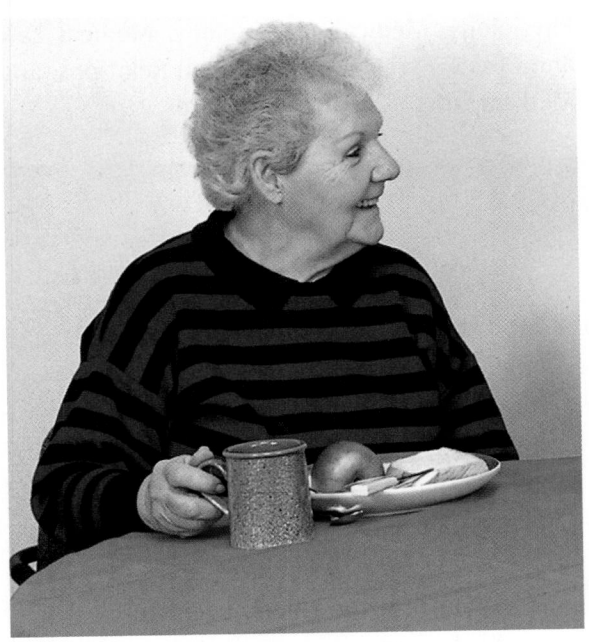

FIGURE 34-2 An older client may add more salt or spices to her food. Sharing mealtime is important to good nutrition and health.

that signal danger in the home. Smoke detectors and carbon monoxide monitors should be in all homes and especially in the homes of the elderly.

Touch

Touch has both physical and emotional aspects. Touch receptors may become less sensitive as a person ages. However, changes in physical sensation are usually related to disorders rather than aging. Peripheral neuropathy can result in an abnormal gait that increases the risk of falling. Neuropathy can affect the client's ability to feel or even notice bruises and cuts. This can lead to a delay in seeking help and getting treatment.

There is a need for touch even in old age. It communicates companionship and caring. Elderly people who are isolated may have a strong need for the emotions connected with touch. Some long-term care facilities have organized sensory groups to help maintain this sense of emotional touch and caring.

Pain

Chronic pain is not a normal part of aging. In the past, older clients' complaints about pain were often ignored, or attributed to a desire for attention, or dismissed as just normal "aches and pains." The medical assistant should ask questions and note signs of pain in the elderly client just as for younger clients. The client should be encouraged to discuss concerns, and the medical assistant may need to use prompting questions. The client may not even know that there are treatment options, or may not want to "bother" anyone by "complaining." The medical assistant needs to use her clinical and therapeutic listening skills to provide quality health care to the aging client.

■ WALKING AND GETTING AROUND

The ability to walk and move the body to perform daily activities is called **mobility.** Both the musculoskeletal system and the nervous system change over the course of a lifetime. For example, joints may become less flexible, thus affecting how fast and how easily a person can move. Skeletal changes, particularly in the vertebrae, can cause postural changes that affect the client's center of gravity and balance (Figure 34-3). Loss of mobility puts the client at greater risk for other health problems. This can become a vicious cycle: decreased physical activity has negative effects on many body systems; in turn, the resulting

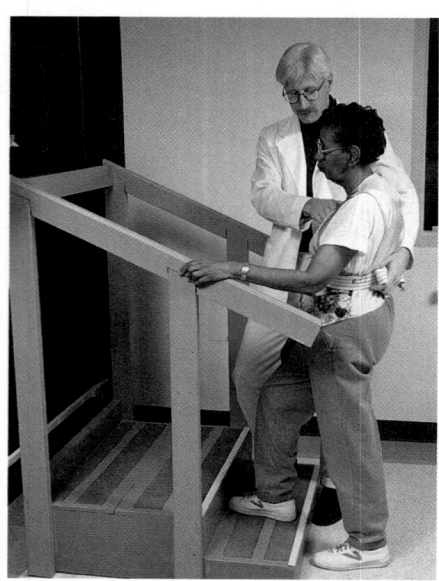

FIGURE 34-3 Learning to use handrails will help the older client balance and stay mobile.

health problems keep the client from maintaining a good level of physical activity.

Immobility and lack of activity are a risk factor for many disorders. Loss of appetite, pressure ulcers, broken bones, constipation, urinary incontinence, kidney stones, breathing difficulties, pneumonia, dehydration, loss of coordination, and loss of balance are all possible complications of immobility. The medical assistant needs to keep this in mind and encourage clients to remain active. The aging process is slowed by regular exercise. A primary goal of health care is to maintain independence of the older client.

BRIDGE TO CAAHEP

This chapter, which discusses the geriatric client, provides information and content related to CAA-HEP standards for Anatomy and Physiology, Medical Terminology, Medical Law and Ethics, Psychology, Communication, Medical Assisting Clinical Procedures, and Professional Components.

ABHES LINKS

This chapter, which discusses the geriatric client, links to ABHES course content for Anatomy and Physiology, Medical Terminology, Medical Law and Ethics, Psychology of Human Relations, and Medical Office Clinical Procedures.

POINTS OF HIGHLIGHT

- The majority of clients who receive care in a medical office setting are elderly.
- Loss of the ability to think, remember, or solve problems is not a normal part of aging.
- Treatment of medical disorders may be more complicated in the elderly client.
- The elderly client may take many different medications each day.
- Absorption, distribution, metabolism, and excretion of medications can all be affected by the aging process and changes in the older person's body.
- Combining OTC medications with prescription medications can be very harmful, especially for the older client.
- Sensory losses or impairments may make it more difficult for the elderly client to successfully and correctly follow health care treatment instructions.
- Immobility and lack of physical activity are a risk factor for many health disorders.

AAMA AREAS OF COMPETENCE

This chapter, which discusses the geriatric client, provides information or content within several areas listed in the Medical Assistant Role Delineation Study. These areas include: administrative, administrative procedures, clinical, fundamental principles, diagnostic procedures, patient(client) care, general transdisciplinary, professionalism, communication skills, legal concepts, and instruction.

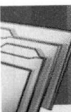 ### STUDENT PORTFOLIO ACTIVITY

The availability of community resources to meet the needs of the elderly is a concern for clients and their families. If you are to work effectively with elderly clients as a medical assistant, it is important for you to be aware of community resources. Visit an adult day care center in the community and write a report about what you discover. In your report, list the available services. Does the center provide transportation, meals, social services, help with medications, and social activities? What is the application process? What are the costs? Is there a waiting list? Make sure that you receive a letter noting the time you spent at the center, or have your observation sheet signed. What attributes of a medical assistant does this activity show the employer? Reflect in writing on this experience in your portfolio.

 ## AMT PATHS

This chapter, which discusses the geriatric client, provides a path to AMT competency in general medical assisting knowledge, anatomy and physiology, medical terminology, medical law, medical ethics, human relations, and patient (client) education.

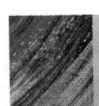 ### APPLYING YOUR SKILLS

An elderly client whom you have known for a while recently forgot an appointment, has been unable to remember many of his medications, and seems to be unclear as to events. These problems with memory, judgment, and behavior are new. Is this a normal part of aging? What should you do about your observation? What information would be helpful to the doctor?

CRITICAL THINKING QUESTIONS

1. How does the aging process affect the absorption of medication?

2. How can impaired vision affect a client's ability to take prescribed medication correctly?

3. What are the four steps necessary for a medication to work successfully in the body?

4. Inactivity in the older client can lead to health problems. Select a body system and tell how immobility can harm that body system.

5. What are OTC medications, and how can they affect the action of prescribed medications?

6. What are some ways in which poor eyesight in an older client might limit self-care activities?

7. Why is use of OTC medication without input from a health care provider a great concern in an elderly client?

8. Go back to the beginning of this chapter and review the Anticipatory Statements. Reread each statement and then indicate whether it is true or false. If the statement is false, rewrite it to make it a true statement.

CLIENT TEACHING PLAN

Instillation of Eyedrops for the Elderly Client

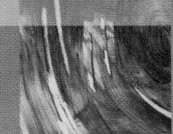

■ What Is to Be Taught:

• Instillation of eyedrops.

■ Objectives:

• Client will instill eyedrops as directed.

■ Preparation Before Teaching:

• Review medication precautions for the eyedrops prescribed.
• Make sure you have a sample eyedrop container to be used for teaching and paper and pen for written instructions.

■ Steps for the Medical Assistant:

1. Gather supplies needed.
2. Introduce yourself to the client.
3. Explain what you are going to teach and why.
4. Demonstrate handwashing technique.
5. Ask the client to wash her hands in the same way.
6. Show the client how to remove the lid or cap from the eyedrop container. Place the lid on a clean area, with the inside of the lid facing up, or ask the client to hold it in her hand to avoid contamination.
7. Ask the client to look up.
8. Tell the client to gently pull down on the lower lid of the eye that will have the drops put in.
9. Instruct the client to line up the eyedrop container with the middle of the lower lid.
10. Guide the client to gently squeeze the container and direct the liquid drops into the lower lid/conjunctiva area. Never let the tip of the container touch the eye.
11. Ask the client to close the eye softly to allow the medication to be absorbed. Remind her that squeezing the eyelids together tightly will press the medication out of the eye.
12. Instruct the client to replace the lid on the container.

13. Tell the client to wash her hands.
14. Remind the client always to read the label on the medicine container, and to keep all medicines out of the reach of children and pets.

■ Special Needs of the Client:

• Look at the client's chart to see if there are any factors that might interfere with the client's ability to instill eyedrops at home.
• Ask the client if there is anything you should know that might affect her ability to instill the eyedrops as directed.

■ Evaluation:

• Client will be able to state the steps of the procedure and list any necessary precautions.
• Client will be able to instill eyedrops with the help of the medical assistant.

■ Further Plans/Teaching:

• Give the client written instructions to refer to at home.
• Give the client the office telephone number and your extension; instruct her to call if she has any questions or concerns.

■ Follow-up:

• Call the client at home the next day and ask if she had any problems or has any questions.

Medical Assistant

Name: _____

Signature: _____

Date: _____

Client

Date: _____

Follow-up Date : _____

CHAPTER 35

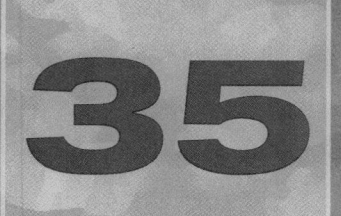

Anticipatory Statements

Read and think about the following statements based upon what you believe now. Decide whether you agree or disagree. Write the word **agree** after the statement if you think the statement is true. Write the word **disagree** after the statement if you think the statement is false. Read the chapter to find out if your current beliefs can be supported.

1. A leading cause of death in young children is accidents.   _____

2. The fastest period of growth for children is the toddler years.   _____

3. Immunizations are a vital part of the well-child visit.   _____

4. Parents should be asked to leave the room when a procedure is being done on a child. _____

Learning Objectives

Upon completion of this chapter, the medical assistant student should be able to:
- Identify the medical assistant's role regarding pediatric clients
- Define a well-child visit
- State the measurements taken at a well-child visit
- Explain the parent's role during a pediatric office visit
- Obtain and record head and chest circumferences of an infant
- Obtain and record the weight and length of an infant

The Pediatric Client

Key Terms

American Academy of Pediatrics National organization that sets guidelines for the practice of pediatricians and the care of children.

anorexia nervosa Eating disorder in which a person starves herself or himself because of a distorted self-image of obesity.

anticipatory guidance Explanation of what to expect from a child at a specific age; given for the purpose of encouraging parents to respond in a helpful way.

chest circumference Measurement around a person's chest; routinely obtained on infants.

developmental level Status (usually related to age) to which the child has grown in skill and function.

head circumference Measurement around a person's head; routinely obtained on an infant.

immunization Process of making a person immune or resistant to a disease; usually done by injection.

pediatrics Medical specialty that oversees the normal growth and development of infants and children and provides care for sick infants and children.

Rinne test Test to compare bone-conduction hearing with air-conduction hearing.

scoliosis Abnormal curvature of the spine; usually discovered during the early childhood years.

vaccination Administration of a preparation of living altered or killed microorganisms for the purpose of protecting a person from a specific disease.

Weber test Hearing test in which a vibrating tuning fork is used. The fork is held against the midline of the top of the head to determine if there is unilateral deafness.

■ INTRODUCTION

Working with children can be professionally rewarding, but it also can be challenging, as there are many special considerations in care of the child. **Pediatrics** is the area of medicine dealing with the growth, development, and care of children. The medical assistant will assist the doctor in performing procedures on pediatric clients. Understanding the basics of growth and development in the child, knowing how to approach and talk with children, and recognizing what is appropriate at different age levels are critical for the medical assistant.

■ OFFICE VISITS

Parents or guardians, as part of their caregiver role, take a child to the pediatrician's office regularly to check on how the child is growing and developing and to receive scheduled immunizations. These visits, called *well-baby* or *well-child visits*, are excellent opportunities for the medical assistant to talk with the parents and offer **anticipatory guidance.** Giving anticipatory guidance means sharing information with the parent about what is normal and what to expect at the child's current stage of development. Teething, toilet training, school success, peer pressure, and rebellious behavior are all common topics of discussion, depending on the child's age and level of development. It is essential that the medical assistant know and recognize the stages of development.

The medical assistant needs to establish a relationship of trust with both the child and the parents. Parental acceptance of the health care provider is often based on how that provider treats the child. A calm, reassuring voice and a nonjudgmental attitude will help in beginning a trusting relationship. Parents will recognize and appreciate the medical assistant's genuine interest in the health of their child. The child will sense the medical assistant's concern through voice and touch. Children and parents have different physical and emotional needs, and it is up to the medical assistant to meet all these needs.

Children often are brought to the pediatrician's office when they are sick. The same principles for care of a well child apply to care of the sick child. A separate waiting room is usually provided for sick children. This helps to protect healthy infants and children from contagious diseases. Thorough cleaning of the waiting room is essential to maintain a safe and healthy environment for the children. There should be no toys that the children will put in their mouths to suck on.

■ VITAL SIGNS

The medical assistant must gain the child's cooperation if he hopes to obtain accurate vital signs and measurements. If a child wiggles or screams and cries, the medical assistant will not be able to hear heart or lung sounds or obtain an accurate temperature or blood pressure reading. The parent can assist the medical assistant by holding the child or talking to the child while the medical assistant performs the procedure.

Head and Chest Circumference

The size of an infant's head, in relation to the size of the child's chest, is an important indicator of normal growth. **Head circumference** and **chest circumference** measurements are taken as part of the well-child visit. The size is obtained by measuring around the infant's head and then chest with a tape measure (Figures 35-1 and 35-2). These numbers are recorded in the client's chart. For accurate measuring, the two ends of the tape measure should meet without twisting or tugging. While obtaining the measurement, ask the parent to talk to the infant to keep him occupied.

Infant Height and Weight

The infant's height and weight are obtained and recorded at each visit. They are important indicators of the infant's growth and nutritional status, and are the basis for calculation of

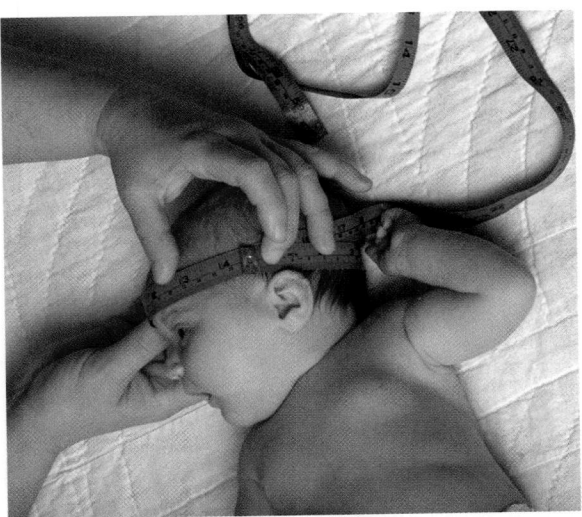

FIGURE 35-1 Measuring the head circumference of an infant.

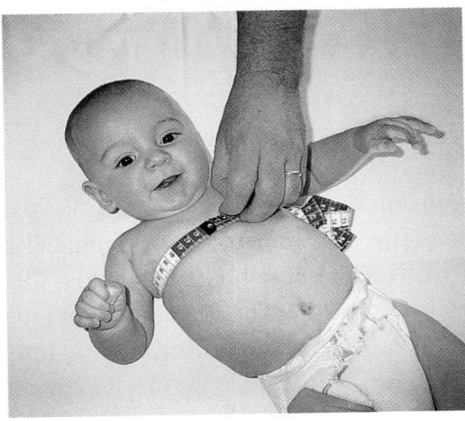

FIGURE 35-2 Measuring the chest circumference of an infant.

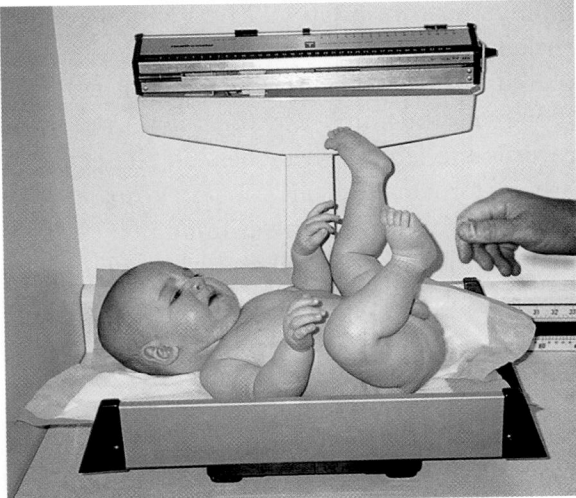

FIGURE 35-3 Measuring the weight of an infant.

gain or loss of even a few ounces can be significant. The parents will usually ask how much the infant weighs and whether that is a good weight for an infant of their child's age. The weight of the infant is often plotted on a pediatric growth chart form, which is kept in the infant client's medical chart.

An infant's height measurement, referred to as the *length* of the infant, is also done while the child is lying down (in the supine position). A tape measure or ruler-type scale can be used for this procedure. The infant's head is placed at the end of the measured markings (Figure 35-4). The infant's parent should gently hold the

dosages of pediatric medicines. If the child becomes sick, the doctor will refer to the infant's chart to find the most recent weight, so that the correct dosage can be prescribed.

To weigh the infant, the medical assistant or parent must remove the infant's clothing. Sometimes a clean diaper is weighed and then put on the infant; this is determined by office policy. To measure the infant's weight, the infant is placed lying down on a baby scale in the supine or dorsal recumbent position (Figure 35-3). First adjust the balance beam that measures pounds; then adjust the beam that measures ounces. The weight measurement must be very accurate, as a

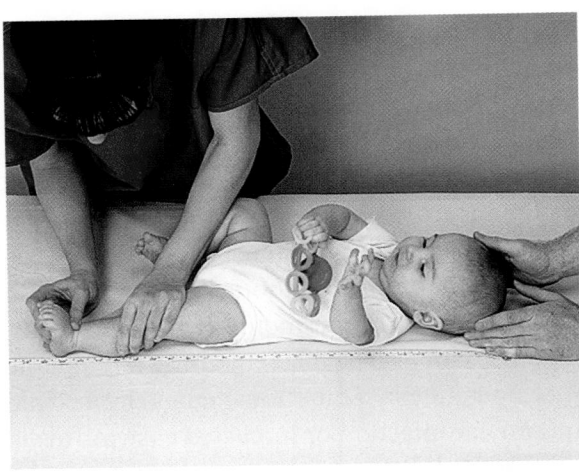

FIGURE 35-4 Measuring the length of an infant.

infant's head in position. The infant's legs are straightened; the heels of the feet are sometimes placed against a board. The medical assistant then reads the number by the infant's heels and records the length, in inches, on the pediatric growth form in the client's chart. Do not leave an infant unguarded on the examination table, as he may roll or wiggle off it. Pick the infant up and hand him to the parent as soon as you are done with the measurement.

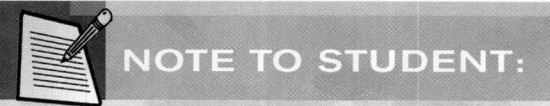

NOTE TO STUDENT:

On the average, an infant can be expected to double the birth length and triple the birth weight by the time he is one year old. For example, a baby who weighed 7 pounds and was 19 inches long at birth will be about 21 pounds and 38 inches long by the baby's first birthday.

Child's Height and Weight

When a child is able to stand independently, the height and weight can be measured using a balance-beam scale (Figure 35-5). The procedure is the same as for an adult (see Chapter 4).

Temperature

The rules that apply to taking the temperature of an adult also apply to the child client; the same kinds of thermometers are used as well. The temperature can be taken by mouth if the child is able to understand and follow directions. This method is usually reserved for children 5 years of age or older. The child must be able to hold the probe in the mouth without biting down. (Do not use a mercury thermometer.) A child's temperature can also be taken by using a tympanic thermometer placed in the ear canal. If the child has an ear infection or impacted earwax, avoid this method. Otherwise, it is a quick, easy, and

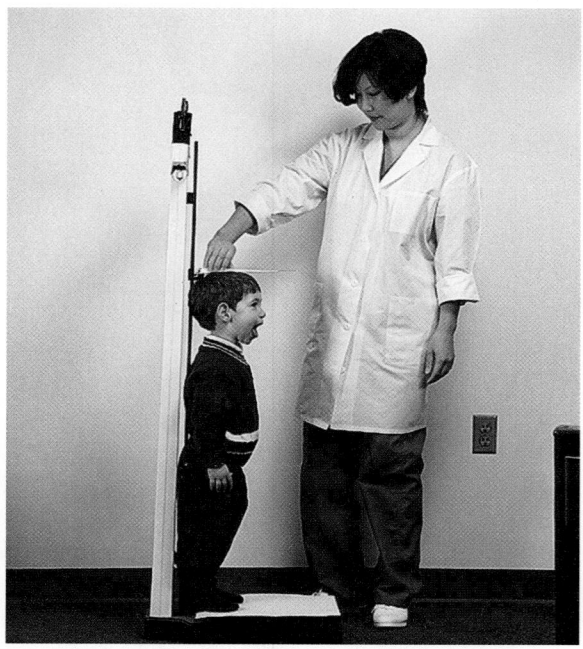

FIGURE 35-5 Measuring the height of a young child.

accurate method. When obtaining an axillary temperature, the thermometer is placed under the arm. The arm must be held against the body for several minutes. The medical assistant must use great caution when taking a rectal temperature. Children may injure themselves by moving too much while the thermometer is inserted. Whatever method is used, the medical assistant must exercise caution.

Pulse

The pulse rate is fastest in the newborn, and decreases as age increases. The average heart rate of a newborn is 110, but decreases to a range of 60 to 100 by time the child is 10 years old. A range of 60 to 100 is the normal range for an adult. The fast heartbeat makes it difficult to count the radial pulse in an infant or young child, so an apical pulse is the preferred method in infants and young children. The medical assistant uses a stethoscope and places it at the apex of the heart. (The apex is found on the left side at the fifth intercostal space, at the midclavicular line.) The apical pulse is counted for one full minute.

Respiration

The respiration rate is fastest in the newborn, and decreases with age until adulthood. In children older than 6, the respiration rate can be counted the same as for an adult. For an infant or a child less than 6 years of age, the medical assistant must watch the rise and fall of the abdomen. One rise as the child inhales and one fall of the abdomen as the child exhales is considered one respiration. It is important to count for one full minute.

Blood Pressure

Blood pressure is not routinely taken on an infant. A pediatric stethoscope should be used on small children. The size of the cuff is important. The cuff size is determined by the size, not the age, of the child. A cuff that is too large will give a false low reading. A cuff that is too small will give a false high reading. As a rule, blood pressure is obtained on children only once a year.

■ SPECIMEN COLLECTION

The collection of urine is a common procedure performed in a pediatrician's office. An older child can provide a urine sample using the same steps as an adult (see Chapter 41). The instruction from the medical assistant should be adjusted to the child's **developmental level.** Depending upon age of development, the parent or medical assistant may need to help the child with urine collection.

For the infant or child who is too young to have urinary control, the procedure is different. The parent can be involved with the procedure. The medical assistant takes the diaper off the infant while the infant is on the examination table. The parent can assist the medical assistant to clean the perineal area and place a clear plastic urine collection bag over the perineum. When applying a collection bag on a female infant, center the opening over the labia. In a male, center the scrotum and penis in the collection bag. A diaper is then put on the infant, covering the collection bag. After urine is collected in the bag, remove the bag carefully, clean the infant as needed, and replace the diaper.

■ IMMUNIZATION

Immunizations or **vaccinations** are part of well-child visits. They are not given if the child is sick at the time of the office visit. The times and numbers of immunizations are scheduled according to guidelines set by the **American Academy of Pediatrics** and office policy as determined by the doctor. Vaccinations are very safe, but, as with any medication or treatment, there is always a risk of side effects. The medical assistant must read the package inserts that come with the medication and keep up to date with information sent

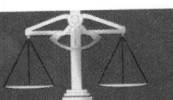

LEGAL/ETHICAL THOUGHTS

The Department of Health and Human Services, a federal agency, states that release of information about pediatric clients to the parents of the minor clients is governed by state laws and other applicable laws.

out from the state's Health Department and the Centers for Disease Control and Prevention. A thorough explanation must be given to the parent before any immunizations are administered. The parent must sign an informed consent form.

Immunizations provide protection against many diseases: measles, mumps, rubella, polio, diphtheria, tetanus, chickenpox, hepatitis, and meningitis. The prevention of disease is an important part of taking care of children. Immunizations protect the individual child and also others in the community. Before immunizations were developed, many infants and children died from these diseases. Families were kept isolated or quarantined to keep others from contracting the disease. State laws vary regarding immunization requirements.

■ VISION AND HEARING TESTING

Other procedures routinely done at well-child visits include vision and hearing tests. To test the child's ability to see clearly, the medical assistant uses a Snellen chart. The medical assistant will find out if the child needs any vision aids, such as glasses or possibly contact lenses. These procedures may be done by the medical assistant in the health office, or at the child's school. The procedures are the same as for adults, with some minor adjustments. If the client is a very young child who has not yet learned to read, the standard Snellen chart may be replaced with a chart that uses shapes, symbols, or the capital letter E pointing in different directions, instead of letters of the alphabet (Figure 35-6). The child names the shape or the direction in which the E points.

Observe for any difficulty in hearing. Note whether the young child turns toward a sound, such as when the medical assistant speaks. Startle reflex in an infant should be noted. The doctor may perform a **Weber test** and/or a **Rinne test** for hearing.

In the Weber test, a vibrating tuning fork is held on top of the head along the midline. In

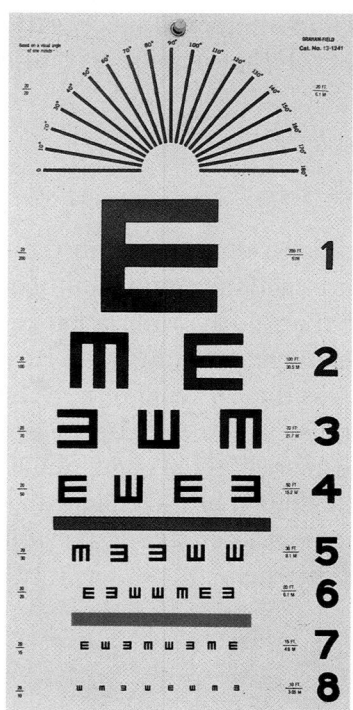

FIGURE 35-6 A Snellen E chart is used for a child who is too young to read a regular Snellen chart. To test visual acuity, the child reads which direction the E is pointing.

some conduction hearing loss, the sound will seem louder in the affected ear. In some hearing loss due to nerve damage, the sound will seem louder in the unaffected ear. In the Rinne test, the vibrating tuning fork is placed on the mastoid process (bone of the skull behind external auditory meatus). When the client can no longer hear the sound then the vibrating fork is held close to the external auditory meatus. It is a normal finding if the client can still hear the sound.

■ DISORDERS IN CHILDREN

Many of the same disorders that affect adults also affect children. The disorders affect the same structures; however, the intensity and course of the disorder may vary depending on the child's age. The treatment may not be the same for children. Certainly, medication formulas and dosages are different from those used with adults. Scoliosis and anorexia nervosa are two disorders that are usually first found during childhood. Often these problems are discovered during the course of routine visits.

Scoliosis

Scoliosis is an abnormal lateral curvature of the spine. In some cases, the cause is congenital. The bones of the spine do not form perfectly, so as the child grows, the vertebrae curve. The spine becomes crooked and the child does not appear to be standing straight. In the majority of cases, though, the cause is unknown. Various treatments are available. A child may need to wear a back brace for several years; if that is the treatment, the medical assistant must give emotional support to both the child and the parents. In other cases, surgery may be done, either to insert metal rods to support the bones or to fuse parts of the vertebrae. It is critical to detect scoliosis at an early stage so that the child can be treated and the condition kept from getting

worse. Although the progression or worsening of a spinal curve can be stopped, the curve can not be completely straightened. Therefore, it is important not to let scoliosis get too advanced. A severe curvature can affect the internal organs.

A scoliosis check is usually done at a well-child visit around the age of 9 or 10. The test is simple. The child stands with his or her back to the medical assistant and bends at the waist (Figure 35-7). The medical assistant looks for any unevenness on either side of the spine. A special ruler is also used in some offices. This is especially helpful if the curve is in the early stages and is hard to find just by looking.

Anorexia Nervosa

Anorexia nervosa is an eating disorder that affects mostly female preteens and teens, although some males suffer from this condition as well. The medical assistant can start assessing a child for anorexia at the age of 9. The medical assistant will talk with the child about self-image and how the child views himself. Questions such as, "Do you like how you look?" and "Who would you want to look like?" are helpful to provide insight into the child's self-perception.

This condition is hard to detect at first. The child may try to hide it from family and friends. If the child is thought to be at risk, or has developed the condition, treatment is aimed at the entire family. A child with this condition has a distorted self-image and sees himself as fat, even though the child may really be very thin. The child will become obsessed with losing weight and begin to starve himself to achieve the goal of being thin. This is a psychological disorder that requires not just medical attention, but also counseling and psychological help. If the condition goes untreated, the child will become malnourished; malnutrition causes irreversible damage to the growing body, including cardiac damage and cessation or delay of the menstrual cycle in females. The members of the health care team need to work together to help a child with this disorder.

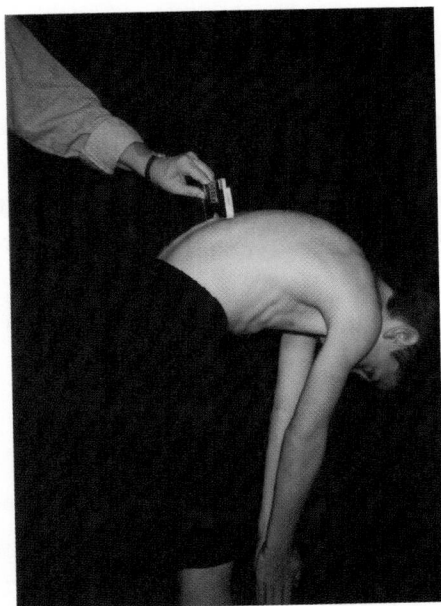

FIGURE 35-7 A medical assistant performing scoliosis screening.

PROCEDURE 35-1

Measuring Infant Chest Circumference

Student Competency Objective: The medical assistant student will obtain and record a measurement of the infant's chest circumference.

Items Needed: Tape measure, paper and pen

Steps:

1. Wash your hands.
2. Get together equipment and supplies.
3. Introduce yourself to the client's parent, even if the parent has brought the child on previous visits to your office. The parent may have forgotten your name. This also helps to establish a provider–client relationship, because it shows the client's parent that you want him to know who you are.
4. Identify the infant client. Ask the parent to state the child's name to establish that this is the right client, and then compare the name given to the name on the chart. It is up to the medical assistant to identify the right client before performing any procedure.
5. Smile at the infant and talk in a soothing, calm voice.
6. Lay the infant on his back on the examination table. If the child is 2 years old or older and cooperative, the child may sit on the table.
7. Ask the parent to help by talking to the infant and gently holding the head.
8. Tell the parent what you are going to do.
9. Place the end marking of the tape measure at the center of the infant's chest, right in line with the infant's nipples. Hold it in place with your finger. Slip the tape measure under the infant's body and bring it around to meet the other end of the tape at the center of the chest.
10. Read the number where the tape measure ends meet. The number may be in centimeters or inches. If in centimeters, read to the nearest 0.01 cm. If in inches, read to the nearest half-inch.
11. Make sure that the parent is holding the infant before you turn to write the number in the infant's chart.
12. Record the procedure in the infant's chart.
13. Wash your hands.

Charting Example:

7/13/20xx   2:30 P.M.   Infant girl—chest circumference 17 in.*

Judy Lowe, S.M.A.

Judy Lowe, S.M.A. (printed name)

*Measurements may be in centimeters or inches, depending on office policy.

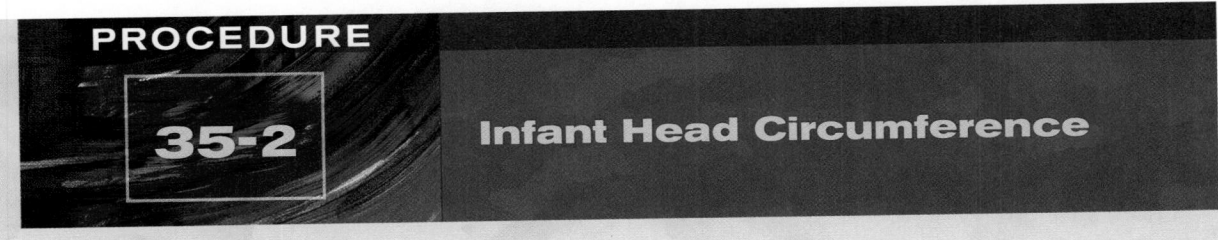

PROCEDURE

35-2

Infant Head Circumference

Student Competency Objective: The medical assistant student will obtain and record a measurement of the infant's head circumference.

Items Needed: Tape measure, paper and pen

Steps:

1. Wash your hands.
2. Get together equipment and supplies.
3. Introduce yourself to the client's parent, even if the parent has brought the child on previous visits to your office. The parent may have forgotten your name. This also helps to establish a provider–client relationship, because it shows the client's parent that you want him to know who you are.
4. Identify the infant client. Ask the parent to state the child's name to establish that this is the right client, and then compare the name given to the name on the chart. It is up to the medical assistant to identify the right client before performing any procedure.
5. Smile at the infant and talk in a soothing, calm voice.
6. Lay the infant on his back on the examination table. If the child is 2 years old or older and cooperative, the child may sit on the table.
7. Ask the parent to help by talking to the infant and gently holding the head.
8. Tell the parent what you are going to do.
9. Wrap the tape measure around the largest part of the infant's head. The tape measure should meet at the middle of the forehead. Do not pull too tightly or stretch the tape measure.
10. Read the number where the tape measure ends meet. The number may be in centimeters or inches. If in centimeters, read to the nearest 0.01 cm. If in inches, read to the nearest half-inch.
11. Make sure that the parent is holding the infant before you turn to write the number in the infant's chart.
12. Record the procedure in the infant's chart.
13. Wash your hands.
14. Infant head circumference is often taken at the same time as the chest circumference. If you are doing both, continue without giving the child to the parent. Give the infant to the parent and record both numbers when both measurements have been completed.

Charting Example:

7/13/20xx   2:40 P.M.   Infant boy—head circumference 40.5 cm.*

Jared Coachmen, S.M.A.

Jared Coachmen, S.M.A. (printed name)

*Measurements may be in centimeters or inches, depending on office policy.

Student Competency Objective: The medical assistant student will measure and record an infant's weight.

Items Needed: Baby scale, paper and pen

Steps:

1. Wash your hands.
2. Get together equipment and supplies.
3. Introduce yourself to the client's parent, even if the parent has brought the child on previous visits to your office. The parent may have forgotten your name. This also helps to establish a provider-client relationship, because it shows the client's parent that you want him to know who you are.
4. Identify the infant client. Ask the parent to state the child's name to establish that this is the right client, and then compare the name given to the name on the chart. It is up to the medical assistant to identify the right client before performing any procedure.
5. Smile at the infant and talk in a soothing, calm voice.
6. Ask the parent to help by talking to the infant.
7. Tell the parent what you are going to do.
8. Remove the client's diaper. Some offices put a clean diaper on the infant and subtract the weight of the diaper from the weight obtained. This is decided by office policy.
9. Lay the infant on his back on the infant scale. If the child is 2 years old or older, and cooperative, the child may sit in the scale. At the point when the child can stand and balance, use the balance beam standing scale.
10. For safety, place one hand very close to but not touching the infant.
11. With your other hand, move the slide on the scale bar marked pounds.
12. Move the slide on the scale bar marked ounces until the beam balances or bounces in the middle.
13. Read the number marked on the pound bar.
14. Read the number marked on the ounce bar.
15. Take the infant out of the scale and make sure that the parent is holding him before turning away to record the weight in the infant's chart.
16. Ask the parent if he has any questions.
17. Clean the scale.
18. Wash your hands.

Charting Example:

5/6/20xx   9:00 A.M.   12-month-old infant brought in by parents for well-child visit. Weight equals 22 pounds, 3 ounces.

Tara McDuffy, S.M.A.

Tara McDuffy, S.M.A. (printed name)

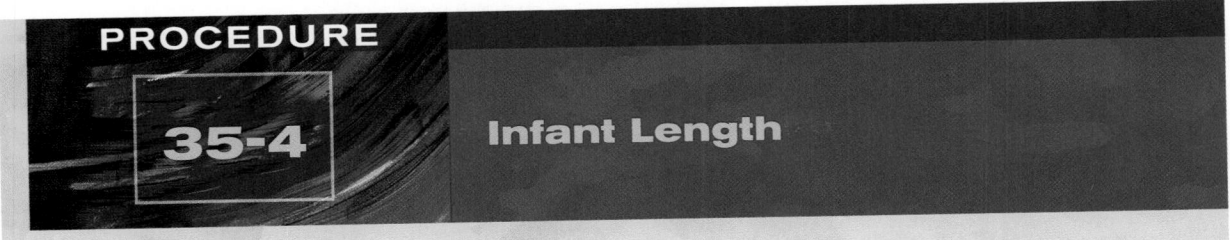

PROCEDURE

35-4

Infant Length

Student Competency Objective: The medical assistant student will measure and record an infant's length.

Items Needed: Baby scale, paper and pen

Steps:

1. Wash your hands.
2. Get together equipment and supplies.
3. Introduce yourself to the client's parent, even if the parent has brought the child on previous visits to your office. The parent may have forgotten your name. This also helps to establish a provider-client relationship, because it shows the client's parent that you want him to know who you are.
4. Identify the infant client. Ask the parent to state the child's name to establish that this is the right client, and then compare the name given to the name on the chart. It is up to the medical assistant to identify the right client before performing any procedure.
5. Smile at the infant and talk in a soothing, calm voice.
6. Tell the parent what you are going to do.
7. Lay the infant on his back on the examination table. Place the infant so that his head lines up at the beginning of the markings on the side of the scale.
8. Ask the parent to help by talking to the infant and gently holding the head.
9. Extend the infant's leg until the foot touches the footboard. If the scale does not have a footboard, use one of your hands as a footboard.
10. Read the number on the ruler to which the infant's feet extend.
11. Make sure that the parent is holding the infant before you turn to record the number in the infant's chart.
12. Ask the parent if he has any questions.
13. Record the procedure in the infant's chart.
14. Wash your hands.

Charting Example:

5/6/20xx   9:00 A.M.   12-month-old infant brought in by parents for well-child visit. Length equals 33½ inches.

Ellen Jackson, S.M.A.

Ellen Jackson, S.M.A. (printed name)

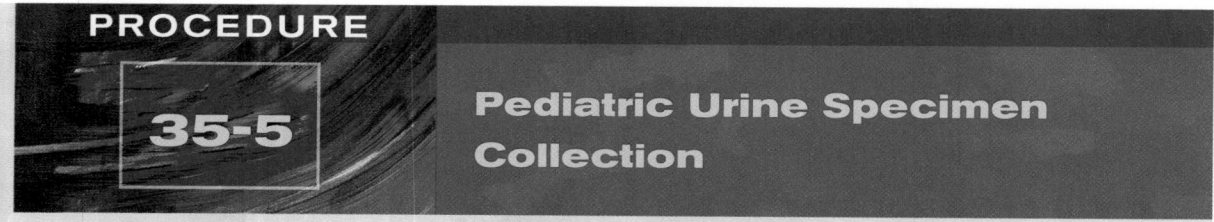

PROCEDURE

35-5

Pediatric Urine Specimen Collection

Student Competency Objective: The medical assistant student will obtain a urine specimen from an infant.

Items Needed: Urine collection bag, gloves, washcloth, towels, soap, water, biohazardous waste bag, lab requisition slip, paper and pen

Steps:

1. Wash your hands.
2. Get together equipment and supplies. Put items needed within reach of the examination table.
3. Introduce yourself to the client's parent, even if the parent has brought the child on previous visits to your office. The parent may have forgotten your name. This also helps to establish a provider–client relationship, because it shows the client's parent that you want him to know who you are.
4. Identify the infant client. Ask the parent to state the child's name to establish that this is the right client, and then compare the name given to the name on the chart. It is up to the medical assistant to identify the right client before performing any procedure.
5. Smile at the infant and talk in a soothing, calm voice.
6. Ask the parent to help by talking to the infant and standing near the infant.
7. Put on gloves.
8. Remove the infant's diaper.
9. Wash the infant's perineum with soap and water. Dry gently.
10. Following the directions on the urine collection bag, place the bag over the infant's perineum (Figure 35–8). For male infants, the center of the bag should be placed over the penis and scrotum. For female infants, the urine bag should be centered over the labia.

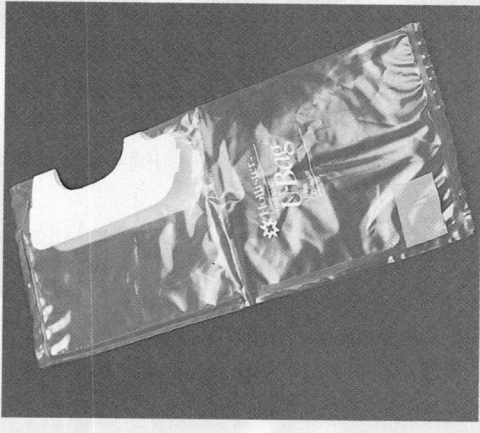

FIGURE 35–8 A pediatric urine collector.

(Continues)

PROCEDURE 35-5 (Continued)

11. Once the bag is in place, gently press the adhesive on the bag so that it adheres to the skin.
12. Carefully place a diaper over the bag.
13. Hand the infant to the parent.
14. Check the bag in 5 minutes and periodically thereafter until urine is present in the bag.
15. When enough urine is in the bag, remove the bag carefully, to avoid spilling urine and to prevent irritation to the infant's skin.
16. Make sure that the parent is holding the infant securely before you proceed to the next step.
17. Place the urine specimen in a container, as indicated by office procedures.
18. Label the specimen container.
19. Discard the collection bag in the biohazardous waste container.
20. Remove your gloves.
21. Ask the parent if he has any questions.
22. Record the amount of urine collected in the client's chart.
23. Wash your hands.

Charting Example:

9/30/20xx   3:00 P.M.   Urine specimen obtained from infant using a pediatric urine collection bag. Specimen labeled, processed, and sent to lab. Parent instructed to call
office for test results.

Nicole Berk, S.M.A.

Nicole Berk, S.M.A. (printed name)

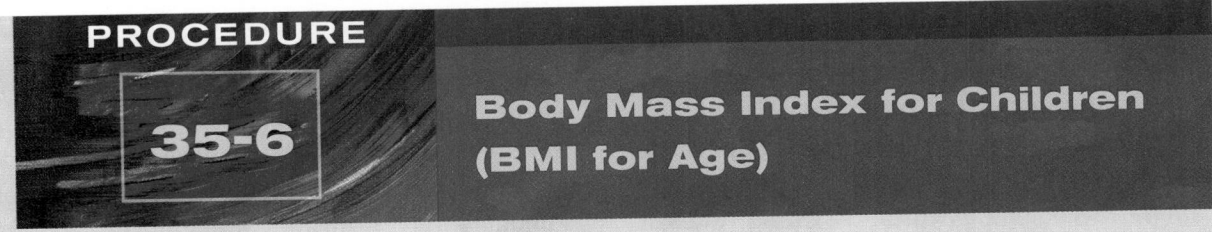

PROCEDURE 35-6
Body Mass Index for Children (BMI for Age)

Student Competency Objective: The medical assistant student will calculate the body mass index (BMI) for a child over the age of 2.

Items Needed: Chart, paper and pen, scale for height and weight (if the child's height and weight are not known and must be measured), BMI formula

Steps:

1. Wash your hands.
2. Get together equipment and supplies.

(Continues)

PROCEDURE 35-6 (Continued)

3. Introduce yourself to the client's parent, even if the parent has brought the child on previous visits to your office. The parent may have forgotten your name. This also helps to establish a provider–client relationship, because it shows the client's parent that you want him to know who you are.

4. Identify the child client. Ask the parent to state the child's name to establish that this is the right client, and then compare the name given to the name on the chart. It is up to the medical assistant to identify the right client before performing any procedure.

5. Obtain the child's height and weight, if not known. (See Procedures 35–3 and 35–4.)

6. If measurements are in pounds and inches, write down the child's weight in pounds (follow office policy).

7. Write down the child's height in inches.

8. Insert these numbers in the correct places in the BMI formula:

   BMI = (weight in pounds / height in inches) × height in inches × 703

9. Work through the formula: Divide the weight in pounds by the height in inches and multiply the result by the height in inches. Take that number and multiply it by 703.

10. If measurements are in kilograms and meters, write down the child's weight in kilograms (follow office policy).

11. Write down the child's height in meters.

12. Insert these numbers in the correct places in the BMI formula:

    BMI = (weight in kilograms / height in meters) × height in meters × 703

13. Work through the formula: Divide the weight in kilograms by the height in meters and multiply the result by the height in meters. Take that number and multiply it by 703.

14. Record the result as the BMI in the child's chart.

 ### BRIDGE TO CAAHEP

This chapter, which discusses the pediatric client, provides information and content related to CAA-HEP standards for Anatomy and Physiology, Medical Terminology, Law and Ethics, Communication, Psychology, Medical Assisting Clinical Procedures, and Professional Components.

 ### ABHES LINKS

This chapter, which discusses the pediatric client, links to ABHES course content for Anatomy and Physiology, Medical Terminology, Medical Law and Ethics, Psychology of Human Relations, and Medical Office Clinical Procedures.

 ### AAMA AREAS OF COMPETENCE

This chapter, which discusses the pediatric client, provides information or content within several areas listed in the Medical Assistant Role Delineation Study. These areas include: clinical, fundamental principles, diagnostic orders, patient (client) care, general transdisciplinary, professionalism, communication skills, legal concepts, and instruction.

 ### AMT PATHS

This chapter, which discusses the pediatric client, provides a path to AMT competency in general medical assisting knowledge, anatomy and physiology, medical terminology, and patient (client) education.

POINTS OF HIGHLIGHT

- Pediatrics is the medical specialty that studies the growth, development, and care of the child.
- An infant's head and chest circumference are routinely measured at a well-baby visit.
- Well-child visits give the medical assistant an excellent chance to give parents anticipatory guidance, which alerts parents as to what to expect at their child's particular stage of growth and development.
- Make the waiting and examination rooms safe and healthy areas for children by keeping these areas clean.
- Measure and record the pediatric client's height and weight at each visit.
- Respiration rates are fastest in newborn babies.
- The medical assistant should watch the rise and fall of the infant's abdomen to count respirations.
- Blood pressure measurement is not routinely done on infants or young children.
- Immunizations are completed during well-child visits at scheduled intervals.
- Scoliosis is an abnormal lateral curvature of the spine.
- Anorexia nervosa is an eating disorder found mostly among girls and young women.

STUDENT PORTFOLIO ACTIVITY

An understanding of the developmental stages of childhood is necessary for medical assistants who work in a pediatric or primary care setting. Plan visits to several preschools and day care facilities. Your observations will help you make the transition from what is learned in the classroom to real life. These experiences will also aid you in offering anticipatory guidance to families, so that parents know what to expect at each developmental stage. Compose a reflection about your experiences and meet with the site contact person for review and signature.

APPLYING YOUR SKILLS

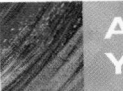

A father and mother have brought in their healthy child for a well-child visit. They are new to the practice and to the area. As part of the first visit, what clinical test must you perform? What will be done before the doctor examines the child? What information do you need to get from the parents? How would you approach this young child? In what ways can you as a medical assistant make a difference? (Remember what you learned about interviewing and welcoming clients in Units 1 and 2.)

CRITICAL THINKING QUESTIONS

1. A mother has brought her infant into the office where you work. As part of the well-child visit, you need to measure the length of the infant. How would you include the mother in this procedure? What would you say? What would you ask her to do to help? Be specific.

2. A 10-year-old girl comes to the office with her mother. During the course of obtaining the history and finding out concerns to be addressed at the visit, you realize that the mother is doing all the talking. What can you do to include the child in the interview process? What are some verbal and nonverbal techniques to help you do this?

3. Establishing trust between the medical assistant and the child is important. Discuss ways to build this trust.

4. Why is it difficult to count the radial pulse in an infant? By which method could you obtain the pulse of an infant?

5. Why are the head and chest circumferences routinely measured at an infant's office visit?

6. A parent asks why he must sign a consent form to have his child receive immunizations. What would you tell this parent?

7. Why are scoliosis checks done at well-child visits beginning when the child is about 10 years old? Why not wait until the parent or child notices any crookedness or unevenness?

8. Identify reasons why anorexia nervosa in its early stages often goes unnoticed by family members.

9. If an infant weighs 8 lbs., 5oz. and is 20 inches long at birth, what do you expect the height and weight to be when the child is 1 year old? How did you reach your answer?

10. In your role as a medical assistant, how do you keep children who have come for well-child visits from being exposed to bacteria or viruses from sick children?

11. Go back to the beginning of this chapter and review the Anticipatory Statements. Reread each statement and then indicate whether it is true or false. If the statement is false, rewrite it to make it a true statement.

Anticipatory Statements

Read and think about the following statements based upon what you believe now. Decide whether you agree or disagree. Write the word **agree** after the statement if you think the statement is true. Write the word **disagree** after the statement if you think the statement is false. Read the chapter to find out if your current beliefs can be supported.

1. An easy way to give medication is by mouth. _____

2. Clients should know the possible side effects of each of their medications. _____

3. It does not matter when the client takes a medication as long as he takes it each day. _____

4. Clients can never get addicted to prescribed medications. _____

5. The Food and Drug Administration helps to protect the American public by regulating what medications can be sold in the United States. _____

Medication and the Client Population

Learning Objectives

Upon completion of this chapter, the medical assistant student should be able to:

- List the rights of clients and medication
- Define the major drug classifications
- State the difference between cream and ointment topical medications
- Identify the common sites for administration of intradermal, subcutaneous, and intramuscular injections
- Explain client factors that might affect the absorption of medications
- Describe the difference between tablets, capsules, and enteric-coated medications

Key Terms

buccal Medications held within the cheek to dissolve.

catheter Hollow tubing that can be inserted and threaded through a vessel such as a vein.

infusion pump Electronic equipment that delivers fluid at a prescribed, set rate.

insertion site Point at which a needle is put into the vein or tissue.

intradermal Within the layers of the skin.

intramuscular Within the muscle layers.

intravenous Within the veins.

metric Uses meter and kilogram as a system for measuring lengths and weights.

over-the-counter (OTC) medication Drugs or medicines that can be purchased without a prescription from a health care provider.

roller clamp A device attached to tubing that can be opened to various degrees or completely closed to regulate the flow of fluid through the tubing.

subcutaneous Under the epidermal and dermal layers of the skin.

sublingual Under the tongue.

syringe Cylinder-shaped instrument, usually made of plastic (sometimes glass), that holds a medication to be injected.

topical Pertaining to the skin or mucous membranes.

tourniquet Springy material resembling a tube that is used to close off blood flow while selecting an insertion site.

INTRODUCTION

Pharmacology is the study of drugs and their actions and effects within and on the human body. Pharmacologists study both what a drug is used for and its side effects. To give quality client care, the medical assistant must understand the basics of pharmacology. This includes being familiar with drug classifications.

The medical assistant's tasks include the preparation and administration of medication. The medical assistant must know the laws regarding prescribing, ordering, administering, dispensing, storing, recording, and discarding drugs. Recordkeeping is an important task with medication administration. The medical assistant must follow the regulations and requirements for handling controlled substances or medications in the office.

The medical assistant will administer medications in different ways in keeping with the scope of practice, federal and state laws, and the medical office policy. Client teaching about medication is a major responsibility of the medical assistant.

PHARMACOLOGY

From pharmacological studies, we learn the effects of drugs and discover which medications work best in which forms for individual clients and their various situations. The medical assistant will need to consider the medication forms to calculate correct dosages for the specific form. Medications are generally given orally, topically, or rectally, or injected through the veins, into muscle, into subcutaneous tissue, or under the skin.

Each drug or medication has specific actions in the body and is used to treat one or more specific conditions. In addition to intended uses, each medication can cause *side effects*, which are unwanted or unintended effects upon the body. Some medications are used in emergency situations. The medical assistant should understand the conditions that might require emergency use of medication.

MEDICATION SOURCES

Substances have been used to treat conditions in humans for centuries. Many medications can be traced to different cultural groups. Some peoples may have used herbs and other substances together within a spiritual ritual. Many of our modern-day medications can be traced to a natural origin in a plant or herb. For example, the drug called digoxin traces its origins back to the foxglove plant. The four main sources of medication are plant, animal, mineral, and synthetic (Figure 36-1).

Plant parts can be used to make medications; thus, it is important to understand which part of the plant is helpful. For example, while the leaf may be an excellent medication, the stem or fruit may be poisonous.

If minerals such as magnesium or zinc are purified, they may be used to treat certain conditions. Antacids may contain magnesium. Topical skin protection medication may contain zinc.

Animal tissue has also been used as medication by humans. For example, insulin, which is used to treat diabetes mellitus, can be obtained from cows or pigs. (Some religious or cultural groups object to use of pig or pork products, so

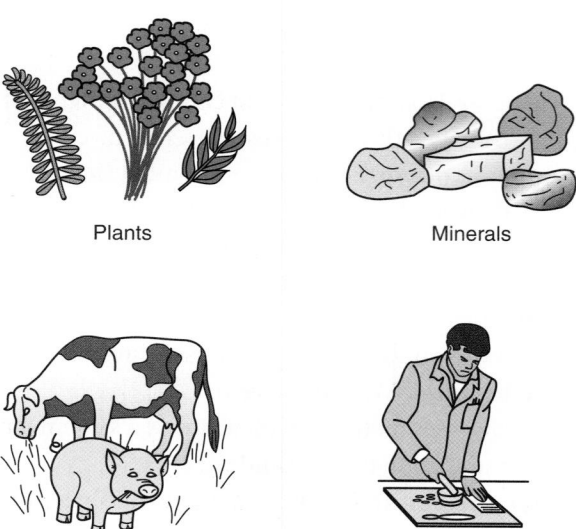

FIGURE 36-1 Sources of drugs.

today some insulin is also made using synthetic means.) Pharmaceutical drug companies can now produce drugs in the laboratory from synthetic sources that have not been harvested from plants or animals. Many antibiotics and pain medications were developed in this way.

■ FORMS OF MEDICATIONS

Medications come in different forms and are administered or given by various methods or *routes*. The most common forms of drug preparations are: oral, topical, transdermal, rectal, injection (veins, through the muscle, subcutaneous, or intradermal), and inhalation.

Oral

An easy way to administer a medication is the oral route. Taking a medication by mouth is also the least expensive. Oral drug forms can be liquid or solid. Solid oral drug forms are tablets, capsules, and lozenges (Figure 36-2). Tablets are medication substances compressed into a small, hard disk or oblong form. Tablets can be marked with a line down the middle, so that the medication can easily be divided in equal halves. Such a tablet is said to be *scored*. Unless it has a coating, a tablet can dissolve quickly in water and leave a bitter taste in the mouth. A coating helps to delay this dissolution and help the client to swallow the tablet. *Enteric-coated* tablets have a special coating that resists being broken down by stomach juices. Medications that are irritating or can cause bleeding are enteric coated. Aspirin may be enteric coated; for a client who must take aspirin regularly, this is a good choice.

In another form, medication granules are placed inside a gelatin covering called a *capsule*. Capsules are designed for easier swallowing. Sustained-release or timed-release capsules are designed to let the medication dissolve and enter the body little by little over time.

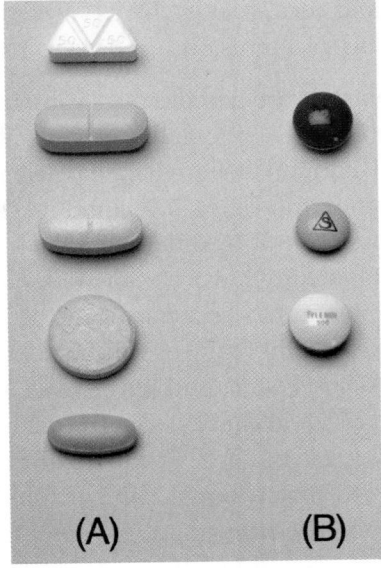
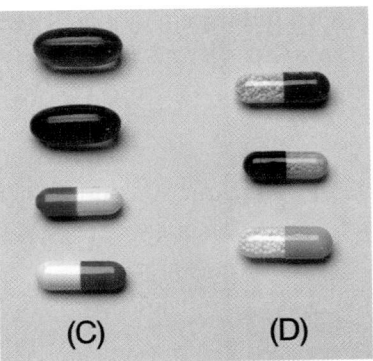

FIGURE 36-2 Oral drug forms. (A) Tablets, scored and unscored, (B) enteric-coated tablets, (C) gelatin capsules, and (D) timed-release capsules.

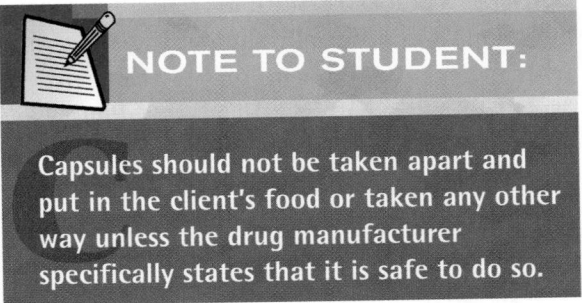

NOTE TO STUDENT:

Capsules should not be taken apart and put in the client's food or taken any other way unless the drug manufacturer specifically states that it is safe to do so.

A *lozenge* is a compressed disk of medication with a flavored coating. It should dissolve in the mouth and not be swallowed whole. It is often used for relief of sore throats.

Liquid oral drug forms are solutions, syrups, elixirs, emulsions, and suspensions:

- *Solutions* are liquids containing medicinal substances completely dissolved within the liquid. The liquid appears clear.
- *Syrups* and *elixirs* are liquid medications. These solutions differ from each other in that elixirs have an alcohol base. It is important to be aware that people who crave alcohol may use elixirs to excess.
- In *emulsions,* oils and fats in water are added to the liquid emulsified in the medicine.
- *Suspensions* are medication granules mixed into a liquid. Unlike solutions, in which the substances are completely dissolved so that the liquid stays clear, particles in suspensions will settle to the bottom when left standing.

NOTE TO STUDENT:

The medical assistant must teach the client to shake a suspension well before each dose is poured, to ensure that each dose has the same amount of medicine in it.

When teaching a client about oral medications, the medical assistant must include special directions if appropriate, such as "swallow only with water," "take on an empty stomach," or "swallow after eating." Read the *Physicians' Desk Reference* (PDR) or other drug reference books carefully for critical information about the use of individual medications.

Topical

Topical medications are applied directly to the skin or mucous membranes. Medication applied to the skin can be in liquid or semisolid form:

- Medicated *lotions* are considered a liquid form. Lotions are best absorbed after a shower or bath while the skin is still damp. This promotes absorption into the skin. Lotions are generally not greasy.
- *Creams* are semisolid preparations that contain medication. A cream is absorbed best when applied to wet or damp skin. It is generally not greasy.
- *Ointments* are similar to creams (Figure 36-3). Ointments have a greasy, oily base to which a medication is added. They are generally applied at night to dry skin to form a barrier protection.

NOTE TO STUDENT:

The medical assistant should teach the client to apply an ointment at night and to be careful with clothing and bedding. Ointments may stain fabrics.

- *Transdermal* medication is applied to the skin in the form of a patch (Figure 36-4). The medication in the patch is absorbed through the skin over a period of time. Depending on the medication, patches can remain in place for hours, a day, or even a week. Transdermal medication is

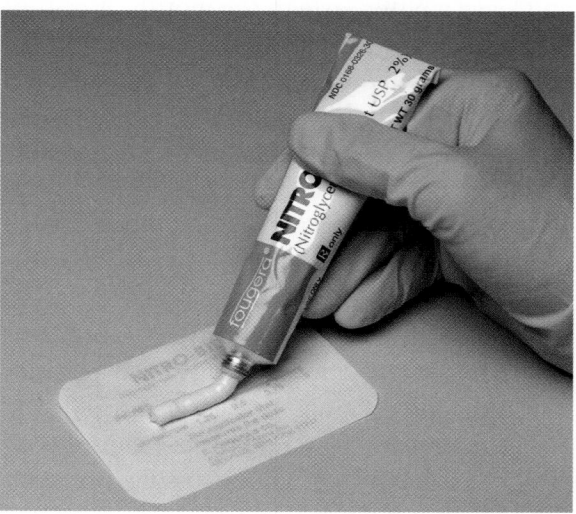

FIGURE 36–3 Topical medication.

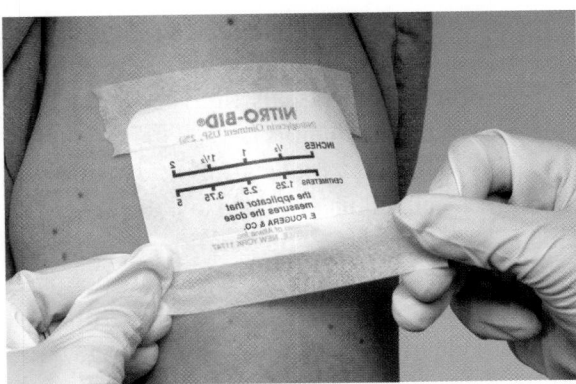

FIGURE 36-4 Patch medication applied to skin.

convenient and easy to use. With less frequent dosing, there is more client cooperation. Nitroglycerin, used to treat cardiac or angina attacks, is available in patch form. Pain medication can also be delivered in this form. Hormones used for hormone replacement therapy, as well as birth control preparations, can be applied in patch form.

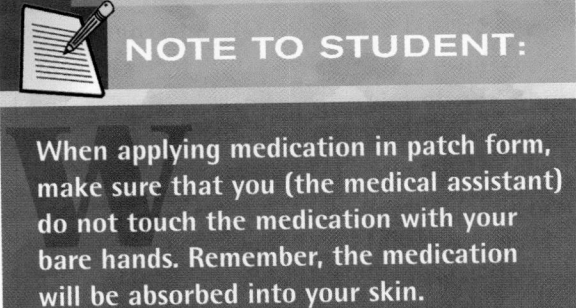

NOTE TO STUDENT:

When applying medication in patch form, make sure that you (the medical assistant) do not touch the medication with your bare hands. Remember, the medication will be absorbed into your skin.

- Medication that is applied to a mucous membrane is considered a topical medication. These include buccal or sublingual tablets; drops for the eye, ear, or nose; vaginal creams or douches; and rectal or vaginal suppositories. **Buccal** means cheek; these tablets are held against the inside of the cheek and allowed to dissolve. They are not swallowed. **Sublingual** means under the tongue; these tablets are placed under the tongue and allowed to dissolve. Nitroglycerin tablets used to treat angina are taken in this way.

- Medicated drops for the eyes, ears, and nose are considered topical because they are absorbed through the mucous membranes. Eyedrops are instilled into the conjunctival sac of the eye. Eardrops are put into the ear or aural canal, and nosedrops are absorbed through the nasal mucous membranes.

- Creams may be inserted into the vagina to treat infections. The medical assistant should instruct the client on the correct way to apply a medicated cream.

- Suppositories are medications shaped into a long cylindrical form. They can be inserted into the vagina or rectum. The medical assistant must instruct the client not to hold suppositories in the hand while getting into position for application. The suppository is made to melt at body temperature, so if it is held in the hand too long, it will melt there.

- A *douche* is a solution used to wash or irrigate the vaginal canal. Some douches, and the overuse of douches in general, can upset the natural balance of flora and pH in the vagina and make a woman more susceptible to infections. Douches prescribed by the doctor should be administered according to the instructions.

Rectal

Rectal suppositories are considered rectal medications although they are intended to have systemic effects. Again, they are designed to melt at body temperature. The medical assistant should know what supplies are necessary to administer rectal medications (Figure 36-5). Lubricant and either a finger cot or glove are needed, whether the medical assistant administers the medication or the client self-administers it. For example, anti-emetic medication is given rectally when the client cannot swallow or is nauseated and cannot keep down oral medication.

Enema solutions are liquids inserted into the rectum. The purpose is usually to act as a

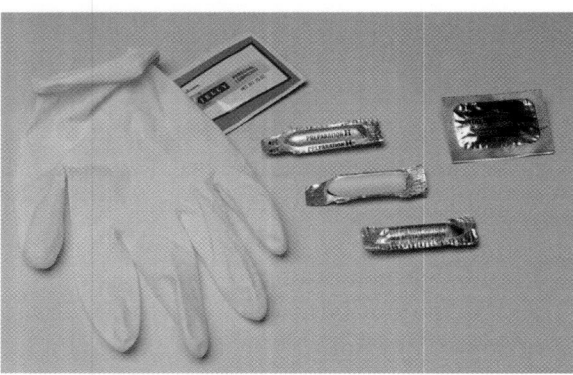

FIGURE 36–5 Supplies for giving rectal medications.

laxative to clear out the lower bowel. Enemas are also part of the preparation for certain tests and examinations of the rectum and colon.

Injection

Injected medication can also be called parenteral medications. *Parenteral* means outside of the digestive tract. Most commonly, these are injections that can be given intravenously (IV), intramuscularly (IM), subcutaneously (SC), or intradermally (ID) (Figure 36-6). These drugs come in various containers, such as ampules or vials (Figure 36-7). Ampules normally contain a single dose, whereas vials often contain multiple doses of the medication.

Intravenous medication is inserted through a vein. This provides fast access to the bloodstream so the medication can work quickly. Intravenous medication can be given by IV push, IV drip, or IV piggyback. In an *IV push,* medicine is put into a **syringe** and injected directly into a vein or IV tubing. An *IV drip* allows the medicine to drip slowly though tubing into a vein. With *IV piggyback,* a medication is given while an IV solution is dripping into the vein at the same time.

Medication can also be injected into a muscle. Medicine is drawn into a syringe with an **intramuscular** needle attached, and then injected at a 90-degree angle straight into the muscle (Figures 36-8 and 36-9). The muscle site depends upon the medication and the health of the client.

Medication that has been drawn up into a syringe with a subcutaneous needle attached is injected at a 45-degree angle into the **subcutaneous** layer (Figure 36-10). This is the layer under the dermis or true layer of the skin.

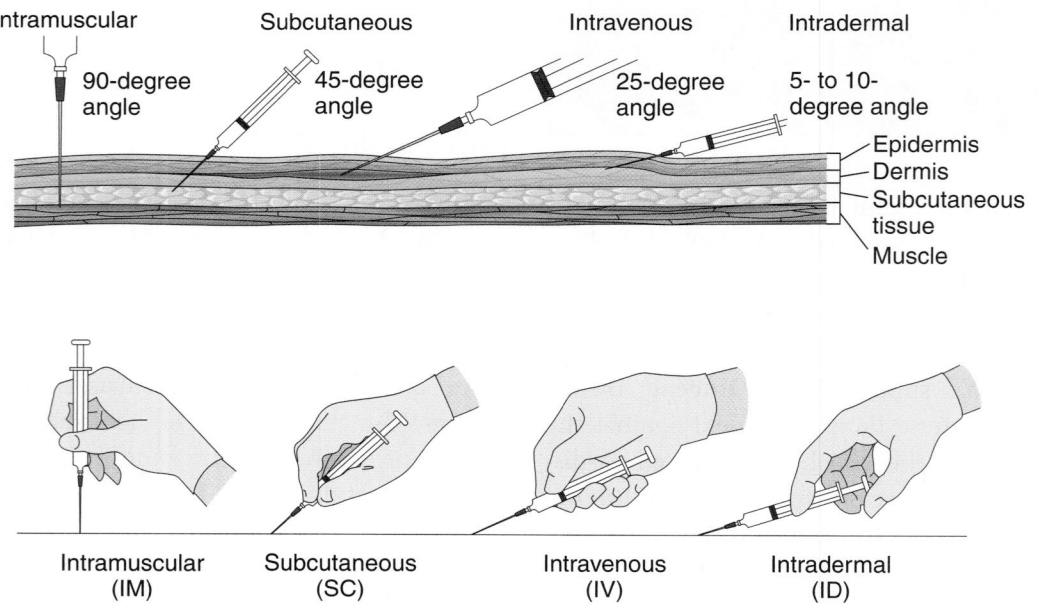

FIGURE 36–6 Angles of injection for intramuscular, subcutaneous, intravenous, and intradermal injections.

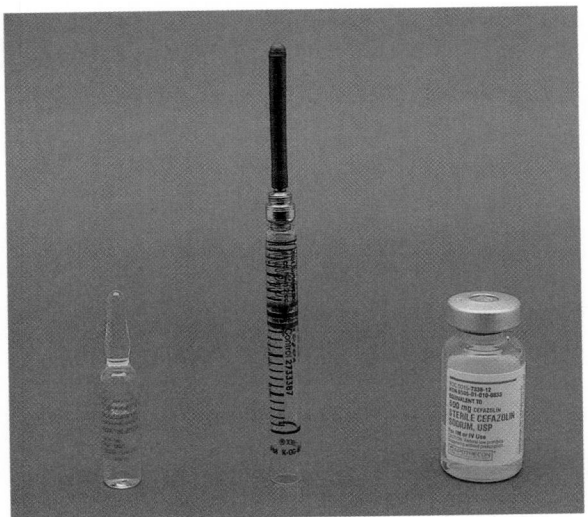

FIGURE 36-7 Ampules and vials of medication for injection.

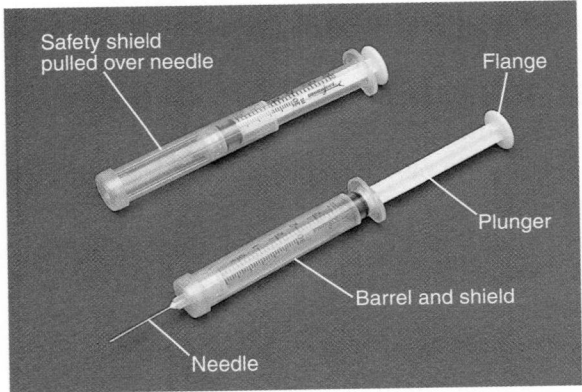

FIGURE 36-8A Parts of a syringe.

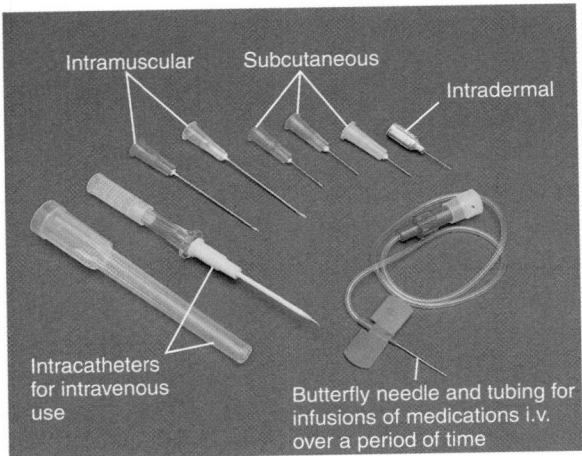

FIGURE 36-8B Various sizes and types of needles; different colored hubs indicate needle gauges.

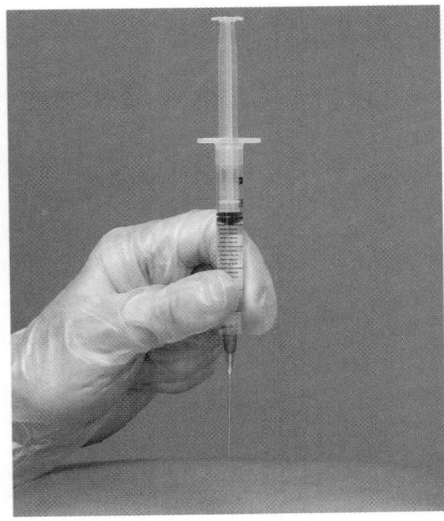

FIGURE 36-9 For an intramuscular injection, medicine is drawn into a syringe and injected after the needle is inserted at a 90-degree angle into the muscle.

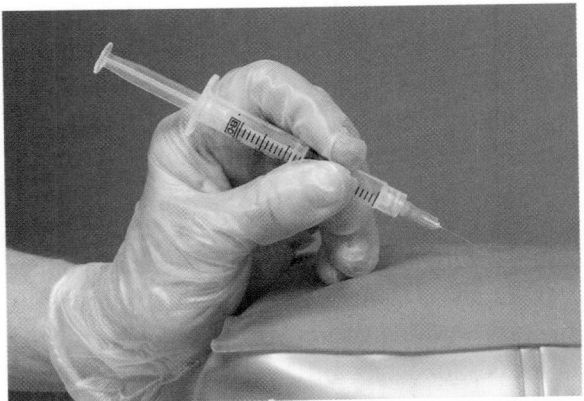

FIGURE 36-10 For a subcutaneous injection, medicine is drawn into a syringe and injected after the needle is inserted at a 45-degree angle under the dermis of the skin.

A needle can be inserted at a 15-degree angle, and a solution injected, right under the skin (Figure 36-11). This is most frequently done for a TB skin test or PPD. It can also be used for **intradermal** allergy skin testing.

Inhalation

Liquid medication can be given by the inhalation method. The liquid is administered in the form of a spray or a mist. It can be a nasal spray or mist, or a spray or nebulizer can direct the mist to the

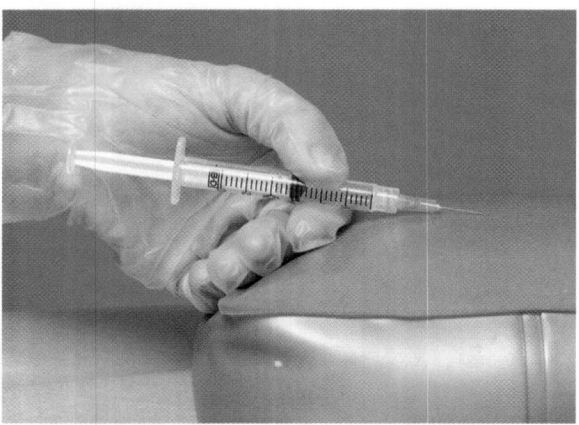

FIGURE 36-11 For an intradermal injection, medicine is drawn into a syringe and inserted at a 15-degree angle under the skin.

lungs through the mouth. A metered-dose inhaler allows a specific number of measured doses. Clients with allergies and asthma often take medications by this method. Clients will need instructions from the medical assistant to correctly self-administer these medicines.

■ INTRAVENOUS THERAPY

Intravenous means through the veins. Inserting a needle into a vein provides quick access to the circulatory system, allowing fluids to flow through or medication to be injected directly into the bloodstream. One of the functions of the circulatory systems is to transport substances throughout the body. The medical assistant should understand the basic theory of IV therapy, which include the purpose, equipment used, site selection, and site maintenance.

Purpose

Intravenous therapy can serve one or more purposes. It can deliver fluid volume to replace fluid that may have been lost due to bleeding, hemorrhaging, or through disorders or surgeries. Different types of fluids can provide hydration, nourishment, or medication. Vitamins and other nutritional support can be given through the veins. Medications are often delivered in this manner. Emergency medications are often delivered by the IV route, such as an IV bolus or IV push (med-

ication that is drawn up into a syringe and inserted into the vein, often through an existing IV tubing line). The medication is delivered over a short period of time (5 to 10 minutes) as the health care provider pushes down on the syringe. This is a fast way to deliver a complete dose directly to the circulatory system. As a result of the direct delivery, the side effects or the effects of an erroneous administration can occur very fast, and be very dangerous or even lethal, compared with other routes. There are strict guidelines regulating which health care providers are permitted to perform IV bolus injections.

Medication may also be delivered through an IV *piggyback*, a small IV bag filled with medication that is attached to the tubing of an existing IV bag. The fluid from the piggyback is allowed to drip through while the flow of solution from the existing bag is closed off. When the medicated solution is finished, the piggyback bag is removed and the flow from the primary, or existing, bag of solution is restarted.

In the past, clients who needed medicine delivered by the IV route were kept hospitalized. As discussed in Chapter 2, hospital stays are now kept as short as possible, and clients (such as those who need antibiotics over a long period of time) are sent home with instructions regarding site maintenance for the administration of IV medications.

Equipment

The medical assistant may need to assemble the equipment and supplies needed to set up an IV. The doctor's order must be compared to the solution or medication to make sure that the fluid selected for administration is in fact the one ordered. The IV bag with the correct solution and tubing is gathered. The correct size needle (have available more than one), safety needle, or **catheter,** along with alcohol wipes, are needed. The needle size depends on the client and the size and integrity of her veins, the site selected, and the solution or medication ordered. Gloves and other personal protective equipment, sterile gauze, towels, nonallergenic tape, bandage scissors, and a biohazardous waste bag should be set out.

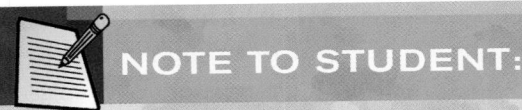

Site Preparation

The health care provider who is preparing the infusion site must wash her hands and correctly identify the client before preparation of the IV site. If it is to be a peripheral IV site, the provider must look at the veins in both the client's arms. The provider should note any bruises, swelling, open areas, or scarring that would eliminate that site for use. If possible, the client's dominant hand and arm (the one that client uses for everyday activities) should be avoided. The **tourniquet** is put on the upper arm and the veins are examined as they dilate. A vein that feels firm and springy is best. The arm selected is supported by a towel placed under it. The site is wiped with an antiseptic solution starting in the center of a circle and working outward. The area is allowed to air-dry. Never blow air on the area, as this contaminates the site. The tourniquet is applied approximately 5 inches above the needle **insertion site.** The designated provider then performs venipuncture, inserts the needle, attaches the tubing and IV solution, secures the administration set in place, and regulates the flow.

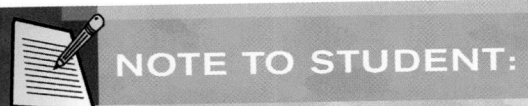

IV Flow Rates

The flow of the solution into the vein can be controlled by a **roller clamp** that is on the tubing or an **infusion pump.** With the roller clamp, the rate is calculated and set by the provider. The clamp then allows the set number of drops to be released. An infusion pump is a piece of electronic equipment that delivers the set amount of solution. Pumps have alarms that sound if something interferes with the rate. (Never ignore an alarm, but do not rely solely on the alarm to signal that something is wrong. Clients must be checked and monitored carefully.)

The flow rate will be decided by the ordering doctor. The person who is responsible for calculating and maintaining the flow rate is specified by governing laws, scope of practice, and facility policy. Maintenance of accurate flow rate is critical to the client's health. A flow rate that is too fast can overload a client's circulatory and respiratory systems. A flow rate that is too slow may not deliver enough medication or solution to help the client. The slow rate may even cause the vein to clot and ruin the site. Any abrupt change in the IV flow can harm the client. A client who is very young, old, or in frail general health is most at risk. Clients who are receiving IV therapy are not in optimal health to begin with, so all should be carefully monitored.

Fluid flows by gravity, so the IV solution bag must be placed at least 36 inches above the venipuncture site. There is a small chamber or container between the bag and tubing that helps to prevent an accidental rush of fluid through the tubing into the client. The client's position can also affect the flow rate. The infusion pump will alarm when the rate changes. A confused client may accidentally cause a change in flow by handling the clamp or just being unaware of activity that might interfere with the flow rate.

Site Maintenance

The IV site must be inspected and cared for to ensure the correct administration of the fluid. This care also maintains a safe, healthy area free from infection. The insertion site of the needle, the dressing, and the skin around the area must all be inspected. The area should be checked for any swelling (fluid might be infiltrating the surrounding tissue), redness, tenderness, or discharge (possible infection or irritation of the site). The client should be instructed to report any pain, tingling, or unusual sensations at the site. The most critical element in maintenance of an IV flow rate and site is close and frequent observation by a competent health care provider.

■ SAFETY OF MEDICATIONS IN THE UNITED STATES

The Pure Food and Drug Act of 1906 was the first law passed to safeguard the American people regarding medicine. It stated that any drug made in the United States must meet a set of basic standards as to strength and quality. The drugs must be pure. If a drug contains any of the addictive drug morphine, that ingredient must be listed on the label. Finally, the law provided for the creation of two official references for approved drugs, *The United States Pharmacopoeia* (USP) and the *National Formulary* (NF). If a person wanted to check if a medicine had met the United States drug standards, she could check these books. In the years since this law was passed, the two reference books have been combined into one, the USP/NF.

People are familiar with the term *FDA-approved.* It is seen on labels of foods and drugs, and it also appears in the media in reference to new drugs being developed or put on the market. If a medicine is to be sold in the United States, it must obtain approval from the Food and Drug Administration (FDA), which was established under the Federal Food, Drug and Cosmetics Act of 1938. Additional parts were added to this law in 1951 and 1965. The familiar words written on prescription bottles—"Caution: Federal law prohibits dispensing without a prescription"—are mandated by this law. This law required that drugs not only be safe and pure, but must also be effective. In other words, the drug must work as the drug company claims it works. This law raised the standards for medications available in the United States.

■ CATEGORIES OF DRUGS

Two major categories of drugs are prescription and **over-the-counter (OTC) medications.** To purchase prescription medication, a client needs a prescription written by a doctor. These medications can be life-saving, but are very potent chemicals. Using prescription medication for disorders that they were not intended for, or at a wrong dosage, can cause bodily harm or even death. Use of prescription medications must be monitored by the pharmacist, the medical assistant, and other health care providers.

Over-the-counter drugs can be purchased without any input, recommendation, or permission from a health care provider. Sometimes these drugs are a lower dose or strength of a prescription medicine. Other OTC drugs are completely different. Even though they can be bought without a prescription, they can cause serious side effects and even death if not used for the right reason or if the correct dosage is not used. The medical assistant must ask the client at each visit about the medications the client is taking. The

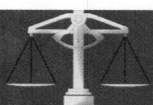

LEGAL/ETHICAL THOUGHTS

The prescribing, dispensing, and administering of medication is regulated by many governmental agencies. Medical assistants must be aware of, keep current with, and obey these laws and regulations.

TABLE 36-1 Schedules of controlled substances.

DRUG CATEGORY	POTENTIAL FOR ABUSE	MEDICAL USE	POTENTIAL FOR DEPENDENCE	EXAMPLES
Schedule I	High	Not accepted for medical use; limited to research	High	Heroin, LSD, marijuana, peyote
Schedule II	High	Accepted for medical use; very restricted	Severe psychic or physical	Amphetamines, morphine
Schedule III	Moderate to low	Acceptable	High psychological	Opioids, barbiturates, some depressants
Schedule IV	Low	Acceptable	Limited physical and psychological	Phenobarbital, propoxyphene
Schedule V	Low	Acceptable	Limited physical and psychological	Codeine in cough syrup

medical assistant must specifically ask about OTC medications, as some people do not consider these medicines to be "real" medications. They think that if it is available without a prescription, the drug must be safe. In reality, OTC medications can be potent and may interact with prescribed medication to cause serious problems. OTC medications are available to treat disorders of every bodily system.

Vitamins are also medications. Clients tend to think that vitamins make a person healthy and are perfectly safe. However, vitamins, especially fat-soluble ones, can build up in the body and become toxic if taken in large amounts. Additionally, vitamins can interfere with prescribed medications. For example, vitamin K helps to clot blood. If the client is taking Coumadin (a blood thinner), too much vitamin K will counteract against the Coumadin and make it useless.

Controlled Substances

Some drugs that have the potential to be abused and cause addiction are called *controlled substances*, as defined by the 1970 Controlled Substances Act. This act put restrictions on drugs that have a potential for addiction and abuse. To prescribe controlled drugs, health care providers must register for and receive a number from the Drug Enforcement Agency (DEA), a federal agency that was also established by the Controlled Substance Act. Limits were also placed on how often certain drugs could be ordered. Drugs that may be addicting or abused are grouped into five levels (Table 36-1): C-I, C-II, C-III, C-IV, and C-V. Level I is the most addictive, with limited medical use, and Level V is the least addictive.

■ GIVING INSTRUCTIONS TO CLIENTS

Working with clients and medications at any step of the process, from phoning in a refill to actually giving a medication to a client, is a major responsibility for the medical assistant. There are six guiding principles for medications and the client (Figure 36-12):

1. Right medicine
2. Right amount

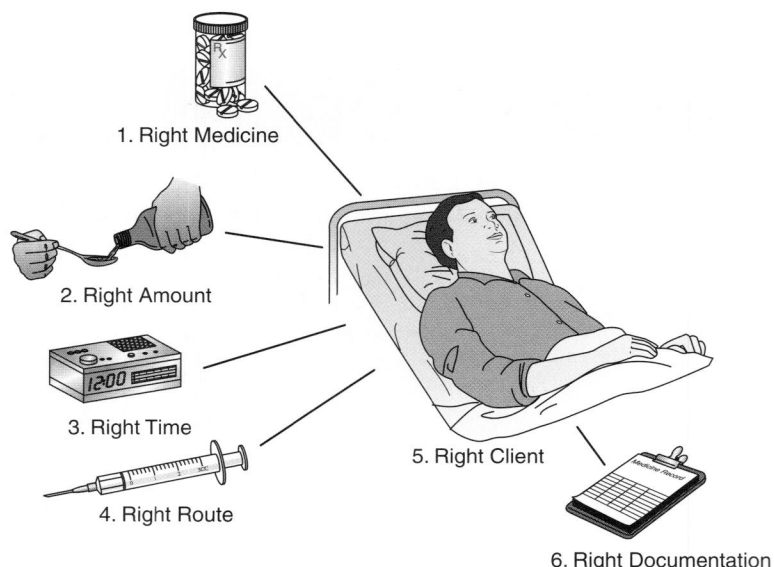

1. Right Medicine
2. Right Amount
3. Right Time
4. Right Route
5. Right Client
6. Right Documentation

FIGURE 36-12 The six rights of clients regarding medications.

3. Right time

4. Right route (way to take the medication)

5. Right client

6. Right documentation

Right Medication

The medical assistant must make sure that the right medicine is being administered. The same steps must be followed each and every time: The name of the drug must be checked in the doctor's orders in the chart. If there is a prescription, check the prescription, making sure that the writing is clear and easily read. If a surgical setup is required, make sure the medicines from the cabinet are the correct ones. If a drug is being administered to a client, read the label three times: once when taking it from the shelf, a second time when comparing it to the doctor's order sheet, and a third time when putting the container back in its place in the cabinet.

Right Amount

Administering the right amount of medication sounds simple, but even a small mistake can cause serious harm or death, especially with children or older adults.

Several different systems are used to measure the amount of medicine to be given. **Metric** and household measures may be used. When calculating a dose and changing it into another system of measurement, it is critical to recheck

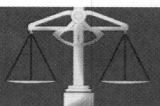

LEGAL/ETHICAL THOUGHTS

Ultimately, the medical assistant who gives a drug is responsible. The person giving the drug is always accountable or liable for her actions.

the number. A second medical assistant or health care worker could check or verify the work. Always know what system of measure is being used.

Often the medical assistant will teach the client to self-administer medicine at home. The client should not be expected to change metric measurements (cc, mL, mg) to household measurements (ounces, teaspoons, tablespoons). Calculate the dose as the client will measure it, and give instructions using terms and measures that the client is familiar with.

Right Time

Timing of medication is very important. There is a potential for serious consequences if the medication is not given or taken at the right time. The prescribed time is calculated so that the medicine will be at the right level in the blood to work at its optimal (best) level. If the level is too high, the medication may become toxic or poisonous to the person. If the level is too low, there may not be enough of the medication in the client's system to work.

When working with clients, make sure that the client knows whether to administer in the morning (A.M.) or evening (P.M.). It makes a difference whether the medicine is ordered every so many hours or so many times a day. For example, every eight hours is not the same as three times a day.

Right Route

There are various ways for medicine to enter the body, called *routes* or *routes of administration*. As discussed, a person can swallow a drug (oral route), spray it into a body opening, or inject it through the skin, into a subcutaneous layer, into a muscle, into a vein, or into a body cavity.

Medicine can be instilled into a body cavity or opening, such as the eyes, ears, nose, mouth, vagina, or rectum. It can also be inhaled. The client's health condition and the characteristics of the medicine will determine which route is ordered. The same medication administered by another route can have drastically different effects on the client. The medical assistant must make sure that the doctor's orders as to the route are followed.

Right Client

Giving the (right) medication to the right client sounds simple, but is a common error. It is the responsibility of the medical assistant administering the medication to correctly identify the client. Always ask the client to state her name; then compare the name with the client's name on the doctor's orders. Never ask the client, "Are you Mr. . . ." or "Ms. . . . ?" The client may not hear well and may just answer yes or nod. Clients almost never question if the medical assistant has the correct person. It is up to the medical assistant to correctly identify the right client.

Right Documentation

Information about medication must be documented accurately and completely. This includes the name of the drug, the route of administration, and the specific instructions for the client. If the medical assistant administers a medication to a client, the documentation must include the date the medicine was given, the time it was administered, the name of the medication given, the amount given, the route by which the medication was given, and any instructions given to the client. The records should include the client's response to the medication, such as relief of pain or side effects noted.

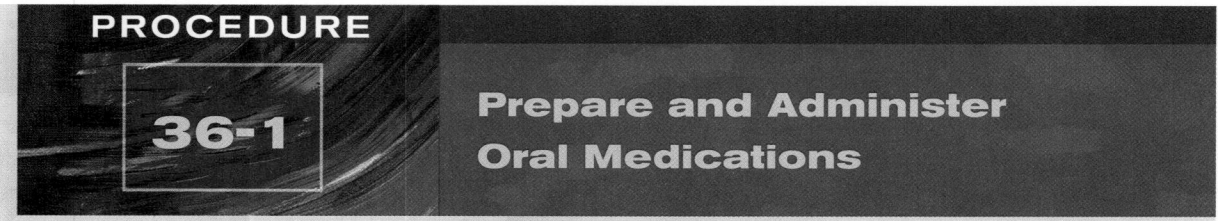

PROCEDURE

36-1

Prepare and Administer Oral Medications

Student Competency Objective: The medical assistant student will set up and give an oral medication.

Items Needed: Oral medication (for lab purposes, very small pieces of candy may be used), water, small paper cup, and small medicine tray

NOTE TO STUDENT:

Review the six rights of clients regarding medications.

Steps:

1. Read the doctor's order for medication.
2. Go to the cupboard in the supply room where the medication is kept.
3. Wash your hands.
4. Place a disposable medication cup on a medicine tray.
5. Find the ordered medication.
6. Check the expiration date.
7. Read the label on the medication and compare it to the doctor's orders.
8. Open the lid of the medicine container and put the lid upside down on a clean surface. (Do not let the rim of the lid touch any surface. If the rim touches anything, it is considered contaminated.)
9. Put the ordered number of tablets or capsules into the lid (Figure 36–13A).
10. Put the contents of the lid into the small, disposable medicine cup that is on the medicine tray (Figure 36–13B).
11. Replace the lid on the container and close it tightly.
12. Compare the medicine container label with the doctor's order as you put the medicine container back on the shelf.
13. Go to the client's examination room.
14. Introduce yourself to the client even if you have seen the client on previous visits to your office. The client may have forgotten your name. This also helps to establish a provider-client relationship, because it shows the client that you want her to know who you are.
15. Identify the client. Ask the client to state her name to establish that this is the right client, and then compare the name given to the name on the chart. Never enter a room and call out a client's name to determine if this person is the correct client. The client may not have heard you clearly and may just nod, smile, or answer yes. Clients almost never question if the medical assistant professional has the right client. It is up to the medical assistant to identify the right client before performing any procedure.
16. Tell the client, in everyday language, what you are going to do.

(Continues)

PROCEDURE 36-1 (Continued)

17. Ask if the client has any questions. If she does, give short and simple answers. Sometimes clients will start (and continue) talking because they are nervous about the procedure.

18. Tell the client that you are going to give her the medicine the doctor ordered.

19. Hand the disposable cup with the tablet(s) or capsule(s) in it to the client. Then hand the client a glass of water.

20. Make sure that the client is able to swallow the tablet(s) or capsule(s). Offer more water as needed.

21. Wash your hands.

22. Chart the medication given in the client's medical record. Be sure to include date, time the medication was given, amount of medication, route, and any client reactions.

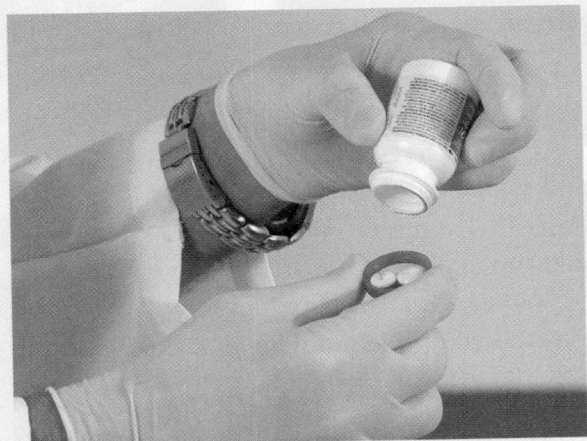

FIGURE 36-13A Pour or shake the ordered number of tablets or capsules into the lid of the medication container.

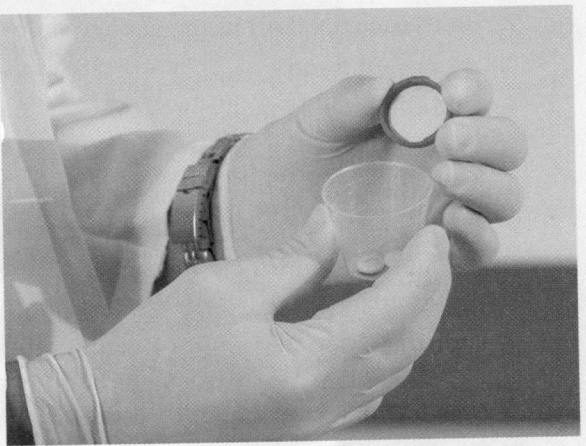

FIGURE 36-13B Pour the tablets or capsules from the lid or cap into the medication cup.

Charting Example:

A Tylenol 325 mg tablet was given to Mr. Smith without problems. You would record the following:

5/10/20xx   10:00 A.M.   Client given Tylenol 325 mg. tablet p.o. with no difficulty swallowing. No complaints offered.

Sally Martin, S.M.A.

Sally Martin, S.M.A. (printed name)

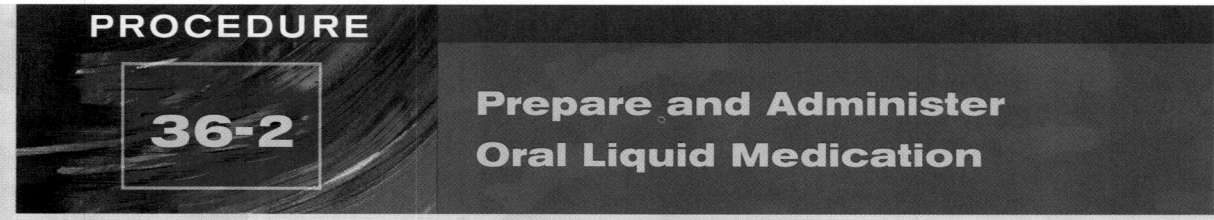

PROCEDURE 36-2

Prepare and Administer Oral Liquid Medication

Student Competency Objective: The medical assistant student will set up and give oral liquid medication.

Items Needed: Oral medication (for lab purposes, use water), small plastic measured medicine cup, small medicine tray

Steps:

1. Read the doctor's order for medication.
2. Go to the cupboard in the supply room where the medication is kept.
3. Wash your hands.
4. Find the ordered medicine.
5. Check the expiration date.
6. Read the label on the medicine container and compare it to the doctor's order.
7. Open the lid of the medicine container and put the lid upside down on a clean surface. Do not let the rim of the lid touch any surface. If the rim touches anything, it is considered contaminated.
8. Pour the ordered amount of liquid into the measured plastic cup (Figure 36–14). Hold the bottle and cup at eye level while you pour, so that you can easily see when you have poured the correct amount.
9. Place the lid back on the container and close it tightly.
10. Compare the medicine container label with the doctor's order as you put the medicine container back on the shelf.
11. Go to the client's examination room.

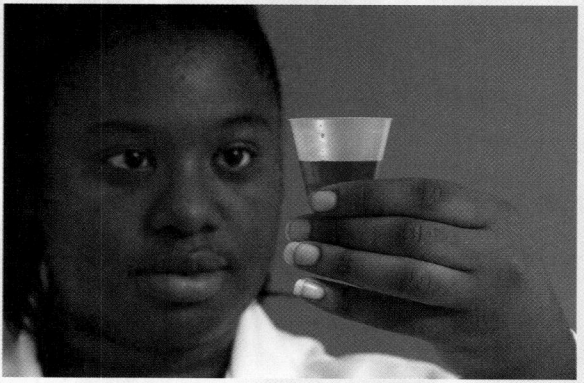

FIGURE 36–14 Pour the right amount of medication into the plastic medicine cup while holding the bottle at eye level and palming the label.

(Continues)

PROCEDURE 36-2 (Continued)

12. Introduce yourself to the client even if you have seen the client on previous visits to your office. The client may have forgotten your name. This also helps to establish a provider–client relationship, because it shows the client that you want her to know who you are.

13. Identify the client. Ask the client to state her name to establish that this is the right client, and then compare the name given to the name on the chart. Never enter a room and call out a client's name to determine if this person is the correct client. The client may not have heard you clearly and may just nod, smile, or answer yes. Clients almost never question if the medical assistant professional has the right client. It is up to the medical assistant to identify the right client before performing any procedure.

14. Tell the client, in everyday language, what you are going to do.

15. Ask if the client has any questions. If she does, give short and simple answers. Sometimes clients will start (and continue) talking because they are nervous about the procedure.

16. Tell the client that you are going to give her the medication the doctor ordered.

17. Hand the plastic measured medicine cup, with the ordered amount of liquid medicine in it, to the client.

18. Make sure that the client is able to swallow the medicine. Check the medication order to see if the client can have water immediately, if desired to help get any bad taste out of her mouth.

19. Wash your hands.

20. Chart the medication given in the client's medical record. Be sure to include date, time the medication was given, amount of medication, route, and any client reactions.

Charting Example:

You gave Tylenol 325 mg liquid to the client without any problems. You would record the following:

      10/28/20xx   2:00 P.M.   Client given Tylenol 325 mg liquid with no difficulty swallowing. No complaints offered.

Jessica Moore, S.M.A.

Jessica Moore, S.M.A. (printed name)

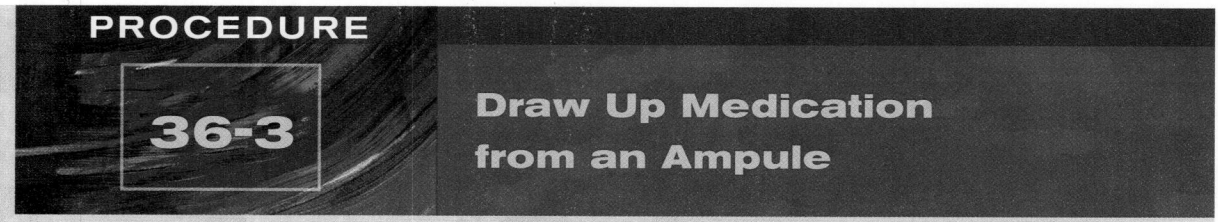

PROCEDURE 36-3 — Draw Up Medication from an Ampule

Student Competency Objective: The medical assistant student will draw up medication from an ampule using a needle and syringe.

Items Needed: Ampule, syringe with needle, filter needle, alcohol wipe, gloves, sharps container

Steps:

1. Read the doctor's order for medication.
2. Go to the cupboard in the supply room where the medication is kept.
3. Wash your hands.
4. Find the ordered medication (in an ampule container).
5. Read the label on the ampule and compare it to the doctor's order.
6. Check the expiration date.
7. Select the correct size needle and syringe, filter needle, and alcohol wipe (Figure 36–15A).
8. Put on gloves.
9. Pick up the ampule and hold it upright. Flick your index finger against the stem of the ampule. This will help to move any air bubbles into the top and make the medication sink to the bottom of the ampule (Figure 36–15B).
10. Grab the stem of the ampule with an alcohol wipe.
11. Pointing the ampule away from your face, snap off the neck of the ampule (Figure 36–15C).
12. Pick up the syringe and needle.
13. Uncap the needle and put the needle into the solution in the ampule.
14. Pull back on the plunger and draw up the ordered amount of solution (Figure 36–15D).
15. Take the syringe and needle out of the solution.
16. Point the needle straight up into the air.
17. Allow air to float to the top of the barrel of the syringe (Figure 36–15E).
18. Push the plunger of the syringe in to get rid of any remaining air.
19. Check the amount of medication in the syringe. If there is more than ordered, push the plunger until the medication is at the correct level, discarding the extra.
20. Change the needle if needed, or put a safety sheath over it.
21. Put the used ampule in a sharps container (Figure 36–15F).
22. Wash your hands.

(Continues)

PROCEDURE 36-3 (Continued)

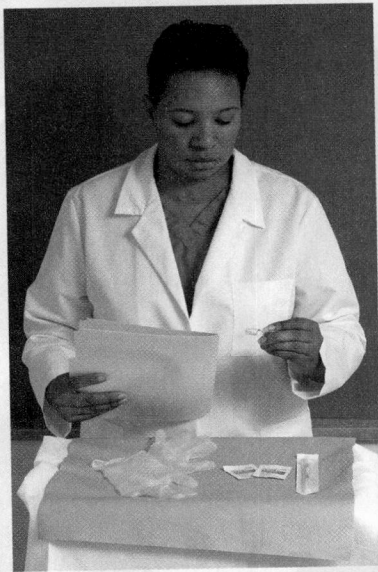

FIGURE 36–15A Assemble the supplies needed to draw up medication from an ampule. Read the label on the ampule, and compare it to the doctor's orders. Select the correct size needle and syringe, filter needle.

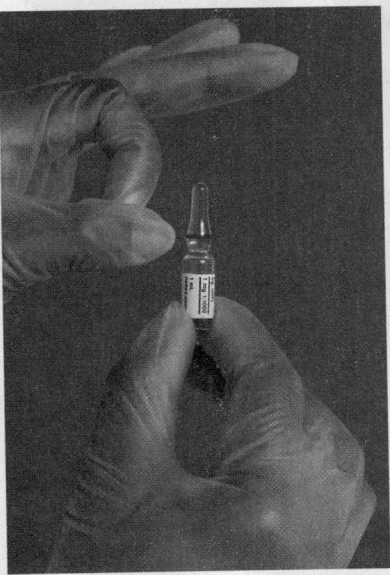

FIGURE 36–15B Flick your finger against the ampule, or tap the ampule so that the contents go to the bottom and any air bubbles to the top.

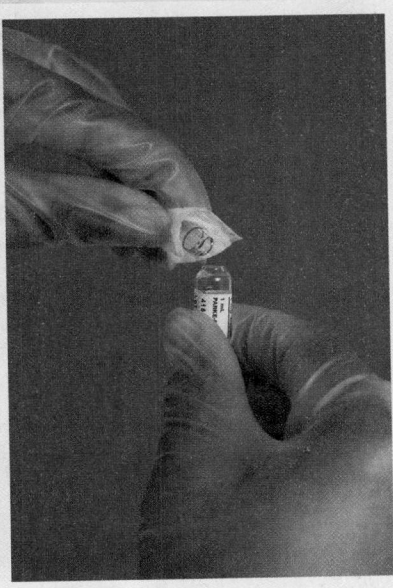

FIGURE 36–15C Using an alcohol wipe, firmly hold the ampule and snap the top at the marked line.

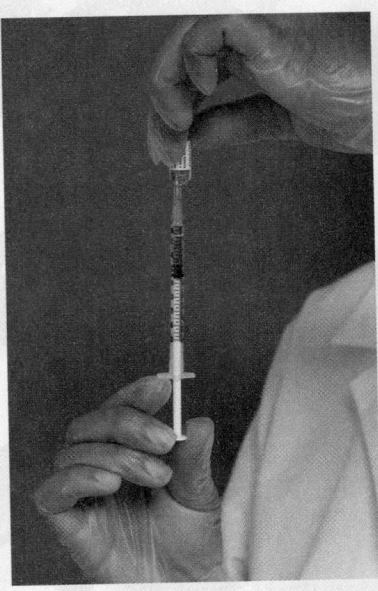

FIGURE 36–15D Draw up medication from the ampule into the syringe.

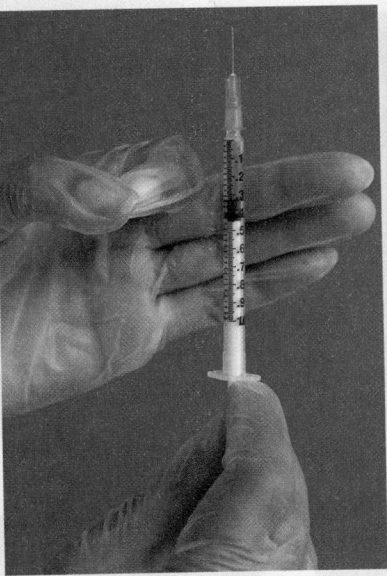

FIGURE 36–15E Remove the syringe and flick your finger against the syringe to move any air to the top.

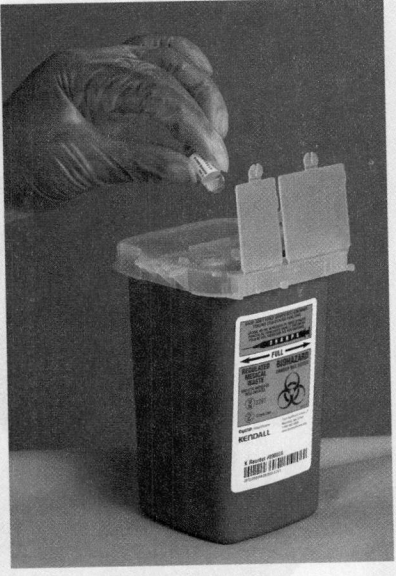

FIGURE 36–15F Discard the used ampule into a sharps container.

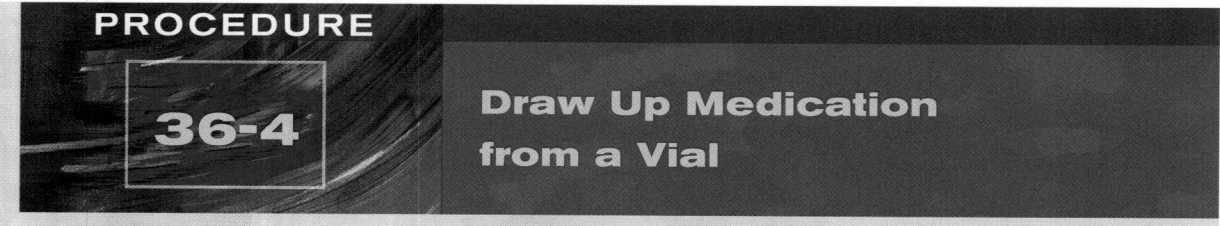

PROCEDURE

36-4

Draw Up Medication from a Vial

Student Competency Objective: The medical assistant student will draw up medication from a vial using a needle and syringe.

Items Needed: Multiple-dose vial, sterile water, alcohol wipes, syringe with needle, filter needle, gloves, sharps container

Steps:

1. Read the doctor's order for medication.
2. Go to the cupboard in the supply room where the medication is kept.
3. Wash your hands.
4. Find the ordered medication.
5. Read the label on the medication container and compare it to the doctor's order.
6. Check the expiration date.
7. Put on gloves.
8. Place the vial on a flat surface.
9. If the vial is new (unused), take off the plastic lid.
10. Rub an alcohol wipe over the rubber covering or port (Figure 36-16A).
11. Pick up the syringe and needle. Pull back the plunger and draw in air until the plunger is at the mark for the amount of medication ordered. Use a filter needle if required (Figure 36-16B).
12. Insert the needle and inject the air into the vial through the rubber covering (Figure 36-16C).
13. Keep the needle above the solution level.
14. With the nondominant hand, hold the vial and needle that has been inserted into the vial and invert them.
15. Keep the vial at eye level.
16. Push the needle into the solution.
17. Pull back on the plunger with the nondominant hand until the solution reaches the ordered line on the syringe (Figure 36-16D).
18. Pull the needle and syringe out of the vial.
19. Hold the syringe with the needle pointing straight up.
20. Flick the barrel of the syringe with your index finger to help any air bubbles rise to the top. Push in the plunger to expel any air.
21. If, after expelling the air, there is not enough medication left in the syringe, insert the needle into the vial again and repeat steps 13–17.
22. Change the needle if needed, or put the safety sheath over it.

(Continues)

PROCEDURE 36-4 (Continued)

23. If you used a multiple-dose vial, store it according to office policy. If it was a single-dose vial, throw it away according to office policy.

24. When you are finished with the syringe and needle, put them into a sharps container.

25. Wash your hands.

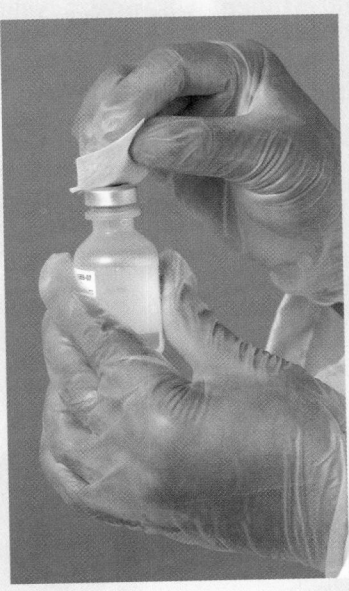

FIGURE 36–16A Wipe the rubber stopper with an alcohol wipe.

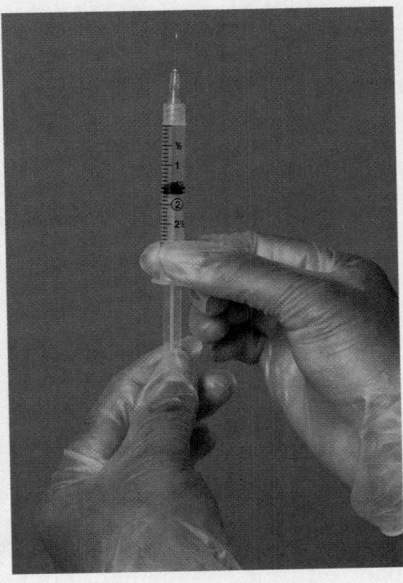

FIGURE 36–16B Put an amount of air into the syringe equal to the amount of medication to be withdrawn from the vial.

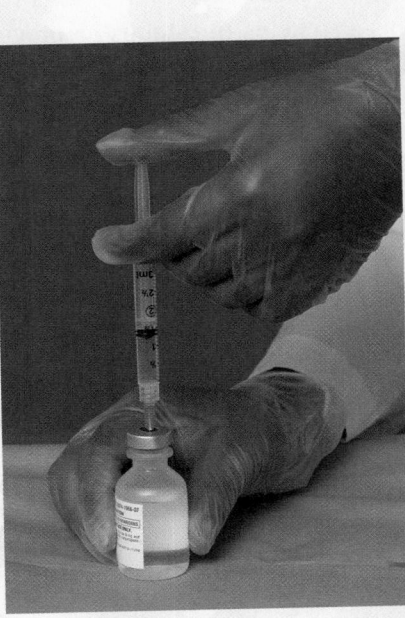

FIGURE 36–16C Inject the air into the vial.

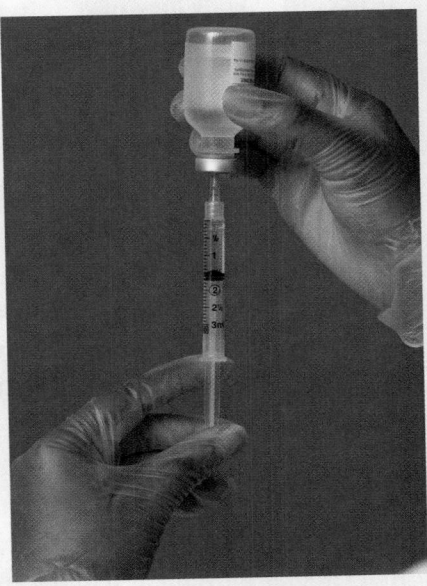

FIGURE 36–16D Turn the vial upside down and withdraw the ordered amount of medication.

PROCEDURE

36-5

Subcutaneous Injection

Student Competency Objective: The medical assistant student will give a subcutaneous injection.

Items Needed: Medication, syringe (subcutaneous syringe, 1–3 mL), needle (25- to 27-gauge needle, 1/2 or 5/8 inch in length), gloves, alcohol wipe, pen, sharps container

Steps:

1. Read the doctor's order for medication.
2. Go to the cupboard in the supply room where the medication is kept.
3. Wash your hands.
4. Find the ordered medication.
5. Read the label on the medication container and compare it to the doctor's order.
6. Check the expiration date.
7. Draw up medication in the syringe following Procedure 36-3 (if the medication is in an ampule) or Procedure 36-4 (if it is in a vial).
8. Check the medication label against the doctor's order again and then put the medication back into the cupboard, or discard a single-dose container.
9. Assemble equipment and supplies.
10. Go to the client's examination room.
11. Introduce yourself to the client even if you have seen the client on previous visits to your office. The client may have forgotten your name. This also helps to establish a provider-client relationship, because it shows the client that you want her to know who you are.
12. Identify the client. Ask the client to state her name to establish that this is the right client, and then compare the name given to the name on the chart. Never enter a room and call out a client's name to determine if this person is the correct client. The client may not have heard you clearly and may just nod, smile, or answer yes. Clients almost never question if the medical assistant professional has the right client. It is up to the medical assistant to identify the right client before performing any procedure.
13. Tell the client, in everyday language, what you are going to do.
14. Ask if the client has any questions. If she does, give short and simple answers. Sometimes clients will start (and continue) talking because they are nervous about the procedure.
15. Put on gloves.
16. Help the client into a comfortable position. The position will depend upon the body site selected for injection. Use anatomical landmarks.
17. Start at the center of where you want to give the injection and wipe with the alcohol wipe in a circular movement (Figure 36-17A).
18. Let the area dry. Do not blow on the area; blowing will contaminate the site.

(Continues)

PROCEDURE 36-5 (Continued)

19. Take the cap off the needle or pull back the safety sheath.

20. With one hand, gently grab up skin and tissue or spread it flat for injection (Figure 36-17B).

21. With the other hand, hold the syringe by the barrel. Do not put your thumb on the plunger yet; if you do, the medication could be injected incorrectly.

22. Insert the needle. Most frequently, it is inserted at a 45-degree angle. If the needle length is 1/2 inch or less, the injection may be given at a 90-degree angle, according to office policy (Figure 36-17C).

23. Let go of the skin.

24. Pull back the plunger to see if any blood comes into the needle. If it does, take out the needle and syringe and start over after drawing up new medication in a new needle and syringe.

25. If no blood enters the syringe, push the plunger in steadily. Do not push fast, as this may cause pain.

26. Take out the needle at the same angle as you put it in.

27. Wipe the area gently with an alcohol wipe.

28. Pull the safety sheath over the needle. If there is no safety sheath, do not recap the needle. Dispose of the needle and syringe in a sharps container (Figure 36-17D).

29. Talk with the client while you observe the client's response to the injection.

30. Take off your gloves.

31. Wash your hands.

32. Record the procedure in the client's chart immediately.

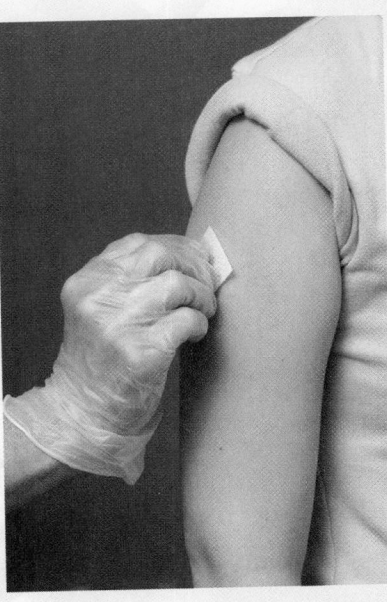

FIGURE 36-17A Select the injection site, and wipe the selected site with alcohol. The outer side of the upper arm is often used.

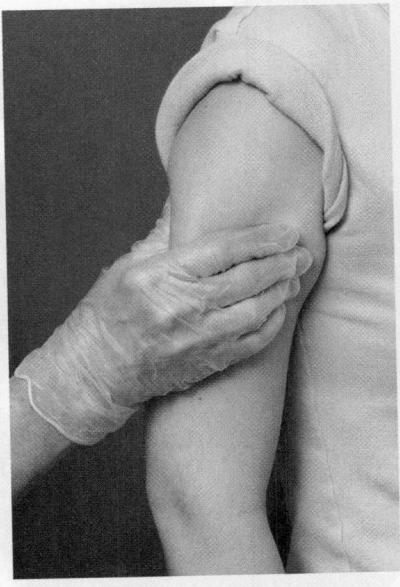

FIGURE 36-17B With your nondominant hand, bunch the skin to hold it steady and find the subcutaneous layer.

(Continues)

PROCEDURE 36-5 (Continued)

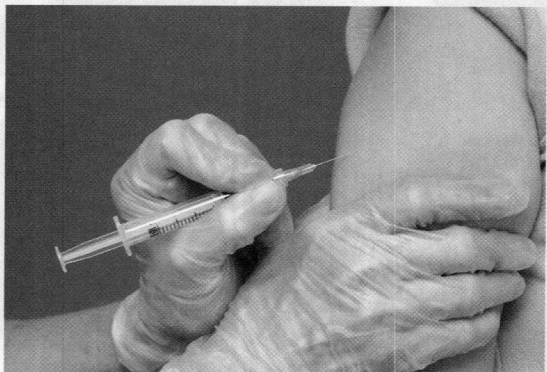

FIGURE 36–17C Hold the syringe at a 45-degree angle, with the bevel of the needle up, and inject the medication.

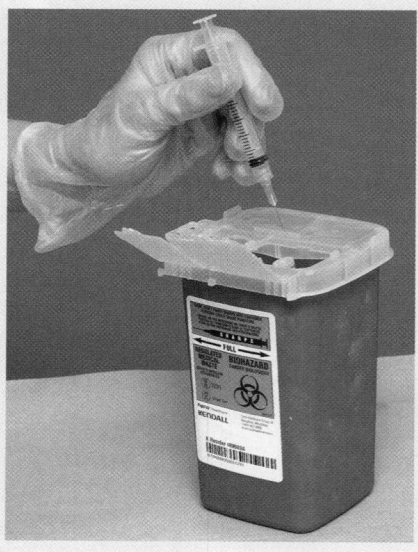

FIGURE 36–17D Dispose of the entire syringe unit in a sharps container.

Charting Example:

You injected 0.5 cc of epinephrine subcutaneously into the client's left arm. You would record the following:

    11/17/20xx   3:15 P.M.   Injected epinephrine 0.5 cc s.c. in client's left arm. No side effects observed. No complaints offered.

    Nina Pollett, S.M.A.

    Nina Pollett, S.M.A. (printed name)

PROCEDURE

36-6   Intramuscular Injection

Student Competency Objective: The medical assistant student will give an intramuscular injection.

Items Needed: Medication, syringe (intramuscular syringe 1–3 mL), needle (21- to 23-gauge, 1 to 1.5 inches long), gloves, alcohol wipe, pen, sharps container

Steps:

1. Read the doctor's order for medication.
2. Go to the cupboard in the supply room where medication is kept.

(Continues)

PROCEDURE 36-6 (Continued)

3. Wash your hands.

4. Find the ordered medication.

5. Read the label on the medication container and compare it to the doctor's order.

6. Check the expiration date.

7. Draw up medication in the syringe following Procedure 36-3 (if the medication is in an ampule) or Procedure 36-4 (if it is in a vial).

8. Check the medication label against the doctor's order again and put the medication container back into cupboard, or discard it if it is a single-dose package.

9. Assemble equipment and supplies.

10. Go to the client's examination room.

11. Introduce yourself to the client even if you have seen the client on previous visits to your office. The client may have forgotten your name. This also helps to establish a provider-client relationship, because it shows the client that you want her to know who you are.

12. Identify the client. Ask the client to state her name to establish that this is the right client, and then compare the name given to the name on the chart. Never enter a room and call out a client's name to determine if this person is the correct client. The client may not have heard you clearly and may just nod, smile, or answer yes. Clients almost never question if the medical assistant professional has the right client. It is up to the medical assistant to identify the right client before performing any procedure.

13. Tell the client, in everyday language, what you are going to do.

14. Ask if the client has any questions. If she does, give short and simple answers. Sometimes clients will start (and continue) talking because they are nervous about the procedure.

15. Put on gloves.

16. Help the client into a comfortable position. The position will depend upon the body site selected for injection. Use anatomical landmarks.

17. Start at the center of where you want to give the injection and wipe it in a circular movement with the alcohol wipe.

18. Let the area dry. Do not blow air on the area; this would contaminate the site.

19. Take the cap off the needle or pull back the safety sheath.

20. Spread the skin where you want to give the injection.

21. With the other hand, hold the syringe by the barrel. Do not put your thumb on the plunger yet; if you do, medication could accidentally be injected before you are ready.

22. Insert the needle at a 90-degree angle (straight down) (Figure 36-18).

23. Let go of the skin.

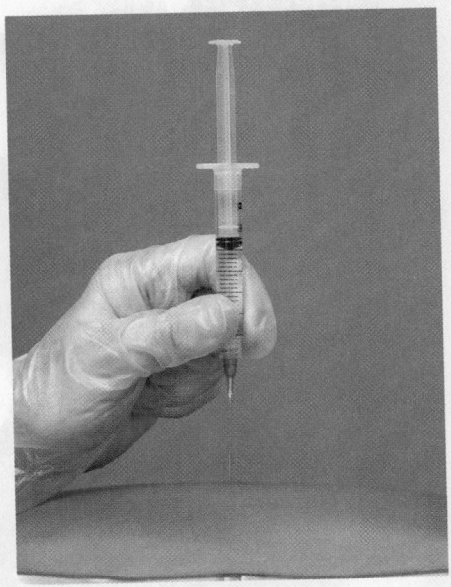

FIGURE 36-18 Hold the needle and syringe at a 90-degree angle and inject the medication.

(Continues)

PROCEDURE 36-6 (Continued)

24. Pull back the plunger to see if any blood comes into the syringe. If it does, take out the needle and start over, drawing up new medication into a new needle and syringe.

25. If no blood enters the syringe, push the plunger in steadily. Do not push fast, as this may cause pain.

26. Take out the needle and syringe at the same angle as you put it in.

27. Wipe the area gently with an alcohol wipe.

28. Pull the safety sheath over needle; if there is no safety sheath, do not recap the needle. Dispose of the needle and syringe in a sharps container.

29. Talk with the client while you observe client's response to the injection.

30. Take off your gloves.

31. Wash your hands.

32. Record the procedure in the client's chart immediately.

Charting Example:
You injected 500 mg of penicillin in the ventrogluteal site on the client's right side. You would record the following:

3/18/20xx	2:17 P.M.	Injected penicillin 500 mg I.M. into right ventrogluteal site. No side effects observed in client. No complaints offered.

James O'Connell, S.M.A.

James O'Connell, S.M.A. (printed name)

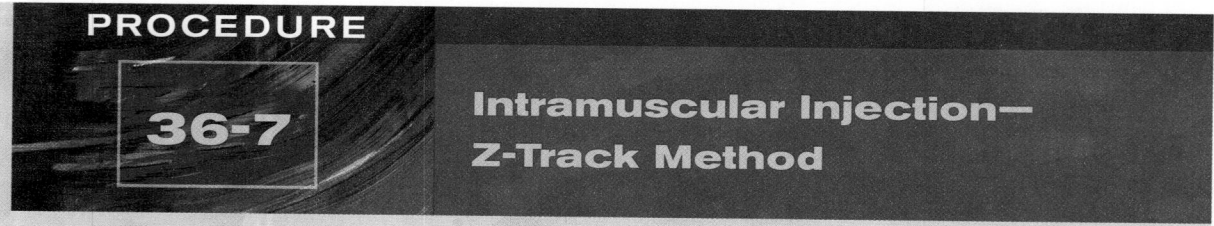

PROCEDURE

36-7

Intramuscular Injection— Z-Track Method

Student Competency Objective: The medical assistant student will give an intramuscular injection using the Z-Track method.

Items Needed: Medication, syringe (intramuscular syringe, 1–3 mL), needle (21- to 23-gauge, 1 to 1.5 inches long), gloves, alcohol wipe, pen, sharps container

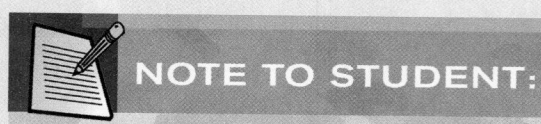

NOTE TO STUDENT:

The Z-Track method is used when the medication can be irritating to the tissue.

Steps:

1. Read the doctor's order for medication.

2. Wash your hands.

3. Go to the cupboard in the supply room where the medication is kept.

4. Find the ordered medication.

(Continues)

PROCEDURE 36-7 (Continued)

5. Read the label on the medication container and compare it to the doctor's order.

6. Check the expiration date.

7. Draw up medication in the syringe following Procedure 36-3 (if the medication is in an ampule) or Procedure 36-4 (if it is in a vial).

8. Check the medication label against the doctor's order again and put the medication back into the cupboard, or discard a single-dose container.

9. Assemble equipment and supplies.

10. Go to the client's examination room.

11. Introduce yourself to the client even if you have seen the client on previous visits to your office. The client may have forgotten your name. This also helps to establish a provider-client relationship, because it shows the client that you want her to know who you are.

12. Identify the client. Ask the client to state her name to establish that this is the right client, and then compare the name given to the name on the chart. Never enter a room and call out a client's name to determine if this person is the correct client. The client may not have heard you clearly and may just nod, smile, or answer yes. Clients almost never question if the medical assistant professional has the right client. It is up to the medical assistant to identify the right client before performing any procedure.

13. Tell the client, in everyday language, what you are going to do.

14. Ask if the client has any questions. If she does, give short and simple answers. Sometimes clients will start (and continue) talking because they are nervous about the procedure.

15. Put on gloves.

16. Help the client into a comfortable position. The position will depend upon the body site selected for injection. Use anatomical landmarks.

17. Start at the center of where you want to give the injection and wipe the site in a circular movement with the alcohol wipe.

18. Let the area dry. Do not blow on the area; this will contaminate the site.

19. Take the cap off the needle or pull back the safety sheath.

20. Pull the skin to the side of the injection site. A Z-Track injection should be given in the gluteal muscle.

21. Pull the skin, subcutaneous layer, and fat into a Z form (Figure 36-19).

22. Hold the syringe by the barrel. Do not put your thumb on the plunger yet; if you do, medication could accidentally be injected incorrectly.

23. Spread the skin taut where you want to give the injection.

24. Insert the needle at a 90-degree angle (straight down) (Figure 36-19).

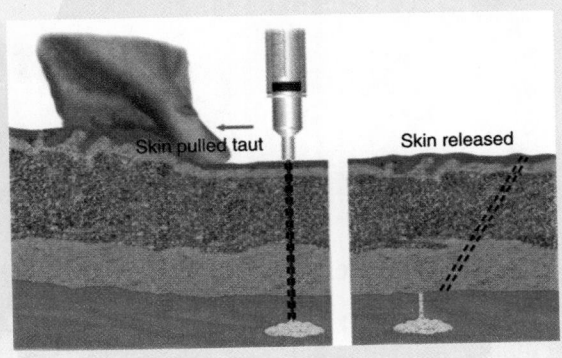

FIGURE 36-19 To give an IM injection using the Z-Track method, pull the skin taut to the side and then release it after the needle is withdrawn.

(Continues)

PROCEDURE 36-7 (Continued)

25. Pull back the plunger to see if any blood comes into the syringe. If it does, take out the needle and syringe and start over, drawing up new medication using a new needle and syringe.

26. If no blood enters the syringe, push the plunger in steadily. Do not push fast, as this may cause pain.

27. Wait a few seconds before taking out the needle and syringe, while still holding the skin taut to the side.

28. Take out the needle and syringe and let the skin return to its normal position. This helps the tissue to close off the path of the needle.

29. Do not rub the injection site.

30. Pull the safety sheath over the needle; if there is no safety sheath, do not recap the needle. Dispose of the needle and syringe in a sharps container.

31. Talk with the client while you observe the client's response to the injection.

32. Take off your gloves.

33. Wash your hands.

34. Record the procedure in the client's chart immediately.

Charting Example:

You give an intramuscular injection of penicillin, 500 mg, in the gluteal muscle using the Z-Track method. You would record the following:

> 6/15/20xx   11:15 A.M.   Injected penicillin 500 mg I.M. using the Z-Track method in the client's (right buttock) gluteal muscle. No side effects observed. No complaints offered.

Susan Morrison, S.M.A.

Susan Morrison, S.M.A. (printed name)

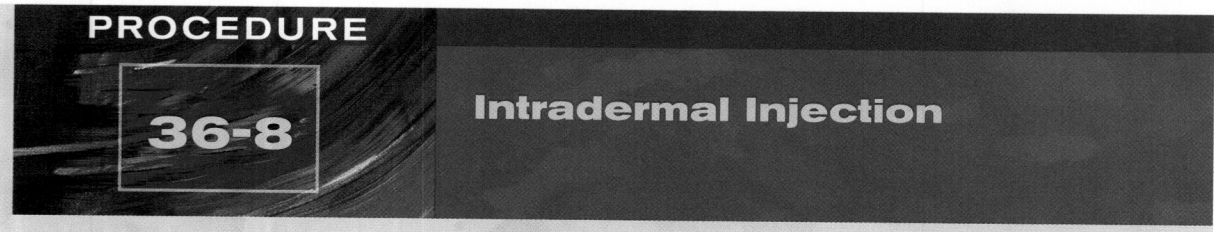

Student Competency Objective: The medical assistant student will give an intradermal injection.

Items Needed: Medication, tuberculin syringe, needle (25- to 26-gauge, intradermal bevel), gloves, alcohol wipes, pen, sharps container

Steps:

1. Read the doctor's order for medication.

2. Go to the cupboard in the supply room where the medication is kept.

3. Wash your hands.

(Continues)

PROCEDURE 36-8 (Continued)

4. Find the ordered medication.

5. Read the label on the medication container and compare it to the doctor's order.

6. Check the expiration date.

7. Draw up medication in the syringe following Procedure 36-3 (if the medication is in an ampule) or Procedure 36-4 (if it is in a vial).

8. Check the medication label against the doctor's order again and put the medication back into the cupboard, or discard a single-dose container.

9. Assemble equipment and supplies.

10. Go to the client's examination room.

11. Introduce yourself to the client even if you have seen the client on previous visits to your office. The client may have forgotten your name. This also helps to establish a provider-client relationship, because it shows the client that you want her to know who you are.

12. Identify the client. Ask the client to state her name to establish that this is the right client, and then compare the name given to the name on the chart. Never enter a room and call out a client's name to determine if this person is the correct client. The client may not have heard you clearly and may just nod, smile, or answer yes. Clients almost never question if the medical assistant professional has the right client. It is up to the medical assistant to identify the right client before performing any procedure.

13. Tell the client, in everyday language, what you are going to do.

14. Ask if the client has any questions. If she does, give short and simple answers. Sometimes clients will start (and continue) talking because they are nervous about the procedure.

15. Put on gloves.

16. Help the client into a comfortable position. The position will depend upon the body site selected for injection. Use anatomical landmarks.

17. Pick an area on the inner side of either forearm.

18. Start at the center of where you want to give the injection and wipe the site in a circular motion with the alcohol wipe (Figure 36-20A).

19. Let the area dry. Do not blow on the area; this will contaminate the site.

20. Take the cap off the needle or pull back the safety sheath.

21. Hold the skin tight and smooth. It will make the injection easier.

22. Hold the needle and syringe at right angles to the skin site.

23. Move the tip of the needle to a 15-degree angle with the bevel (slanted part of needle tip) pointing up. This angle is almost horizontal.

24. Insert the needle just under the top layer of skin (Figure 36-20B).

25. Push the plunger and inject the medication slowly. A small wheal or raised area should form around the needle point (Figure 36-20C).

26. Take out the needle at the same angle.

27. Do not rub the area.

28. Tell the client not to rub or scratch the area.

29. Pull the safety sheath over the needle. If there is no safety sheath; do not recap the needle.

(Continues)

PROCEDURE 36-8 (Continued)

30. Dispose of the needle and syringe in a sharps container.
31. Talk with the client while you observe the client's response to the injection.
32. Remind the client not to rub or scratch the area.
33. Take off your gloves.
34. Wash your hands.
35. Record the procedure in the client's chart immediately.

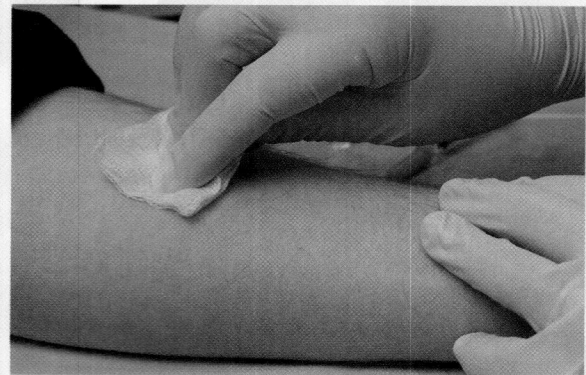

FIGURE 36–20A Cleanse the site with alcohol.

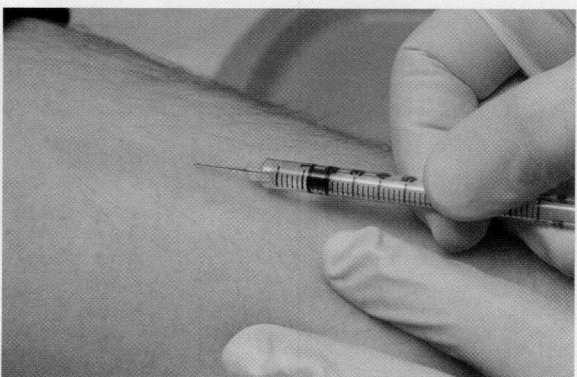

FIGURE 36–20B Hold the needle at a 10- to 15-degree angle, with the bevel of the needle up.

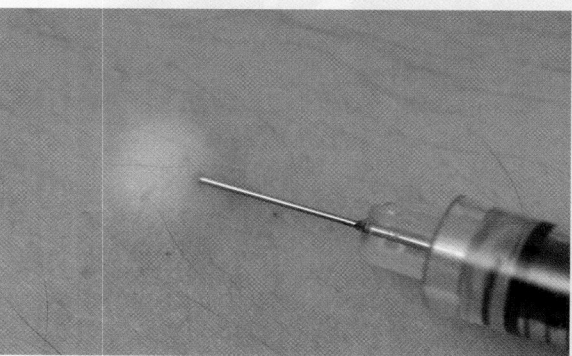

FIGURE 36–20C Inject the medication slowly. A small raised area will form around the needle point.

Charting Example:

You injected 0.3 mL of PPD solution under the skin on the client's right forearm. You would record the following:

7/10/20xx   4:15 P.M.   Injected 0.3 mL of PPD solution intradermally into inner aspect of right forearm. No side effects observed. Instructed client not to rub or scratch wheal or raised area and to return in two days to the medical office for "reading" of the results.

Thomas Burns, S.M.A.

Thomas Burns, S.M.A. (printed name)

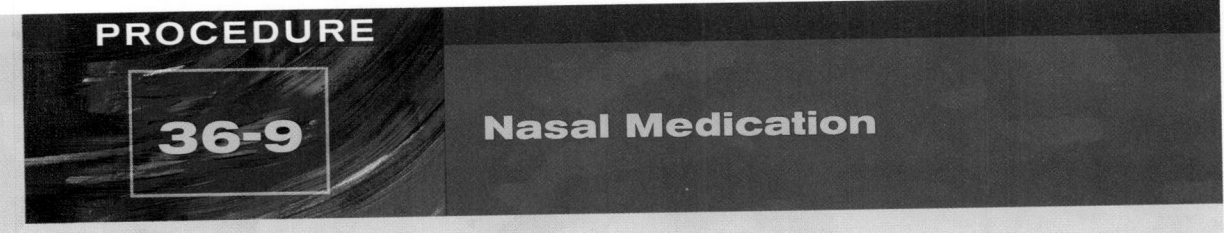

PROCEDURE

36-9

Nasal Medication

Student Competency Objective: The medical assistant will administer nasal medication.

Items Needed: Medication, doctor's order, gloves, tissues, pen, paper

Steps:

1. Wash your hands.
2. Assemble equipment and supplies.
3. Check the medication three times, comparing it to the doctor's order.
4. Introduce yourself to the client even if you have seen the client on previous visits to your office. The client may have forgotten your name. This also helps to establish a provider–client relationship, because it shows the client that you want her to know who you are.
5. Identify the client. Ask the client to state her name to establish that this is the right client, and then compare the name given to the name on the chart. Never enter a room and call out a client's name to determine if this person is the correct client. The client may not have heard you clearly and may just nod, smile, or answer yes. Clients almost never question if the medical assistant professional has the right client. It is up to the medical assistant to identify the right client before performing any procedure.
6. Tell the client, in everyday language, what you are going to do.
7. Ask if the client has any questions. If she does, give short and simple answers. Sometimes clients will start (and continue) talking because they are nervous about the procedure.
8. Ask the client to lie back on the examination table.
9. Place a pillow under the client's shoulder.
10. Support the client's neck (Figure 36–21A).
11. Put on gloves.
12. Hold the medication straight up above the nostril (do not touch the nostril with the dropper tip). Administer one drop at a time, up to the ordered numbered of drops (Figure 36–21B).
13. Repeat step 12 with the other nostril.
14. Instruct the client to remain lying down for a few minutes.
15. Wipe any excess moisture away from the skin or around the nose.
16. Assist the client to a sitting position.
17. Ask if the client has any questions.
18. Help the client get off the exam table.
19. Take off your gloves.
20. Wash your hands.
21. Record the procedure in the client's chart immediately.

(Continues)

PROCEDURE 36-9 (Continued)

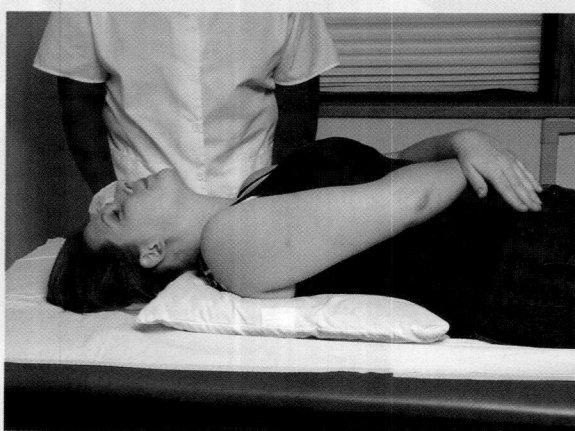

FIGURE 36-21A With the client lying on the examination table, place a pillow under the client's shoulder and support the neck.

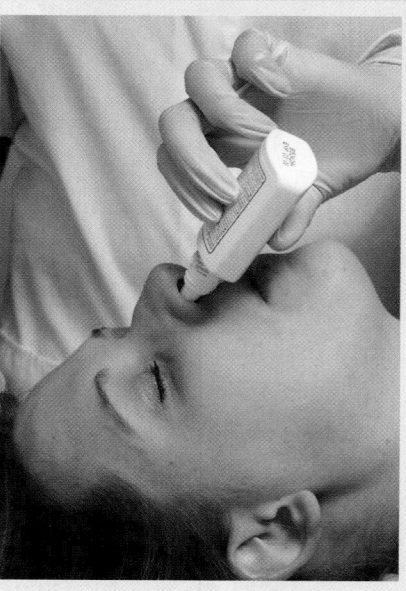

FIGURE 36-21B Holding the medication above the nostril, administer the medication.

 **NOTE TO STUDENT:**

When administering nasal spray: Instead of lying down, ask the client to sit. Hold the spray at the tip of the nostril and spray as the client breathes in. Repeat with the other nostril. Do not let the container tip touch the nasal area or any skin surface. The other steps remain the same.

Charting Example:

2/16/20xx   10:30 A.M.   Administered nasal medication to client. Two drops in each nostril. Answered client's questions.

Sandra Williams, S. M. A.

Sandra Williams, S.M.A. (printed name)

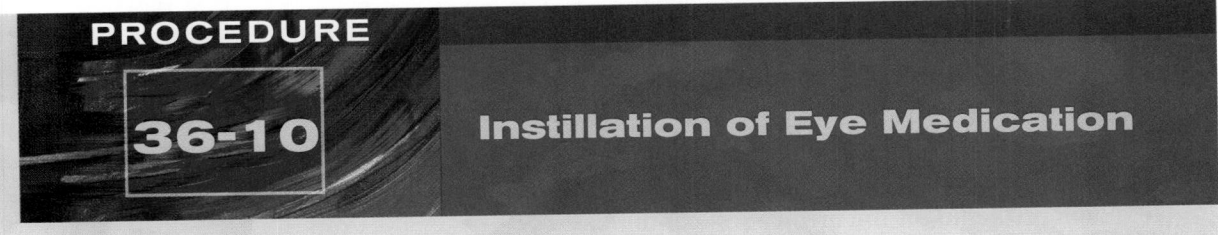

PROCEDURE 36-10   Instillation of Eye Medication

Student Competency Objective: The medical assistant student will set up and give ophthalmic (eye) medication.

Items Needed: Ophthalmic medication, dry cotton balls, paper and pen for charting

Steps:

1. Read the doctor's order.
2. Go to the medication cupboard.
3. Wash your hands.
4. Find the correct medication.
5. Check the expiration date.
6. Compare the label on the medication container with the doctor's order.
7. Assemble equipment and supplies.
8. Introduce yourself to the client even if you have seen the client on previous visits to your office. The client may have forgotten your name. This also helps to establish a provider–client relationship, because it shows the client that you want her to know who you are.
9. Identify the client. Ask the client to state her name to establish that this is the right client, and then compare the name given to the name on the chart. Never enter a room and call out a client's name to determine if this person is the correct client. The client may not have heard you clearly and may just nod, smile, or answer yes. Clients almost never question if the medical assistant professional has the right client. It is up to the medical assistant to identify the right client before performing any procedure.
10. Tell the client, in everyday language, what you are going to do.
11. Ask if the client has any questions. If she does, give short and simple answers. Sometimes clients will start (and continue) talking because they are nervous about the procedure.
12. Open the eye medication container.
13. Hold the medication in your hand to avoid contamination.
14. Have the client sit or lie down.
15. Ask the client to look up.
16. Gently pull down on the lower lid of the eye into which you will instill the drops (Figure 36-22A).
17. Line up the eyedrop container at the middle of the lower lid (Figure 36-22B).
18. Gently squeeze the container and direct the liquid drops into the lower-lid conjunctival area.

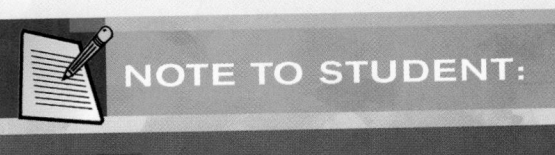

NOTE TO STUDENT:

Never let the tip of the container touch the eye.

(Continues)

PROCEDURE 36-10 (Continued)

19. Instruct the client to close the eye gently to allow the medication to be absorbed. Make sure the client does not squeeze the eyelids together tightly, as this will force the medication out of the eye (Figure 36–22C).
20. Replace the lid on the medication container.
21. Hand the client a dry cotton ball to remove extra moisture.
22. Wash your hands.
23. Record the procedure in the client's chart immediately.

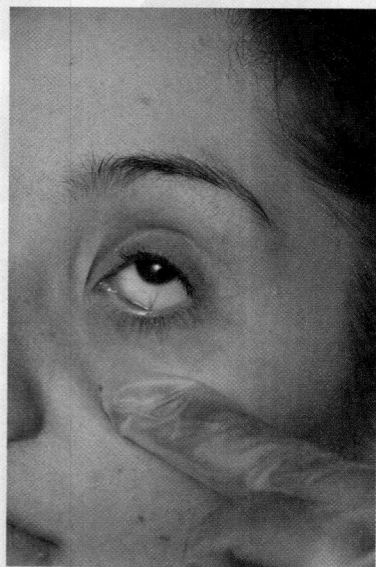

FIGURE 36–22A With the client looking up, gently pull the lower lid of the client's eye down and slightly out.

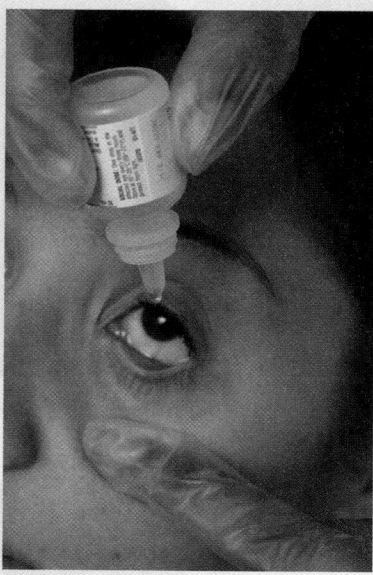

FIGURE 36–22B Line up the eye drop container at the middle of the lower lid and allow a drop of the liquid medication to fall into the lower conjunctiva.

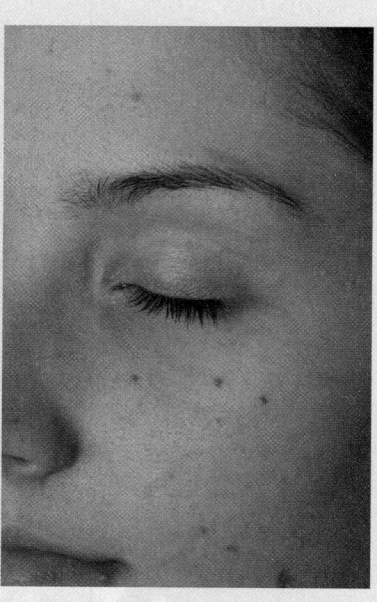

FIGURE 36–22C Ask the client to close the eye gently to allow the medication to be absorbed. Caution the client not to squeeze the lids together.

Charting Example:

2/23/20xx   9:15 A.M.   Two drops of ophthalmic medication instilled in client's left eye (O.S.). No discomfort or complaint offered by client.

James Evans, S.M.A.

James Evans, S.M.A. (printed name)

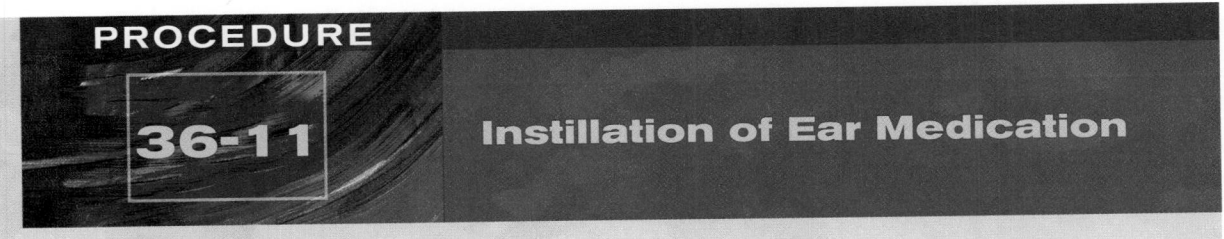

PROCEDURE

36-11   Instillation of Ear Medication

Student Competency Objective: The medical assistant student will set up and give otic (ear) medication.

Items Needed: Otic medication, dry cotton balls, paper and pen for charting

Steps:

1. Read the doctor's order.
2. Go to the medication cupboard.
3. Wash your hands.
4. Find the correct medication.
5. Compare the label on the medication container with the doctor's order.
6. Check the expiration date.
7. Assemble equipment and supplies.
8. Introduce yourself to the client even if you have seen the client on previous visits to your office. The client may have forgotten your name. This also helps to establish a provider-client relationship, because it shows the client that you want her to know who you are.
9. Identify the client. Ask the client to state her name to establish that this is the right client, and then compare the name given to the name on the chart. Never enter a room and call out a client's name to determine if this person is the correct client. The client may not have heard you clearly and may just nod, smile, or answer yes. Clients almost never question if the medical assistant professional has the right client. It is up to the medical assistant to identify the right client before performing any procedure.
10. Tell the client, in everyday language, what you are going to do.
11. Ask if the client has any questions. If she does, give short and simple answers. Sometimes clients will start (and continue) talking because they are nervous about the procedure.
12. Ask the client to sit with the head tilted toward the unaffected ear.
13. Straighten the ear canal of the affected ear. This is done by gently pulling the external ear upward and backward for adults and children over 3 years old (for children under the age of 3, pull the external ear downward and backward). This step will help the medication to reach all parts of the ear canal (Figure 36-23A).
14. Place the tip of the otic medication container in the ear canal without touching the ear canal (Figure 36-23B).
15. Gently squeeze the correct number of drops along the side of the ear canal without touching the ear canal.
16. Tell the client to remain in this position for 2 to 3 minutes.
17. Loosely place a cotton ball into the external ear of the affected ear.
18. Wash your hands.
19. Record the procedure in the client's chart immediately.

(Continues)

PROCEDURE 36-11 (Continued)

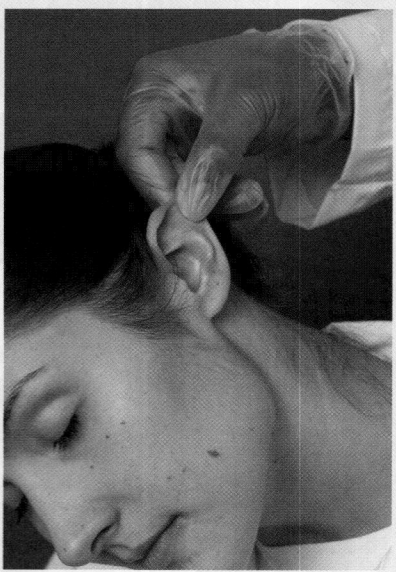

FIGURE 36-23A With client's head tilted toward the unaffected ear, straighten the ear canal of the affected ear.

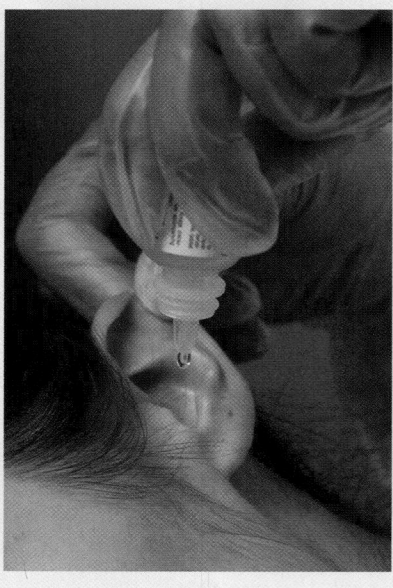

FIGURE 36-23B Administer the medication in the ear, being careful not to touch the ear canal with the medication container.

Charting Example:

5/16/20xx   11:30 A.M.   Three drops of medication into client's right ear. Client remained in position for two minutes without complaint.

Miranda Jacobs, S.M.A.

Miranda Jacobs, S.M.A (printed name)

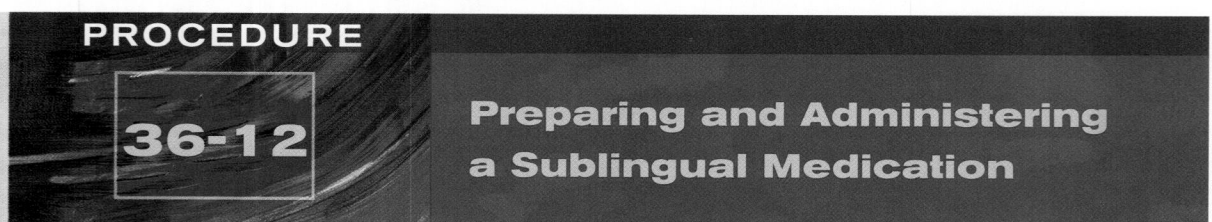

PROCEDURE
36-12
Preparing and Administering a Sublingual Medication

Student Competency Objective: The medical assistant student will set up and give sublingual medication.

Items Needed: Sublingual medication, disposable cup, paper and pen for charting

Steps:

1. Read the doctor's order.
2. Go to the medication cupboard.
3. Wash your hands.

(Continues)

PROCEDURE 36-12 (Continued)

4. Find the correct medication.
5. Compare the label on the medication container with the doctor's order.
6. Check the expiration date.
7. Assemble equipment and supplies.
8. Introduce yourself to the client even if you have seen the client on previous visits to your office. The client may have forgotten your name. This also helps to establish a provider–client relationship, because it shows the client that you want her to know who you are.
9. Identify the client. Ask the client to state her name to establish that this is the right client, and then compare the name given to the name on the chart. Never enter a room and call out a client's name to determine if this person is the correct client. The client may not have heard you clearly and may just nod, smile, or answer yes. Clients almost never question if the medical assistant professional has the right client. It is up to the medical assistant to identify the right client before performing any procedure.
10. Tell the client, in everyday language, what you are going to do.
11. Ask if the client has any questions. If she does, give short and simple answers. Sometimes clients will start (and continue) talking because they are nervous about the procedure.
12. Instruct the client not to swallow the medication, but allow it to dissolve under the tongue.
13. Hand the client the sublingual medication in the disposable cup.
14. Tell the client to place the medication under her tongue.
15. Stay with the client until the medication has dissolved completely.
16. Wash your hands.
17. Record the procedure in the client's chart immediately.

Charting Example:

4/08/20xx   3:00 P.M.   Sublingual medication administered to client. Remained with client until medication completely dissolved.

Trent Michaels, S.M.A.

Trent Michaels, S.M.A. (printed name)

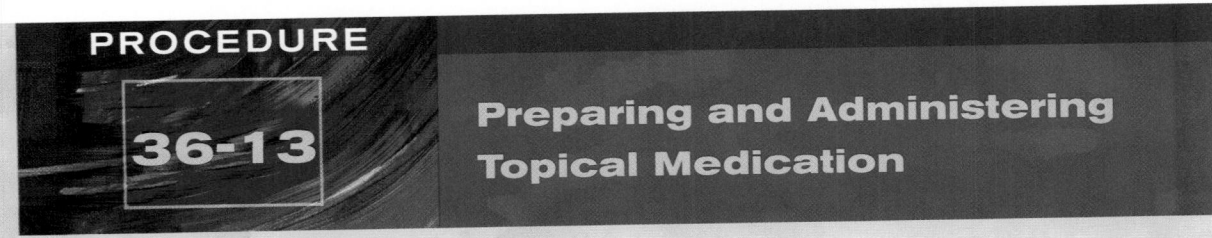

PROCEDURE

36-13   Preparing and Administering Topical Medication

Student Competency Objective: The medical assistant student will set up and give topical medication.

Items Needed: Topical medication, gloves, cotton swab or tongue blade, pen and paper for charting

(Continues)

PROCEDURE 36-13 (Continued)

Steps:

1. Read the doctor's order.
2. Go to the medication cupboard.
3. Wash your hands.
4. Find the correct medication.
5. Compare the label on the medication container with the doctor's order.
6. Check the expiration date.
7. Assemble equipment and supplies.
8. Introduce yourself to the client even if you have seen the client on previous visits to your office. The client may have forgotten your name. This also helps to establish a provider-client relationship, because it shows the client that you want her to know who you are.
9. Identify the client. Ask the client to state her name to establish that this is the right client, and then compare the name given to the name on the chart. Never enter a room and call out a client's name to determine if this person is the correct client. The client may not have heard you clearly and may just nod, smile, or answer yes. Clients almost never question if the medical assistant professional has the right client. It is up to the medical assistant to identify the right client before performing any procedure.
10. Tell the client, in everyday language, what you are going to do.
11. Ask if the client has any questions. If she does, give short and simple answers. Sometimes clients will start (and continue) talking because they are nervous about the procedure.
12. Put on gloves.
13. Check the skin area where the medication will be applied (Figure 36-24A).
14. Squeeze medication onto a large cotton swab or tongue blade (Figure 36-24B). (A tongue blade may be harsh and cause client discomfort. Only use a blade if so directed by the doctor.)
15. Start applying topical medication from the center of the selected area and working outward in a circle (Figure 36-24C).
16. Leave the application area open to the air unless the doctor orders differently.
17. Remove your gloves.
18. Wash your hands.
19. Record the procedure in the client's chart immediately.

 NOTE TO STUDENT:

Do not rub back and forth over the area with the swab. In addition to contamination, this motion often irritates the client's skin and causes it to become itchy.

(Continues)

PROCEDURE 36-13 (Continued)

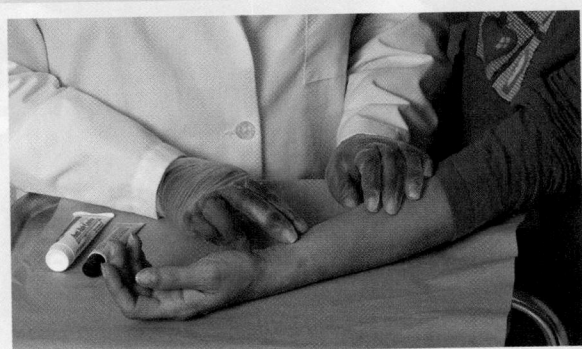

FIGURE 36-24A Check the skin around the area in which you will apply the medication on the client.

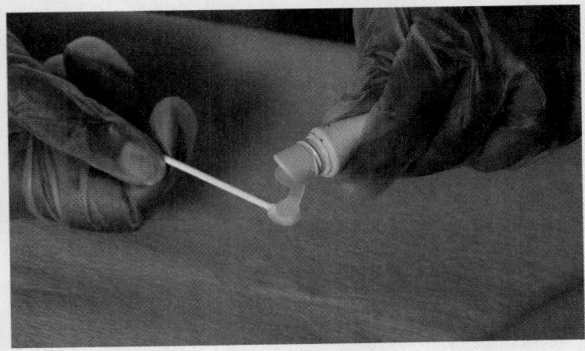

FIGURE 36-24B Use a large cotton swab to apply the medication. A tongue blade may be used if directed by the doctor.

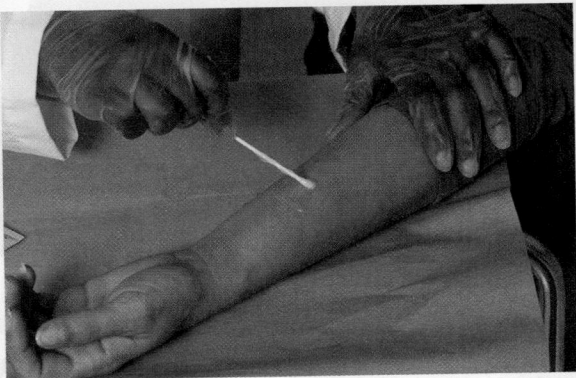

FIGURE 36-24C Apply the topical medication from the center of the area in a circular motion.

Charting Example:

11/15/20xx   8:30 A.M.   Applied topical medication to the left forearm. Area was red and irritated. Client did not complain of additional discomfort after application of medication.

Dominque Pae, S.M.A.

Dominque Pae, S.M.A. (printed name)

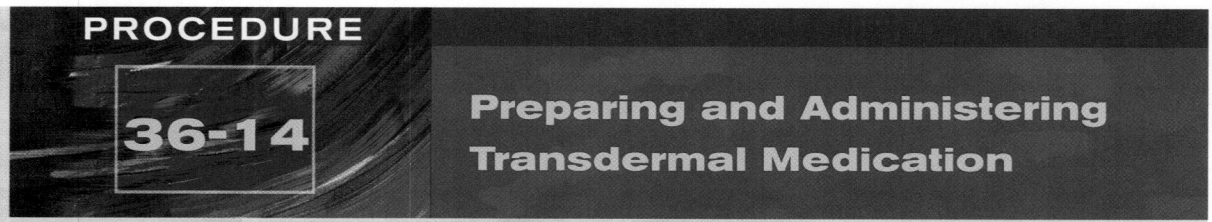

PROCEDURE

36-14

Preparing and Administering Transdermal Medication

Student Competency Objective: The medical assistant student will set up and give transdermal medication.

Items Needed: Transdermal (patch) medication, gloves, pen and paper for charting

Steps:

1. Read the doctor's order.
2. Go to the medication cupboard.
3. Wash your hands
4. Find the correct medication.
5. Compare the label on the medication container with the doctor's order.
6. Check the expiration date.
7. Assemble equipment and supplies.
8. Introduce yourself to the client even if you have seen the client on previous visits to your office. The client may have forgotten your name. This also helps to establish a provider-client relationship, because it shows the client that you want her to know who you are.
9. Identify the client. Ask the client to state her name to establish that this is the right client, and then compare the name given to the name on the chart. Never enter a room and call out a client's name to determine if this person is the correct client. The client may not have heard you clearly and may just nod, smile, or answer yes. Clients almost never question if the medical assistant professional has the right client. It is up to the medical assistant to identify the right client before performing any procedure.
10. Tell the client, in everyday language, what you are going to do.
11. Ask if the client has any questions. If she does, give short and simple answers. Sometimes clients will start (and continue) talking because they are nervous about the procedure.
12. Choose the area to place the medicated patch. Select an area where the skin is dry and clear of any irritation. Good candidate sites are the chest, the back, behind an ear, or the upper arm.
13. Put on gloves.
14. If an old patch is still on the client, remove it. Do not place the new patch at the same spot.
15. Open the package by peeling it apart according to the manufacturer's instructions (Figure 36–25A).
16. Do not touch the medicated part of the patch.
17. Place the transdermal patch at the selected site. Gently but firmly press the edges down, starting at the center (Figure 36–25B).
18. Remove your gloves.

(Continues)

PROCEDURE 36-14 (Continued)

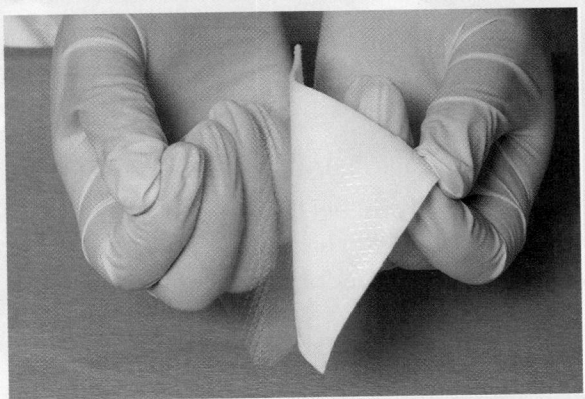

FIGURE 36–25A Following the manufacturer's instructions, open the package containing the transdermal medication.

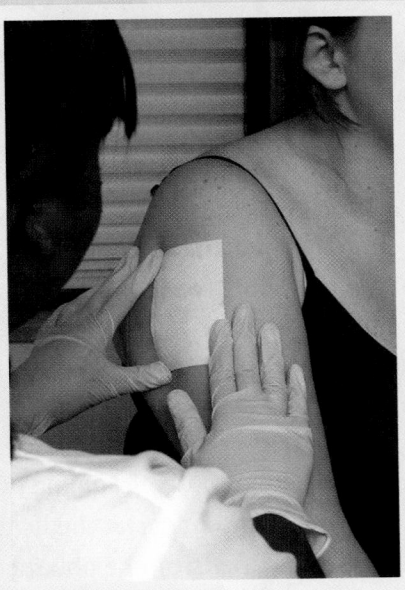

FIGURE 36–25B Apply the transdermal patch.

19. Wash your hands.
20. Record the procedure in the client's chart immediately.

Charting Example:

01/22/20xx   11:35 A.M.   Applied transdermal patch medication to right upper arm. Removed old patch from left upper arm.

Brandon Dominio, S.M.A.

Brandon Dominio, S.M.A. (printed name)

BRIDGE TO CAAHEP

This chapter, which discusses medication and the client population, provides information and content related to CAAHEP standards for Anatomy and Physiology, Medical Terminology, Medical Law and Ethics, Psychology, Communication, Medical Assisting Clinical Procedures, and Professional Components.

ABHES LINKS

This chapter, which discusses medication and the client population, links to ABHES course content for Anatomy and Physiology, Medical Terminology, Medical Law and Ethics, Psychology of Human Relations, Medical Office Clinical Procedures, and Pharmacology.

AAMA AREAS OF COMPETENCE

This chapter, which discusses medication and the client population, provides information or content within several areas listed in the Medical Assistant Role Delineation Study. These areas include: administrative, administrative procedures, clinical, fundamental principles, diagnostic orders, patient (client) care, general transdisciplinary, professionalism, professional communication skills, legal concepts, instruction, and operational functions.

POINTS OF HIGHLIGHT

- Pharmacology is the study of drugs (medications) and their effects on the body.
- Medication sources include plants, animals, minerals, and synthetics (man-made materials and components).
- Medications can be taken by mouth, put on the skin (topical or transdermal), inhaled through the nose or mouth, inserted into the rectum or vagina, or injected into the veins, muscles, subcutaneous layer, or under the skin (intradermally).
- The oral route is the most common and least expensive route for administration of medication.
- Solid oral drug forms include tablets, capsules, and lozenges.
- Solutions, syrups, elixirs, emulsions, and suspensions are examples of liquid oral forms of medications.
- The injection route of administration is also known as the parenteral route.
- Two major categories of medication are prescription and over-the-counter (OTC).
- OTC medications can be obtained by the consumer without a prescription or guidance by a doctor or other health care professional.
- Controlled substances are drugs that have the potential to be abused and cause addiction.
- The 1970 Controlled Substances Act defined controlled substances and established the Drug Enforcement Agency.
- The Food and Drug Administration regulates the manufacture and sale of drugs in the United States.
- There are six guiding rules for medication: (1) right medicine, (2) right amount, (3) right time, (4) right route, (5) right client, (6) right documentation.

 AMT PATHS

This chapter, which discusses medication and the client population, provides a path to AMT competency in general medical assisting knowledge, anatomy and physiology, medical terminology, medical law, medical ethics, human relations, patient (client) education, and clinical medical assisting.

STUDENT PORTFOLIO ACTIVITY

Design a teaching aid for self-administration of medication at home by clients. Make sure to take into account the needs and abilities of elderly clients and clients with any special needs. Ask your instructor to review your teaching aid. Place it in your portfolio as an example of meeting an individual client's needs.

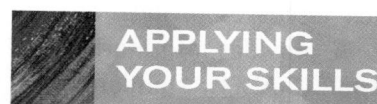 **APPLYING YOUR SKILLS**

While you are working with a client, she casually mentions that she has been taking vitamins to improve her health. You are aware that this client also takes prescription medications. What do you need to know? What questions would you ask? What do you do with the information? Why is this important to know for the client's health care and outcome?

CRITICAL THINKING QUESTIONS

1. A client has been prescribed an ointment medication that is to be applied to a large area of the client's skin at night. Think about what you have learned about the characteristics of ointments. What instructions would you give to the client regarding when to apply this medication to the skin? What would you say about the client's clothing and bedding?

2. The doctor prescribed enteric-coated aspirin for a client who needs to take it on a regular basis for pain control. The client complains to you that it costs more than regular aspirin tablets. Why would the doctor prescribe enteric-coated medication? Why might it be better for the client?

3. A client has been prescribed medication that is in a timed-release capsule form. Why should the capsule not be taken apart?

4. What will happen if a client holds a suppository in the hand too long before inserting it? Why?

5. Why is it important to ask about OTC medications when questioning a client about medications? Why might a client not tell you about OTC medications she uses unless specifically questioned?

6. A client tells you about a new drug that she read about in the newspaper. The FDA has not approved it for use yet. She does not understand the reason for the delay. What do you tell her about the role of the FDA?

7. The doctor has prescribed a medication in a suspension form. You are asked to teach the client about the medication. What is important for you to include in teaching about suspensions?

8. What do you tell a caregiver who will apply a transdermal medication patch to the client once a day? What is important for the caregiver to know about the application process?

9. Your instructor tells you to check medication three times before administering it to a client. A fellow student comments that once should be enough. What do you say?

10. You observe a health care professional drawing up medication into a syringe. The uncovered needle accidentally touches the countertop. What do you do?

11. Go back to the beginning of this chapter and review the Anticipatory Statements. Reread each statement and then indicate whether it is true or false. If the statement is false, rewrite it to make it a true statement.

Anticipatory Statements

Read and think about the following statements based upon what you believe now. Decide whether you agree or disagree. Write the word **agree** after the statement if you think the statement is true. Write the word **disagree** after the statement if you think the statement is false. Read the chapter to find out if your current beliefs can be supported.

1. An inactive lifestyle is a risk factor for cardiovascular disorders. _____

2. Breakfast is the most important meal of the day. _____

3. Obesity is a major health problem in the United States. _____

4. Vitamins in any amount are always safe to take. _____

5. Smoking has been linked not only to cancer but also to many other disorders. _____

Healthy Lifestyle in the Primary Client Population

Learning Objectives

Upon completion of this chapter, the medical assistant student should be able to:

- List ways to live a healthy lifestyle
- Understand how to address the topic of risky behaviors
- Identify various types of risky behavior
- Describe the physical and mental benefits of living a healthy lifestyle
- Explain the importance of the concept of moderation in a healthy lifestyle

Key Terms

antioxidant effects Change free radicals from harmful substances, which can change DNA and increase a person's cancer risk, into nonharmful substances.

emphysema Chronic pulmonary condition with impaired gas exchange due to damaged alveoli.

endorphins Chemicals produced by the brain that help lessen pain perception.

lifestyle The typical way in which a person lives his life.

medical clearance Statement by doctor that no known condition exists that would prevent participation in an activity such as surgery or exercise.

nicotine Addictive ingredient in tobacco.

sedative Substance that quiets, soothes, or tranquilizes.

■ INTRODUCTION

Understanding the elements of a healthy lifestyle, and how to include them in one's own life, is knowledge that the medical assistant should not only be aware of but also practice and share with clients. Proper care and treatment of the body are essential to healthy living. One of the medical assistant's major responsibilities to clients is instructing them on how to live a healthy life by taking proper actions and avoiding risky behaviors. Understanding how to care for the body properly, both physically and mentally, should be part of the medical assistant's knowledge. Nutrition, eating the right foods in the right amounts, getting physical exercise, reducing harmful stress, and avoiding risky behaviors (such as smoking, excessive drinking, and abusing drugs) are the main focus of the medical assistant's instruction to clients on how to live a healthy lifestyle.

■ NUTRITION AND EXERCISE

Two of the most important issues to address, when meeting with or teaching a client, are nutrition and exercise. Healthy **lifestyle** choices are essential to a person's mental and physical well-being. It is crucial that people know which habits promote a healthy lifestyle and which do not. Just as essential as knowledge of the organ system and the functions of the body is knowledge of proper treatment of the self to keep the body healthy. The role of the medical assistant includes instructing clients on how to practice or incorporate healthy choices into everyday life.

A first point is that being "healthy" does not mean eating distasteful foods and spending countless hours in the gym every day. Many people have the misconception that the only way to be healthy is to restrict themselves to an extremely low-calorie or low-carbohydrate diet and overdo physical exercise, possibly to the point of burnout, exhaustion, or injury. However, these are neither the best options nor the healthiest. Once the person goes off the diet or

stops exercising, he is at high risk of gaining back any weight lost, and usually ends up adding even more extra pounds.

Rather than extreme dieting or physical exercise, changing one's lifestyle provides more successful results for long-lasting general health. It is imperative to eat properly. This does not mean starving yourself or eliminating sweets completely from your diet. Sweets should be eaten in moderation. Eating a variety of foods, including a plentiful amount of fruits and vegetables, has beneficial **antioxidant effects.** The medical assistant should know the proper amounts and suggested servings from the five major food groups (Figure 37-1).

As for the physical aspect, one can make minor changes in everyday routines that make a major difference. Even small increases in activity during everyday activities (separate from a specific exercise routine) have been shown to have positive effects on health. For instance, rather than taking the elevator at work, take the stairs. Park the car farther away and walk the extra feet to a store or office, or leave the car at home and walk to a nearby intended destination. These small changes in habits can help incorporate exercise into a daily routine. Gardening, weeding, lawn mowing, and car washing are additional ways to burn extra calories, improve blood flow, and also save money that would otherwise have been spent paying someone else to do these tasks! Also, adding a brisk walk three or four times a week for 30 to 40 minutes can significantly improve one's overall health.

As more and more conveniences become available, allowing less physical exertion to accomplish everyday activities, people must either adjust their caloric intake or find other ways to burn calories. As sedentary lifestyles increase, so does the rate of obesity.

If the client wishes to start exercising, it is important for the medical assistant to assist the client in creating an exercise program specific to and appropriate for that client. Before any exercise program is begun, the doctor should give **medical clearance** to the client. For example, if the client has high blood pressure or needs to

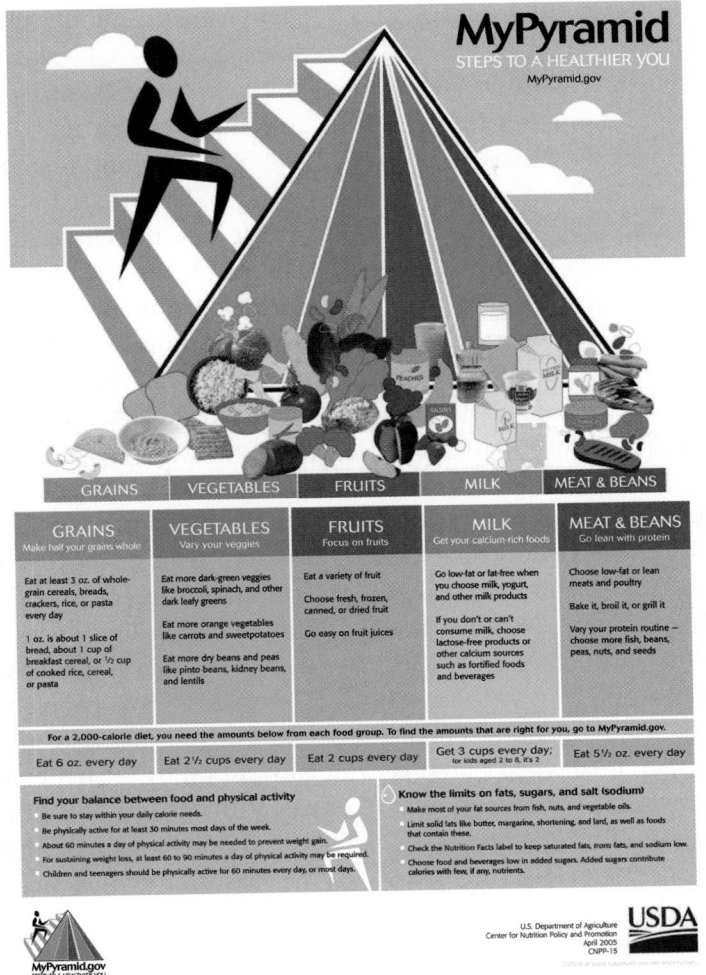

FIGURE 37-1 The Food Pyramid (Courtesy of the U.S. Department of Agriculture).

lose weight to prevent diabetes, the medical assistant must make the program client-specific. Older clients may not be able to sustain the same rigorous exercise as a younger client would. The medical assistant also needs to inform the client that it is important to ease into any exercise program and build up strength. Doing too much too soon is likely to lead to injury, exhaustion, and ultimately failure to achieve the intended goal. Adequate stretching and cooling down are key to any exercise program.

Included with proper nutrition and exercise is proper hydration (drinking at least eight glasses of water a day) and elimination of unhealthy habits such as excess drinking, cigarette smoking, and drug abuse. The medical assistant needs to make sure the client is aware of healthy habits and the benefits they bring to overall health.

■ SMOKING

One unhealthy habit that the medical assistant needs to discuss with the client is cigarette smoking, which is also a major public health issue. Long-term smoking can cause permanent, irreversible damage to the alveoli of the lungs and is the major cause of **emphysema** and lung cancers. Because cigarettes contain **nicotine**, users become addicted to them. Therefore, the best choice is never to start smoking—cigarettes or any other tobacco product. With smoking, prevention is the key to a healthy lifestyle. The medical assistant should be aware of the potential dangers to clients' health from smoking. The medical assistant has a responsibility to inform clients of these potential dangers. If a client is already a smoker, the medical assistant should inform the client about the various ways to quit smoking and offer assistance in finding programs that will aid the client.

If a client does wish to terminate this deadly habit of smoking, he has several routes to choose from. The first is to quit smoking "cold turkey," or, in other words, to completely stop smoking all at once without taking any nicotine into the body from any outside sources. This is usually the most difficult path, because the addicted body responds negatively when its supply of nicotine is cut off. Another way to make the process easier is to use a nicotine patch. With this method, a small, medicated patch is put on the skin, through which it releases timed, measured amounts of nicotine into the body. This is a step-by-step process that feeds the body small amounts of nicotine over time. This way the shock of withdrawal is less dramatic for the body, and it is easier for the person to quit smoking successfully. Nicotine gum works the same way, but delivers the medication in the form of chewing gum instead of a patch.

■ SECONDHAND SMOKE

Secondhand smoke is another major threat to clients' health. Secondhand cigarette smoke is even worse for the nonsmoker than for the smoker, as the smoker is inhaling through a filter on the cigarette. Persons inhaling smoke from another person's cigarette are exposed to unfiltered smoke. Secondhand smoke has been linked to an increase in bronchitis and pneumonia, as well as fluid buildup in the middle ear, especially in children who are exposed to secondhand smoke. Nonsmokers can develop lung cancer from exposure to secondhand smoke. It also harms the blood vessels and heart, even

increasing the chance of having a heart attack. Secondhand smoke in a house where there are young children increases the children's risk of respiratory problems.

In this situation, the client is being harmed by a problem created through another person's choice, not the client's own unhealthy choice. Therefore, the medical assistant needs to deal with this issue in a different way. The medical assistant must first find out if the client is at risk of exposure to secondhand smoke. Perhaps the client lives with a relative or friend who smokes, or is constantly around a person who smokes. In this case, the client may feel that he cannot control other people's actions, but the medical assistant can encourage the client to limit the amount of time he spends with smokers, and to stay away from places that allow smoking where the air is clouded with smoke. If the client does know people who smoke, he should inform those people of the dangers and various ways to quit that he learned from the medical assistant.

The danger of secondhand smoke is one of the reasons that many restaurants have specific sections set aside for smoking, and state and federal governments have passed laws restricting smoking in public places. Some states have banned smoking entirely in bars, restaurants, and public workplaces.

■ ALCOHOL

Alcohol is a **sedative** drug. If too much alcohol is ingested in a short period of time, the person may become intoxicated. Alcohol temporarily impairs the drinker's senses and judgment; while drunk, a person may lose his normal inhibitions and act foolishly and recklessly. Becoming intoxicated can have deadly consequences. People who operate motor vehicles while in this state put not only themselves but also others at risk: Many deadly car crashes have resulted from drunk driving. This is why state laws prohibit driving by anyone who has more than a certain alcohol level in the bloodstream. The police use several methods to test people who are suspected of driving while under the influence of alcohol. Two common methods are the breathalyzer test, which uses an instrument to measure the amount of alcohol in the breath, and the straight-line walking test, which shows whether the person's sense of balance is impaired.

The medical assistant needs to address the topic of alcohol use with the client. First, the medical assistant should check for any signs of alcoholism, a condition that includes dependency on having one or more drinks every day and a tendency to use alcohol as a means to solve all problems. Usually, specific signs of alcoholism are detected by asking a series of questions designed to reveal whether a person has a problem with alcohol. For example, the medical assistant could ask the following:

- How do you feel about your drinking?
- How do others feel about your drinking?
- Does anyone ever complain or make you feel guilty about your drinking?
- Do you ever drink first thing in the morning?
- How often do you feel that you "need a drink?"

Alcohol Abuse

Alcoholism (alcohol abuse) is a problem that affects both the person who drinks and the other people in his life. Many families are torn apart by a parent's abuse of alcohol. It can cause a person to be violent toward a spouse and even children. Sometimes the parent loses a job because of a problem with alcohol, a situation that creates even more tension in the family. People usually lose the respect of friends, family, and society when their alcohol abuse becomes obvious and undeniable.

There are many causes of alcoholism. Alcoholism is associated with heredity and family history: if a parent had a problem with alcohol, that person's children have a higher risk of abusing alcohol themselves. People also abuse alcohol when they feel a loss of control in their lives.

Many alcoholics have lost their jobs or loved ones, and self-medicate to dull their emotional pain. Alcohol may also be used as a stress reliever, if a person is under pressure for a long time. Some who become alcoholics start drinking when they are young, simply because their friends are drinking, and then become addicted to alcohol.

Although alcohol can be dangerous when not used responsibly, many people are able to enjoy alcohol while still maintaining control and not becoming addicted to it. Many people enjoy beer, wine, and spirits with meals, during social occasions or the holidays, or on special occasions. Alcohol is a part of many cultures' traditions. Some studies even indicate that having one glass of wine a day can actually improve one's health. The medical assistant needs to stress to the client that the key to drinking alcohol is *moderation*. Excessive drinking, either in frequency or amount, should be avoided.

If the medical assistant does suspect that a client has a problem with alcohol, he should discuss it with the client and inform the client about programs that can help treat the problem. The medical assistant must first inform the doctor about any observations that suggest an alcohol problem. The doctor will determine if the client really does have a problem, and then define a course of treatment and action. There is no cure for alcoholism, so it is something the client will have to struggle with for the rest of his life. However, the medical assistant can make recommendations on where to go for help. The Alcoholics Anonymous program has been very helpful for many people, and is a good starting place when clients are seeking help with their alcohol problems.

Also, the medical assistant can give other helpful suggestions. For example, if a person is trying to stop drinking, it is better for him to stay away from places and events where alcohol is served, to avoid temptation. The client could also seek help from family members, who can offer support and encouragement through words and by removing any alcoholic substances from the client's reach. (Remember confidentiality and privacy; you must obtain permission from the client before you speak with family members about the client's health matters, including alcoholism.)

DRUGS

It is the medical assistant's responsibility to address the topic of drug abuse with clients. Drug abuse can cause permanent damage to the body and mind, and frequently is fatal. There are two forms of drug abuse: use of illegal drugs and abuse of prescription medications. People begin abusing drugs for a variety of reasons and may start at any age.

Teenagers may use illegal drugs because of peer pressure. Early experimentation with illicit drugs often leads to a downward spiral. For example, many teenagers try marijuana while under the misconception that it is harmless. Marijuana causes the user to experience a euphoric "high," but it also impairs sensation and judgment, just like alcohol. It is unsafe to operate a vehicle while under the influence of marijuana, because the sensory and judgmental impairments can lead to deadly accidents. Marijuana injures the brain, and the smoke is more physically harmful than cigarette smoke. As with alcohol, users build a tolerance to marijuana, so that they need more to reach the same high they initially got from the drug. Therefore, it is called a *gateway* drug: many people who start off using only marijuana become dissatisfied and begin using other, stronger, more dangerous drugs, such as crack cocaine and heroin, in search of a better high.

However, crack cocaine and heroin are extremely dangerous, and in some cases first use of the drug is fatal. In addition to the horrendous havoc these substances cause in the body and mind, many people overdose (take more than the body can handle at one time) and die. If they are lucky enough to make it to a hospital in time and survive, most likely they will have brain damage and loss of bodily functions. Unfortunately, few people who overdose on drugs are taken to the hospital. Either they are alone when they take the drugs or the people with them are also incapable of getting help.

The deadly side effects of illegal drugs should aid in motivating the medical assistant to talk about drug abuse with the client. The medical assistant has a responsibility to clients to make sure they are doing all they can to live a healthy lifestyle. The medical assistant needs to find out if the client is taking any illegal drugs or has a problem with prescription pills. Sometimes people become addicted to prescription pills after taking them for a legitimate purpose: to deal with pain from an injury or some other medical condition. Addiction must be addressed immediately. If the medical assistant believes that a client is addicted to illegal or prescription drugs, he must speak with the physician and share the information. The client's health and life are the first concern. Other health care providers could unknowingly become involved in the client's abuse of prescription drugs.

Drug abuse is not only unhealthy, but also illegal. A person with a drug habit is risking both his life and his freedom. Users could be charged with possession of or trafficking in illegal drugs. Furthermore, illegal drugs are expensive. Many people who sustain a drug habit for a long period of time have financial trouble. If a person's current job does not bring in enough to support the drug habit, the person often turns to illegal means to obtain more money.

It is crucial that the addicted client receive help to stop taking drugs, so the medical assistant should facilitate the provision of this help. However, the medical assistant may run into some problems while addressing this topic. Even when the medical assistant is positive that a client has been or is currently abusing drugs, the client may still deny it. In this situation, the medical assistant must not abandon the effort to get help for this client. Rather, he needs to talk with the client and demonstrate, clearly and in great depth, the effects of drug abuse on the mind, body, personal relationships, and mortality. It is important for the medical assistant to enlist the help of the physician, who will decide upon and direct a treatment plan.

■ MENTAL HEALTH

The other aspect of healthy living is the maintenance of good mental health, which can directly affect physical health. The world is changing rapidly. Technology is advancing at an ever-increasing pace. Nevertheless, the improvements in industry and inventions that claim to make life easier can actually add more unhealthy stress to everyday life. Too much stress can cause unhealthy side effects. In a society that constantly demands more, people can break down under the pressure.

Women, for example, currently face more stress than ever before. Many women experience both the pressure of running a household and caring for a family, and also the stress of pursuing a career and balancing both . Men are being asked to take on nontraditional roles within the family. This stress often affects not only the mental state but also the physical state. Too much stress and lack of adequate rest can wreak havoc on the body. Finding time to complete all the tasks people are taking on is becoming more of a challenge. If medical assistants are to ensure the well-being of their clients, they have to emphasize the importance of exercise and rest as ways to reduce the amount of harmful stress in clients' lives. The body strives to maintain homeostasis (balance), mentally as well as physically.

Exercise and Stress

As stated earlier, exercise is vital to a healthy lifestyle. It keeps the body in shape and assists body functions to work properly. However, the benefits of exercise are not purely physical: it has mental benefits as well. While working out or exercising, the body relieves built-up stress and tension. Exercise has a tremendous ability to clear the mind and elevate a person's mood. Exercise such as running can help the body release helpful **endorphins.** Exercise should be one of the first things the medical assistant suggests to clients as a means of reducing stress.

The Medical Assistant's Role in Client Mental Health

The medical assistant should find out what is causing particular stress for the client. There might be only one major stressor, or a client may be subject to a buildup of smaller stresses that combine to make everyday life nearly intolerable. The medical assistant usually finds the answer to this question by taking time to talk with the client and discover what is causing him concern. Maybe the client is unable to pinpoint the stress himself. In that case, talking with the medical assistant may help clients sort through their thoughts and find a clearer path to healthy choices.

The medical assistant can approach the topic by asking the following questions:

- Do you have to cook meals, clean the house, and wash dishes on your own, without help?
- Do you feel that there is never enough time to get done everything you need to do in a day?
- Do you cancel or skip recreational activities, such as going out with friends, because you have too much work?

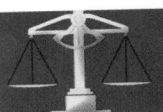

LEGAL/ETHICAL THOUGHTS

To be able to make informed decisions regarding healthy lifestyle choices, clients need to be provided with up-to-date, current, and accurate health information. This ethical duty of the medical assistant can also become a legal issue if the client is not informed about healthy behaviors and develops certain preventable conditions.

- Do you feel that there is no one you can call on to help run an errand, or watch the children, when you have a schedule conflict?
- Do you take work home at night?
- Do you spend evenings thinking about what happened at work or what will happen tomorrow?
- Do you feel obligated to always say yes when you are asked to help out?
- Do you have trouble falling asleep at night?

If the client answers yes to any of these questions, ask the client to describe the situation. The medical assistant must share this information with the doctor, who can explore these concerns in more detail with the client. The doctor can determine any treatment options. The inability to deal with stress can have a negative effect on the client's health. Unrelieved stress can cause physical damage to the body as well as be a most uncomfortable emotional state. It can interfere with the prognosis or outcome of other medical problems that are being treated.

Rest and Stress

The medical assistant should also explain to the client the importance of rest. Although society may view taking a break or vacation from everyday hassles as weak or selfish, the body still requires an adequate amount of rest. Sleep is the body's opportunity to restore vitality and repair damage. It is a way for the body to be refreshed. Without this time of rest, the body's functions will begin to slow down and eventually stop working. Everyday tasks will require more effort to complete, and thus cause even more stress and work for the person. The medical assistant should also inquire about the client's sleep habits. For example, the medical assistant should find out if the client has any trouble falling asleep or staying asleep through most of the night. Many sleep disturbances or problems, including one form of insomnia, are caused by stress.

An easy way to determine sleep hygiene is simply to ask the client to describe his routine when preparing to go sleep. The client might not understand, or state that he does not have a routine. Some specific questions may help elicit that information:

- Do you drink pop, coffee, or alcohol in the evening?
- Do you have a bedtime snack?
- Do you take a shower or warm bath in the evening?
- In the evening, do you work on projects that you brought home in your bedroom?
- On the average, how many hours do you sleep each night?
- Do you get up during the night?

The medical assistant should share this information with the physician, who can then relate these responses to other aspects of the client's mental and physical health.

Identifying Stressors

Besides exercise and rest, the medical assistant should help the client identify the stressful elements in his life. Stress is a major threat to a client's health and well-being. It is more difficult to detect than smoking or alcohol abuse, because it builds up slowly, but it is equally important for the medical assistant to address. Mental well-being is just as critical to living a healthy lifestyle as physical health.

This identification can also be done by talking with the client. For example, maybe the client is stressed from balancing a career and running a household. Once stressors are identified, the medical assistant may be able to assist the client to decide on steps to reduce the stress. For example, perhaps the client could have a family discussion and ask the spouse and other family members to share in the household responsibilities and duties.

 BRIDGE TO CAAHEP

This chapter, which discusses healthy lifestyle in the primary client population, provides information and content related to CAAHEP standards

POINTS OF HIGHLIGHT

- Healthy lifestyle choices are important to a client's physical and mental well-being.
- The medical assistant's role includes working with clients to guide them in making healthy choices.
- Nutrition and exercise are important parts of healthy living.
- Smoking is a major risk factor for many disorders.
- Alcoholism and drug abuse affect not only the individual but also entire families.
- Stress and the client's reactions to it are major factors in both physical and mental health.
- Sleep and rest are essential for a person to function effectively.

for Anatomy and Physiology, Medical Terminology, Communication, Medical Assisting Clinical Procedures, and Patient (Client) Care.

 ## ABHES LINKS

This chapter, which discusses healthy lifestyle in the primary client population, links to ABHES course content for Anatomy and Physiology, Medical Terminology, Medical Law and Ethics, Psychology, Medical Office Clinical Procedures, Communication, and Professional Components.

 ## AAMA AREAS OF COMPETENCE

This chapter, which discusses healthy lifestyle in the primary client population, provides information or content within several areas listed in the Medical Assistant Role Delineation Study. These areas include: clinical professionalism, patient (client) care, general transdisciplinary, fundamentals principles, diagnostic orders, communication, legal concepts, and instruction.

 ## AMT PATHS

This chapter, which discusses healthy lifestyle in the primary client population, provides a path to AMT competency in general medical assisting knowledge, anatomy and physiology, medical terminology, medical law, medical ethics, human relations, and patient (client) education.

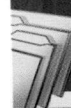 ## STUDENT PORTFOLIO ACTIVITY

Gather information on and make a list of reputable local health-related facilities and resources, such as workout centers, exercise activities, nutritional centers, counseling agencies, and so on. Review the list so that you are familiar with each place and know which places are best for which needs of people. (For example, some gyms are designed for older people; others are more child-centered.) Being able to offer clients this information makes the first step on the path of living a healthy lifestyle easier. What qualities does this project show that the medical assistant possesses?

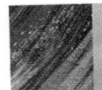 ## APPLYING YOUR SKILLS

A smoker who has not quit smoking has heard about the harmful effects of secondhand smoke. What suggestions can you make so that this smoker can protect his family from the effects of secondhand smoke?

CRITICAL THINKING QUESTIONS

1. How could the medical assistant help a client who expresses an interest in quitting smoking or cutting down the number of cigarettes smoked each day?

2. In addition to denial, what other problems might the medical assistant face while addressing the topic of drug abuse with a client?

3. How might the medical assistant encourage healthy lifestyle habits, such as proper nutrition and exercise, to a client who is limited by food allergies or limited physically by the need to use a wheelchair?

4. What are some causes of stress that are present today but were not 15 years ago? What are some stressors that were present 15 years ago but are not today?

5. What advice might the medical assistant offer to encourage or assist the client who wants help for an alcohol problem?

6. Think about an issue that might become a public health concern in the next few years. How will it affect you as a medical assistant? As a health care professional, how can you get involved to help?

7. What do you say to the client who excitedly talks about a new diet that will help him lose a great deal of weight within two weeks? What is the chance of long-term weight loss with this plan?

8. What can a client do to become more active when a membership in a gym or a participation in an organized class is not possible?

9. You understand that a client is at risk of respiratory disorders due to secondhand smoke. What steps could you share with the client to decrease his risk?

10. Why is rest so important? How can lack of sleep hurt a client?

11. Go back to the beginning of this chapter and review the Anticipatory Statements. Reread each statement and then indicate whether it is true or false. If the statement is false, rewrite it to make it a true statement.

CLIENT TEACHING PLAN

Get In Shape and Attain a Healthy Weight

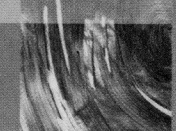

What Is to Be Taught:

- How to get in shape and attain a healthy weight through recommended nutrition and exercise.

Objectives:

- Client will learn and perform steps necessary to achieve a realistic weight and stay in shape so as to maintain good health and reduce health risks.

Preparation Before Teaching:

- Review the steps necessary for the client to achieve and maintain a healthy weight. These include healthy eating habits, beneficial exercise, and elimination of risky behaviors such as smoking and excess drinking.
- Gather any diagrams, charts, or other materials that would be useful in helping to explain the importance of balanced nutrition and exercise.

Steps for the Medical Assistant:

1. Wash your hands.
2. Gather supplies needed.
3. Introduce yourself to the client.
4. Explain what you are going to teach and why. Explain that the client will be taught how to

successfully achieve better health by making a few lifestyle changes.

5. Explain to the client that both nutrition and exercise are key to staying healthy.
6. Discuss with the client various ways to incorporate healthy eating habits into his diet. This includes drinking an adequate amount of water (at least eight glasses of water a day). Help the client figure out which foods are best to avoid and which are best to eat. For example, fruits and vegetables are important parts of a healthful diet. Especially if the client has high blood pressure, advise him to stay away from sodium-filled foods such as canned soup and crackers.
7. Inform the client that portion sizes make a difference as well.
8. Tell the client to keep a food journal (see Table 37-1) and record what he eats and how much he eats every day. Sometimes people do not realize how much they actually eat until they write it down on paper.
9. Explain to the client that exercise is critical to health. It not only helps to take weight off, but also keeps the heart, mind, and other parts of the body working well.
10. Inform the client that eliminating health hazards is important too, as well as a healthy

TABLE 37–1 Sample food journal.

1/25/20xx	FOOD & SERVINGS
Breakfast	One 8 oz. glass of orange juice. One piece of toast lightly buttered. One cup of cereal and half a cup of skim milk. One banana.
Lunch	One 8 oz. glass of skim milk. Turkey sandwich with one piece of cheese, lettuce, and a slice of tomato. Side salad with light Italian dressing.
Dinner	16 oz. of ice water. Chicken. One serving of potatoes. One serving of green beans. Salad greens selection with croutons.
Evening snack	Two cups of light air-popped popcorn.

(Continues)

CLIENT TEACHING PLAN (Continued)

diet and exercise. Smoking, excess drinking, not wearing a seat belt, and not using sunscreen to protect the skin against harmful rays are all health hazards that should and can be eliminated.

11. Ask the client if he has any questions or comments about what you have discussed.

Special Needs of the Client:

- Look at the client's chart to see if there are any factors that could interfere with the client's ability to take steps toward healthy nutrition or exercise. For example, if the client has a mobility impairment, the medical assistant may need to discuss alternative ways to get exercise.

Evaluation:

- Client will take the recommended steps to stay healthy.
- Client's weight, blood pressure, and cholesterol levels will all improve.
- Client will record in food journal what he eats every day, so that he can keep track and make sure he gets all the recommended nutrition.

Further Plans/Teaching:

- Show the client how to use a blank, spiral-bound notebook as a food diary. At the next visit, have

the client bring his food diary with him. Entries since the last visit should have been recorded in the diary.
- Offer the client encouragement and let him know that he can call the medical assistant at the office if he has any questions or concerns.

Follow-up:

- At the client's next visit, check the client's weight, blood pressure, and cholesterol levels. Ask the client how he feels, not just physically but mentally as well.
- Check the client's food journal and make comments or suggestions for improvement if necessary.
- Offer encouragement.

Medical Assistant

Name: _____

Signature: _____

Date: _____

Client

Date: _____

Follow-up Date : _____

CHAPTER 38

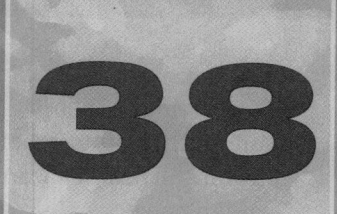

Anticipatory Statements

Read and think about the following statements based upon what you believe now. Decide whether you agree or disagree. Write the word **agree** after the statement if you think the statement is true. Write the word **disagree** after the statement if you think the statement is false. Read the chapter to find out if your current beliefs can be supported.

1. Medical assistants can assist the doctor in minor office surgery.   _____

2. As long as clean technique is used; minor office surgery need not be done using sterile technique.   _____

3. The medical assistant can change a client's dressing.   _____

4. Some common procedures use disposable sterile setups.   _____

5. A medical assistant should be able to name and describe frequently used surgical instruments.   _____

Minor Surgery

Learning Objectives

Upon completion of this chapter, the medical assistant student should be able to:

- Identify the medical assistant's role in preparing clients for minor office surgery
- Explain the difference between medical asepsis and surgical asepsis
- List five precautions that a medical assistant can take to maintain surgical asepsis during a sterile procedure
- Describe the purpose of thumb forceps, hemostatic forceps, tissue forceps, dressing forceps, and sponge forceps
- State five guidelines for caring for surgical instruments
- Explain the purpose of each step in putting on and taking off sterile gloves

Key Terms

abscess Specific area or localized site that contains pus made up of dead bacteria, blood, and tissue.

autoclave Machine used to sterilize instruments and medical items.

biopsy Removal of a small piece of tissue to use for diagnostic testing.

contamination Process of becoming dirty or infected with microorganisms.

curette Scraping instrument with a ring or loop on one end.

cyst A closed, defined area, like a pouch or sac, that contains liquid, dead cells, and/or waxy material.

forceps Instruments used to hold or grab tissue or blood vessels.

incision A clean, neat cut, such as that made by a scalpel.

medical asepsis Techniques used to decrease the number and transmission of pathogenic organisms.

ratchets Notches on an instrument that hold the instruments closed or open at a specific degree.

scalpel Surgical knife used to make incisions.

sebaceous Refers to sebum, an oily, waxy substance, secreted by certain glands.

speculum An instrument used to open or enlarge an area for easier viewing.

surgical asepsis Sterile techniques.

suture Thread used to sew or bring together tissue in surgical procedures.

■ INTRODUCTION

With the changing health care environment, many procedures that were once performed only in hospitals are now routinely being performed in medical offices. Which procedures will be performed in a medical office is determined by the type of medical practice, the regulating body, and state and federal laws. As a rule, surgical procedures performed in the office do not involve general anesthesia, where the client is completely unconscious. Office surgeries normally do not enter into the major body cavities.

The health of the client is also a factor in determining where procedures are performed. If a client has certain health problems, such as respiratory or cardiac disorders, a surgical procedure that is usually done in the office may be done in a hospital or same-day surgical unit, where additional personnel and equipment are available in case of problems.

■ ROLE OF THE MEDICAL ASSISTANT IN MINOR SURGERY

The medical assistant will prepare the client for the procedure. The medical assistant's clinical tasks include setting up the room and establishing a sterile field with the instruments needed for the procedure. Assistance with the actual clinical procedure is done according to the scope of practice and the doctor's office policy. After the procedure, the medical assistant will complete client care by giving discharge and postproce-

dure instructions. After the client has left, the medical assistant will clean the environment and dispose of waste in biohazardous waste containers (Figure 38-1). If the instruments are for one-time use only, they will be disposed of in sharps containers according to regulations. Otherwise, the instruments will be sanitized and sterilized. The room will be cleaned and disinfected.

■ COMMON PROCEDURES

The medical assistant can expect certain surgeries to be done in a medical office setting. **Biopsies** are routinely performed in the office. In a biopsy, a small piece of tissue is removed and sent as a sample to a lab to be examined for signs of disease or pathology.

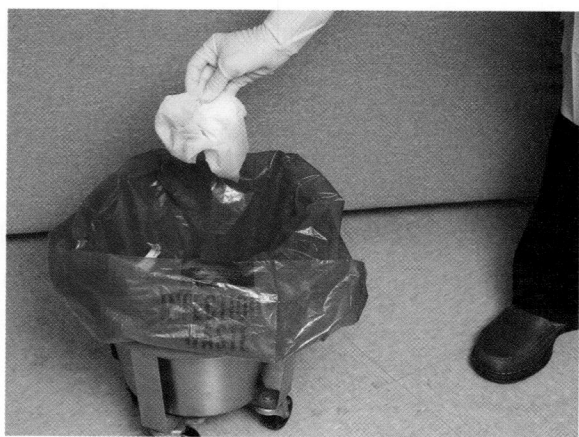

FIGURE 38–1 After a procedure, the medical assistant will clean and sterilize the room, removing waste into a biohazardous waste container.

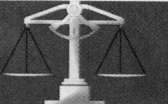

LEGAL/ETHICAL THOUGHTS

Before any procedure is done, the client needs to understand what it involves, and know the benefits and risks of the proposed procedure, as well as alternatives. These must be explained so that the client can give informed consent for a procedure or surgery. A student should never sign as a witness on an informed consent form.

Sebaceous cysts are often removed. This involves making an **incision** (cut) with a **scalpel** and then removing the cyst. Stitches are often needed to close the incision. Similarly, an incision and drainage procedure may be done to relieve a localized infection. An **abscess** may have to be drained to allow an area to heal. The doctor will make an incision, drain the contents of the abscess, and then cover the incision with a sterile dressing. As part of discharge instructions, the medical assistant will teach the client how to care for the dressing and surgery site.

Often a client who has had surgery in a hospital setting will come to the office thereafter, within a week or so after the operation, for removal of **sutures** (stitches). If this occurs frequently in a particular office practice, disposable suture-removal kits are kept in the office. If this is so, the medical assistant will not have to clean, sterilize, and package the suture-removal setup.

■ SURGICAL HANDWASHING

Good handwashing is the single most important activity to prevent the spread of harmful microorganisms. In most settings, the handwashing technique is called *medical handwashing* or *clean technique.* For surgical procedures, more intensive handwashing is required, called *surgical handwashing* or *surgical technique.* Medical handwashing is done to promote **medical asepsis.** Surgical handwashing is done to promote **surgical asepsis.** The medical assistant practices medical asepsis at all times, to maintain a clean environment that is free from **contamination.** Medical asepsis includes practices done after a procedure to prevent the spread of bacteria and other pathogens. In addition to handwashing, surfaces are dusted and cleaned and rooms are kept well ventilated. These practices, in combination, are used to maintain a safe, healthy environment.

Surgical handwashing is done before procedures are begun, to prevent harmful microorganisms from entering the client's body.

Surgical technique is used when a wound or open area of the body is being treated. Sterile technique is also used when piercing the skin with an injection needle. When a sterile body cavity, such as the urinary bladder, is catheterized, the procedure must be done with strict sterile technique.

Surgical handwashing is done for 5 to 6 minutes, compared to the 2 minutes needed for medical handwashing (Figures 38-2A–D). In addition to hands and wrists, the medical assistant must wash up to the elbows. During sterile-technique rinsing, the hands are held up. This is the opposite of medical handwashing, where the fingertips must point down. A nail brush and cuticle stick are used to clean the nails. Lotion should not be applied after surgical handwashing. The ingredients in many lotions react with the latex in gloves and allow microorganisms to penetrate the gloves. The medical assistant should use only approved lotions.

Guidelines for practicing surgical asepsis include:

- Wash hands before putting on sterile gloves.
- Once the hands are gloved, keep your hands elevated. Never let your hands hang down at your sides. Anything below your waist is considered contaminated.
- Never touch a nonsterile item with a sterile-gloved hand.
- When a sterile tray is set up, a one-inch imaginary border around the sterile field is considered contaminated (Figure 38-3). The *sterile field* is the area where the sterile items are set out. Never let nonsterile objects touch, get into, or pass over the area (Figure 38-4). The part of the drape that hangs over the edge of the tray is considered contaminated.
- Never reach over the sterile field.
- Never pass nonsterile items over the sterile field (Figure 38-5).
- Never turn your back on the sterile field.
- If an item becomes wet, it is considered nonsterile. If any of a poured solution splashes onto the sterile field, the entire

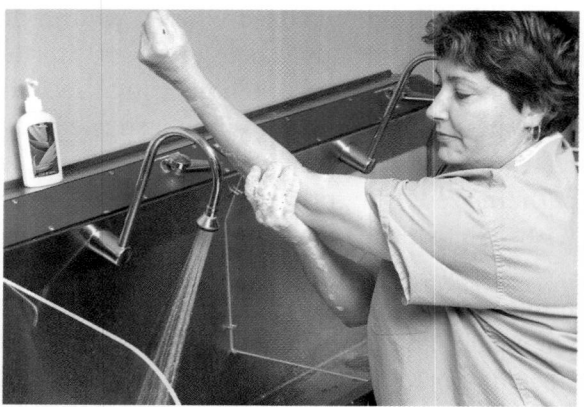

FIGURE 38-2A In surgical asepsis, the medical assistant must wash up to the elbows. Work soap into a lather, rubbing the palms, backs of hands, and between fingers, and being sure to keep hands above waist level.

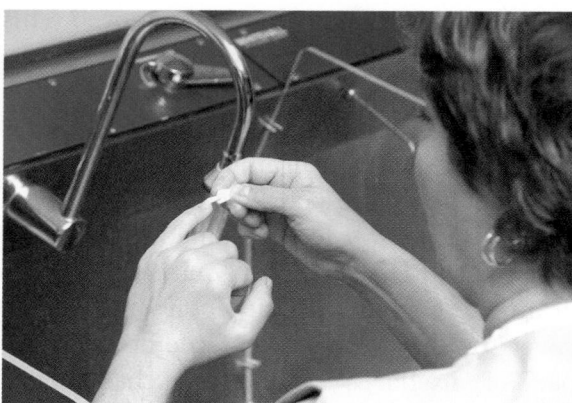

FIGURE 38-2B Use a stick to clean underneath the fingernails.

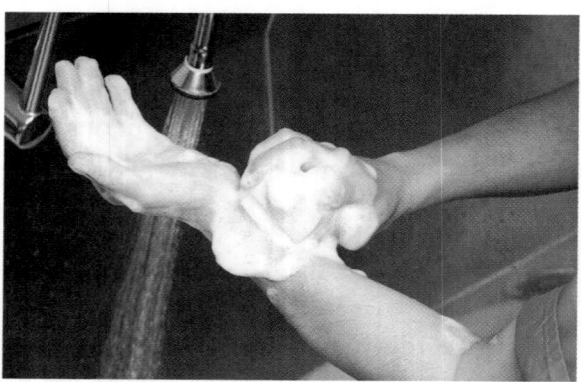

FIGURE 38-2C Scrub the palms, backs of hands, fingernails, wrists, and forearms.

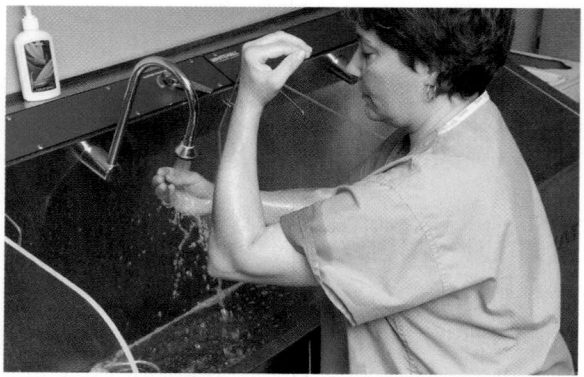

FIGURE 38-2D Rinse off the soap, keeping hands above waist level and higher than the elbows.

field is considered contaminated. Wet areas attract microorganisms and allow them to penetrate barriers.

- When pouring a solution, make sure the rim of the bottle does not touch the container that the solution is being poured into.

- The outside of a sterile dressing package is not sterile. Only the contents of the package are sterile.

- The contents of a sterile package are dropped onto the sterile field after the package is opened. Carefully drop the item or items onto the sterile field. An item

should not be tossed on top of another item that is already on the tray.

- If you are not sure whether sterile technique was broken and an item was contaminated, always considered it contaminated and do not use it.

- The maintenance of a sterile field is the responsibility of the medical assistant. Always be alert, watching yourself and others, to maintain the sterility of the area. If anyone or anything seems to have broken sterile technique, it is up to the medical assistant to speak up. The safety of the client depends on it!

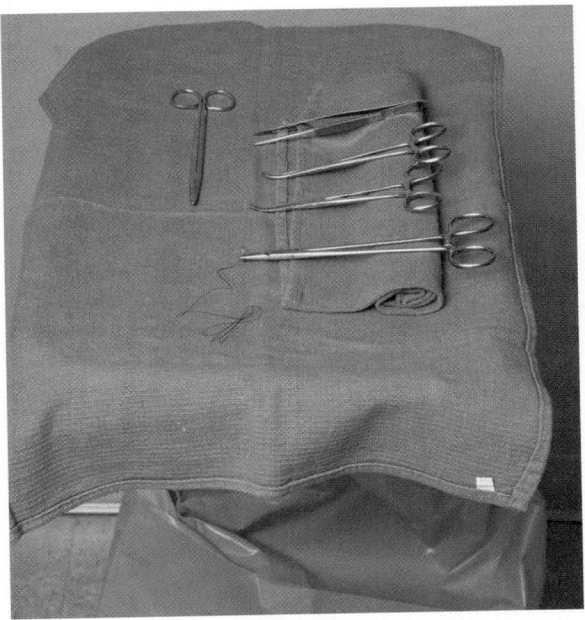

FIGURE 38-3 After a surgical tray is set up, nothing should be placed within one inch of the edge of the tray, as this area is considered contaminated.

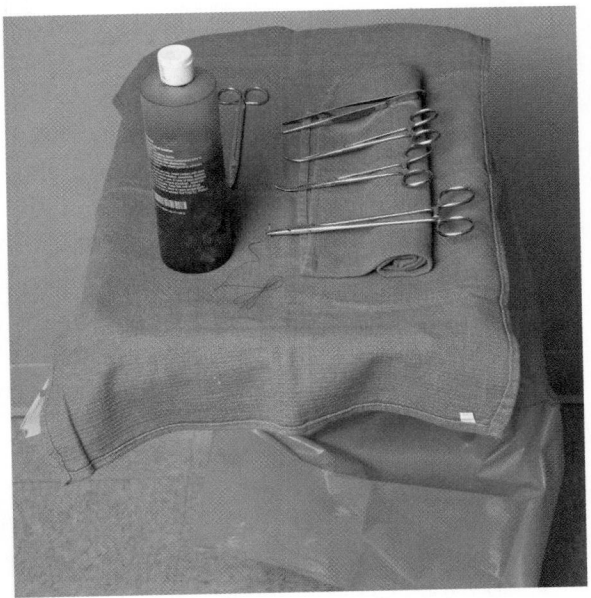

FIGURE 38-4 Do not place nonsterile objects on or into the sterile field.

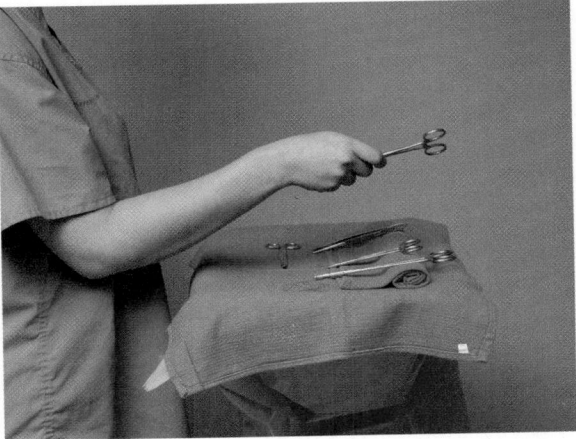

FIGURE 38-5 When a sterile field is set up, never reach over it or pass a nonsterile object over the field.

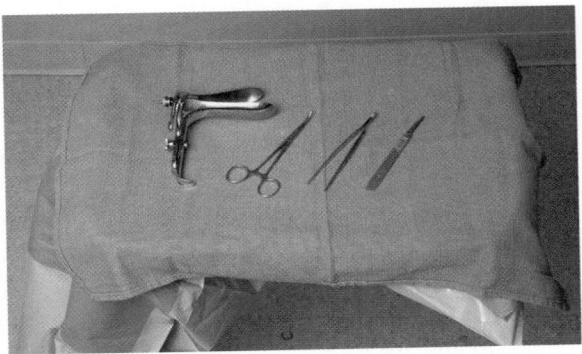

FIGURE 38-6 Surgical instruments commonly found in the medical office are speculums, scissors, forceps, and scalpels.

■ SURGICAL INSTRUMENTS

The instruments used for minor office surgery will vary according to the type of practice.

Depending on need, there may be less variety but more of the same types of instruments. For example, a surgeon removes sutures postoperatively in the office and so she will need suture removal instruments. A dermatologist will need instruments to perform skin biopsies and scrapings. It is up to the medical assistant to become familiar with the instruments needed in her place of employment.

There are major kinds of instruments that are used in many different medical specialties. Medical assistants should recognize these instruments by name, sight, and usage. Scalpels, forceps, scissors, and speculums are tools commonly found in the office (Figure 38-6).

Scalpels

Scalpels are small knives designed for use in surgery. One side is a sharp blade edge; the opposite side is convex (curves outward). The standard scalpel handle can be fitted with different blades. The blades are identified by numbers. Different-sized handles are often identified by number.

Curettes

Curettes may be used both in surgery and in office procedures. These instruments have a ring or loop end that is used to scrape tissue. Curettes are most often used in gynecological procedures such as dilation and curettage (D & C), in which the cervix is dilated and tissue scraped out. The doctor may also use a curette to aid in the removal of cerumen (earwax).

Forceps

Forceps are used to grasp. Within each grouping of forceps, there are many individual kinds designed for a specific use in a specific situation or for a specific purpose. The types of forceps are too numerous to list.

Forceps are named according to their use. For example, hemostat forceps are used to stop bleeding; that is, to keep a blood vessel clamped off. Tissue forceps hold tissue. Similarly, thumb forceps can pick up and hold tissue. Splinter forceps are sharp-pointed forceps used to remove splinters or foreign objects from tissue. Splinter forceps look like the tweezers that are used to remove hair. Sponge forceps are used to grab surgical sponges, so the ends are shaped like rings. Dressing forceps are used to pick up and apply or remove dressings. Transfer forceps, commonly found in the medical office, are used to transfer or carry something from one sterile container to another. Needle holders are used to hold a needle and keep it from slipping; these forceps look like wide hemostat forceps.

Clamps are similar to forceps. The most common is the towel clamp. It is attached to the sterile drapes, which are then attached to another drape.

Scissors

Scissors are used for cutting. Just as there are different types of scissors for the home (such as kitchen, meat, paper, and dressmaking scissors), there are various types of scissors for surgery. These are sharp instruments, but each type has a varying degree of sharpness. Operating scissors are used to cut through tissue. Suture scissors are specially designed for cutting sutures or stitches. Ordinary household scissors will not cut through suture material. Bandage scissors are one of the most versatile instruments. A medical assistant may even want to own a pair of bandage scissors. These are used to cut dressings or tape. The bandage scissors have a large, blunt edge that can slip between the dressing and the client's skin. The blunted tip prevents the user from nicking or cutting the client's skin under the bandage.

Speculums

A **speculum** opens or makes wider a body opening or cavity, to allow better visualization of the internal parts. A speculum opens to different sizes and can be locked into place. Speculums are named after the specific body area for which they were designed, such as the nasal speculum that allows better visualization of the inside of the nose. The medical assistant who works in a gynecologist's office will often work with vaginal speculums. Vaginal speculums are inserted into the vagina to hold the area open, allowing the doctor to examine the internal structure, take samples, or perform procedures. These instruments come in various sizes from small to large. They are used in almost all pelvic examinations.

■ PARTS OF INSTRUMENTS

When selecting an instrument for use in a procedure, in addition to remembering its name and recognizing its appearance, it is helpful to be able to identify key parts of the instrument. Correct terms are important in describing instrument parts (Figure 38-7). Handles are shaped for the user to operate the instrument

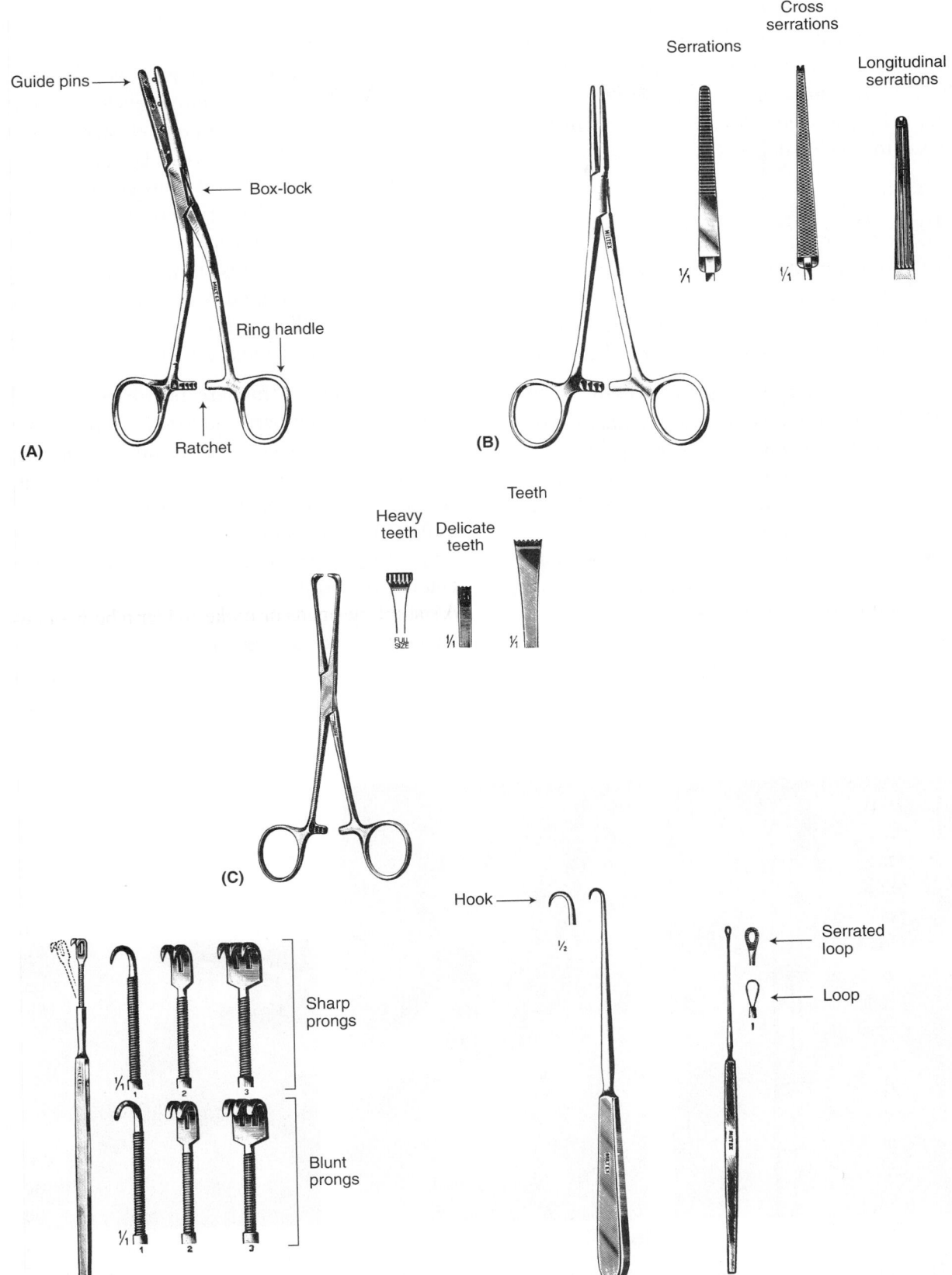

FIGURE 38-7 Structural features of instruments: (A) ratchets, ring handle, pins, and box-locks; (B) serrations; (C) teeth; (D) prongs, hooks, and loops. (Courtesy of Miltex, Inc.)

either by squeezing the handles with the thumb and finger, called *thumb handles;* or by putting fingers and thumb inside the ring, called *ring handles.* **Ratchets** are notches on the instrument. The ratchets allow the instrument to be closed to varying degrees of tightness.

■ CARE OF INSTRUMENTS

All instruments must be handled carefully. Always follow the manufacturer's directions for use and care of any instrument or equipment. These are some general guidelines for the medical assistant:

- Handle all instruments with care.
- Do not grab several instruments together. Some instruments have sharp edges and may cut your hands. Bunching them together may also nick, chip, or dull the working edges of the instruments.
- Sharp instruments should be kept separate, or the cutting edge may become dull and ruin the instrument.

- Keep open instruments that can close in a closed position at the first notch.
- Clean instruments as soon as possible to keep blood and contaminants from drying and becoming stuck on the instrument.
- Look at each instrument before cleaning to make sure that it is in good working condition and that there are no nicks, scratches, or dull areas.
- Never use an instrument for anything other than what it was designed for.
- Always follow procedure when cleaning and sterilizing instruments.

Instruments that are not disposable are sanitized and sterilized. *Sanitization* is the cleaning of instruments to remove any visible dirt, blood, or body secretions. The steps in sanitization include rinsing, sudsing with a detergent, and then rinsing off the detergent (Figure 38-8). Sometimes instruments are soaked in a solution before the sanitization process. The medical assistant needs to become familiar with office policy regarding sanitation for instruments.

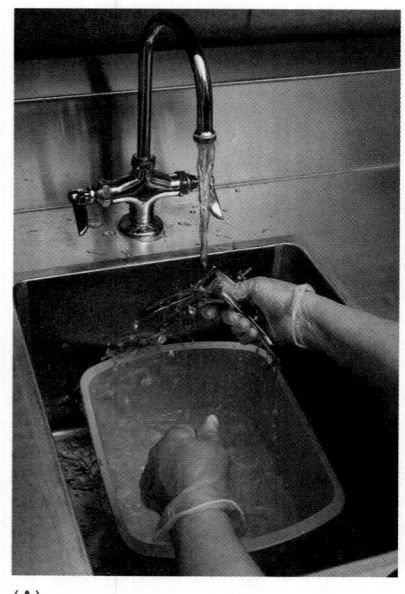
(A)

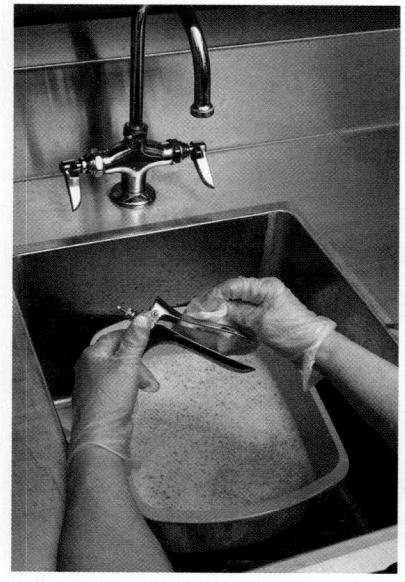
(B)

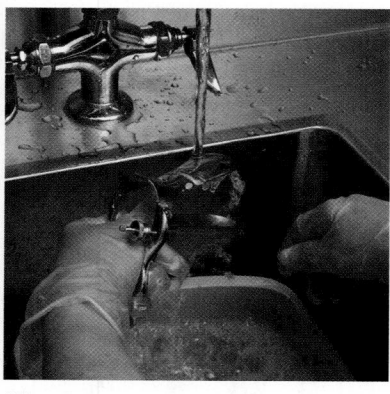
(C)

FIGURE 38-8 Sanitize an instrument by first (A) rinsing, then (B) sudsing it with a detergent, and finally (C) rinsing off the detergent.

Sterilization is the removal or killing of all microorganisms. An object is either sterile or it is not. In the medical office, instruments and objects are frequently sterilized in an **autoclave,** a machine that uses steam to destroy microorganisms (Figure 38-9). Manufacturer's directions must be followed when using the autoclave to ensure sterilization, but there are a few common principles to remember. The items to be sterilized must be sanitized first. Items cannot be placed in the autoclave with matter such as blood or tissue on them. Instruments must be packed and placed in the autoclave loosely, as the steam must be able to circulate around them freely. The sterilization process in the machine is timed, but the medical assistant must wait until the correct temperature is reached before starting the timer. Finally, the items must be completely dry before they are removed from the autoclave.

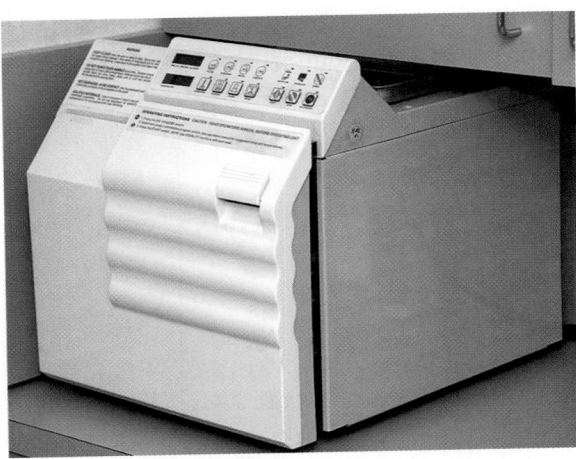

FIGURE 38-9 An autoclave in a medical office

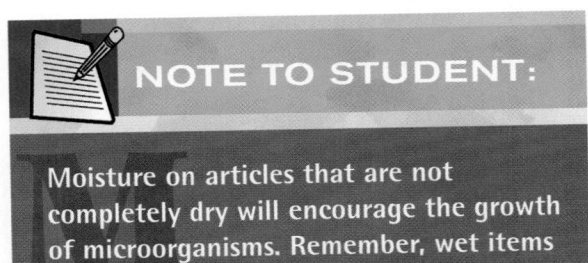

NOTE TO STUDENT:

Moisture on articles that are not completely dry will encourage the growth of microorganisms. Remember, wet items are always considered contaminated.

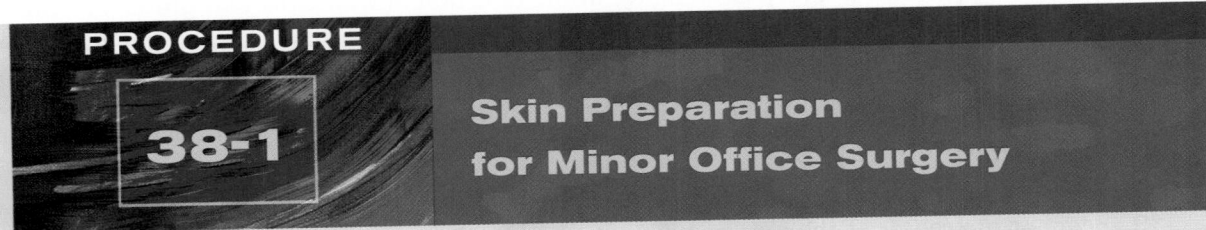

PROCEDURE

38-1

Skin Preparation for Minor Office Surgery

Student Competency Objective: The medical assistant student will prepare a client's skin for minor office surgery.

Items Needed: Soap, water, sterile water, antiseptic solution, 4 x 4 gauze pads, gloves, towels, drape, razor with safety blade, scissors, forceps, small container such as emesis basin, biohazardous waste container

Steps:

1. Wash your hands.
2. Assemble equipment and supplies.
3. Introduce yourself to the client even if you have seen the client on previous visits to your office. The client may have forgotten your name. This also helps to establish a provider–client relationship, because it shows the client that you want her to know who you are.

(Continues)

PROCEDURE 38-1 (Continued)

4. Identify the client. Ask the client to state her name to establish that this is the right client, and then compare the name given to the name on the chart. Never enter a room and call out a client's name to determine if this person is the correct client. The client may not have heard you clearly and may just nod, smile, or answer yes. Clients almost never question if the medical assistant professional has the right client. It is up to the medical assistant to identify the right client before performing any procedure.

5. Tell the client, in everyday language, what you are going to do.

6. Ask if the client has any questions. If she does, give short and simple answers. Sometimes clients will start (and continue) talking because they are nervous about the procedure.

7. Ask the client to remove clothing as necessary to expose the area to be prepped. Help as needed and maintain privacy.

8. Help the client into the correct position on the examination table.

9. Place drapes around the area.

10. Put on gloves.

11. Dip a gauze pad into a soapy solution.

12. Wipe the client's skin only once with each gauze pad and then dispose of the pad into the basin.

13. Look at the area to be shaved. If the hair is long, you will need to cut it before shaving the area.

14. Cut hair carefully so as not to cut or nick the skin.

15. Shave the area with a safety razor. Shave in the direction in which the hair grows. Pull on the skin below the area being shaved. This will help to keep the skin taut and smooth, to ensure a clean, even shave without nicks (Figure 38-10A).

16. Rinse soap and any remaining hair off with a sterile gauze pad and sterile water.

17. Dry the area with sterile gauze.

18. Using sterile forceps, dip gauze into an antiseptic solution (Figure 38-10B).

19. Begin at the center of the area being prepped.

20. Move the antiseptic-soaked gauze in a circle, working from the center of the area into bigger and bigger circles. Do not go back and forth or change direction (Figure 38-10C).

21. Place a sterile drape over the prepped area.

22. Tell the client not to touch the area.

23. Discard disposable items in a biohazardous waste bag container.

24. Place other items and instruments in an appropriate place to be sanitized and sterilized.

25. Remain in the room with the client. Talk with client to reassure, comfort, and distract her as appropriate.

26. Assist the doctor as needed.

(Continues)

PROCEDURE 38-1 (Continued)

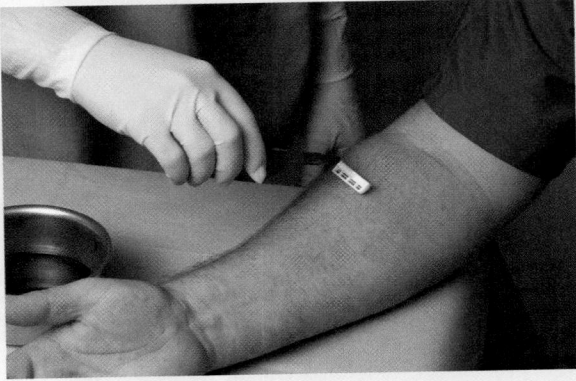

FIGURE 38-10A Shave the affected area with a safety razor and dry it with sterile gauze.

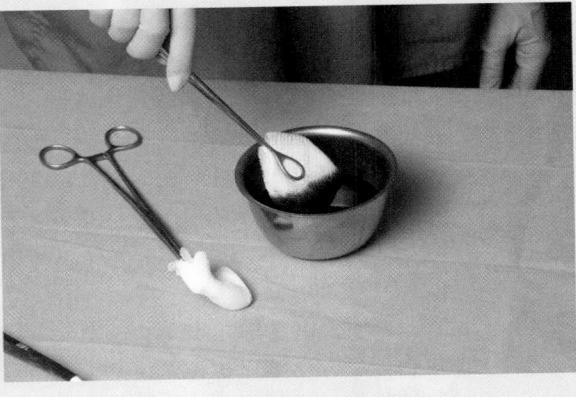

FIGURE 38-10B Dip gauze into the antiseptic solution using sterile forceps.

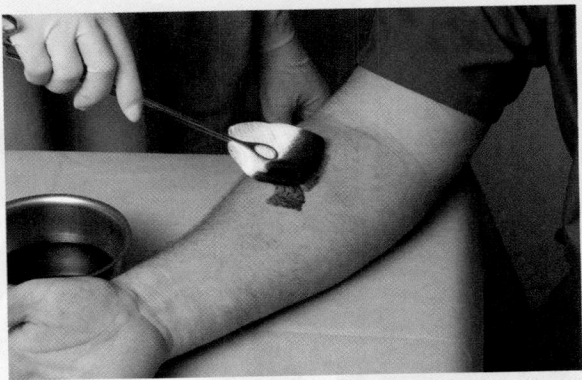

FIGURE 38-10C Start in the center of the affected area and move in a circular motion, gradually making a bigger circle circumference.

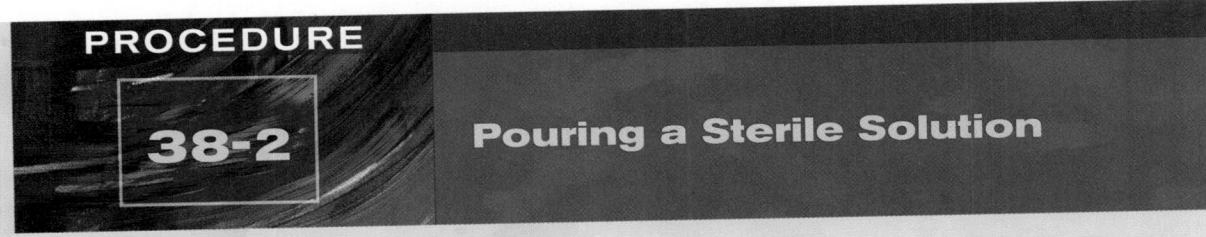

PROCEDURE 38-2 — Pouring a Sterile Solution

Student Competency Objective: The medical assistant student will pour a sterile solution into a sterile container.

Items Needed: Sterile solution, sterile container, sterile towel on a sterile tray or field

Steps:
1. Wash your hands.
2. Assemble equipment and supplies.

(Continues)

PROCEDURE 38-2 (Continued)

3. Read the label on the bottle to make sure that you have the right solution.

4. Check the expiration date on the bottle. Do not use the solution if the expiration date has passed. Discard the outdated solution and use a new bottle.

5. Pick up the solution. Make sure that you palm the label (Figure 38-11A). To palm the label means to hold the bottle with the palm of your hand over the label. This will prevent any solution that might drip from running down the side and blurring the words on the label.

6. Take the cap off the solution bottle with your other hand, being careful not to touch the inside of the cap.

7. Place the cap on a flat surface with the open side up. The rim should not touch any flat surface. The cap may also be held in the hand. If you do this, hold the cap right side up. Do not touch the inside of the cap.

8. Pour a small amount of the solution into a separate container. This rinses the lip of the solution container and helps to wash out any contaminants on the rim.

9. Approach the sterile field.

10. Pour the correct amount of solution into the sterile container, being careful not to let the rim of the solution bottle touch the sterile container. Pour slowly to avoid spilling or splashing the solution on the sterile field. Wetness will contaminate the sterile field (Figure 38-11B).

11. Do not reach over or touch any part of the sterile field. Be careful that the front of your uniform does not touch the sterile field.

12. Put the cap back on the sterile solution bottle, using sterile technique.

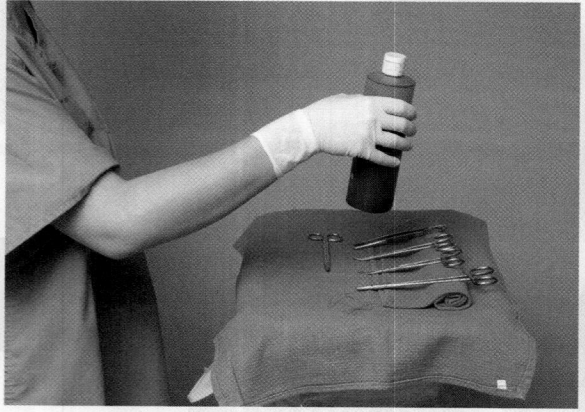

FIGURE 38-11A Pick up the sterile solution, palming the label.

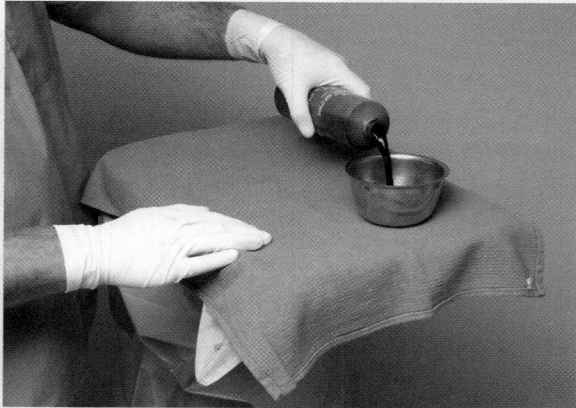

FIGURE 38-11B Pour the solution into a sterile container on the sterile field, being careful not to spill or splash the solution onto the sterile field.

PROCEDURE

38-3

Sterile Dressing Application

Student Competency Objective: The medical assistant student will apply a sterile dressing using sterile technique.

Items Needed: Sterile field setup, sterile gauze pads in the size needed for the specific situation, sterile forceps, sterile antiseptic solution, sterile container for solution, disposable examination gloves, sterile gloves, tape, bandage scissors, hazardous waste container, cotton balls, creams or ointments as ordered by doctor

Steps:

1. Wash your hands.
2. Assemble equipment and supplies.
3. Introduce yourself to the client even if you have seen the client on previous visits to your office. The client may have forgotten your name. This also helps to establish a provider-client relationship, because it shows the client that you want her to know who you are.
4. Identify the client. Ask the client to state her name to establish that this is the right client, and then compare the name given to the name on the chart. Never enter a room and call out a client's name to determine if this person is the correct client. The client may not have heard you clearly and may just nod, smile, or answer yes. Clients almost never question if the medical assistant professional has the right client. It is up to the medical assistant to identify the right client before performing any procedure.
5. Tell the client, in everyday language, what you are going to do.
6. Ask if the client has any questions. If she does, give short and simple answers. Sometimes clients will start (and continue) talking because they are nervous about the procedure.
7. Ask the client about any allergies to tapes or adhesives.
8. Reassure the client and instruct her not to move during the procedure.
9. Set up the sterile field (Figure 38-12A).
10. Place the waterproof bag away from the sterile field, but close enough to where you will be working that you can reach it easily, without crossing over the sterile field.
11. Put on sterile gloves.
12. Look at the client's wound.
13. Look for any signs of infection (redness, swelling, purulent matter) or other drainage. Note the type and amount of any drainage observed.
14. Using forceps, pick up sterile dressings (Figure 38-12B).
15. Put the sterile dressing over the area, using the forceps or your other sterile-gloved hand.
16. Take off the sterile gloves.
17. Dispose in biohazardous waste container.

(Continues)

PROCEDURE 38-3 (Continued)

18. Using tape or elastic bandage, secure the gauze to the client's skin. Make sure the tape strips are even and smooth. If using an elastic bandage, make sure that it is smooth and does not twist or bind (Figure 38–12C).

19. Teach the client the proper care of the gauze dressing. The dressing should be kept clean and dry. Include other instructions from the doctor. Tell the client to call the doctor if there is any swelling, pain, or discharge through the gauze dressing.

20. Ask the client if she has any questions.

21. Help the client to get off the examination table.

22. Clean the area according to regulations and office policy.

23. Wash your hands.

24. Record the procedure in the client's chart immediately.

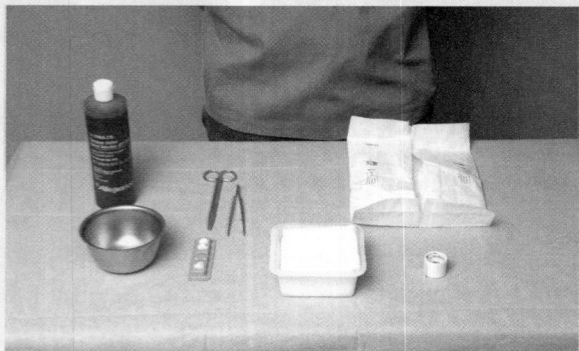

FIGURE 38–12A Assemble the items needed to apply a sterile dressing, and set up the sterile field.

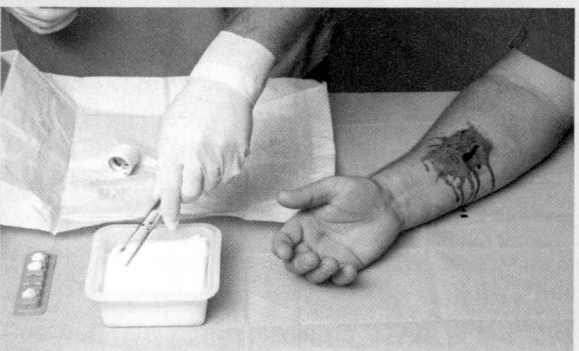

FIGURE 38–12B Apply gloves and pick up the sterile dressing, using forceps.

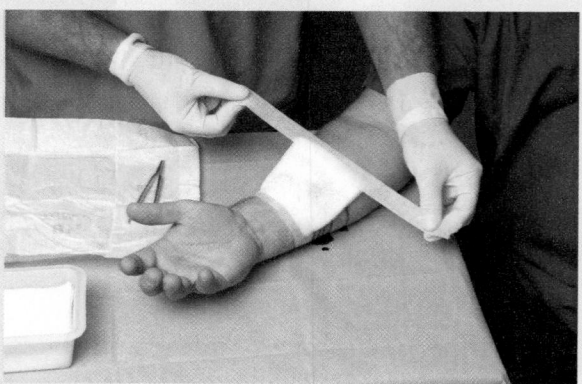

FIGURE 38–12C Secure the gauze to the skin, using tape or an elastic bandage.

Charting Example:

02/03/20xx   4:10 P.M.   Sterile dressing applied to right forearm. Area noted to be red and open. No drainage or odor noted.

Robin Kirnick, S.M.A.

Robin Kirnick, S.M.A. (printed name)

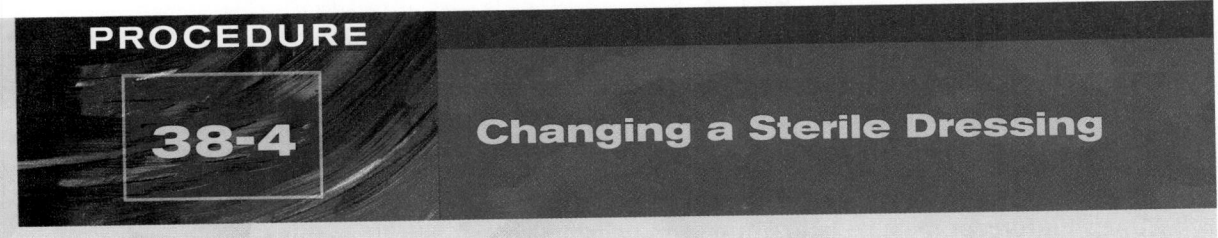

PROCEDURE

38-4

Changing a Sterile Dressing

Student Competency Objective: The medical assistant student will change a sterile dressing using sterile technique.

Items Needed: Sterile field setup, sterile gauze pads in the size needed for the specific situation, sterile forceps, sterile antiseptic solution, sterile container for solution, disposable examination gloves, sterile gloves, tape, bandage scissors, waterproof waste bag, biohazardous waste container, cotton balls, any creams or ointments ordered by doctor

Steps:

1. Wash your hands.
2. Assemble equipment and supplies.
3. Introduce yourself to the client even if you have seen the client on previous visits to your office. The client may have forgotten your name. This also helps to establish a provider–client relationship, because it shows the client that you want her to know who you are.
4. Identify the client. Ask the client to state her name to establish that this is the right client, and then compare the name given to the name on the chart. Never enter a room and call out a client's name to determine if this person is the correct client. The client may not have heard you clearly and may just nod, smile, or answer yes. Clients almost never question if the medical assistant professional has the right client. It is up to the medical assistant to identify the right client before performing any procedure.
5. Tell the client, in everyday language, what you are going to do.
6. Ask if the client has any questions. If she does, give short and simple answers. Sometimes clients will start (and continue) talking because they are nervous about the procedure.
7. Set up the sterile field.
8. Pour sterile solution.
9. Place the biohazardous waster container away from the sterile field, but close enough to where you will be working so that you can reach it easily without crossing over the sterile field.
10. Reassure the client and instruct her not to move during the procedure.
11. Put on disposable examination gloves.
12. Remove the old dressing gently.
13. Place the soiled dressing in the biohazardous waste container without touching the sides of the container (Figure 38–13A).
14. Do not pass the old dressing over the sterile field.
15. Look at the wound.
16. Look for any signs of infection (redness, swelling, purulent matter) or other drainage. Note the type and amount of any drainage observed.

(Continues)

PROCEDURE 38-4 (Continued)

17. Take off your contaminated gloves according to Procedure 3-4.
18. Wash your hands.
19. Put on sterile gloves according to Procedure 3-3.
20. Using forceps, pick up gauze or cotton balls moistened with the sterile antiseptic solution (Figure 38-13B).
21. Clean the wound area, starting at the center and working outward.
22. Put used gauze into the biohazardous waster container.
23. Put the sterile gauze over the area, using the forceps or your sterile-gloved hand (Figure 38-13C).
24. Take off the sterile gloves according to Procedure 3-4.

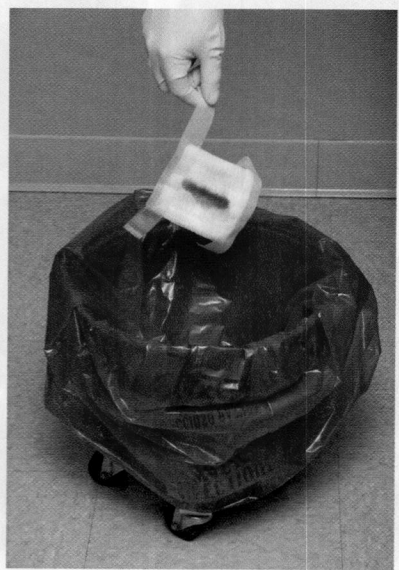

FIGURE 38-13A Remove the old dressing and place it in a biohazardous waste container.

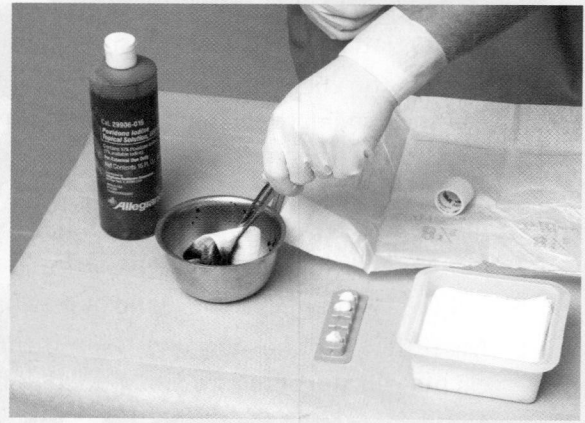

FIGURE 38-13B Using forceps, pick up and moisten gauze with a sterile antiseptic solution.

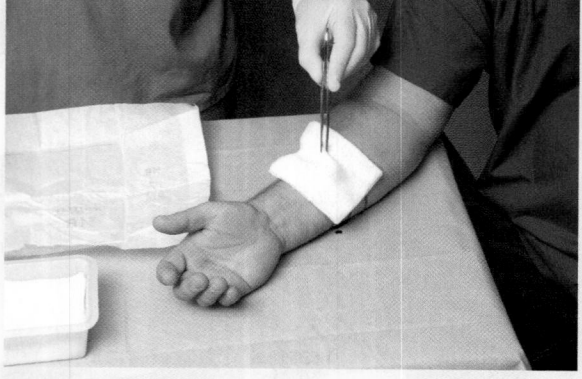

FIGURE 38-13C Using forceps, apply the sterile gauze over the area.

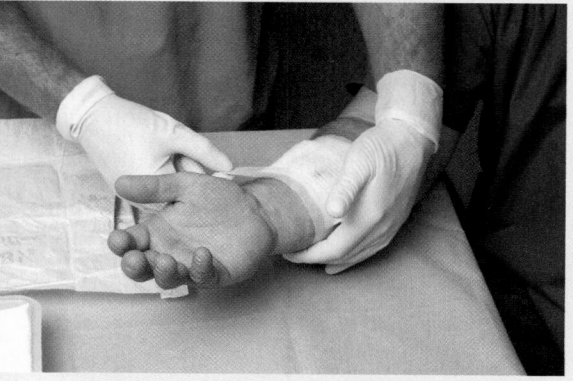

FIGURE 38-13D Secure the gauze to the skin, using tape or an elastic bandage.

(Continues)

PROCEDURE 38-4 (Continued)

25. Using tape or elastic bandage, secure the gauze to the skin. Make sure the tape strips are even and smooth. If using an elastic bandage, make sure that it is smooth and does not twist or bind (Figure 38-13D).
26. Teach the client the proper care of the gauze dressing. The dressing should be kept clean and dry. Include other instructions from the doctor. Tell the client to call the doctor if there is any swelling, pain, or discharge through the gauze dressing.
27. Ask the client if she has any questions.
28. Help the client to get off the examination table.
29. Dispose of contaminated items in the biohazardous waste container.
30. Clean the room according to regulations and office policy.
31. Wash your hands.
32. Record the procedure in the client's chart immediately.

Charting Example:
You performed a sterile dressing change on a client's left arm, and saw only a small amount of clear drainage. You would record the following :

3/22/20xx   2:45 P.M.   Removed gauze dressing from client's left arm. Small amount of clear drainage noted. Area washed with antiseptic solution. Sterile dressing applied. Instructed client to keep area clean and dry and to call the doctor if any pain, swelling, or discharge noted.

Samuel Keegan, S.M.A.

Samuel Keegan, S.M.A. (printed name)

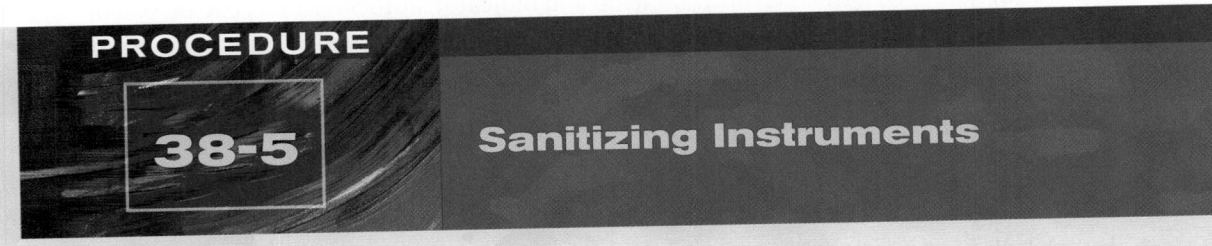

PROCEDURE 38-5   Sanitizing Instruments

Student Competency Objective: The medical assistant student will sanitize instruments.

Items Needed: Instruments to be sanitized, sink, running water, soaking solution, basins, soft brush, gauze, cleaning solution, gloves, mask, gown

Steps:
1. Wash your hands.
2. Assemble equipment and supplies.
3. Put on gloves.
4. Rinse the instruments and then use the cleaning solution.

(Continues)

PROCEDURE 38-5 (Continued)

5. Look closely at the instruments for any defect.
6. Open hinged instruments.
7. Use a soft brush or gauze to clean grooves, joints, hinges, ratchets, and any uneven surfaces where microorganisms might be difficult to remove.
8. Rinse instruments again thoroughly.
9. Leave all instruments in their open positions.
10. Dry thoroughly.
11. Remove your gown, mask, and gloves.
12. Wash your hands.

NOTE TO STUDENT:

If the instruments cannot be sanitized immediately, rinse them and put them in a soaking solution to keep contaminating matter from becoming hard and drying on the instruments. Rinse off the soaking solution before sanitization.

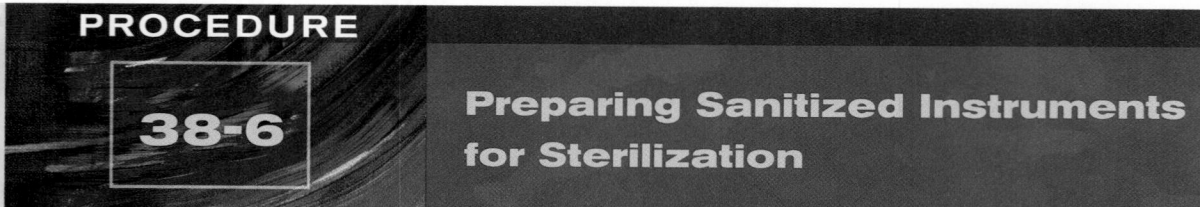

PROCEDURE 38-6

Preparing Sanitized Instruments for Sterilization

Student Competency Objective: The medical assistant student will prepare sanitized instruments for sterilization.

Items Needed: Sanitized items, sterilization wrap and indicator, autoclave tape, cotton ball or gauze, marker (if items are to be placed in a pack, a list of items should be available for comparison)

Steps:
1. Wash your hands.
2. Assemble equipment and supplies.
3. Open all instruments to allow complete penetration of steam.
4. Lay a cloth on the bottom of the tray; larger items should be laid down first.
5. Place items in order of use for a specific pack, to prevent accidental contamination during the sterilization procedure.
6. Put gauze or a cotton ball between the tips of any sharp hinged instruments.
7. Take the bottom edge of the wrapper and fold it over the article.
8. The corner of this edge is then folded back.
9. Take the right side of the wrapper and fold it over.
10. The corner of this side is then folded back.
11. Take the left side of the wrapper and fold it over.
12. The corner of this side is then folded back.

(Continues)

PROCEDURE 38-6 (Continued)

13. Take the last corner of the wrapper and fold it over.
14. Tape the last corner with autoclave tape or tuck the edge under the other corners before taping, depending on office policy.
15. Seal the package with sterilization tape.
16. Write the items included on the tape.
17. Write the date and your initials on the tape.

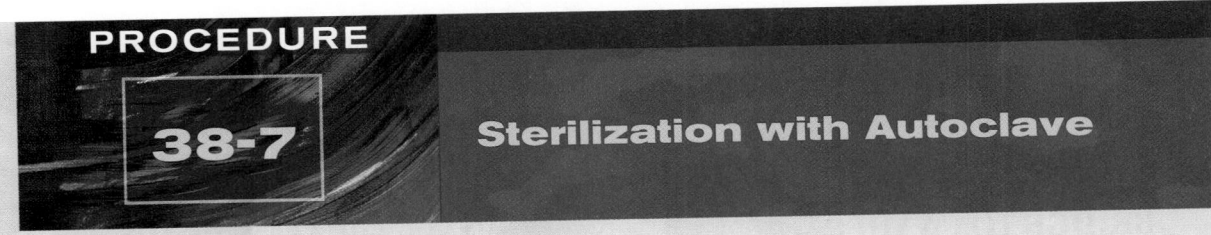

PROCEDURE

38-7   Sterilization with Autoclave

Student Competency Objective: The medical assistant will sterilize items using an autoclave.

Items Needed: Sanitized items, wrapped packs for sterilization, sterilization tape, distilled water, manufacturer's manual for autoclave machine

Steps:
1. Wash your hands.
2. Assemble equipment and supplies.
3. Read the manual to familiarize yourself with the particular machine you will be using.
4. Look at the water level indicator, making sure that water is at the "fill" line.
5. Place small packs in the autoclave, keeping packs and articles separate from each other and away from the sides of the machine. (This helps promote circulation of steam within the machine.)
6. Containers should be laid on their sides, with the lids ajar or removed.
7. Put an indicator in the middle of the items to be sterilized.
8. Close the autoclave door securely.
9. Turn on the machine.
10. Set the timer when the temperature gauge reaches the required temperature.
11. Vent the chamber when the cycle is complete.
12. Allow items to dry.
13. Remove items when cooled.
14. Check the sterilizer indicator.
15. Place items in a clean, dry area. Packs are considered sterile for 30 days, unless they are opened, become wet, or are damaged.
16. Clean and service the autoclave according to the manufacturer's directions. The manufacturer's manual should be kept near the machine; easily available to those who operate the machine.

POINTS OF HIGHLIGHT

- Minor surgical procedures are often performed in the medical office.
- The medical assistant's role will include setting up sterile fields, cleaning up after procedures, and assisting the doctor during procedures.
- Handwashing is the single most important activity to prevent the spread of harmful microorganisms.
- Surgical handwashing varies from handwashing for medical asepsis.
- Common instruments used in minor office surgeries are scalpels, forceps, scissors, and speculums.
- The maintenances of sterile technique by all involved in the minor office procedure is the responsibility of the medical assistant.

 ### BRIDGE TO CAAHEP

This chapter, which discusses minor surgery, provides information and content related to CAAHEP standards for Anatomy and Physiology, Medical Terminology, Medical Law and Ethics, Communication, Psychology, Medical Assisting Clinical Procedures, and Professional Components.

 ### ABHES LINKS

This chapter, which discusses minor surgery, links to ABHES course content for Medical Terminology, Medical Law and Ethics, Psychology of Human Relations, Medical Office Clinical Procedures, and Medical Laboratory Procedures.

 ### AAMA AREAS OF COMPETENCE

This chapter, which discusses minor surgery, provides information or content within several areas listed in the Medical Assistant Role Delineation Study. These areas include: administrative procedures, clinical, fundamental principles, diagnostic orders, patient (client) care, general transdisciplinary, professionalism, communication skills, legal concepts, and instruction.

 ### AMT PATHS

This chapter, which discusses minor surgery, provides a path to AMT competency in general medical assisting knowledge, anatomy and physiology, medical terminology, medical law, medical ethics, human relations, patient (client) education, clinical medical assisting, asepsis, sterilization, instruments, minor surgery, and laboratory procedures.

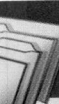

STUDENT PORTFOLIO ACTIVITY

During your clinical observations and externship experiences, you will have the opportunity to observe and/or assist with minor surgical procedures. In advance, compile a list of procedures that were discussed in class. When in the clinical settings, check off and date the procedures that you observed or assisted with. Ask your clinical supervisor to sign your list on the same day, after completion of the procedure. Be sure to make a copy of this list when you have completed your clinical learning experiences and place it in your portfolio. An employer can use this convenient log to verify that you have practical as well as theoretical knowledge from the classroom.

APPLYING YOUR SKILLS

During the course of setting up for a minor surgical procedure in the office, you observe another medical assistant reaching over the sterile field, thus breaking surgical technique. You are not sure if she actually touched any of the items on the tray. What do you do?

CRITICAL THINKING QUESTIONS

1. How would you know when to use surgical asepsis instead of medical asepsis? What are some reasons for using surgical asepsis? Give an example of a client situation in which you would need to use surgical asepsis.

2. The doctor has decided to perform a biopsy on a client. The client asks you to explain this. What do you say? What should the client expect?

3. Speculums are used to open body areas. For what examinations or procedures might you use speculums? What are two common speculums used in medical offices?

4. You overhear another health care professional tell a client that there is nothing to worry about, as only minor office surgery is being done. What do you say?

5. You work in a surgeon's office. She is deciding whether to switch from reusable instruments to disposable ones. What are some advantages of a disposable suture kit?

6. Why must a medical assistant be familiar with the surgical instruments used in an office?

7. What are some factors that might determine whether a procedure is done in a hospital setting or an office setting?

8. What determines the amount of assistance the medical assistant gives the doctor during minor office surgery? Where would you find this information?

9. You pour a sterile solution and splash some on the sterile field. The field is then considered contaminated. Why, as the wetting is from a sterile solution?

10. Your instructor tells you about surgical handwashing. Another student asks why it is necessary: "Aren't good handwashing techniques enough?" Your instructor asks you to answer that question. What do you say?

11. Go back to the beginning of this chapter and review the Anticipatory Statements. Reread each statement and then indicate whether it is true or false. If the statement is false, rewrite it to make it a true statement.

CLIENT TEACHING PLAN

First Aid for Cuts and Abrasions

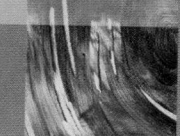

■ What Is to Be Taught:

- First Aid steps for the treatment of minor cuts and abrasions.

■ Objectives:

- Client will be able to treat minor cuts and abrasions in a safe, clean way.

■ Preparation Before Teaching:

- Review information about cuts, abrasions, lacerations, and other conditions in which the skin is broken.
- Look over the First Aid steps for identifying and treating minor skin cuts and abrasions.
- Gather pictures of cuts and abrasions to help illustrate your verbal description; samples of sprays, creams, and lotions for demonstration purposes; and paper and pen for notes and instructions.
- Make sure the area is free from distractions while you are teaching.

■ Steps for the Medical Assistant:

1. Wash your hands.
2. Gather supplies needed.
3. Introduce yourself to the client.
4. Explain what you are going to teach and why.
5. Explain what is considered a minor cut or abrasion. Show diagrams and pictures as illustrative examples.
6. Tell the client that one of the most important things to remember is to *remain calm.*
7. Wash your hands.
8. Ask the client to wash her hands.
9. Select an area such as the client's inner forearm.
10. Gently wash the selected area with warm water and antibacterial soap.
11. Spray antiseptic on the area.

12. Allow the area to air-dry. Do not blow on the area; it can be contaminated with bacteria from the nose and mouth.
13. Put on a sterile bandage. The gauze part of the bandage must be large enough to cover the cut or abrasion. The sticky part should not touch the open or abraded area.
14. After your demonstration, ask the client to repeat these steps.
15. Wash hands when completed.
16. Remind the client to call the doctor if she is in doubt about any steps or has concerns about the injury.

■ Special Needs of the Client:

- Look at the client's chart to see if there are any factors that might interfere with the client's ability to decide if an injury is minor and carry out the First Aid steps.
- Ask the client if there is anything you should know that might affect her ability to do these First Aid steps.

■ Evaluation:

- Client will be able to perform First Aid steps for treating a minor cut or abrasion after demonstration by the medical assistant.

■ Further Plans/Teaching:

- Instruct the client to call the doctor if she is in doubt as to whether something is a minor injury, or if a certain situation seems different.
- Tell the client that if, after a few days, the area appears red, swollen, or tender, or if there is a discharge from the area, she should call the doctor for further instructions.

■ Follow-up:

- Review the First Aid steps at the next office visit.

(Continues)

CLIENT TEACHING PLAN (Continued)

Medical Assistant

Name: _____

Signature: _____

Date: _____

Client

Date: _____

Follow-up Date: _____

Anticipatory Statements

Read and think about the following statements based upon what you believe now.
Decide whether you agree or disagree. Write the word **agree** after the statement if you
think the statement is true. Write the word **disagree** after the statement if you think the
statement is false. Read the chapter to find out if your current beliefs can be supported.

1. Clients who are on certain medications are at
   risk of choking because of a reduced gag reflex.   _____

2. The symptoms of a heart attack are the
   same in males and females.   _____

3. Good Samaritan laws apply only to doctors.   _____

4. The medical assistant's primary responsibility
   when a client experiences a seizure is to keep the
   client safe and free from injury.   _____

5. Direct pressure is not helpful in stopping bleeding.   _____

Medical Office Emergencies and First Aid

Learning Objectives

Upon completion of this chapter, the medical assistant student should be able to:

- List basic guidelines for action in emergency situations
- Identify three sources of bleeding
- Explain safety steps for a client who is having a seizure
- State possible differences in heart attack symptoms between males and females
- State what information is included in an incident report
- Describe safety practices to prevent poisoning in the home

Key Terms

abdominal thrusts Procedure to aid in the removal of a foreign body airway obstruction (FBAO) in adults and children over one year of age; also called the *Heimlich maneuver* or *subdiaphragmatic abdominal thrusts.*

cardiac arrest Often called "heart attack"; condition in which vital organs are deprived of blood when heart action and circulation stop or are interrupted.

cardiopulmonary resuscitation (CPR) Procedure to restore spontaneous circulation in a person.

epilepsy Disorder in which periodic misfiring of the electrical system of the brain results in a convulsion and/or partial or total loss of consciousness.

leadership The ability of a person to guide and direct others with influence and authority.

proximal Near the center or center point.

seizure Sudden misfiring of the electrical rhythm of the central nervous system.

■ INTRODUCTION

Situations can arise in the office that require quick thinking and action to ensure the health and safety of clients and staff. Within a client-centered health care setting, clients depend on health care professionals, including medical assistants, for help. The universal emergency medical identification symbol helps everyone recognize the proximity of medical help (Figure 39-1). Whatever the problem or emergency, following basic guidelines will aid the medical assistant.

■ BASIC GUIDELINES

Emergency situations demand specific, immediate responses made in an efficient and safe manner. For example, an individual who is experiencing a convulsive seizure needs a specific reaction by the health professional. This response is not the same as the care given to an individual who is experiencing symptoms of a **cardiac arrest.** Each situation requires a different, specific plan of action. It is critical that the medical assistant understand what happens in the body when a client experiences a problem that is classified as an emergency. The medical assistant must be competent in giving care in response to emergency situations.

The two guiding principles in all situations are calmness and preparedness. The medical

assistant's skills will be useless if he cannot remain calm. Upset and excitability will directly and negatively affect the medical assistant's decision-making abilities. Preparedness is necessary to carry out a plan of action. Time is a critical factor in emergencies, and the medical assistant must have the skills and be ready to perform the procedures required.

Keep Calm

The medical assistant is a health care professional and, as such, must take a **leadership** role in any health care situation. The medical assistant must assess the situation, quickly develop a plan of action, and keep everyone involved calm.

Be Prepared

Preparedness is key in meeting client needs in any situation. First, the medical assistant must have a basic understanding and knowledge of the human body and its responses in dangerous situations. For example, when a person gets cut severely and bleeds profusely, the body automatically responds to protect itself from excessive blood loss by blood clotting and possibly shock reactions. A medical assistant's understanding of the body's automatic responses will enable him to predict what might happen and how to respond to help the client's body stop the bleeding.

The office policies and procedures manual will guide all personnel as to how to handle an emergency. Every office should have a book with step-by-step instructions and a listing of items needed for all procedures performed in that office. This book or manual also includes procedures during an emergency; it outlines the steps to be followed when a crisis situation arises. It will specify everyone's tasks, who should be notified or informed, and what paperwork is to be completed. A policy manual helps to tell the medical assistant who is responsible for what actions.

Every staff person in the medical office should know his own role and how to respond

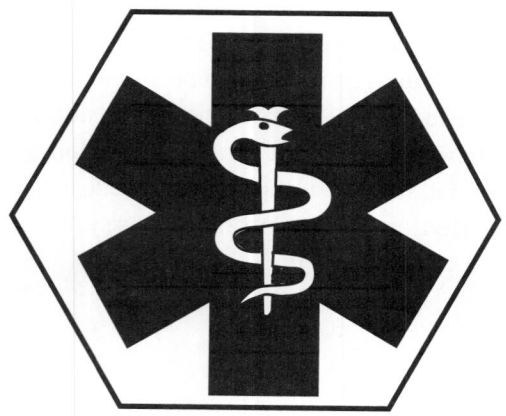

FIGURE 39-1 The universal emergency medical identification symbol.

appropriately to a crisis. The middle of an emergency is not the time to be figuring out office policy. Each staff member should read and become familiar with the office manuals when first hired. Periodically afterward, each staff member must review the policies and procedures. The manuals also have to be reviewed and updated. It might be the medical assistant's task to review and then meet with the physician to keep the information in the office manuals current. The medical assistant would then share this information with other office personnel.

LEGAL ISSUES

Clients have a right to care that is delivered in a quick, efficient, and competent manner. Federal laws establish many mandatory reporting and notification rules. They specify what situations must be reported and to whom the report is sent. The state will also have a set of laws governing issues of professional competence, although these laws vary from state to state. Education laws regarding scope of practice govern all health team members. Local laws or health departments may establish rules or issue guidelines as well. Finally, the doctor will establish guidelines and rules for the particular office.

Good Samaritan laws have been enacted to protect persons who help others in an emergency situation. For example, if a medical assistant sees a motor vehicle accident and begins to assist before the emergency medical service team arrives, that medical assistant is protected from legal liability by the Good Samaritan law. Of course, the medical assistant must have acted in a responsible, prudent manner if he is to claim this legal protection.

In the office, the medical assistant must thoroughly document the emergency situation and enter the information into the client's chart. The client's chart or medical record is a legal document. It details the actions of the doctor and other health care providers, and may be used to transmit information to other providers. Therefore, it is crucial that information be recorded promptly and accurately.

In addition to the note in the client's chart, an incident form is completed after any emergency. Office policy will specify what information must be included and who is to receive the report (or a copy of the report). Common in most incident reports are:

- Date of the incident
- Name of the person who was injured, hurt, or taken ill
- Address of that person
- Status of the person (client, visitor, staff member, etc.)
- Name, title, and position of each health care provider involved
- Action(s) taken
- Medications given: to whom, how much, route by which the medicine was administered, and by whom it was administered
- Name of physician involved
- Where the client went after the emergency action: home, ambulance, hospital, other
- Who accompanied the client after the emergency action, and condition of the client at that point
- Names of persons who accompanied the client
- Printed name and signature of person who wrote the incident report

EQUIPMENT

Regulatory agencies and other groups that oversee a particular health care setting help decide what equipment must be available. The type of medical practice will influence the need for or mandate of additional equipment. Equipment must be in good working order and easily accessible. All personnel must know where the equipment is stored and how to operate the equipment. (The medical assistant is often the person who calls for service checks on equipment.) Telephones must be easily locatable and accessible quickly. All personnel must know which paramedics respond to 9-1-1 calls and any other local emergency telephone numbers and codes.

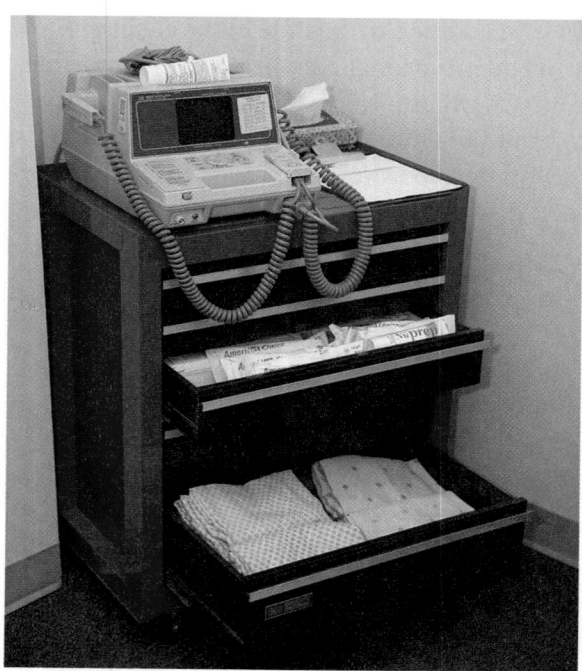

FIGURE 39-2 A medical crash cart with defibrillator.

Fire extinguishers must be checked regularly. All personnel must know the location of the extinguishers and how to operate them. The competency of all staff with fire equipment, fire doors, and evacuation procedures must be documented. Office policy will determine how frequently competency is assessed.

Many office settings have portable oxygen equipment readily available. A medical emergency cart or crash cart must be inspected frequently to make sure that no medicine has expired (Figure 39-2). An expired medicine must be replaced immediately. The contents of the drawers should be checked against the master list attached to the cart. The health care providers must know where the cart is kept and what is in each drawer, because clients' lives depend on it.

■ EMERGENCY STATUS

What is an emergency? Who needs to be seen immediately? Who can wait? Should 9-1-1 be called? Making these informed decisions takes knowledge, training, and experience. In a medical office setting, the medical assistant often is the first to meet the client and become involved in a problem situation. In addition to general medical knowledge and experience, there are some basic guidelines to help the medical assistant:

- Always check for an open airway.
- Determine if the client is experiencing problems with breathing.
- Can the client speak?
- Are there chest noises when the client inhales or exhales?
- Can the client stand, or is the client leaning or sitting down to breathe?

Bleeding

Bleeding can be slight and stop without any help from the medical assistant. At the other extreme, excessive bleeding from an artery can result in death in a matter of minutes. It is important to determine the source of the bleeding. Bleeding may occur from an artery, vein, or capillary. Blood from an artery will be bright red and spurt. Blood from a vein will look dark red, and the amount will depend on the size of the vein and the depth of the wound. Most often, wounds cause capillary bleeding, in which the blood appears to ooze from the wound. Direct pressure will help to stop such bleeding until a doctor can assess if stitches and additional treatment are necessary (Figure 39-3).

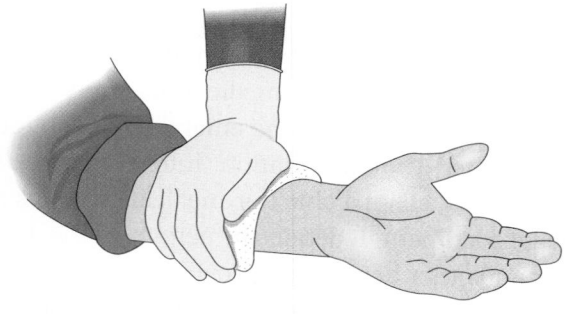

FIGURE 39-3 Apply direct pressure to help stop bleeding.

The medical assistant should have gloved hands and a sterile gauze dressing to apply directly over the site of a bleeding injury. If the bleeding is severe and does not respond to direct pressure, pressure should be applied to one of the body's pressure points (Figure 39-4). The pressure point selected is the one **proximal** to the bleeding area; in other words, the pressure point that is closest to the center of the body and the site of injury. This will prevent blood from rushing to the open area.

Bleeding may be external or internal. External bleeding, as described earlier, can be seen. The source of internal bleeding, which occurs inside the body, can be more difficult to find. The client may not be aware that he is bleeding, but will show some signs indicating internal bleeding. The client may have a fast, weak pulse and take shallow breaths. He may feel dizzy or light-headed. As the blood loss increases, the client may act restless and express feelings of anxiety or impending disaster.

Heart Attack

A heart attack is caused by a blockage of blood flow to the heart. There are risk factors that increase a person's chance of having a heart attack:

- Stress
- Diets high in fat, cholesterol, and sodium
- Low activity and lack of exercise

A person who is of normal weight, exercises regularly, and seems outwardly healthy may still experience a heart attack. Quick response and proper treatment can help to save lives. The medical assistant must know the warning signs of a heart attack and respond quickly and competently. The classic symptoms of crushing pain, or pressure, in the middle of the chest, pain that travels down the left arm and/or into the jaw, and extreme perspiration are not always present during a heart attack. The "classic" symptoms seem to happen more frequently in men than in women. Symptoms in a woman can be vague, such as pain in the back between the shoulder blades. Because women's heart attack symptoms are frequently nonspecific, and can be attributed to other causes, women have a higher morbidity and mortality rate from cardiac emergencies.

If you, as a medical assistant, suspect that someone is having a heart attack, activate the emergency response system. A large facility may have a "code team" to respond to such calls. In a small office, call 9-1-1 or other local emergency number. The medical assistant should know the correct procedure for his place of employment. If the client has stopped breathing, begin **cardiopulmonary resuscitation (CPR)** (see Procedures 39-1 and 39-2).

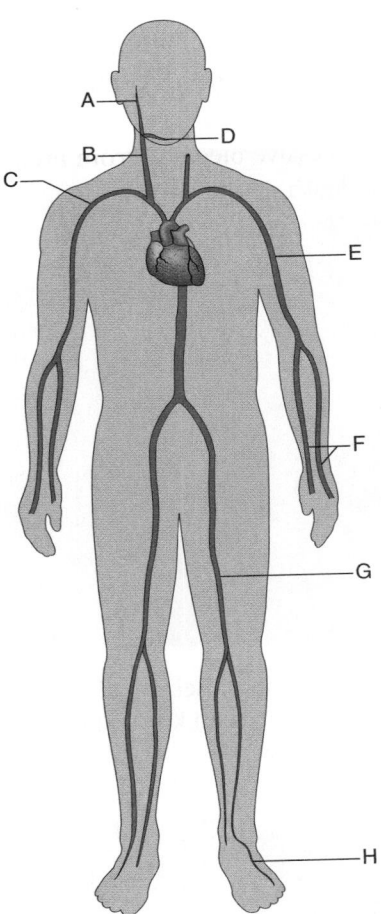

FIGURE 39–4 If bleeding continues after applying direct pressure, place pressure on the closest pressure point. (A) Temporal artery. (B) Carotid artery. (C) Subclavian artery. (D) Facial artery. (E) Brachial artery. (F) Radial artery. (G) Femoral artery. (H) Dorsalis pedis artery.

Choking

Choking can happen at any time and in any situation. The medical assistant must recognize the emergency and help to prevent respiratory and cardiac arrest (Figure 39-5). Adults frequently choke in restaurants while eating, drinking, and talking. Some factors increase the risk of choking, including: drinking alcohol, laughing while eating, attempting to swallow large pieces of food, and taking certain medications that depress the gag reflex. Children often choke on objects they have put into their mouths. Remember, infants and young children learn about the environment by touching and tasting. Parents and caregivers must become aware of dangerous objects and make sure their homes are as safe as possible to prevent accidents—this is literally a matter of life and death.

In the event of choking, the medical assistant must be prepared to assess the situation and give **abdominal thrusts** (also called the Heimlich maneuver) to a conscious adult. The procedure is different for infants and unconscious adults (see Procedures 39-6, 39-7, and 39-8).

Seizures

A **seizure** is uncontrolled electrical activity in the brain. Seizures can be caused by a fever or high temperature associated with any infectious process, by a head injury, or by a seizure disorder such as **epilepsy.** There are different forms of seizures, each of which appears different to the observer. The medical assistant's primary responsibility is to keep the client safe and protected from injury (Figure 39-6). Remove objects and people from the client's vicinity, to

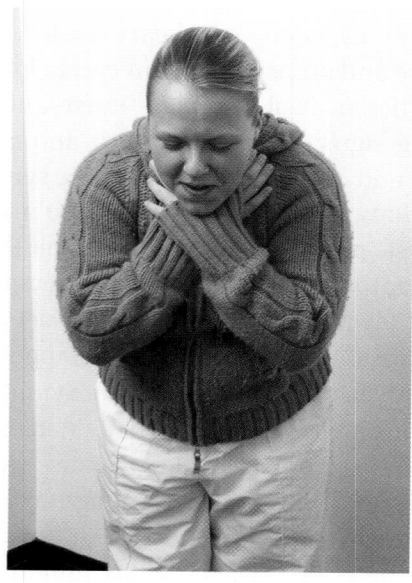

FIGURE 39-5 The universal sign for choking.

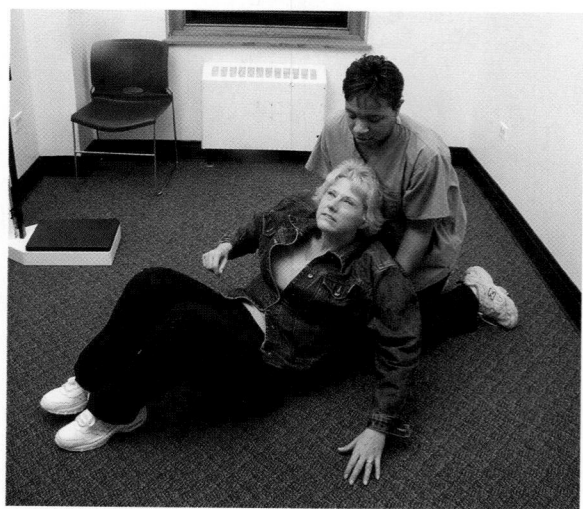

FIGURE 39-6 During a seizure, the medical assistant should focus on keeping the client protected from injury.

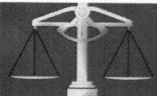

LEGAL/ETHICAL THOUGHTS

Medical assistants are health care professionals who can give First Aid. The Good Samaritan laws help legally protect individuals who provide first aid to victims in emergency situations, such as a motor vehicle accident, before highly trained emergency medical personnel arrive.

avoid injury. Never try to put a tongue blade or anything in the seizing client's mouth; this could easily obstruct the airway or otherwise injure the client. When the seizure is over, the client will be exhausted and need to sleep.

Poisoning

Safety and the prevention of poisoning are critical issues, especially in the case of children. Most children are curious, and very young children learn about the environment by putting objects into their mouths. Older children may be attracted by the color of a substance, its scent, or the shape or color of the container. The medical assistant needs to instruct clients on how to make their homes safe and prevent accidental poisonings. When teaching a client about poisoning, the following information should be included:

- Keep all medicines, even over-the-counter medications, vitamins, and herbs, out of the reach of children. Keep medicines in tamper-resistant, childproof containers.
- Keep all cleaning products and any other chemicals in their original containers.
- Keep household chemicals and cleaning products in a locked cabinet, not under a kitchen or bathroom sink. Store all cleaning products away from where food is kept.
- Keep the poison control number near or on the telephone.

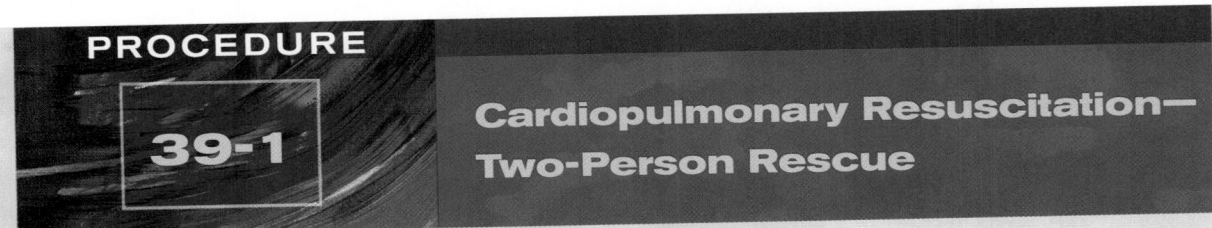

PROCEDURE 39-1

Cardiopulmonary Resuscitation— Two-Person Rescue

Student Competency Objective: Two medical assistant students will demonstrate CPR on a training mannequin while being observed by a certified instructor.

Items Needed: Training mannequin, gauze squares, alcohol wipes, gloves, barrier respiratory devices

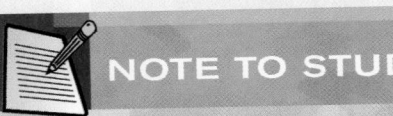

NOTE TO STUDENT:

The word client is substituted for mannequin to simulate a real situation. This procedure is never practiced on a real person.

Steps:

1. Shake the client and shout, "Are you okay?" to determine if the client is unresponsive.
2. If there is no response, one rescuer activates the emergency medical services (EMS) system.
3. Place the client on the floor or other hard, flat surface.
4. Rescuer One kneels at the client's side to give chest compressions.
5. Rescuer Two kneels by the side of the client's head. Rescuer Two will stay at the client's head to do rescue breathing, open the airway, monitor the carotid pulse (Figure 39-7A).
6. Open the client's airway using the head-tilt, chin-lift maneuver or the jaw-thrust method (Figure 39-7B).
7. Look, listen, and feel for breath and breathing.
8. If the client is not breathing, keep his head in the head-tilt or jaw-thrust position.

(Continues)

PROCEDURE 39-1 (Continued)

9. Pinch the client's nostrils closed.

10. Rescuer Two puts his mouth over the client's mouth (or uses a barrier device, if available).

11. Give two slow breaths (each two seconds long). Take a breath in between two slow breaths (Figure 39-7C).

12. Observe the client for chest rise.

13. Turn your head to the side to listen and feel for return of air while looking for chest rise.

14. Check for the carotid pulse (on the side of the neck) with your index and middle finger. At the same time, watch for signs of circulation, breathing, coughing, or movement. This should take no longer than 10 seconds (Figure 39-7D).

15. If circulation signs are observed but no breathing, give rescue breathing (1 breath every 5 seconds, or 10 to 12 breaths per minute).

16. If there is no sign of circulation (pulse), Rescuer One starts chest compressions. To find the correct position for hand placement, start at the lower edge of the client's rib cage and follow it with your finger to the notch or V at the center of the chest. Put two fingers above the notch. Place the heel of the hand that is closest to the client's head over the other hand and interlace and lock fingers. Hold fingers off the client's chest.

17. Rescuer One positions himself on his knees, with shoulders directly over his hands, which are on the client's sternum.

18. Keep arms straight and press down on the client's chest ($1\frac{1}{2}$ to 2 inches) and then release (Figure 39-7E).

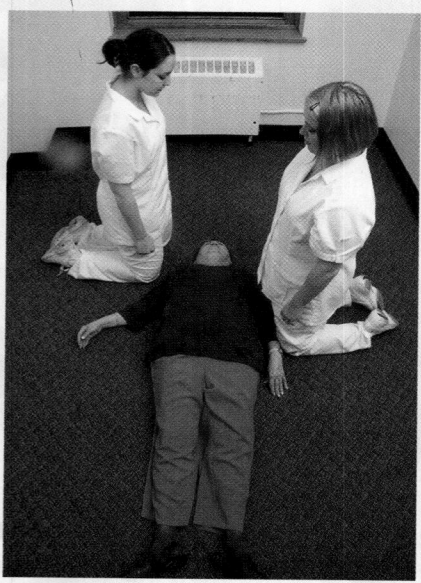

FIGURE 39-7A In two-person CPR, one medical assistant kneels at the client's side and prepares for chest compressions. The other medical assistant kneels by the client's head and prepares to open the airway and perform rescue breathing.

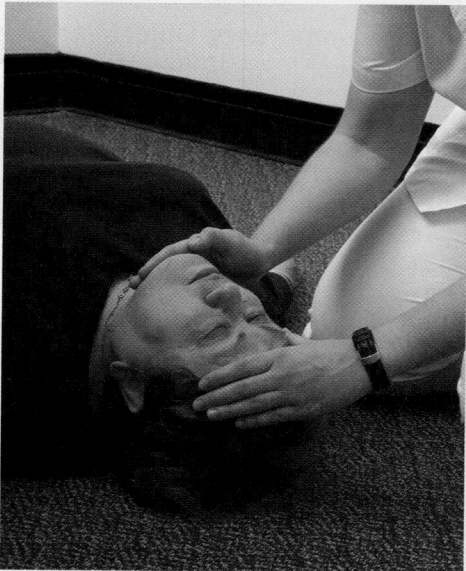

FIGURE 39-7B The second medical assistant opens the client's airway by tilting the head and lifting the chin.

(Continues)

PROCEDURE 39-1 (Continued)

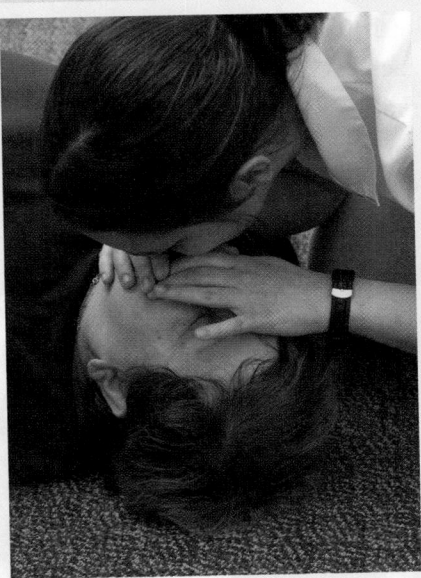

FIGURE 39-7C The second medical assistant gives the client two slow breaths, while keeping the client's nostrils closed.

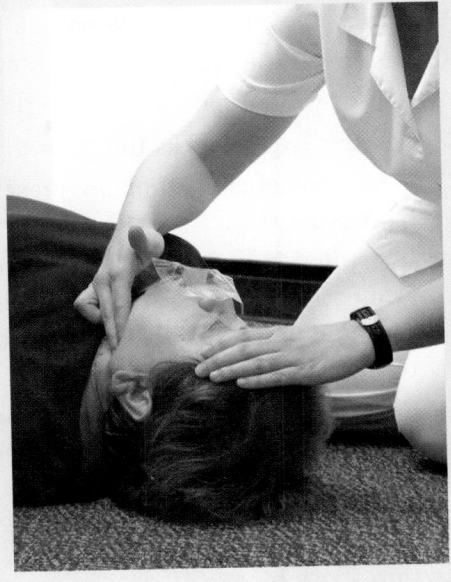

FIGURE 39-7D The second medical assistant listens for the client's breath to return, then checks the carotid pulse. Both medical assistants should look for signs of movement and chest rise in the client.

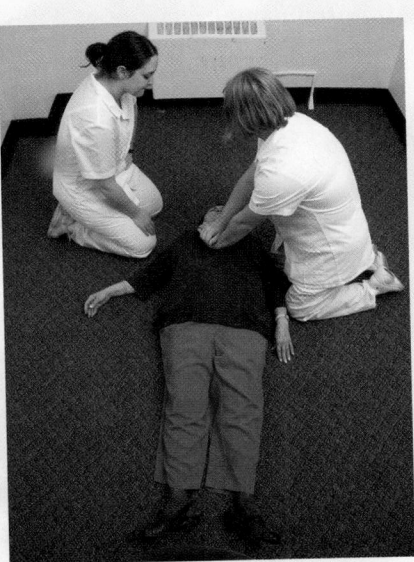

FIGURE 39-7E Keeping the arms straight, the first medical assistant presses down on the client's chest, then releases the compression.

(Continues)

PROCEDURE 39-1 (Continued)

19. Repeat the chest compression 15 times (rate will be 100 compressions per minute).
20. Rescuer Two gives the client 2 slow breaths after each cycle of 15 compressions.
21. Repeat the cycle of 15 compressions and 2 slow breaths (15:2) four times.
22. Rescuer Two rechecks the carotid pulse and looks for signs of circulation and breathing.
23. If no signs of circulation are present, resume the cycle, beginning with chest compressions by Rescuer One.
24. If circulation is observed but no signs of breathing, Rescuer Two gives rescue breathing (1 breath every 5 seconds, or 10 to 12 per minute). Once you have started CPR, you must continue until the client recovers or another person takes over, such as emergency medical technicians (EMTs).
25. Clean the mannequin thoroughly with alcohol wipes. Some mannequins have disposable parts; follow directions for cleaning these.
26. Wash your hands.
27. Record the procedure immediately.

Charting Example:

1/9/20xx 9:00 A.M. Client collapsed. Unresponsive and no signs of breathing or circulation. EMS activated. CPR administered for four minutes until EMTs took over. Client transported via ambulance to Charity Hospital at 9:30 a.m.

Norma Wilson, S.M.A.

Norma Wilson, S.M.A. (printed name)

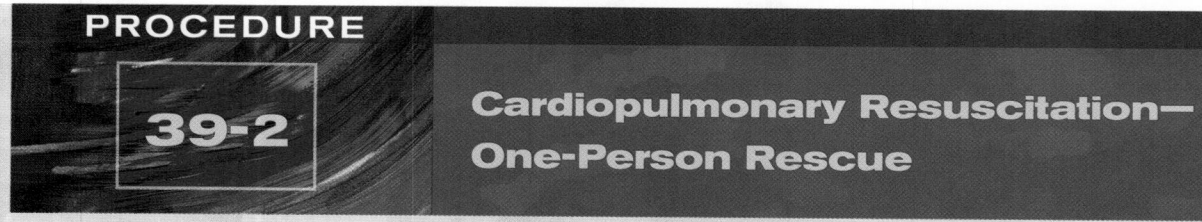

PROCEDURE

39-2

Cardiopulmonary Resuscitation— One-Person Rescue

Student Competency Objective: The medical assistant student will demonstrate CPR on a training mannequin while being observed by a certified instructor.

Items Needed: Training mannequin, gauze squares, alcohol wipes, gloves, barrier respiratory devices

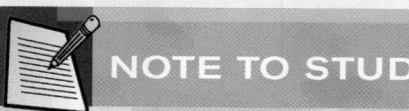

NOTE TO STUDENT:

The word client is substituted for the word mannequin to simulate a real situation. This procedure is never practiced on a real person.

Steps:

1. Shake the client and shout, "Are you okay?" to determine if the client is unresponsive.
2. If there is no response, activate the EMS system.

(Continues)

PROCEDURE 39-2 (Continued)

3. Place the client on the floor or other flat, hard surface.

4. Kneel at the side of the client's head (Figure 39-8A).

5. Open the client's airway, using the head-tilt, chin-lift maneuver or jaw-thrust method (Figure 39-8B).

6. Look, listen, and feel for breath and breathing.

7. If the client is not breathing, keep his head in the head-tilt or jaw-thrust position.

8. Pinch the client's nostrils closed.

9. Put your mouth over the client's mouth (or use a barrier respiration device, if available).

10. Give two slow breaths (each two seconds long). Take a breath in between the two slow breaths.

11. Observe the client for chest rise.

12. Turn your head to the side to listen and feel for the return of air while looking for chest rise (Figure 39-8C).

13. Check for the carotid pulse (at the side of the neck) with your index and middle finger. At the same time, watch for signs of circulation, breathing, coughing, or movement. This should take no longer than 10 seconds.

14. If circulation signs are observed, but there is no breathing, give rescue breathing (1 breath every 5 seconds, or 10 to 12 breaths per minute).

15. If no sign of circulation (pulse) is present, begin chest compressions. To find the correct position for hand placement, start at the lower edge of the client's rib cage and follow it with your finger to the notch or V at the center of the chest. Put two fingers above the notch. Place the heel of the hand that is closest to the client's head over the other hand and interlace and lock fingers. Hold fingers off the client's chest.

16. Kneel with your shoulders over your hands, which are over the client's sternum.

17. Keep your arms straight and tight.

18. Press down on the client's chest (1½ to 2 inches) and release (this is one chest compression) (Figure 39-8D).

19. Repeat the compression 15 times (at a rate of 100 compressions per minute).

20. Give the client 2 slow breaths after each cycle of 15 compressions.

21. Do not move from where you are positioned by the client's head.

22. Repeat the cycle of 15 compressions and 2 slow breaths (15:2) four times.

23. Recheck the carotid pulse and observe for signs of circulation and breathing.

24. If no signs of circulation are present, resume the cycle, beginning with chest compressions.

25. If circulation is observed but there are no signs of breathing, give rescue breathing (1 breath every 5 seconds, or 10 to 12 per minute). Once you have started CPR, you must continue until the client recovers or another person takes over, such as emergency medical technicians.

26. Clean the mannequin thoroughly with alcohol wipes. Some mannequins have disposable parts; follow directions for cleaning these.

27. Wash your hands.

28. Record the procedure immediately.

(Continues)

PROCEDURE 39-2 (Continued)

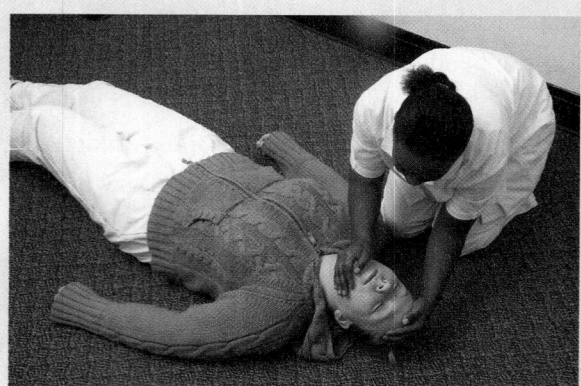

FIGURE 39-8A Begin one-person CPR by kneeling at the side of the client's head.

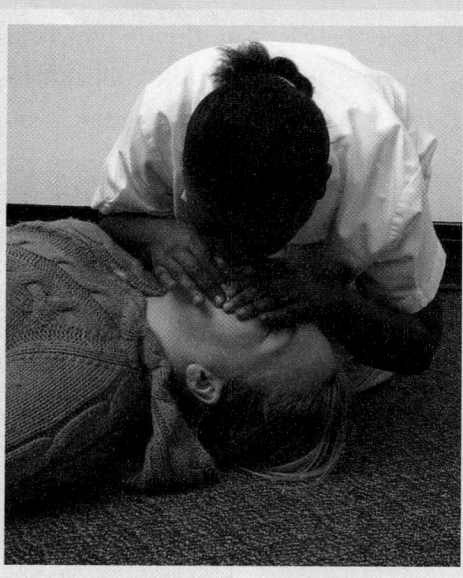

FIGURE 39-8B Open the client's airway.

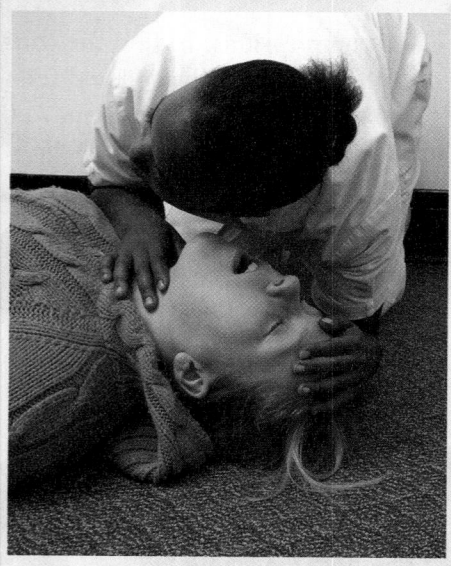

FIGURE 39-8C After giving rescue breaths, turn your head to the side to listen for the client's breathing to return and watch for the chest to rise.

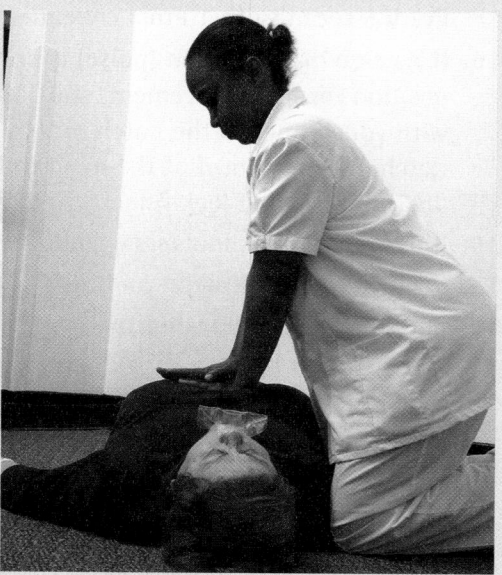

FIGURE 39-8D If there is no sign of movement from the client, begin chest compressions.

Charting Example:

1/9/20xx   9:00 A.M.   Client collapsed. Unresponsive and no signs of breathing or circulation. EMS activated. CPR administered for four minutes until EMTs took over. Client transported via ambulance to Charity Hospital at 9:30 a.m.

Norma Wilson, S.M.A.

Norma Wilson, S.M.A. (printed name)

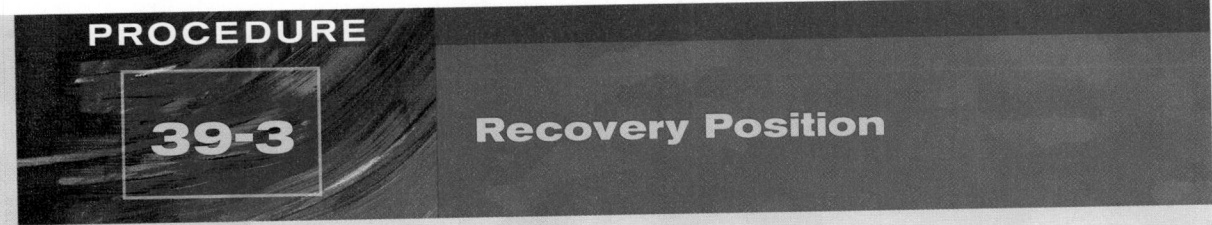

PROCEDURE

39-3

Recovery Position

Student Competency Objective: The medical assistant student will position an unresponsive client who is breathing and has signs of circulation.

Items Needed: Flat, firm surface (floor)

Steps:

1. Kneel next to the client.
2. Straighten the client's legs.
3. Using the arm that is nearest you, bend the client's arm at the elbow.
4. Place the forearm of that arm near the client's head, with the palm facing up.
5. Put the client's other arm across his chest (Figure 39–9A).
6. Place your hand on the back of the client's leg that is farthest from you, about 2 to 3 inches above the knee (Figure 39–9B).
7. Pull the thigh up toward the client's body.
8. Grab the client's shoulder that is farthest away from you with your other hand.
9. In a smooth motion, roll the client onto his side toward you (Figure 39–9C).

NOTE TO STUDENT:

The recovery position is used for the unresponsive person who is breathing and has signs of circulation and in whom there are no signs of trauma. This position helps to keep the airway open.

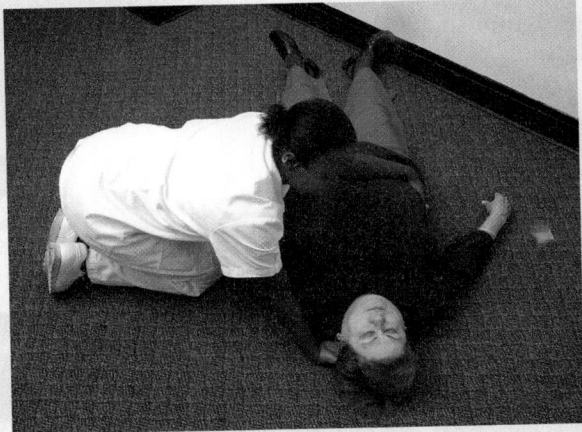

FIGURE 39–9A The medical assistant begins to place the client into recovery position. Kneeling next to the client, place one of the client's arms near his head, with the palm facing up. The other arm is placed across the client's chest.

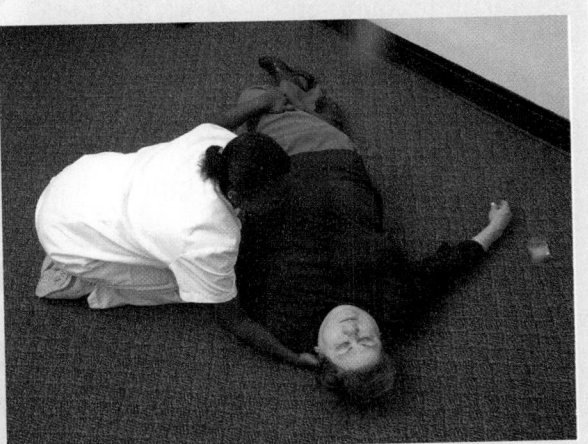

FIGURE 39–9B Place your hand on the back of the client's leg (the one farthest away from where you are kneeling), approximately 2 to 3 inches above the knee, and pull the thigh upward, toward the client's body.

(Continues)

PROCEDURE 39-3 (Continued)

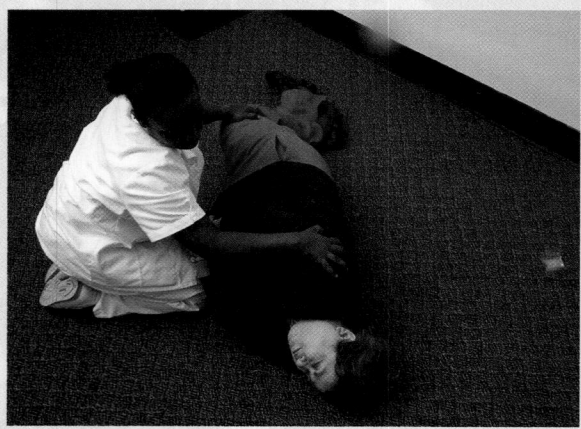

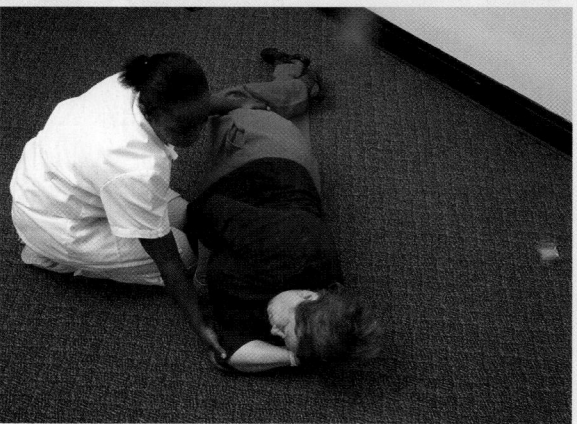

FIGURE 39–9C With your other arm, hold onto the client's shoulder (the one farthest away from where you are kneeling), and roll the client onto the side of the body, toward you.

FIGURE 39–9D Tilting the client's head back, position the client's hand underneath the cheek.

10. Make sure that the hip and knee of the client's uppermost leg are flexed and at right angles. If not, adjust them.

11. Tilt the client's head back to keep the airway open.

12. Take the client's uppermost hand and place it under his cheek (with the back of the hand against the cheek) (Figure 39–9D).

13. Look, listen, and feel for breathing and circulation.

14. If breathing or circulation stops, begin CPR (see Procedure 39–2).

Charting Example:

3/16/20xx   10:30 A.M.   Client found on floor, unresponsive but with signs of breathing and circulation present. Client placed in recovery position. Doctor notified.

Jose Cordaro, S.M.A.

Jose Cordaro, S.M.A. (printed name)

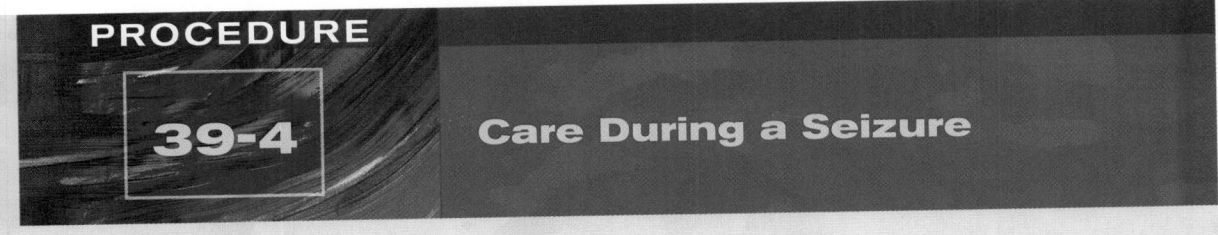

PROCEDURE

39-4

Care During a Seizure

Student Competency Objective: The medical assistant will demonstrate care for a client who is having a generalized seizure.

Items Needed: Firm, hard surface

Steps:

1. Gently assist the client to the floor, if he is not already seizing on the floor (Figure 39–10A).
2. Move objects away from the client, to avoid accidental contact injuries.
3. Check your watch to note the time.
4. Remove bystanders and provide privacy.
5. Call the physician.
6. Observe characteristics of the seizure, such as tremors in the arms and/or legs, vocalizations, and duration of the seizure.
7. After the seizure is over, position the client on his side in the recovery position (Figure 39–10B).

Charting Example:

4/23/20xx   3:45 P.M.   Client was observed stiffening while sitting in chair in exam room. Assisted to floor, objects moved, doctor notified. Seizure lasted for two minutes with tonic-clonic movements of arms and legs. After seizure, vital signs: BP-140/90, P-88, R-20. Client was positioned on side after seizure ended.

Krista Jones, S.M.A.

Krista Jones, S.M.A. (printed name)

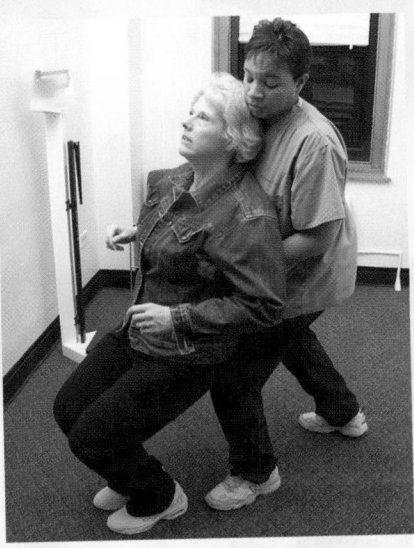

FIGURE 39–10A Assist the client to the floor to prevent injury.

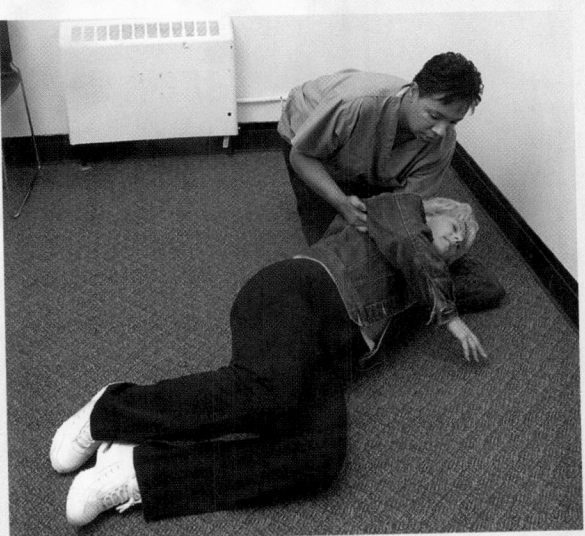

FIGURE 39–10B Move the client into the recovery position after the seizure is completely over.

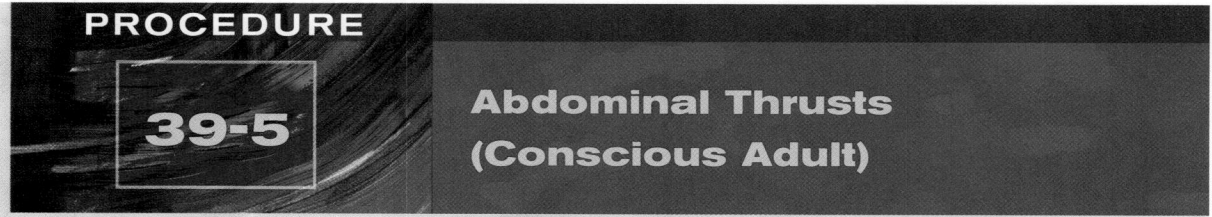

PROCEDURE

39-5

Abdominal Thrusts (Conscious Adult)

Student Competency Objective: The medical assistant student will perform abdominal thrusts to relieve a foreign body airway obstruction.

Items Needed: Mannequin

Steps:

1. Ask the person, "Are you choking?" "Can you speak?" (If person does not or cannot respond, continue the steps of this procedure.)

2. Tell the person that you will help him and that you need to stand behind him. A person who is desperate for your help may think you are turning away when you move behind him, and may try to circle around you.

3. Stand behind the choking person.

4. Place one foot between the person's feet (Figure 39–11A). This will help you to safely lower the person to the floor if he becomes unconscious and limp.

5. Place your arms around the client's abdomen, locking one hand over the other fist on the upper abdomen (stay away from the lower sternum or xiphoid) (Figure 39–11B).

6. Pull inward and upward sharply to give an abdominal thrust. Repeat abdominal thrusts until the object is expelled or the person becomes unresponsive. If the client stops breathing and shows no signs of circulation, start CPR (see Procedure 39–2).

NOTE TO STUDENT:

Chest thrusts instead of abdominal thrusts should be done on pregnant women and obese individuals.

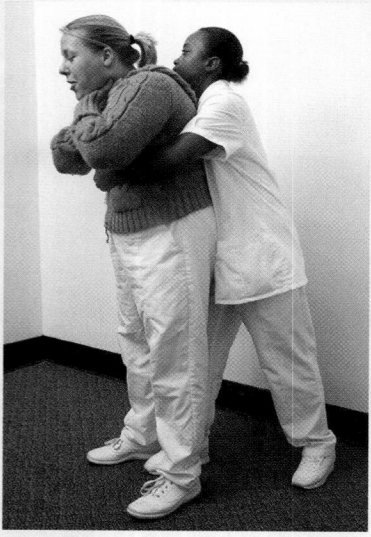

FIGURE 39–11A Position yourself behind the choking client with one foot between the client's feet.

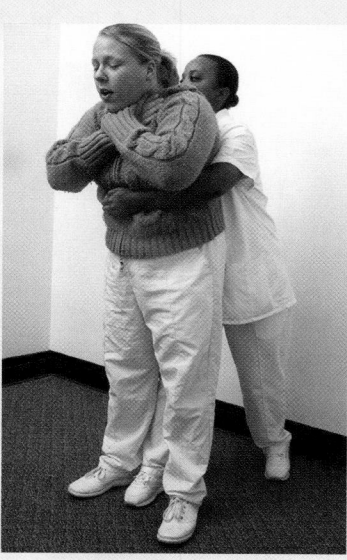

FIGURE 39–11B Initiate abdominal thrusts on the client.

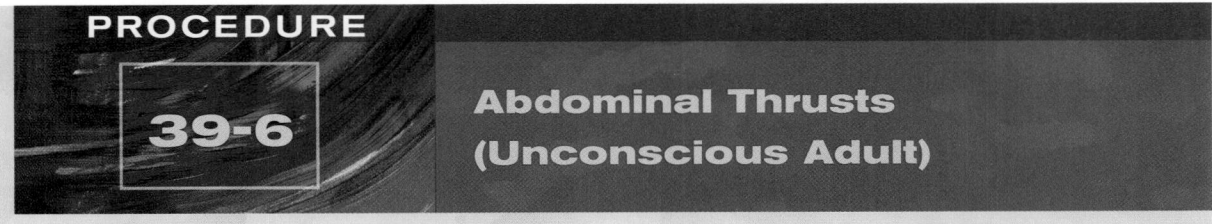

PROCEDURE

39-6

Abdominal Thrusts (Unconscious Adult)

Student Competency Objective: The medical assistant student will perform abdominal thrusts to relieve a foreign body airway obstruction.

Items Needed: Mannequin

Steps:

1. Activate the emergency response system (most likely 9-1-1).
2. Open the client's airway with the tongue-jaw lift (Figure 39-12A).
3. Sweep your finger through the client's mouth to remove any foreign objects (Figure 39-12B).
4. Open the client's airway and try to ventilate (give rescue breaths) (Figure 39-12C). If the client's chest does not go up, then do steps 5 through 8.
5. Reopen the client's airway and try again.
6. If the client's chest still does not rise, give five abdominal thrusts. Make sure to avoid the lower sternum (xiphoid process) (Figure 39-12D).
7. Repeat until rescue breathing is effective.
8. When the airway has been successfully cleared, and the client has signs of circulation and breathing, put the client in the recovery position.

> **NOTE TO STUDENT:**
>
> A person may become unresponsive while you are performing abdominal thrusts, or may already be unresponsive when you arrive.

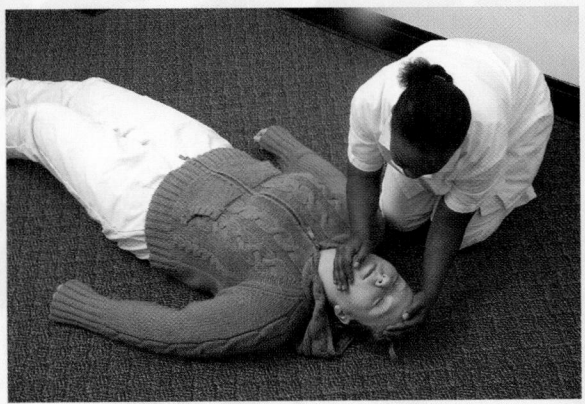

FIGURE 39-12A When a client is unconscious, open the client's airway using the tongue-jaw lift.

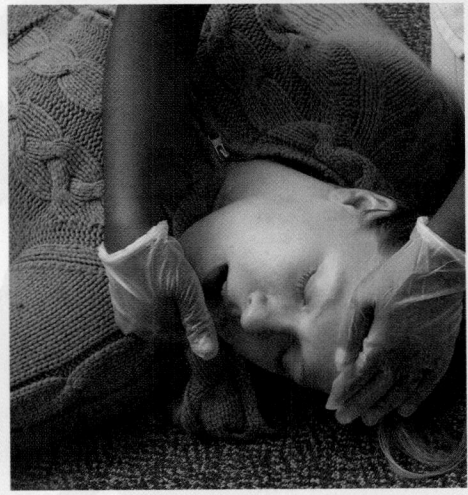

FIGURE 39-12B Remove any foreign objects from a client's mouth using a sweeping motion with your finger.

(Continues)

PROCEDURE 39-6 (Continued)

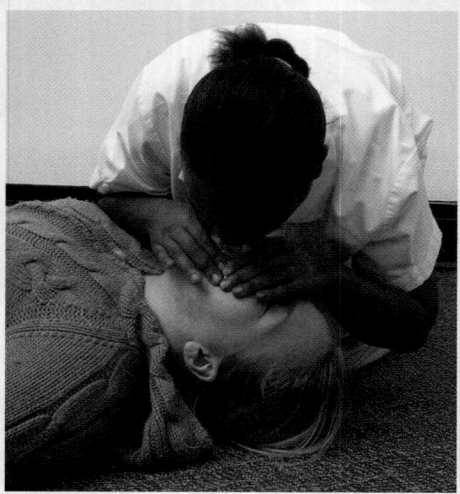

FIGURE 39–12C Initiate rescue breathing and look for the client's chest to rise.

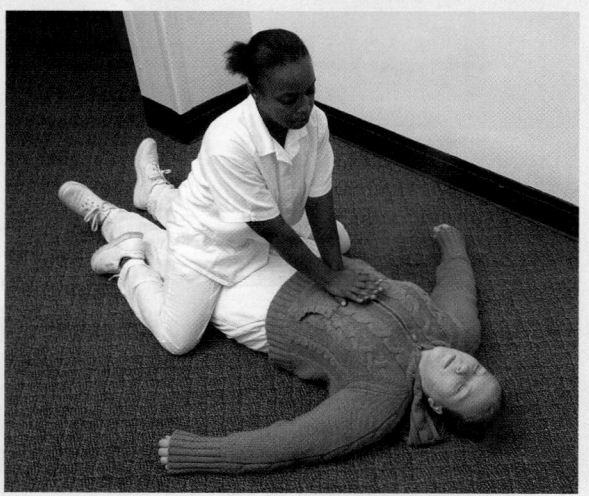

FIGURE 39–12D When rescue breathing attempts have been unsuccessful, give the client 5 abdominal thrusts.

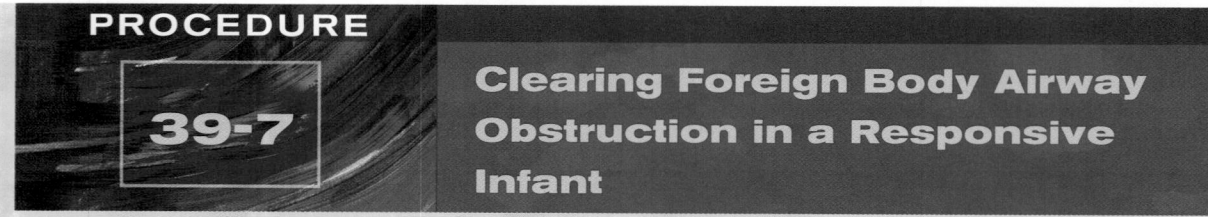

PROCEDURE 39-7

Clearing Foreign Body Airway Obstruction in a Responsive Infant

Student Competency Objective: The medical assistant student will dislodge a foreign body obstruction from an infant (mannequin).

Items Needed: Knowledge of rescue procedure, infant mannequin

Steps:
1. Look at the infant for difficulty in breathing, weak cough, and weak or no cry.
2. Pick up the infant. Support the infant's head and abdomen on the palm of your hand and forearm.
3. Give five back blows with the heel of your hand (Figure 39-13A).
4. Turn the child over and give five chest thrusts. Use only two fingers on the chest (Figure 39-13B).
5. Repeat steps 3 and 4 until the foreign body is expelled or the infant becomes unresponsive.
6. If unresponsive, initiate Procedure 39-8.

(Continues)

PROCEDURE 39-7 (Continued)

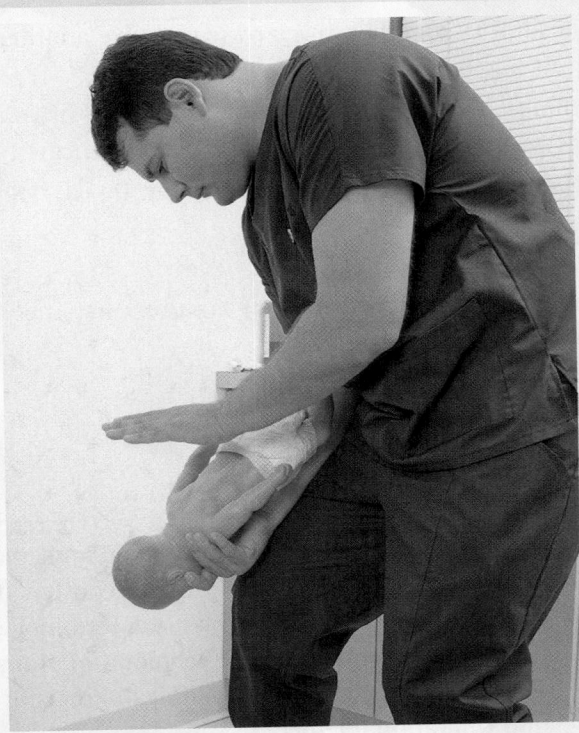 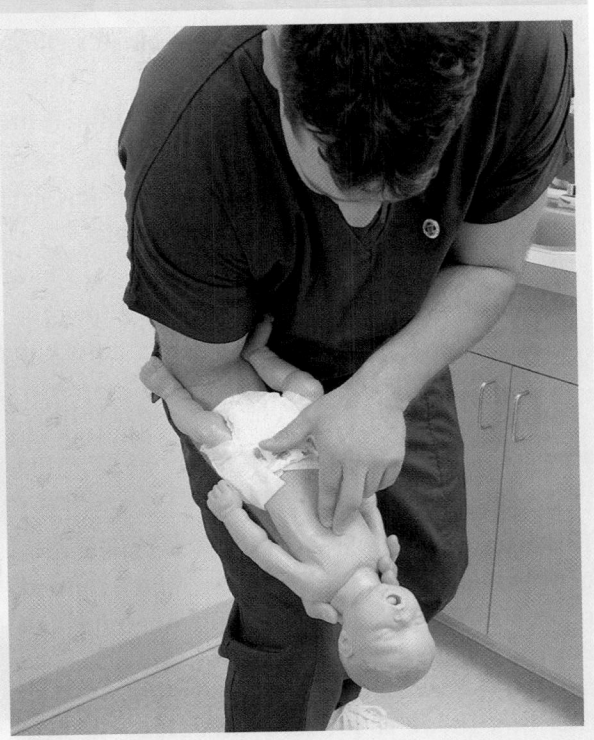

FIGURE 39–13A Hold the infant, supporting the head in the palm of your hand and the abdomen on your forearm. Give five back blows using the heel of your hand.

FIGURE 39–13B Turn the infant and give five chest thrusts, using only two fingers on the infant's chest.

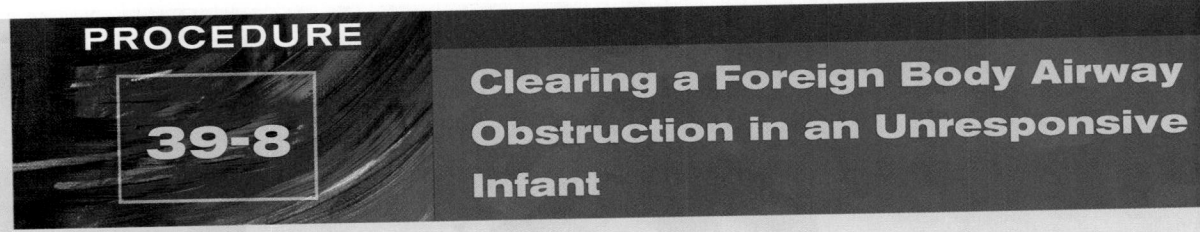

PROCEDURE 39-8   Clearing a Foreign Body Airway Obstruction in an Unresponsive Infant

Student Competency Objective: The medical assistant student will dislodge a foreign body obstruction from an unresponsive infant (mannequin).

Items Needed: Knowledge of rescue procedure, infant mannequin

Steps:

1. Establish unresponsiveness. (This is not necessary if the infant was conscious and became unresponsive while you were attempting to dislodge the foreign body.)
2. If another person is available, send that person to activate the emergency response system.
3. Open the client's airway and check for breathing.

(Continues)

PROCEDURE 39-8 (Continued)

4. Give rescue breaths. If the client's chest does not rise, reopen the airway and give another rescue breath.

5. If unsuccessful (the client is still not breathing), give five back blows with the heel of your hand and then five chest thrusts. Use only two fingers on the chest for the chest thrusts.

6. Open the airway with a tongue-jaw lift. If you see the foreign body, remove it. Do NOT do a blind finger sweep on an infant.

7. Repeat steps 3–6 until rescue breathing is effective. Continue CPR as needed.

8. If you are alone and cannot remove the airway obstruction within one minute, carry the infant with you as you activate the emergency response system.

 ## BRIDGE TO CAAHEP

This chapter, which discusses first aid and emergencies, provides information and content related to CAAHEP standards for Anatomy and Physiology, Medical Terminology, Medical Law and Ethics, Psychology, Communication, Medical Assisting Administrative Procedures, Medical Assisting Clinical Procedures, and Professional Components.

 ## ABHES LINKS

This chapter, which discusses first aid and emergencies, links to ABHES course content for Anatomy and Physiology, Medical Terminology, Medical Law and Ethics, Psychology of Human Relations, Medical Office Clinical Procedures, and Operational Functions.

POINTS OF HIGHLIGHT

- Staying calm is important in any health care situation.
- To meet client needs effectively and appropriately, the medical assistant must always be prepared.
- Good Samaritan laws are designed to protect individuals who render assistance in an emergency situation.
- Office policy and regulations determine what is included in an incident report.
- Direct pressure helps to stop bleeding from wounds.
- Quick response in treatment can save a person's life during a heart attack.
- The medical assistant's primary role during a client's seizure is to protect the client from injury.
- Much can be done to prevent accidental poisoning in the home.
- CPR can be administered by either one or two people. Practice and recertification are most important in maintaining CPR skills.

AAMA AREAS OF COMPETENCE

This chapter, which discusses first aid and emergencies, provides information or content within several areas listed in the Medical Assistant Role Delineation Study. These areas include: clinical Fundamental Principles, Diagnostic Orders, patient (client) care, general transdisciplinary, communication, legal concepts, instruction, professionalism, and Operational Functions.

 ## AMT PATHS

This chapter, which discusses first aid and emergencies, provides a path to AMT competency in general medical assisting knowledge, anatomy and physiology, medical terminology, and patient (client) education.

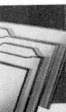 ### STUDENT PORTFOLIO ACTIVITY

CPR certification is required by most clinical places of employment. Check with your school or community health agencies to find a class. Register, attend, and complete a First Aid course for health care providers. Place a copy of your First Aid certification in your portfolio to demonstrate competency beyond the minimum required.

 ### APPLYING YOUR SKILLS

Preparedness is key in meeting client needs in any situation. Explain the importance of being prepared and how the medical assistant can have a direct, positive effect on health outcomes in an emergency situation. Give examples to support your points.

CRITICAL THINKING QUESTIONS

1. You are a newly hired medical assistant in a large practice setting. You read through the manuals to familiarize yourself with the office policies and procedures. You do not find any that cover emergency situations, such as what actions to take and who to notify. When you ask another staff member, he says he does not know, but tells you not to worry, as there has never been an emergency in the office and he is sure someone would know what to do. What would you do? What are your responsibilities?

2. A client slides and falls on a slippery spot on the floor, created by snow brought into the waiting room on people's boots. You go over to assist the client. What basic guidelines should you follow in assessing the situation and helping the client? What steps would you take after the client has been assisted? What would be a good follow-up plan?

3. Explain how the Good Samaritan law protects medical assistants from legal liability.

4. A client is bleeding from a deep cut on the arm. How do you stop the bleeding? What are some safety precautions you should take?

5. Why do women have a higher morbidity and mortality rate from heart attacks?

6. You suspect that a client may be having a heart attack. What do you do?

7. A client experiences a seizure in the waiting room. How do you respond?

8. Describe some ways to make a home safer and avoid accidental poisonings.

9. Different equipment must be available depending on the health care setting. How do you know what should be available? Where do you look for sources of information?

10. Why are the observation skills of a medical assistant so important while a client is experiencing a seizure?

11. Go back to the beginning of this chapter and review the Anticipatory Statements. Reread each statement and then indicate whether it is true or false. If the statement is false, rewrite it to make it a true statement.

CLIENT TEACHING PLAN

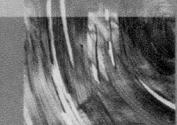

Prevention of Falls with Walkers

◼ What Is to Be Taught:

• How to care for a walker to prevent falls or accidents.

◼ Objectives:

• Client will be able to examine walker and observe safety considerations when using the walker.

◼ Preparation Before Teaching:

• Review information about the different types of walkers and the specific parts of a walker.
• Make sure you are able to explain the purpose of using a walker, as well as safety issues with walkers, to the client.
• Get together materials such as a diagram of a walker, walker used for teaching, and paper and pen.
• Make sure the area is free from distractions while you are teaching.

◼ Steps for the Medical Assistant:

1. Wash your hands.
2. Gather supplies needed.
3. Introduce yourself to the client.
4. Explain what you are going to teach and why.
5. Explain to the client that a walker can help to increase his ability to ambulate (walk). This in turn will help to maintain his independence and ability to carry out activities of daily living. Stress that this can happen only if the walker is kept in good working order and the client uses it safely.
6. Show the client the sample walker. Point to each part while stating the name of the part and its function (Figure 39-14A).
7. While the walker is folded, point out the tips of each leg of the walker. Each tip should remain dry to prevent slipping. (If the tips get wet when the walker is used outside, be sure to dry them off right away.)

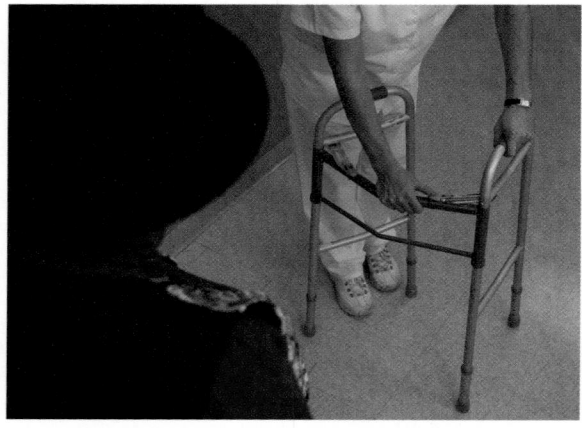

FIGURE 39-14A The medical assistant teaches the client about each part of the walker.

8. Ask the client to touch the tips on the sample walker. The tips should be even and firm. Explain to the client that if the tips wear down or become uneven, the walker will be off balance and dangerous to use.
9. Open the walker and snap it into the locked position.
10. Release the lock and refold the walker.
11. Ask the client to open and lock the walker and then to release the lock and refold it.
12. Show the client the correct position for standing with the walker (Figure 39-14B).
13. Instruct client to stand with the walker. Help him place his hands in the correct position.
14. Instruct the client to stand in the middle of the walker. Explain to the client that if he stands too far forward, he will lose his balance and fall forward. If he is too far back, he will lose control and the walker will slip away from him.
15. Give the client a few additional points to remember. The walker is intended to guide and assist with balance. The client should not use it to pull himself up out of chairs. Do not lean on it so that it must support his weight unevenly.

(Continues)

CLIENT TEACHING PLAN (Continued)

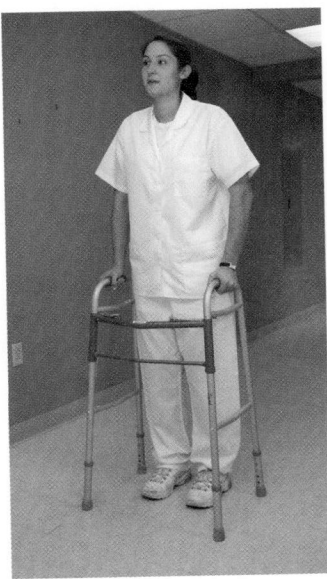

FIGURE 39-14B The medical assistant demonstrates the correct standing position for using a walker.

16. Give the client written instructions to use for a reference at home.

■ Special Needs of the Client:

* Check the client's chart for any factors that might interfere with the client's ability to care for the walker and use it safely.
* Ask the client, before and after the demonstration, if there is anything you should know that might affect his ability to use and care for the walker.

■ Evaluation:

* Client is able to tell you the purpose of walkers.
* Client is able to demonstrate the safety checks and how to stand with the walker safely.

■ Further Plans/Teaching:

* Ask the client if he has any questions or needs any additional information.

■ Follow-up:

* At the next visit, check the client's walker.
* Observe the client while he is using the walker.
* Ask the client to demonstrate safety checks. Review the steps again if needed. Encourage the client to continue using his walker safely and caring for it properly.

Medical Assistant

Name: _____

Signature: _____

Date: _____

Client

Date: _____

Follow-up Date: _____

UNIT SIX

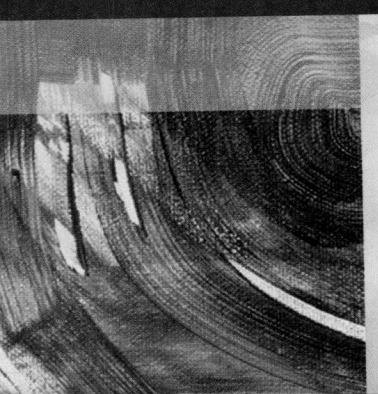

Diagnostics and Clinical Laboratory

In the final unit, the medical assistant is introduced to diagnostic and clinical laboratory testing. As noted in Unit Two, laboratory tests are a critical part of the client examination, as the results help the doctor to correctly diagnose and treat clients. This unit investigates the most common diagnostic and clinical laboratory tests in more detail. Tests identified in earlier units are highlighted in terms of the medical assistant's role. Client-centered care before, during, and after these testing procedures is explained.

The unit includes an examination of basic principles and purposes of laboratory testing, as well as types of laboratories where tests are performed and the medical assistant's role in testing and lab work. Safety of the client and health care worker and accuracy of testing are emphasized in all activities. Urinalysis, common blood tests, blood chemistry, cardiac diagnostic laboratory procedures, and diagnostic and therapeutic radiology are all covered, and the medical assistant's role in client preparation for and during testing is presented.

At the end of each chapter, you will be given a health care situation or client problem to solve by using what you have learned in the chapter and by applying your critical thinking skills. Sample client teaching plans illustrating teaching opportunities for the medical assistant are found in many chapters. You can use these in working with your clients and change them to meet individual client needs.

CHAPTER 40

Anticipatory Statements

Read and think about the following statements based upon what you believe now. Decide whether you agree or disagree. Write the word **agree** after the statement if you think the statement is true. Write the word **disagree** after the statement if you think the statement is false. Read the chapter to find out if your current beliefs can be supported.

1. Attitude of health care workers is most important in preventing accidents in the laboratory. _____

2. Medical assistants often work in physician's office laboratories. _____

3. Quality control is part of a medical assistant's responsibility in the laboratory setting. _____

4. The purpose of OSHA is to protect the employer. _____

5. Laboratory testing is done only to find disease. _____

Learning Objectives

Upon completion of this chapter, the medical assistant student should be able to:

- Identify the medical assistant's role in the physician's office laboratory
- Discuss the purpose of laboratory tests
- Identify the types of laboratories
- Describe the provisions of CLIA
- State seven safety guidelines for the medical assistant to follow in the laboratory
- Explain what OSHA is and its role in the health care setting
- Explain the idea of quality control and quality assurance in the clinical laboratory

Physician Office Laboratory

Key Terms

automated method Method of testing specimens by means of instruments that both perform tests and complete mathematical calculations to yield results.

baseline Starting point or beginning set of measurements or observations that are used as a basis of comparison with future data.

Clinical Laboratory Improvement Amendments of 1988 (CLIA) Federal law and associated regulations that govern all testing facilities.

manual method Method of testing in which handling of specimens and calculation of results is done by the individual laboratory worker, by hand.

Material Safety Data Sheet (MSDS) A manufacturer's document setting out directions for use and storage of a substance, identifying hazards, and specifying measures for emergency handling of the product; also, an employer's listing of potentially hazardous substances that a worker might encounter on the job.

microscope Optical instrument that uses lenses to enlarge or magnify a specimen.

Occupational Safety and Health Administration (OSHA) Organization that regulates workplace safety and protects the health and safety of workers.

personal protective equipment (PPE) Equipment that helps to keep workers safe from and avoid contact with hazardous materials. Examples of PPE are gloves, gowns, masks, and face shields.

quality control Procedures and systems to ensure that test results are reliable and accurate.

reference laboratory Laboratories that do complex testing; many rules and regulations govern these facilities.

specimen Small amount of tissue used for examination and testing.

■ INTRODUCTION

An important part of client-centered care is knowledge and correct use of laboratory tests. The tests may be started in the physician's office or other health center facility, and are usually completed in either a physician's office laboratory or another type of laboratory. The client is the reason laboratory tests are performed, so policies and procedures are established with the client as the focus. All safety guidelines are established to guard the worker and ensure the safety of the client.

The medical assistant's role in the physician's office laboratory depends on several factors. First, the medical assistant must always work within the scope of practice set by state (and sometimes federal) law. Second, the policy of a facility will determine what tasks the medical assistant performs. A major task of the medical assistant in laboratory testing is client preparation. The client needs to know what tests are to be done (and why), what is going to happen, what to expect during the testing, and how to prepare herself for the test.

In some laboratories, the medical assistant performs the test, in addition to recording and reporting the results. State and federal laws and regulatory governing bodies also specify what tasks the medical assistant may perform.

■ PURPOSE OF LABORATORY TESTS

There are several reasons why laboratory tests are ordered. Although laboratory tests are just one part of a physical examination, they are extremely important: Decisions that affect the client's life are made based on the results of these tests, so accuracy is critical. The medical assistant needs to understand the process and follow all directions carefully to ensure accurate test results.

Screening

Screening laboratory tests are used to discover abnormal conditions or disorders. For example,

simple diagnostic tests, such as capillary blood finger sticks, can be used to screen large numbers of people for diabetes. Urine tests and blood work are ordered as part of a physical. These are often called *routine tests.* **Baseline** values, as well as the early stages of disorders, can be found through these tests. Baseline or routine tests are generally used as a starting point with which to compare future tests. In other words, baseline tests are used to determine what is normal for that client.

Clinical Diagnosis

Laboratory tests are also ordered to aid in both clinical and differential diagnosis. When a client comes to the office, the doctor gathers information from the client and reviews data obtained by the medical assistant. The doctor bases a diagnosis on the client's signs and symptoms. However, laboratory tests are usually needed to confirm the diagnosis made on the clinical findings.

Differential Diagnosis

A client may have signs and symptoms that are common in several different disorders. A laboratory test may help the doctor to learn which disorder this client has, so that appropriate treatment can be started. A differential test answers the question: "Does the client have disorder A, or is it disorder B?"

Tracking Progress

Once a diagnosis is made, the doctor must continue to watch how the disorder progresses in the client. Does the disorder follow the usual course? Is anything else going on? Laboratory tests are another tool to help the doctor monitor the effects of the disorder and any treatment.

Treatment

When a doctor orders treatment, many questions remain: Is the treatment helping? Is the client's health getting better, worse, or staying the same? Is the treatment the best one for the client? Laboratory tests will show if the treatment is being effective. Should the doctor increase or decrease the amount of medication? Should she completely change the treatment plan? Laboratory tests can help doctors make the right decisions.

TYPES OF LABORATORIES

Regulatory agencies governing laboratories and testing facilities specify what tests may be performed, under what conditions, where they may be performed, and who may perform the tests. Laboratories can be grouped according to the complexity or the type of tests that are permitted to be performed in the laboratory. The three groups are: waived or simple, moderately complex, and highly complex. These groups are based on classifications established by the **Clinical Laboratory Improvement Amendments of 1988 (CLIA).** CLIA set forth federal regulations that govern all testing facilities.

The Physician's Office Laboratory

Waived (simple or low-complexity) tests may be done in the physician's office laboratory (POL). The medical assistant commonly works in a POL. Each POL will keep a list of tests that can be performed there. The medical assistant must strictly follow that list. Remember, as a professional, the medical assistant must work within the scope of the profession. Some tests commonly done in a POL include certain urine and blood tests. Urinalysis, using a reagent strip or tablet, is one of the tests most frequently performed in POL. Blood **specimens** are often obtained and then tested on site. Hematology tests, such as getting baseline readings of the number of red blood cells and white blood cells, are routinely done. The medical assistant can test blood for glucose using a glucometer. Stool samples are examined for blood. Pregnancy tests are frequently done in a POL. Test kits are used to test blood cholesterol level. Rapid strep

tests, in which throat swabs are tested for Streptococcus bacterial infections, are also common.

The medical assistant needs to understand all of the steps required for testing. These steps include: understanding the order, correctly obtaining or collecting the specimen, labeling and processing the specimen, testing the specimen, recording the test results, and, finally, reporting the results. The test kits, instructions for use, and supplies used may differ or change depending on office policy and the manufacturer of the kits. To maintain competency, the medical assistant must always keep up with new changes, rules, and regulations. Learning is a lifelong process.

A **microscope** is a piece of equipment commonly found in a medical laboratory, including a POL (Figure 40-1). Microscopes allow a person to view organisms and structures that are too small to be seen with the naked eye. Students are often first introduced to microscopes in anatomy, physiology, microbiology, or other science classes. A microscope is a valuable and

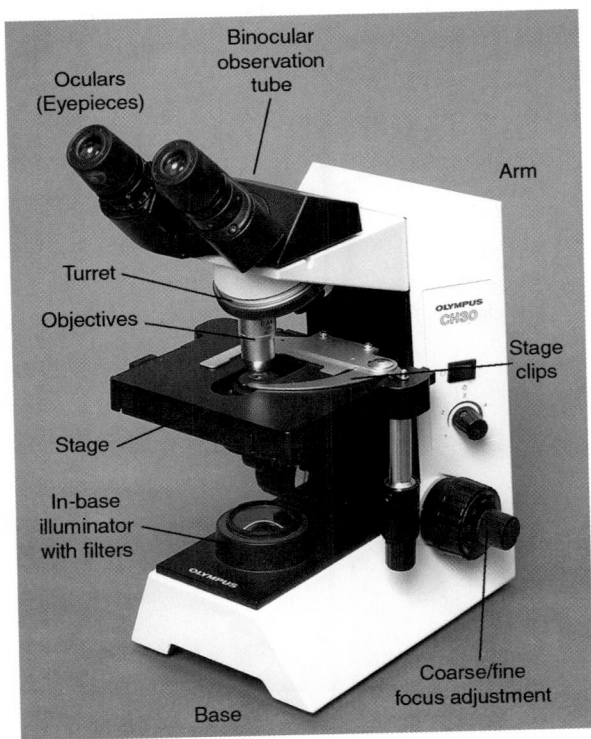

FIGURE 40-1 The microscope is an important piece of equipment in the laboratory.

delicate instrument. The medical assistant must follow the manufacturer's instructions for use and care of a microscope.

The POL will supply care and use instructions specific to the microscope used there to keep it in good working order. However, some general rules for the care of a microscope include:

- Always carry the microscope using two hands (never try to carry other items at the same time) (Figure 40-2).
- Avoid banging the microscope into objects.
- Set the microscope down gently.
- Clean the microscope after each use by following the directions. Never use anything other than the required lens cleaner and paper.
- Cover the microscope when it is not in use.
- Make sure the microscope is in a safe, secure place, to avoid accidental damage.

Additional Types of Laboratories

"Moderately complex" laboratories perform more detailed and involved tests. There are more rules governing this type of laboratory. People

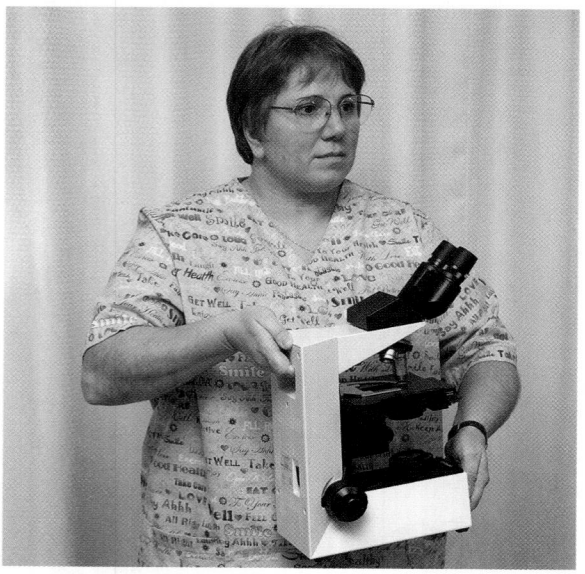

FIGURE 40-2 Carry a microscope safely, with one hand under the base and the other hand firmly grasping the arm of the microscope.

who work in these laboratories must have more education and training than workers in POLs, because they have more responsibilities. "Highly complex" testing laboratories, also called **reference laboratories,** are the labs where the most difficult and technical tests are performed. As the complexity and difficulty of the tests increase, so do the rules and regulations guiding the facilities that perform these tests: highly complex means highly regulated.

All types of laboratories must maintain quality control and have quality assurance policies and procedures. This is critical to ensure accuracy of testing and results. Health care decisions for clients depend on these lab results. The safety of both client and worker must be guarded.

■ MANUAL AND AUTOMATED TESTING

Laboratory testing is sometimes done by the **manual method,** which means that a laboratory worker does the testing, applies the theory, and performs the mathematical calculations. The medical assistant must be thoroughly knowledgeable and accurate to avoid errors and incorrect test results when using the manual method. With an **automated method** of testing, a testing instrument or machine tests the sample and does the mathematical calculations to arrive at the test results. This process is quicker, and there is less chance of error with an automated method. However, the medical assistant must strictly follow the manufacturer's directions to ensure accurate functioning of an automated system. Automated systems are becoming more common in all facilities.

There is a close relationship between the medical office setting and clinical testing laboratories, even when the medical assistant works in an office setting that does not perform any tests on site. In these settings, the medical assistant still has a role in laboratory testing. The medical assistant must understand the purpose of the test. The medical assistant usually must prepare the client for the test, and sometimes must obtain the sample. The specimen must be properly labeled, processed, and sent to the correct laboratory. The complex laboratory may do the testing, but the report of the results will come back to the medical office. When the report is received, the medical assistant must promptly inform the doctor of the findings. The medical assistant must report all findings and file them correctly. The receipt and reporting of laboratory results are done according to office policy. It is up to the medical assistant to know and follow all policies and procedures.

■ OCCUPATIONAL SAFETY AND HEALTH ADMINISTRATION

The primary purpose of the **Occupational Safety and Health Administration (OSHA)** is to ensure the safety and health of all workers. This applies to all places of employment, not just laboratories or medical offices. OSHA sets standards and rules that all employment settings must follow. If a facility is inspected and found not to be following even one regulation, the office can be cited and penalized with a monetary fine. Other restrictions may also be placed on a noncompliant facility. Following the regulations and guidelines established by OSHA helps to ensure worker safety.

There are environmental controls as well as worker controls. Environmental facility controls are those pertaining to the structure of the building (again, designed to protect the worker). Eyewash stations (Figure 40-3), hoods on testing shelves and benches (Figure 40-4), safety hoods, proper ventilation, adequate lighting, and safe storage and seating all contribute to the well-being of the worker. The employer must provide **personal protective equipment (PPE)** (Figure 40-5). It is not the responsibility of the worker to supply these items. Face masks, face shields, gloves, and gowns are all examples of PPE that protects the worker's body. Safety rules for the worker also prohibit food or drink in the laboratory, both to prevent accidental injury to the worker and possible contamination of specimens.

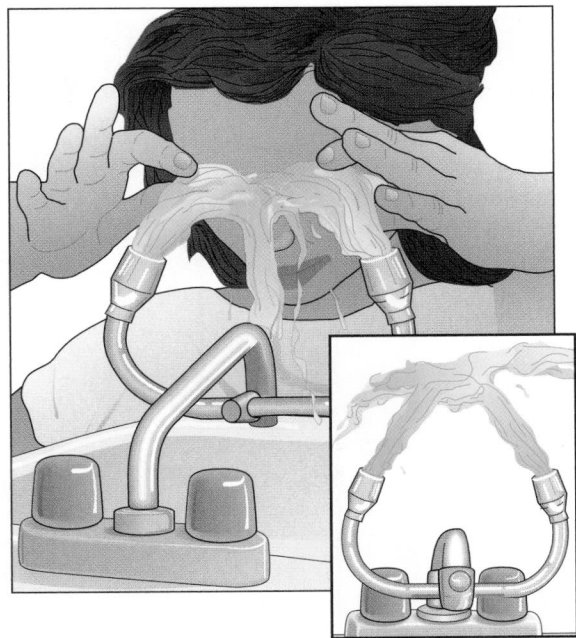

FIGURE 40-3 An eyewash station allows quick flushing in case of accidental contamination.

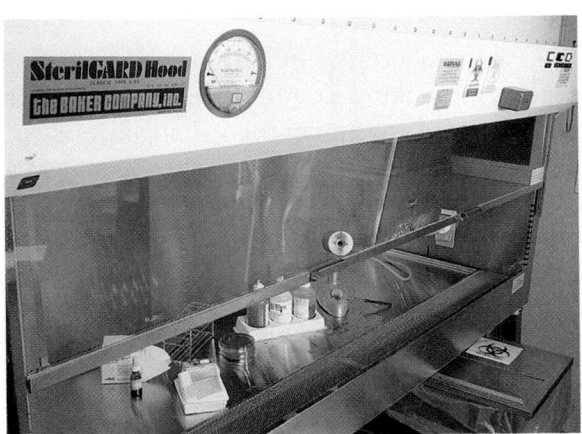

FIGURE 40-4 Safety hood in laboratory.

Nevertheless, all these built-in safety structures, and all the personal protective equipment provided, are only as good as the worker who uses them. Worker behavior and attitude are the keys to maintaining safety—for the worker and everyone else—in any setting. The worker who does not use gloves exposes herself and clients to disease or injury. The worker who does not properly close and store testing supplies, liquids, or equipment endangers not only herself but also all the other workers who use those materials.

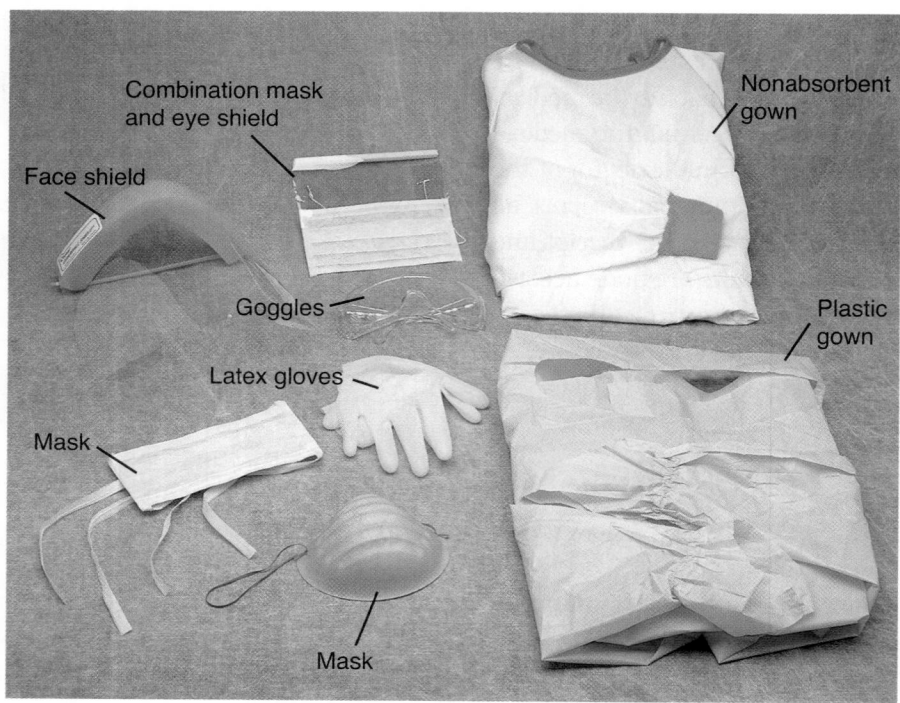

FIGURE 40-5 Personal protective equipment.

In the laboratory, **quality control** refers to a process for making sure that the test results are reliable and accurate. For this to happen, all steps along the way must be done correctly and in a safe manner. Quality control ranges from preparing the client to the final stage of giving the client the test results. Laboratories must have quality control policies and procedures that are strictly followed. These procedures always include use of a control sample to make sure that all equipment and materials are working properly. Manufacturers include instructions with their products, and these directions must be followed. Equip-ment must be checked periodically to make sure it is in good working order. This is sometimes called *instrument calibration.* Any expired testing supplies, such as reagents, must be disposed of according to the laboratory policy. Specific laboratories will establish additional regulations as part of a quality control program. Any testing facility must demonstrate continued compliance with both external and internal regulations.

Quality assurance is often maintained through a series of policies and procedures. A committee may oversee the program, making sure that the procedures are actually being fol-

LEGAL/ETHICAL THOUGHTS

Accurate coding of all procedures and tests performed in the laboratory is required. Complete documentation must support the tests and procedures that are billed to the client and/or third-party payers. Medical assistants must keep current with coding numbers and protocols, as the requirements for reimbursement are continually evaluated and revised.

lowed correctly. Are the policies followed? Who is responsible? If a problem occurs, what steps are taken to prevent it from happening again? Laboratories may require that each worker earn continuing education credits or attend a specific number of classroom hours to keep up to date with current technology and any changes in policy. This ultimately benefits the client. Each worker's competence is monitored and evaluated according to lab policy. This is the work of the committee and also the responsibility of every worker in the laboratory.

■ MEDICAL ASSISTANT LABORATORY SAFETY CONCERNS

The medical assistant working in a laboratory must be aware of safety issues and take steps to maintain a safe work environment. Hazards in the laboratory can be classified as physical, biological, or chemical dangers. *Physical hazards* can be caused by broken instruments or malfunctioning equipment. *Biological hazards* can cause disease. *Chemical hazards* include exposure to or contact with dangerous substances, such as acids or fumes from chemicals. A facility often has a written list of potential hazards found at its site. It will also have available the **Material Safety Data Sheet (MSDS)** from each manufacturer of products and supplies used in the facility. These detailed information sheets should be read by all employees (Figure 40-6). Equipment, supplies, and room areas where biohazardous materials are found are labeled with the universal biohazard symbol. This warns individuals to take the necessary precautions.

The following are some general rules and basic guidelines for working in the laboratory.

- *Never* eat, drink, or smoke in the laboratory.
- Keep hands away from eyes and mouth, to avoid accidental contact with harmful substances.
- Keep pens and pencils out of the mouth and off the face.

- Wear a lab coat over your street clothes or uniform.
- Wash hands frequently; always wash hands before putting on gloves and after removing gloves.
- Refrain from inhaling laboratory fumes.
- Wear gloves, masks, goggles, and other appropriate PPE whenever there is a chance of contact with potentially harmful substances.
- Read the manufacturer's instructions (MSDS) for safe handling of supplies and equipment.
- When pouring liquids, palm the label; pour at eye level and recap containers securely.
- Check supplies and instruments for broken glass pieces or chips. Follow office policy and directions when disposing of broken or damaged items.
- Dispose of needles and syringes in a sharps container.
- Use biohazardous waste containers for contaminated items.
- Be aware of the location of eyewash stations and First Aid equipment.
- Know where fire and chemical extinguishers are located and how to use them.
- Report any work-related incidents.
- Follow all manufacturers' safety precautions.
- Be alert and aware of your surroundings.

 **NOTE TO STUDENT:**

All the engineering and environmental safety precautions provided by the employer will not mean anything without a safety-conscious attitude on the part of workers. The medical assistant must make safety a top priority in all work situations.

MATERIAL SAFETY DATA SHEET

I – PRODUCT IDENTIFICATION

COMPANY NAME: We Wash Inc.

ADDRESS: 5035 Manchester Avenue
         Freedom, Texas 79430

Tel No:	(314) 621-1818
Nights:	(314) 621-1399
CHEMTREC:	(800) 424-9343

PRODUCT NAME: Spotfree

Product No.: 2190

Synonyms: Warewashing Detergent

II – HAZARDOUS INGREDIENTS OF MIXTURES

MATERIAL:	(CAS#)	% By Wt.	TLV	PEL
According to the OSHA Hazard Communication Standard, 29CFR 1910.1200, this product contains no hazardous ingredients.		N/A	N/A	NA

III – PHYSICAL DATA

Vapor Pressure, mm Hg: N/A
Evaporation Rate (ether=1): N/A
Solubility in H_2O: Complete
Freezing Point F: N/A
Boiling Point F: N/A
Specific Gravity H_2O=1 @25C: N/A

Vapor Density (Air=1) 60–90F: N/A
% Volatile by wt N/A
pH @ 1%   Solution 9.3–9.8
pH as Distributed: N/A
Appearance: Off-White granular powder
Odor: Mild Chemical Odor

IV – FIRE AND EXPLOSION

Flash Point F: N/AV

Flammable Limits: N/A

Extinguishing Media: The product is not flammable or combustible. Use media appropriate for the primary source of fire.

Special Fire Fighting Procedures: Use caution when fighting any fire involving chemicals. A self-contained breathing apparatus is essential.

Unusual Fire and Explosion Hazards: None Known

V – REACTIVITY DATA

Stability - Conditions to avoid: None Known

Incompatibility: Contact of carbonates or bicarbonates with acids can release large quantities of carbon dioxide and heat.

Hazardous Decomposition Products: In fire situations heat decomposition may result in the release of sulfur oxides.

Conditions Contributing to Hazardous Polymerization: N/A

FIGURE 40–6 A material safety data training sheet (Courtesy of POL Consultants, 2 Russ Farm Way, Delanco, NJ 08075; (856) 824–0800).

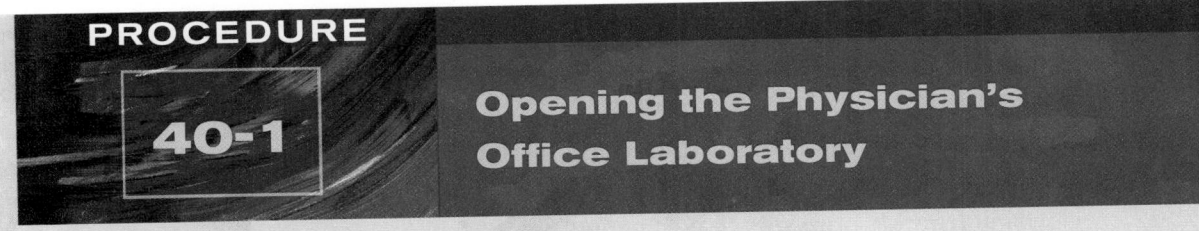

PROCEDURE

40-1

Opening the Physician's Office Laboratory

Student Competency Objective: The medical assistant student will open the physician's office laboratory.

Items Needed: Key or password codes to gain clearance to laboratory or equipment

Steps:

1. Unlock the door and turn on the lights. Arrive early enough to allow time for equipment to warm up before the first client is scheduled to arrive or the first test is scheduled to be run.

2. Wash your hands.

3. Review messages on the answering machine.

4. See if there are any fax messages.

5. Look over the activities on the day's schedule.

6. Shut off special ultraviolet lights.

7. Walk the area and switch machines on.

8. Make sure to switch machines from standby or energy-save mode to ready.

9. Take from the refrigerator any supplies that must be at room temperature for use.

10. Record on the appropriate forms the temperature readings on any equipment that must be at a certain temperature to work.

11. Put on gloves, gown, and mask (PPE) according to protocol.

12. Go through the daily control checks and record the results according to the laboratory's quality assurance policy.

13. Check the labels of disinfectants for expiration dates.

14. Make sure containers are filled and ready for use that day.

15. Make sure work surfaces that will be used that day are clean.

16. Check supplies and discard any outdated supplies according to safety standard precautions.

17. Reorder supplies as needed.

18. Arrange supplies on shelves with the newest items at the back. This helps to avoid waste from expired supplies.

19. Sign your name, the date, and the time in the appropriate record when finished with these tasks.

NOTE TO STUDENT:

To make opening and closing a POL go smoothly and safely, you should first familiarize yourself with office procedures and policies and any special or unique practices in the particular office lab. Make sure to ask questions before you are assigned this task. You will be on your own, and failure to complete the task competently can have a great impact on all the clients that day and on the other workers in the POL.

(Continues)

PROCEDURE 40-1 (Continued)

20. Look over the tests scheduled for the day.
21. Assemble items that will be needed for these tests, to stay organized and save time. (This also helps to cut down on mistakes.)
22. Review any requests or results that came in since closing the day before.
23. Inform the doctor of any new requests or results.
24. Write test results in charts per laboratory/office policy.
25. Check the sheet that lists weekly tasks.
26. Compare the weekly list to today's date.
27. Complete tasks as required.
28. Sign your name, the date, and the time on the laboratory sheet.
29. Begin the day's client testing and procedures.

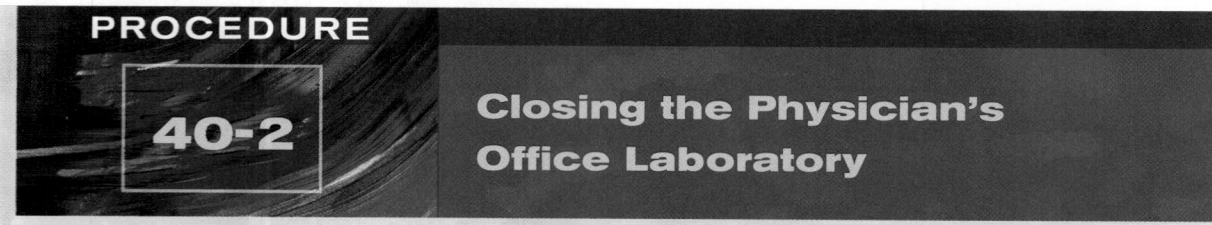

PROCEDURE
40-2
Closing the Physician's Office Laboratory

Student Competency Objective: The medical assistant student will close the physician's office laboratory.

Items Needed: Key or password code to close, lock, and shut down clearance to laboratory and equipment

Steps:

1. Using the correct form, list the activities that should be done the next day after opening the POL. Remember, you may not always be the one to reopen the laboratory. It is critical to be as clear as possible for the worker whose responsibility it will be to perform that task. This will help to prevent mistakes.
2. Send out any samples that must go to more specialized laboratories.
3. Store properly any samples that will be tested the following day.
4. Get an authorization or "all clear" from the doctor before shutting off the machines or switching to standby.
5. Put away supplies.
6. Check supplies that were received or opened that day and make sure that these supplies are dated and signed.
7. Pick up and straighten up the lab area.
8. Discard waste according to safety standard precautions.
9. Clean and sterilize equipment and supplies as necessary.
10. Clean and disinfect surfaces where lab tests are done.

(Continues)

PROCEDURE 40-2 (Continued)

11. Put medical waste into biohazardous waste containers.
12. Discard biohazardous waste container according to regulations.
13. Shut off machines or change them to power save or standby.
14. Replace items that are in low supply.
15. Check fax communications and any last messages.
16. Turn on the answering machine.
17. Wash your hands.
18. Put on special ultraviolet lights.
19. Turn off any other lights.
20. Close and lock doors and access to laboratory equipment.

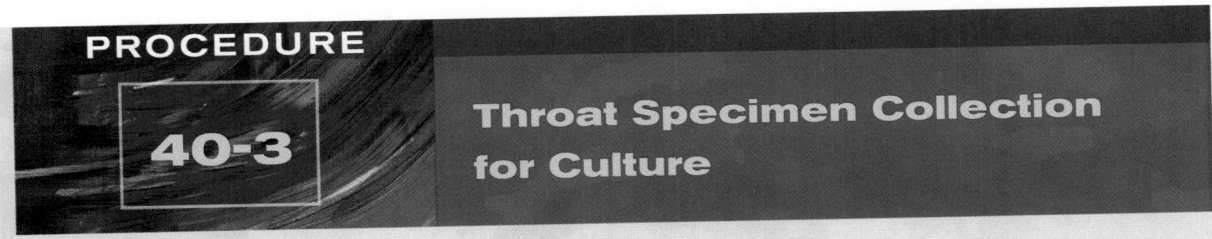

PROCEDURE 40-3

Throat Specimen Collection for Culture

Student Competency Objective: The medical assistant student will obtain a throat specimen for culture.

Items Needed: Tongue blade, sterile specimen container, sterile swab (sometimes included with specimen container), gloves, face mask, lab request form, label for specimen, pen light or examination light, biohazardous waste container, pen and paper

Steps:

1. Wash your hands.
2. Assemble equipment and supplies.
3. Introduce yourself to the client even if you have seen the client on previous visits to your office. The client may have forgotten your name. This also helps to establish a provider–client relationship, because it shows the client that you want her to know who you are.
4. Identify the client. Ask the client to state her name to establish that this is the right client, and then compare the name given to the name on the chart. Never enter a room and call out a client's name to determine if this person is the correct client. The client may not have heard you clearly and may just nod, smile, or answer yes. Clients almost never question if the medical assistant professional has the right client. It is up to the medical assistant to identify the right client before performing any procedure.
5. Tell the client, in everyday language, what you are going to do.
6. Ask if the client has any questions. If she does, give short and simple answers. Sometimes clients will start (and continue) talking because they are nervous about the procedure.
7. Ask the client to sit on the examination table.

(Continues)

PROCEDURE 40-3 (Continued)

8. Adjust the light if using an examination light.

9. Put on gloves and a face mask.

10. Take the sterile swab out of the sterile container.

11. Ask the client to open the mouth and say, "Ahhh."

12. Press on the middle of the client's tongue with a tongue blade.

13. Gently place the swab at the back of the client's throat. Firmly touch with the swab any red, inflamed, or white areas, such as at the tonsillar area. Turn the swab constantly while obtaining the specimen; this uses all areas of the swab for maximum specimen (Figure 40-7A).

14. Keep the client's tongue down with the tongue blade.

15. Take the swab out of the client's mouth. Keep the tongue depressed to avoid getting saliva on the throat specimen.

16. Put the swab into the sterile container immediately (Figure 40-7B). (Follow the directions on the container.)

17. Label the specimen container with the client's name, date, client's identification number, the part of throat from which the specimen was obtained, and other requested or required information (Figure 40-7C).

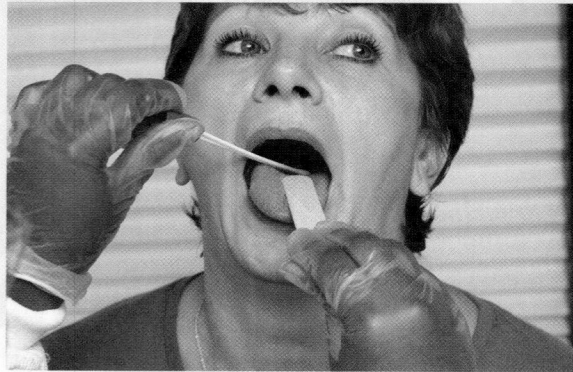

FIGURE 40-7A To obtain a throat culture, hold the client's tongue down with a tongue depressor, and place the swab at the back of the client's throat.

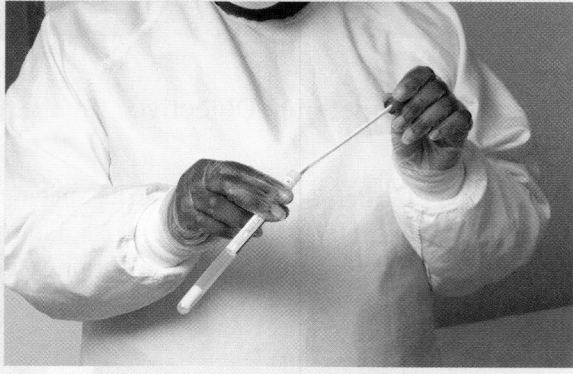

FIGURE 40-7B After removing the swab from the client's mouth, immediately place it into a sterile container.

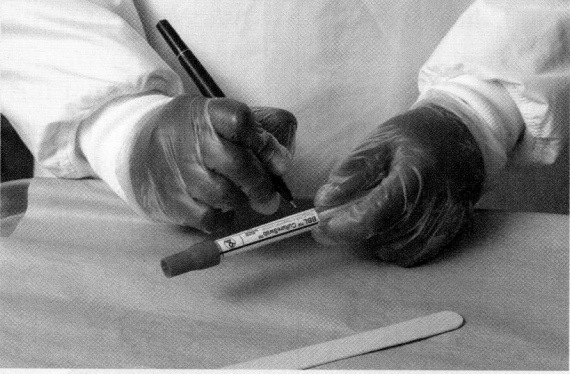

FIGURE 40-7C Prepare the container to be sent to the laboratory for testing. Make sure to label the container with all appropriate information.

(Continues)

PROCEDURE 40-3 (Continued)

18. Ask the client if she has any questions.
19. Dispose of equipment and supplies according to office policy.
20. Remove your gloves and face mask.
21. Wash your hands.
22. Record the procedure in the client's chart immediately.
23. Store and send the specimen to a laboratory for testing.

Charting Example:
9/28/20xx   9:30 A.M.   Swabbed client, throat tonsillar area to obtain specimen. Specimen obtained, labeled, and sent to lab.

Sandra Wilcox, S.M.A.

Sandra Wilcox, S.M.A. (printed name)

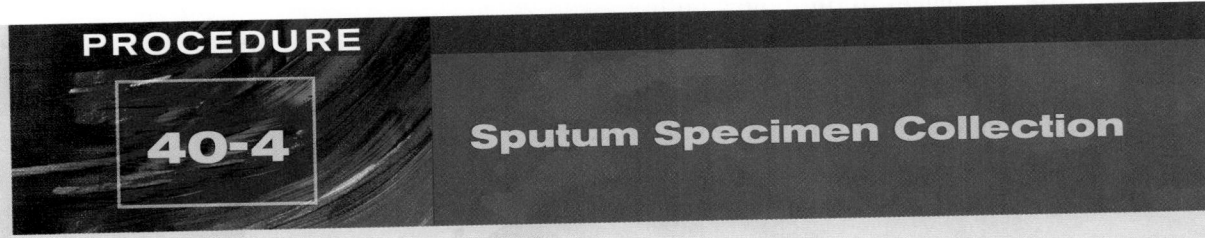

PROCEDURE 40-4 Sputum Specimen Collection

Student Competency Objective: The medical assistant student will collect a sputum specimen for culture.

Items Needed: Sterile specimen container, gloves, face mask or shield, gown, pen, paper, biohazardous waste container, lab request form and label

Steps:
1. Wash your hands.
2. Assemble equipment and supplies.
3. Introduce yourself to the client even if you have seen the client on previous visits to your office. The client may have forgotten your name. This also helps to establish a provider-client relationship, because it shows the client that you want her to know who you are.
4. Identify the client. Ask the client to state her name to establish that this is the right client, and then compare the name given to the name on the chart. Never enter a room and call out a client's name to determine if this person is the correct client. The client may not have heard you clearly and may just nod, smile, or answer yes. Clients almost never question if the medical assistant professional has the right client. It is up to the medical assistant to identify the right client before performing any procedure.
5. Tell the client, in everyday language, what you are going to do.
6. Ask if the client has any questions. If she does, give short and simple answers. Sometimes clients will start (and continue) talking because they are nervous about the procedure.

(Continues)

PROCEDURE 40-4 (Continued)

7. Ask the client to rinse the mouth well.

8. Put on gloves, gown, and face mask or face shield.

9. Instruct the client to breathe deeply and cough deeply (Figure 40–8A).

10. Tell the client to use the abdominal muscles to help cough up secretions from the lower lungs.

11. Tell the client to expectorate (spit) sputum directly into the specimen container.

12. Instruct the client not to touch the inside of the container.

13. Ask the client to avoid getting sputum on the side of the container (Figure 40–8B).

14. Immediately take the container from the client, observing standard precautions as you do so.

15. Put the lid on the container.

16. Complete the label and lab request form, including name, date, and client's identification number.

17. Instruct the client to rinse the mouth.

18. Ask the client if she has any questions.

19. Dispose of used items according to office policy.

20. Remove gloves, gown, and face mask or shield.

21. Wash your hands.

22. Send the specimen to a laboratory for testing.

23. Record the procedure in the client's chart immediately.

Charting Example:

10/13/20xx   2:30 P.M.   Assisted client with sputum specimen collection. Thick yellow sputum collected. Sent to lab.

James Hughes, S.M.A.

James Hughes, S.M.A. (printed name)

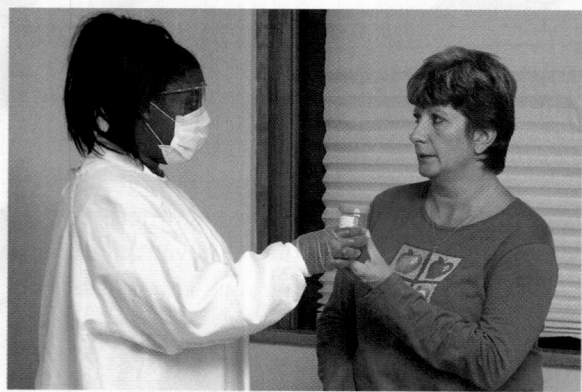

FIGURE 40–8A Instruct the client on proper sputum collection, and hand the sterile container to the client.

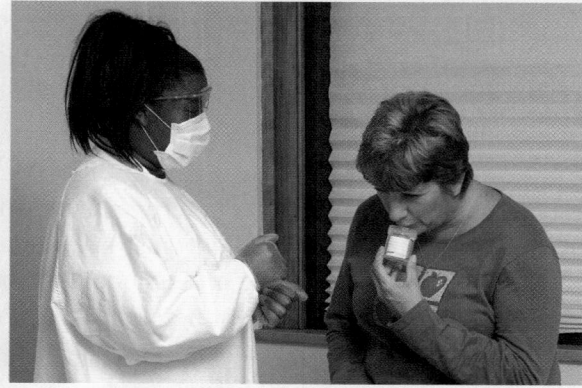

FIGURE 40–8B Tell the client to expectorate without touching the inside of the container or getting sputum on the sides of the container.

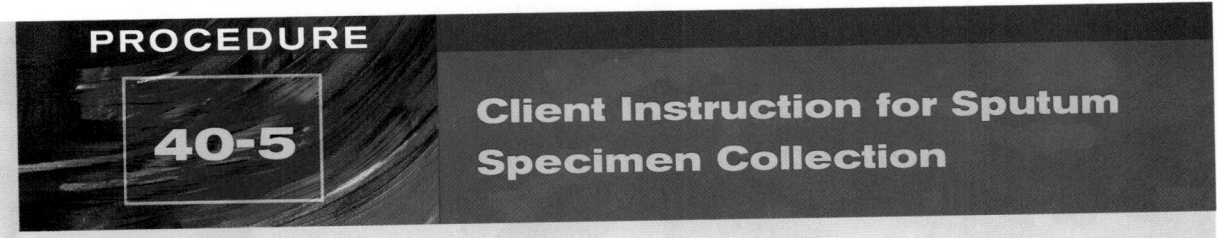

PROCEDURE 40-5

Client Instruction for Sputum Specimen Collection

Student Competency Objective: The medical assistant student will teach a client how to obtain a sputum specimen for testing.

Items Needed: Sterile specimen container, client instruction sheet (either preprinted or hand-written), label, laboratory request form, paper and pen

Steps:

1. Wash your hands.
2. Assemble equipment and supplies.
3. Introduce yourself to the client even if you have seen the client on previous visits to your office. The client may have forgotten your name. This also helps to establish a provider-client relationship, because it shows the client that you want her to know who you are.
4. Identify the client. Ask the client to state her name to establish that this is the right client, and then compare the name given to the name on the chart. Never enter a room and call out a client's name to determine if this person is the correct client. The client may not have heard you clearly and may just nod, smile, or answer yes. Clients almost never question if the medical assistant professional has the right client. It is up to the medical assistant to identify the right client before performing any procedure.
5. Tell the client, in everyday language, what you are going to do.
6. Ask if the client has any questions. If she does, give short and simple answers. Sometimes clients will start (and continue) talking because they are nervous about the procedure.
7. Tell the client that a first morning, productive cough sputum is best.
8. Using the teaching supplies, show the client how to remove the lid and not contaminate the specimen. Remind the client not to touch the inside of the container and not to get sputum on the sides of the container.
9. Tell the client not to let saliva get into the container.
10. Instruct the client to breathe deeply, cough deeply, and expectorate sputum from the lower lungs into the container.
11. Tell the client to put the lid on the container immediately after expectorating.
12. Remind the client to wash her hands after obtaining the sputum specimen.
13. Tell the client to fill in the information on the label of the container and lab request form, including name, date, and time of specimen collection.
14. Instruct the client to take the sputum specimen to the office or lab as directed by the doctor. Make sure to tell the client to refrigerate the specimen if the specimen cannot be delivered to the testing site within two hours.
15. Give written, step-by-step instructions to the client.
16. Ask the client if she has any questions.

(Continues)

PROCEDURE 40-5 (Continued)

17. Wash your hands.
18. Record the procedure in the client's chart immediately.

Charting Example:

4/12/20xx   8:30 A.M.   Client instructed with step-by-step directions to obtain a sputum specimen at home. Instructed to bring specimen to lab immediately. Answered client's questions. Written instructions given.

Virginia McIsaac, S.M.A.

Virginia McIsaac, S.M.A. (printed name)

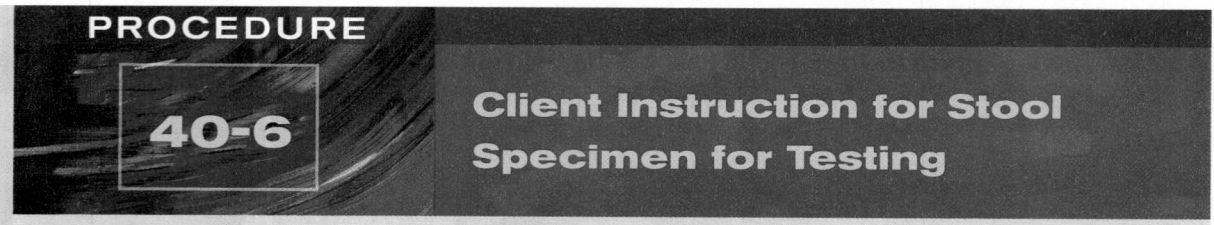

PROCEDURE

40-6   Client Instruction for Stool Specimen for Testing

Student Competency Objective: The medical assistant student will teach a client to obtain a stool specimen for testing.

Items Needed: Stool specimen container, tongue depressors (sometimes a commercial specimen kit contains all the items needed), client instruction sheet (either preprinted or handwritten), label, laboratory request form, paper and pen

Steps:

1. Wash your hands.
2. Assemble equipment and supplies.
3. Introduce yourself to the client even if you have seen the client on previous visits to your office. The client may have forgotten your name. This also helps to establish a provider-client relationship, because it shows the client that you want her to know who you are.
4. Identify the client. Ask the client to state her name to establish that this is the right client, and then compare the name given to the name on the chart. Never enter a room and call out a client's name to determine if this person is the correct client. The client may not have heard you clearly and may just nod, smile, or answer yes. Clients almost never question if the medical assistant professional has the right client. It is up to the medical assistant to identify the right client before performing any procedure.
5. Tell the client, in everyday language, what you are going to do.
6. Ask if the client has any questions. If she does, give short and simple answers. Sometimes clients will start (and continue) talking because they are nervous about the procedure.
7. Instruct the client to obtain stool or feces from the next bowel movement.
8. Inform the client to urinate first; no urine should be mixed with the stool specimen.

(Continues)

PROCEDURE 40-6 (Continued)

9. Show the client how to use the kit or how to use the tongue depressor and specimen container to obtain a stool specimen.

10. Tell the client that nothing but stool or feces should be in the container. This includes toilet paper.

11. Instruct the client to put the lid on the container immediately after putting the specimen in the container.

12. Remind the client to wash her hands after obtaining a stool specimen.

13. Fill out the label with the client's name; have the client fill in the date and time the specimen was collected.

14. Complete the laboratory request form with the required information.

15. Tell the client to bring the specimen container to the office or lab as directed by the doctor within two hours after obtaining the specimen (if this is not possible, the specimen must be refrigerated).

16. Give the client written instructions for reference at home.

17. Ask the client if she has any questions.

18. Record the procedure in the client's chart immediately.

Charting Example:

5/16/20xx   3:00 P.M.   Instructed client with step-by-step directions to obtain a stool specimen at home and to bring to office as directed by doctor. Gave written instructions and answered client's questions.

Timothy Balk, S.M.A.

Timothy Balk, S.M.A. (printed name)

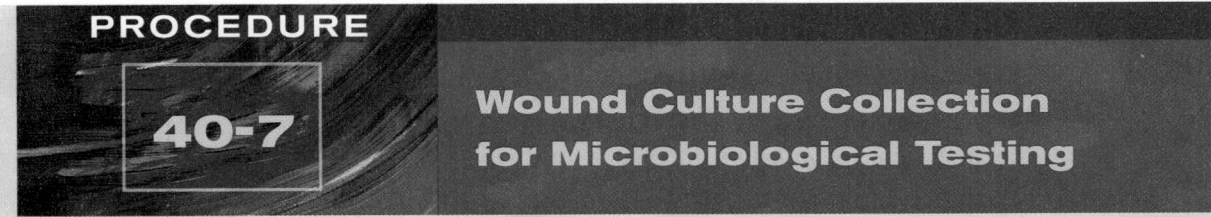

PROCEDURE
40-7
Wound Culture Collection for Microbiological Testing

Student Competency Objective: The medical assistant student will collect a specimen from a wound for microbiological testing.

Items Needed: Culture tube, swab, gloves and other PPE (such as mask, gown, and eye protection as needed), sterile gauze, sterile saline solution, cleansing agent, alcohol wipes, biohazardous waste container

Steps:

1. Wash your hands.

2. Assemble equipment and supplies.

(Continues)

PROCEDURE 40-7 (Continued)

3. Introduce yourself to the client even if you have seen the client on previous visits to your office. The client may have forgotten your name. This also helps to establish a provider-client relationship, because it shows the client that you want her to know who you are.

4. Identify the client. Ask the client to state her name to establish that this is the right client, and then compare the name given to the name on the chart. Never enter a room and call out a client's name to determine if this person is the correct client. The client may not have heard you clearly and may just nod, smile, or answer yes. Clients almost never question if the medical assistant professional has the right client. It is up to the medical assistant to identify the right client before performing any procedure.

5. Tell the client, in everyday language, what you are going to do.

6. Ask if the client has any questions. If she does, give short and simple answers. Sometimes clients will start (and continue) talking because they are nervous about the procedure.

7. Reassure the client and instruct her not to move during the procedure.

8. Put on gloves and other PPE as needed.

9. Look at the wound and note its size, color, and smell (if any).

10. Using the sterile saline solution, rinse the wound if you noted pus or other drainage. (This helps ensure that the specimen is taken from within the wound.)

11. Using the sterile gauze, gently dry the area.

12. Dispose of the used gauze in the biohazardous waste container.

13. Remove contaminated gloves, wash your hands, and put on clean gloves.

14. Pick up the sterile swab.

15. With one gloved hand, hold the wound area. With the other gloved hand, rotate the swab over the wound, being careful not to wipe the edges of the wound. (You want to collect organisms from within the wound, not the surface of the skin.)

16. Put the swab in the culture tube.

17. Label the tube and fill out other lab forms.

18. Ask the client if she has any questions.

19. Send the wound culture specimen to the lab.

20. Clean the area. Remove your PPE and wash your hands.

21. Record the procedure in the client's chart immediately.

Charting Example:

10/14/20xx   11:15 A.M.   Obtained wound specimen from client's right forearm as ordered. Wound 1" by 2" with moderate amount of drainage; no odor noted. Specimen obtained, labeled, and sent to lab per doctor's order. Client instructed to call doctor at the end of the week for test results.

Susan Maloney, S.M.A.

Susan Maloney, S.M.A. (printed name)

BRIDGE TO CAAHEP

This chapter, which discusses the physician office laboratory, provides information and content related to CAAHEP standards for Anatomy and Physiology, Medical Terminology, Medical Law and Ethics, Psychology, Communication, Medical Assisting Administrative Procedures, Medical Assisting Clinical Procedures, and Professional Components.

ABHES LINKS

This chapter, which discusses the physician office laboratory, links to ABHES course content for Anatomy and Physiology, Medical Terminology, Medical Law and Ethics, Psychology of Human Relations, Medical Office Clinical Procedures, Medical Laboratory Procedures, Operational Functions, and Career Development.

AAMA AREAS OF COMPETENCE

This chapter, which discusses the physician office laboratory, provides information or content within several areas listed in the Medical Assistant Role Delineation Study. These areas include: administrative, administrative procedures, clinical, fundamental principles, diagnostic orders, patient (client) care, general transdisciplinary, professionalism, communication skills, legal concepts, instruction, and operational functions.

AMT PATHS

This chapter, which discusses the physician office laboratory, provides a path to AMT competency in general medical assisting knowledge, anatomy and physiology, medical terminology, medical law, medical ethics, human relations, patient (client) education, clinical medical assisting, asepsis, sterilization, instruments, and laboratory procedures.

POINTS OF HIGHLIGHT

- Reasons for performing laboratory tests include screening for abnormal conditions, making differential diagnoses of disorders, and monitoring progress or treatment.
- Medical assistants frequently work in physician's office laboratories.
- The Clinical Laboratory Improvement Amendments of 1988 are federal laws and regulations that govern all facilities that conduct laboratory testing for health care clients.
- Laboratories can be grouped according to the type of testing performed. The three types are waived or low complexity, moderate complexity, and high complexity.
- Quality control is a process to make sure that test results are reliable and accurate.
- Quality assurance is safeguarded through a series of policies and procedures that are consistently followed by all workers at the site.
- Accuracy in all the steps of the laboratory testing process must be maintained to ensure that test results are valid; these results ultimately affect client outcomes.
- The medical assistant's attitude and behavior regarding safety are the most important factor in maintaining a safe work environment.

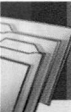

STUDENT PORTFOLIO ACTIVITY

Find out when job fairs and informational meetings are scheduled at your school. Check for additional locations of job fairs in your community. At these settings you can find out about prospective employers. They will be able to tell you about current openings and the skills they need in employees. This allows you to form an initial impression of a particular employer's setting and whether those jobs match your skills and interests. Afterward, review your portfolio in light of employers' comments about what they look for in employees.

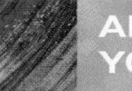

APPLYING YOUR SKILLS

You have been hired to work as a medical assistant in a POL. How could you find out your role and responsibilities as a medical assistant in this type of work setting? What resources would you use? What qualities of a medical assistant are helpful in this setting?

CRITICAL THINKING QUESTIONS

1. How would a medical assistant find out what tests are performed in a POL?

2. What are the reasons for laboratory testing?

3. Explain how the Occupational Safety and Health Administration affects the medical assistant's work in the POL.

4. What does CLIA mean, and what is the purpose of CLIA?

5. Why do POLs have to institute and practice quality control measures?

6. Why is the attitude of the medical assistant who works in a clinical laboratory so important to the safety of the environment?

7. Laboratory testing may be done for screening. What does this mean? Give an example.

8. How does CLIA relate to your role as a medical assistant?

9. If a medical assistant works in an office setting that does not perform laboratory testing, what role will that medical assistant play in the laboratory testing process?

10. You see a fellow laboratory worker throw contaminated items into a wastebasket. How do you respond? Who does this unsafe action affect?

11. Go back to the beginning of this chapter and review the Anticipatory Statements. Reread each statement and then indicate whether it is true or false. If the statement is false, rewrite it to make it a true statement.

Anticipatory Statements

Read and think about the following statements based upon what you believe now. Decide whether you agree or disagree. Write the word **agree** after the statement if you think the statement is true. Write the word **disagree** after the statement if you think the statement is false. Read the chapter to find out if your current beliefs can be supported.

1. Dark-yellow urine indicates disease.   _____

2. Urine is rarely tested in the doctor's office.   _____

3. Only a lab worker can test urine.   _____

4. A urine specimen should be refrigerated unless tested immediately.   _____

5. Urinalysis can provide important information about the working of the kidneys and urinary system.   _____

Learning Objectives

Upon completion of this chapter, the medical assistant student should be able to:

- List the three main reasons for urine testing
- Define the types of urine testing
- Identify methods of urine specimen collection
- Explain urethral catheterization
- Demonstrate testing of a urine specimen using a reagent strip
- State five safety practices when collecting, labeling, and processing urine specimens
- Develop a teaching plan and teach another person how to obtain a urine specimen at home for testing

Urinalysis

Key Terms

clean-catch Method of collecting a urine sample; reduces the possibility of contamination from the area near the urinary meatus.

double-voided Method of collecting urine sample that involves voiding or urinating twice.

gestational Pertains to pregnancy.

glucose tolerance test (GTT) Test to determine the metabolism of glucose in the body.

phenylketonuria (PKU) Disorder in which the amino acid phenylalanine cannot be changed to tyrosine. Untreated, PKU can lead to severe cognitive impairments. Screening is done within a few days after birth.

postprandial After a meal; some urine specimens are collected at a specific time after the client has eaten.

random In urine testing, refers to a sample taken at any time of the day.

reagent test strip Plastic or cardboard strips that have chemicals within; used to test for substances in the urine.

refractometer Instrument used to measure the specific gravity of urine; uses a light, prism, and scale.

renal threshold Level at which a substance begins to "spill over" from the kidney into the urine.

specimen Sample or part representing the whole of a tissue or substance.

urinalysis Testing of a sample of urine; may include physical, chemical, and/or microscopic examinations.

urinometer Instrument used to measure specific gravity of urine; uses a float with a stem and a scale.

■ INTRODUCTION

The collection, processing, and testing of urine is one of the most frequently performed procedures in the medical office. The medical assistant will take part in some or all of the steps involved. The collection of urine is a simple and almost always noninvasive procedure, because a urine **specimen** is easily attainable. Routine urine tests yield valuable information and are relatively inexpensive to process.

■ URINE TESTS

Urine tests are used to screen for, diagnose, and monitor disorders. There are three major types of urine tests: random, timed, and eight-hour. The type of test will determine what kind of urine specimen is to be used and how it is collected.

Random Tests

Random testing of urine specimens is frequently performed in the physician's office. No special client preparation is needed before testing. Random testing of urine is useful to check if a substance or indicator is present, so this kind of testing is often done for routine screening and to screen for use of illegal drugs.. This type of test is not helpful to determine a specific amount of a substance over time.

Timed Tests

Timed urine tests are selected when it is important to check for a substance or find the amount of a substance within a specified range of time. In these tests, urine is collected at specific times or intervals. An example of a timed test is the *two-hour postprandial* specimen. **Postprandial** means after meals. This test is frequently done to determine glucose metabolism. The client eats a meal high in carbohydrates. This meal can be at any time of the day. Two hours later, a urine specimen is collected. Tests are run on the urine specimen for glucose. The purpose of the postprandial test is to diagnose diabetes mellitus.

Glucose Tolerance Test. A related timed test is the **glucose tolerance test (GTT)**. After the client fasts for 12 hours, a urine specimen is collected. Following this, the client drinks a glucose solution. Urine is collected at the timed intervals of one-half hour, one hour, and two hours after the client drinks the glucose solution. If the client is slow to metabolize the glucose, additional samples will be obtained at three hours and four hours. Blood samples are also collected during this test. This test is used to diagnose diabetes mellitus. It is also used to check for **gestational** diabetes. Clients with other endocrine disorders may also have abnormal test findings.

Double-Voided Tests. **Double-voided** means that two specimens are collected, separated by an exact amount of time. This is done to check for the concentration of a substance. The second specimen collected is the freshest specimen and best reflects the concentration of the substance being examined. Glucose and ketones are most frequently checked with this type of specimen collection.

Eight-Hour Tests

First morning specimens are the third type of urine specimen. These are also called *eight-hour specimens, overnight*, or *early morning specimens.* The urine collected is the first urine void of the morning. Concentration of substances in the urine is usually greatest at this time. It is important that this be an eight-hour specimen. If the client gets up during the night to urinate, the accuracy of the test will be affected. The urine will not have contained the substances for the required time period, so the result will not accurately reflect the substances excreted. A first morning urine specimen is the preferred method when performing a urine pregnancy test. Human chorionic gonadotropin (hCG) is a hormone secreted by the placenta shortly after conception. Because this hormone is most concentrated in the first morning voided urine, this test detects the level and can confirm or rule out pregnancy. This urine test can be performed even before the first missed menstrual period.

A 24-hour urine specimen is a timed test that looks not only at the concentration of a substance, but also at the volume of urine excreted. The specimen is collected over an exact 24-hour time period. These tests are normally performed in a reference laboratory. However, the medical assistant will need to instruct the client regarding the collection steps.

Timed tests may also be ordered for a specific time of day when the targeted substance is normally at its highest amount.

■ METHODS OF COLLECTION

Methods or ways to collect urine are chosen depending on the test ordered, the client, and the clinical setting. Certain tests necessitate a particular method of collection. Client factors also play a role. Is the client able to follow directions? Is there a problem with mobility (for example, will the client need assistance in the bathroom)? In what kind of setting is the collection taking place (a physician's office, a clinic, or a laboratory)? Will the specimen be tested on site or sent out? All these factors will determine the method of collection and the instructions that the client will receive from the medical assistant.

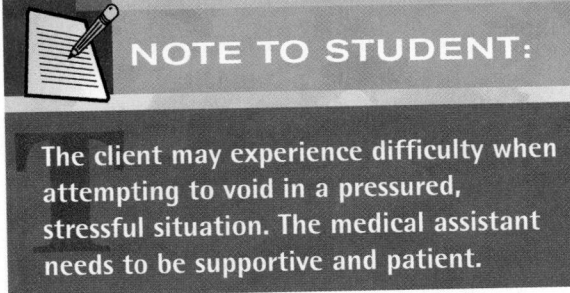

NOTE TO STUDENT:

The client may experience difficulty when attempting to void in a pressured, stressful situation. The medical assistant needs to be supportive and patient.

Random

A random or routine collection is a simple, easy way of collecting a urine specimen; this method is often used in a doctor's office. The client does not need to do anything special in preparation for the collection. The client is given a nonsterile container and asked to go to the bathroom and urinate into the container.

Clean-Catch

The **clean-catch** method is sometimes referred to as *midstream specimen collection*. Clean-catch collection may be required for various reasons. For example, a client is suspected of having a urinary tract infection, and a urine sample is needed to determine the specific antibiotic that should be used to treat the infection. In this case, it is essential to test bacteria from the bladder and not the surrounding areas. Client factors may also necessitate use of this method. For example, if the client is experiencing menstrual bleeding or any vaginal discharge, the clean-catch method is used to avoid contamination by the discharge. To collect a clean-catch urine specimen, the urinary meatus must be thoroughly cleansed. This is done to avoid contamination of the urine specimen by organisms at the urinary meatus. The client begins to urinate and then stops. This gets rid of any urine present in the distal urethra. The client then takes the sterile container and voids about 3 to 4 ounces of urine into it. The client finishes urinating into the toilet (see Procedure 41-1).

24-Hour

The amount of a substance excreted in the urine can vary throughout the day. To get the most accurate results, it is often necessary to collect all of the urine excreted over a 24-hour period. For example, the client is in the office at 10:00 a.m. and the doctor wants the test to begin immediately. The client is asked to void and discard the urine in the toilet. The 24-hour test is then said to have begun at 10:00 a.m. All the urine expelled over the next 24 hours is collected and saved. At 10:00 a.m. the next day, the client voids and saves that sample to complete the 24-hour collection. The laboratory will

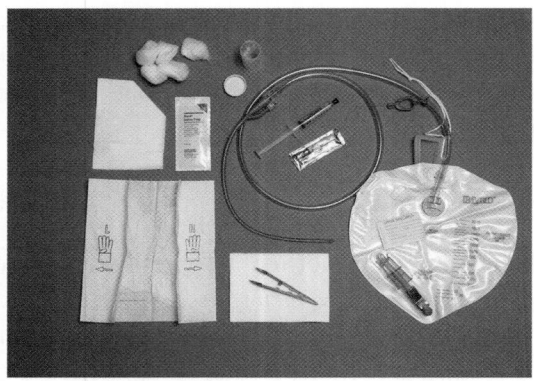

FIGURE 41-1 Urinary catheter.

record the amount or volume of urine and then begin the analysis of substances.

Urethral Catheterization

A sterile urinary catheter (tube) may be inserted into the urinary bladder to collect a urine specimen; this is called a *urethral catheterization* (Figure 41-1). Catheterization must be done using strict sterile technique to avoid causing an infection. This collection method is used when a client cannot void or cannot give a sample using a less invasive method.

■ URINE SPECIMEN PROCESSING

The medical assistant needs to follow guidelines when processing the collected urine specimen.

Container

The type of container used is determined by the test ordered. The most common type of container for routine urine collection is a small plastic container with a lid (Figure 41-2A). The container holds about 100 to 200 mL of urine. The lid should be a screw-on type, to make a good seal and prevent leaking or splashing when the cap is placed on the container. For clean-catch specimens, these plastic containers often come sealed in a clear plastic wrap. The container also has a sticky tab sealing the lid to the container. If the seal is broken, the container

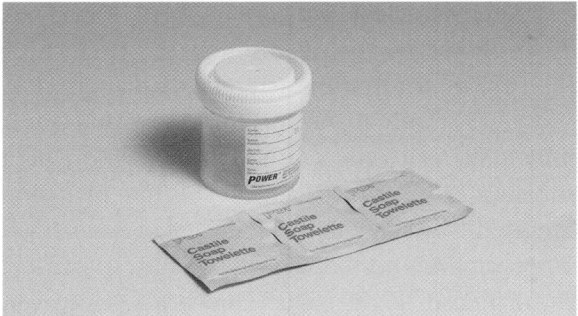

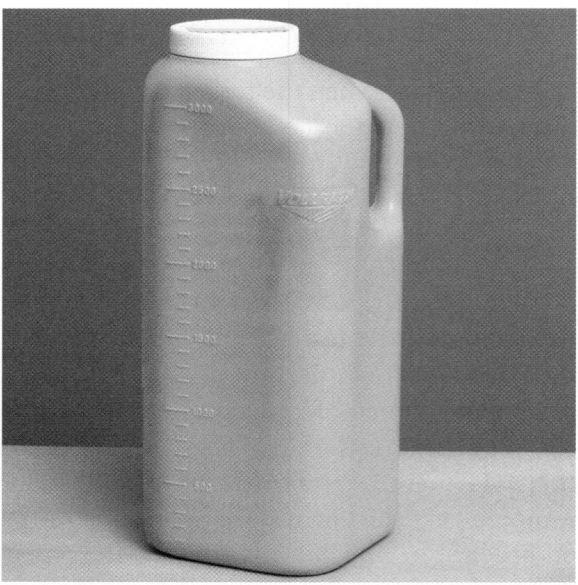

FIGURE 41-2 Urine collection containers: (A) Clean-catch method (B) 24-hour method.

should not be used, because sterility cannot be guaranteed. A 24-hour urine collection container is usually a dark-colored (because it must be resistant to light), plastic container similar to a gallon jug (Figure 41-2B). A preservative may be inside the container. In addition to a screw-on lid, the rim or edge of the container must be wide (wide mouth) to avoid spilling urine. These large containers hold about 3,000 mL.

Labeling

It is critical to label or mark the container immediately upon collection of a urine specimen. The client's name, the date, the time of collection, and the collection method should be written on the label (Figure 41-3). If the specimen is to be sent to an outside laboratory, a requisition slip

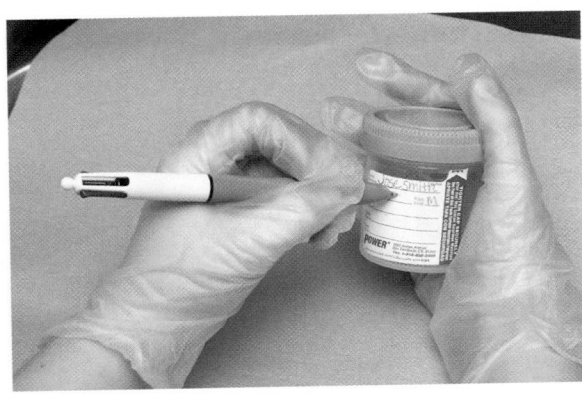

FIGURE 41-3 Label the urine collection container with the client's name, date, time, and collection method used.

must also be completed. Always label the container, not the lid. If the lid is labeled, the urine container will no longer have any identification on it when the lid is removed. If the urine specimen is to be sent to a laboratory outside the physician's office or specimen collection setting, more people are involved in the process. Extra steps must be taken to ensure that the transition from the client to the testing facility is smooth, so that the test results will be an accurate reflection of the client's urinary system functioning.

■ URINALYSIS

One of the most commonly performed urine tests is the **urinalysis.** A complete urinalysis or examination of urine consists of three separate examinations, although sometimes only certain factors or properties are examined. To be complete, the urinalysis must include physical, chemical, and microscopic examinations.

Physical Examination

The physical examination of urine involves assessment or testing without chemicals or a microscope. Four properties or characteristics of urine are examined: (1) color, (2) clarity, (3) odor, and (4) specific gravity.

Color. The normal color of urine falls within the yellow range. Urine may look very slightly yel-

low; sometimes it may appear almost colorless. The urine may also be a very dark yellow. Any shade of yellow between the two extremes can fall in the normal range. Several factors can affect the color of the urine but not indicate disease. For example, a client voids right before coming into the examination room. He then drinks a glass of water so that he can give a urine sample before the visit is over. The urine sample will appear almost colorless, looking like water. One way to avoid this is to request that clients check with the medical assistant before using the bathroom, in case a sample is needed.

Clarity. The *clarity* of urine refers to the appearance of the urine. Urine should look clear or transparent. You should be able to look through the urine and see an object behind it. The appearance of urine is described as clear, slightly cloudy, cloudy, or very cloudy. Each office will have guidelines to help the medical assistant decide what falls in each of these groups. Urine must be looked at while it is still fresh. Healthy urine can become cloudy if left standing. Several factors may cause urine to look cloudy. Blood, red blood cells, white blood cells, bacteria, sperm, lipids (fat), mucous threads, and other contaminants in the urine may cause cloudiness. Any freshly voided urine that is cloudy should undergo additional tests.

Odor. The odor of urine is not considered a diagnostic test, but is done as part of the physical examination of urine. Freshly voided healthy urine has a characteristic slight odor. If the urine sample is concentrated, the odor will be stronger. If the urine sample is left standing for a while, it will smell like ammonia, because of the breakdown of urea by bacteria. Foods can cause different smells to the urine. For example, asparagus can cause a musty smell. Certain conditions can also cause distinctive odors. Foul-smelling urine may indicate an infection. A fruity odor may be present in a person who has diabetes mellitus. **Phenylketonuria (PKU)** may cause a mousy odor. A maple-syrup smell is found with maple syrup urinary disease.

Specific Gravity. Specific gravity compares the weight of urine with an equal amount of distilled water (pure water). Urine contains both water and dissolved substances. The dissolved substances give urine its weight. Testing for specific gravity can show how well the kidneys concentrate urine. The specific gravity of distilled water is 1.000. The normal specific gravity of urine ranges from 1.005 to 1.030, but can vary greatly. The amount of fluid a person drinks and his resulting state of hydration will affect the urine specific gravity: the more fluid, the less concentration of dissolved substances and therefore a lower number; the less fluid, the more concentration of dissolved substances and therefore a higher number. The time of day may affect the test. Normally the urine is more concentrated in the first morning void, because the urine has stayed in the bladder all night.

Diseases or disorders may affect the urine specific gravity. If the kidneys cannot concentrate the urine, the specific gravity will be down. Low specific gravity occurs with diabetes insipidus, chronic renal insufficiency, and malignant hypertension. Hepatic disease, adrenal insufficiency, diabetes mellitus, and congestive heart failure can cause a high urine specific gravity reading. In addition, if a person is dehydrated, the urine will be more concentrated and thus yield a high specific gravity number. This can happen with vomiting, diarrhea, and sustained fever.

The medical assistant can test the specific gravity of urine using one of three methods: a reagent strip, a **urinometer,** or a **refractometer.** Only a drop of urine is needed when using a **reagent test strip** to test for specific gravity (Figure 41-4). After obtaining a urine sample, the medical assistant dips the reagent strip into the urine and quickly takes it out. Often these strips are called *dipsticks*. After waiting the required number of seconds, the medical assistant compares the color on the spot marked "specific gravity" with the accompanying color chart. A much greater amount of urine is needed when using a urinometer. At least 15 mL of urine are placed in a cylinder. The urinometer is then placed in the cylinder with a spinning motion,

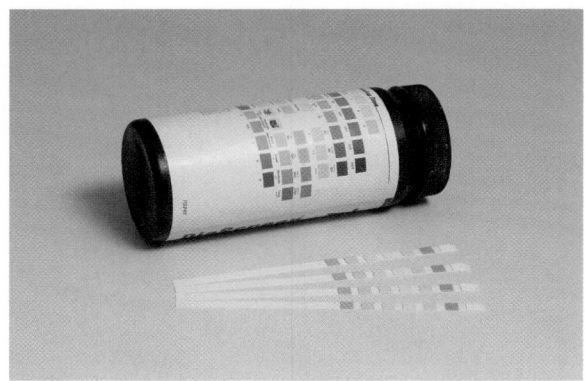

FIGURE 41-4 Chemical reagent dip strips with color-coded chart.

and the number on the stem at the curvature of the liquid is read. In contrast, the refractometer uses only a drop of urine (Figure 41-5). This commonly used method employs a scale to obtain the specific gravity number (Figure 41-6). This method uses the speed of light traveling through air compared with light traveling through urine to calculate the specific gravity.

Chemical Examination

When the medical assistant has completed the physical examination, a chemical examination of the urine specimen is done. Many substances can be present in the urine, in varying

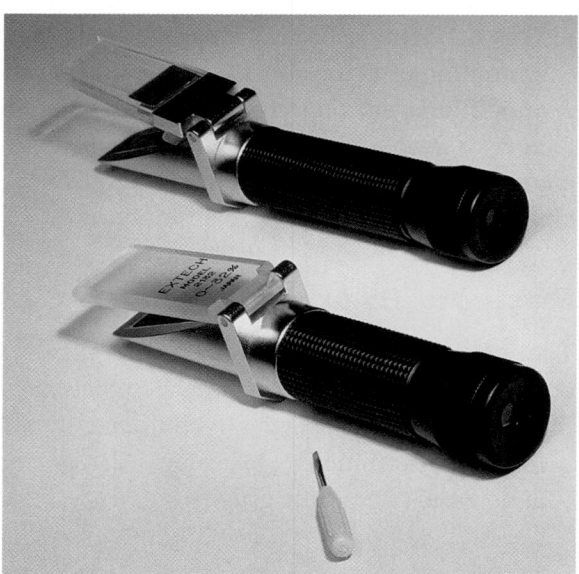

FIGURE 41-5 Refractometer.

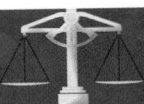

LEGAL/ETHICAL THOUGHTS

The medical assistant may enter results from urine testing into the computer. To preserve confidentiality, always make sure that the computer screen is positioned so that others cannot view the client's information.

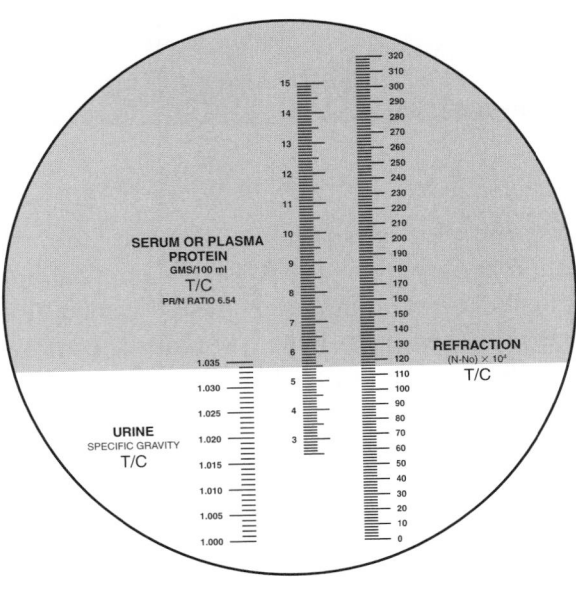

FIGURE 41-6 Specific gravity as viewed through a refractometer.

amounts. The presence, absence, or amount of a specific chemical can help detect or diagnose many disorders. Testing for many substances has become simplified with the use of chemical reagent strips. These thin, narrow plastic strips have different-colored, square pads along the strip, each marked with the name of a substance. After the medical assistant obtains a urine sample from the client, he dips the strip into the urine and then quickly removes it. Each pad is compared with the corresponding pad on a color chart provided by the test-strip manufacturer. The strips must be cared for and stored properly, as light, moisture, and heat can damage the strips and make the results unreliable.

Chemical reagent strips can be used to test for pH, glucose, proteins, ketones, blood, biliru-

bin, urobilinogen, nitrite, and leukocytes (white blood cells).

The *pH* refers to the acidity or alkalinity of the urine. The lower the number; the more acidic the urine. Conversely, the higher the number, the more alkaline or basic the urine. Normal urine pH ranges from 5 to 8, with a reading of 7 considered neutral. Normal urine is slightly acidic, and a reading of 6 is very common. The urine must be freshly voided or the reading can be falsely high. A very alkaline reading from a freshly voided urine sample may indicate an infection of the urinary tract.

The kidneys filter and reabsorb glucose. Normal urine should contain no glucose. If all the glucose cannot be absorbed and the level of glucose in the blood rises too high, glucose will "spill over" into the urine. At this point the glucose has reached the **renal threshold.** Glucose in the urine is called *glycosuria.* The most common cause of glycosuria is diabetes mellitus.

Increased amounts of protein in the urine are usually a sign of a disorder. Kidney disease and urinary tract infections can cause a high amount of protein in the urine. This condition is called *proteinuria.* A temporary increase in protein in the urine can be caused by pregnancy or strenuous physical exercise.

Ketones should not be found in normal urine. The presence of ketones means that the body is burning more fat than is normal. Uncontrolled diabetes, a starvation diet, or a fad diet extremely high in fat are possible causes of this finding.

Blood is not normally found in urine. The presence of blood can mean that there has been an injury to the urinary tract, or that the client has a kidney disorder, an infection, or cancer.

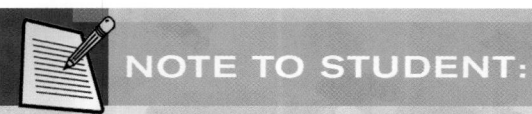

NOTE TO STUDENT:

Blood may be found in the urine of a woman during her menstrual flow when the urine sample has been contaminated by blood from vaginal menstrual flow. The urine test will have to be repeated when the woman's menstrual period is over, to avoid missing any disorder or false positives from the menstrual blood.

Normally, bilirubin is processed in the liver and excreted into the bile. Certain disorders of the liver, such as hepatitis, stones, or cirrhosis, may cause bilirubin to be found in the urine. This is called *bilirubinuria*. Bilirubin is changed to urobilinogen in the intestines by the action of bacteria. An increase in bilirubin will also mean an increase in urobilinogen. In addition to liver disorders, congestive heart failure and infectious mononucleosis may also cause an increase of urobilinogen in the urine.

The presence of nitrite in the urine, as detected by the reagent test strip, often indicates a urinary tract infection. Nitrites are formed from nitrates by the action of bacteria.

A positive test for leukocytes (white blood cells) usually signals a lower urinary tract infection or an infection or inflammation in the kidneys.

NOTE TO STUDENT:

When obtaining a urine specimen from a female client, it is best to use the clean-catch method. Secretions from the vagina may contain leukocytes, which would give a false positive reading.

Microscopic Examination

Microscopic examination of the urine sediment often confirms the results of the physical and chemical examinations. A freshly voided, first morning specimen is best because it contains the highest concentration of sediments. The urine is centrifuged in preparation for testing. Several structures can be examined during this testing. The examiner looks for red blood cells, white blood cells, epithelial cells, casts, and crystals. Mucous threads, bacteria, yeast cells, parasites, and spermatozoa may also be found. Entry-level medical assistants would not likely perform a microscopic examination of urine.

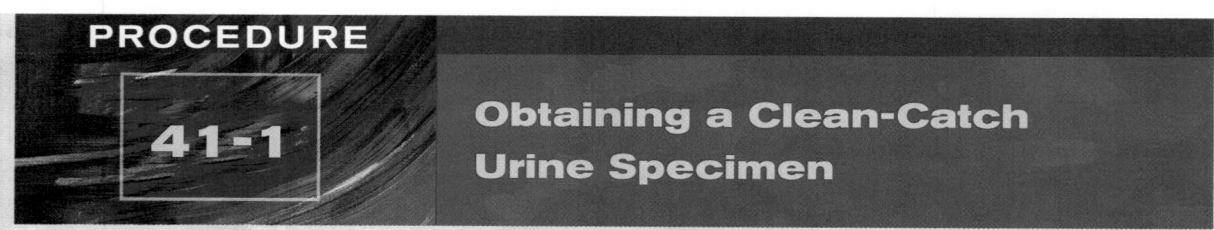

PROCEDURE 41-1

Obtaining a Clean-Catch Urine Specimen

Student Competency Objective: The medical assistant student will obtain a clean-catch urine specimen.

Items Needed: Sterile wipes or sterile cotton balls, antiseptic, sterile urine container

Steps:

1. Wash your hands.
2. Read the doctor's order.
3. Assemble equipment and supplies.

(Continues)

PROCEDURE 41-1 (Continued)

4. Introduce yourself to the client even if you have seen the client on previous visits to your office. The client may have forgotten your name. This also helps to establish a provider-client relationship, because it shows the client that you want him to know who you are.

5. Identify the client. Ask the client to state his name to establish that this is the right client, and then compare the name given to the name on the chart. Never enter a room and call out a client's name to determine if this person is the correct client. The client may not have heard you clearly and may just nod, smile, or answer yes. Clients almost never question if the medical assistant professional has the right client. It is up to the medical assistant to identify the right client before performing any procedure.

6. Tell the client, in everyday language, what you are going to do.

7. Ask if the client has any questions. If he does, give short and simple answers. Sometimes clients will start (and continue) talking because they are nervous about the procedure.

If the client is a female, give her the needed items and tell her to do steps 8 through 21:

8. Wash hands.

9. Spread the labia apart with one hand.

10. Take a cotton ball with antiseptic solution, or an antiseptic wipe, and wipe down on one side of the meatus from front to back, using only a single stroke. (The front-to-back single pass helps to keep microorganisms from the rectal area from getting into the cleaned urinary area.)

11. Throw away the used cotton ball or wipe.

12. Take another cotton ball or wipe and wipe down the other side of the meatus from front to back, again using only a single stroke.

13. Throw away the used cotton ball or wipe.

14. Take a third cotton ball or wipe and wipe down the middle of the meatus, from front to back.

15. Throw away the used cotton ball or wipe.

16. Rinse the area with sterile cotton balls.

17. Throw away the used cotton balls.

18. Hold the labia apart and void a small amount of urine into the toilet. (This helps to wash away any remaining bacteria.)

19. Take the sterile container and bring it into the urine stream while continuing to urinate.

20. Void the last small amount of urine into the toilet.

21. Put the cap on the sterile container when finished.

If the client is male, give him the needed items and tell him to do steps 22 through 34:

22. Wash hands and remove underpants.

23. Retract the foreskin of the penis.

24. Take a cotton ball with antiseptic solution or an antiseptic wipe and wipe in a circular motion away from the urinary meatus.

25. Throw away the used cotton ball or wipe.

(Continues)

PROCEDURE 41-1 (Continued)

26. Take another cotton ball or wipe and wipe again in a circular motion.
27. Throw away the used cotton ball or wipe.
28. Take a third cotton ball or wipe and wipe again in a circular motion.
29. Throw away the used cotton ball or wipe.
30. Keep the foreskin retracted.
31. Void a small amount into the toilet.
32. Take the sterile container and bring it into the urine stream while continuing to urinate.
33. Void the last small amount of urine into the toilet.
34. Put the cap on the sterile container when finished.

The medical assistant then completes steps 35 to 39, whether the client is male or female:

35. With gloves on, label and test or process the urine specimen as directed by office policy.
36. Clean the area, following standard precautions.
37. Remove your gloves.
38. Wash your hands.
39. Record the procedure in the client's chart immediately.

Charting Example:

8/13/20xx   8:30 A.M.   Instructed client to obtain a clean-catch urine sample while at office. Reviewed steps with client. Handed client items to wash and sterile specimen container for urine. Clean-catch urine sample obtained, labeled, and sent to lab. Client given instructions to call office for test results in three days.

Valerie Fitzgerald, S.M.A.

Valerie Fitzgerald, S.M.A. (printed name)

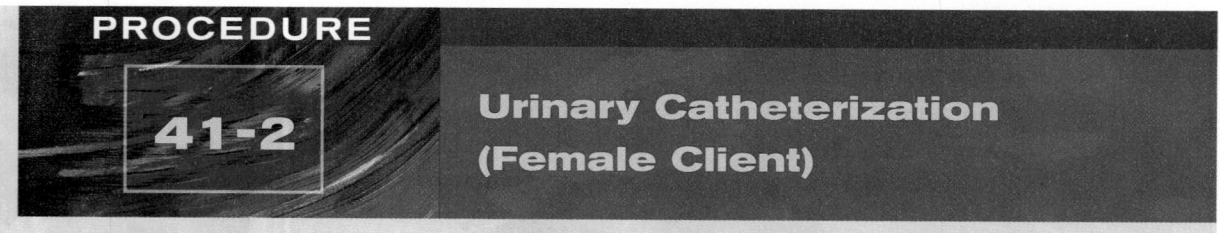

PROCEDURE 41-2

Urinary Catheterization (Female Client)

Student Competency Objective: The medical assistant student will perform a urinary catheterization on a female client.

Items Needed: Catheter tray with #14 or #16 Fr. catheter, sterile gloves, antiseptic solution, urine specimen container, lubricant, biohazardous waste container, paper and pen

Steps:

1. Wash your hands.
2. Assemble equipment and supplies.

(Continues)

PROCEDURE 41-2 (Continued)

3. Introduce yourself to the client even if you have seen the client on previous visits to your office. The client may have forgotten your name. This also helps to establish a provider–client relationship, because it shows the client that you want her to know who you are.

4. Identify the client. Ask the client to state her name to establish that this is the right client, and then compare the name given to the name on the chart. Never enter a room and call out a client's name to determine if this person is the correct client. The client may not have heard you clearly and may just nod, smile, or answer yes. Clients almost never question if the medical assistant professional has the right client. It is up to the medical assistant to identify the right client before performing any procedure.

5. Tell the client, in everyday language, what you are going to do.

6. Ask if the client has any questions. If she does, give short and simple answers. Sometimes clients will start (and continue) talking because they are nervous about the procedure.

7. Ask the client to remove her clothing from the waist down.

8. Assist the client onto the examination table as needed.

9. Position the client in the dorsal recumbent position (on back with feet flat on table and knees bent).

10. Open the catheter tray and place it between the client's legs.

11. Put on sterile gloves.

12. Take a sterile drape from the catheter tray and place it under the client's buttocks. Do not contaminate your gloves while doing this.

13. Open the antiseptic wipes and lubricant. Squeeze lubricant onto the tip of the catheter. (You do not have to pick up the catheter to put lubricant on it.)

14. Using your nondominant hand, gently spread the labia apart to expose the urinary meatus. (Your hand must remain in position until catheterization is complete, because that hand is now contaminated.)

15. Pick up forceps and grab an antiseptic wipe.

16. Starting at one side of the urinary meatus, wipe from top to bottom in one stroke. Wipe once and discard the used wipe.

17. Pick up another antiseptic wipe with the forceps.

18. Go to the other side of the urinary meatus and wipe from top to bottom. Wipe once and discard the used wipe.

19. Pick up another antiseptic wipe with the forceps.

20. Wipe from top to bottom down the center of the urinary meatus.

21. Using the sterile gloved hand, pick up the catheter. Keep the labia separated at all times.

22. Gently insert the catheter tip 2 or 3 inches into the urinary meatus.

23. When urine begins to flow, hold the catheter in place with the hand that had been keeping the labia open.

24. Place the sterile specimen container under the drainage tip of the catheter.

25. Fill the container with 30 mL of urine.

26. Allow the rest of the urine to drain into the collection tray.

(Continues)

PROCEDURE 41-2 (Continued)

27. Remove the catheter by pulling it out gently.

28. Remove the collection tray from between the client's legs and tell her that she can relax her position.

29. Note the amount of urine that drained into the collection tray.

30. Discard the extra urine, following standard precautions.

31. Take off your gloves and wash your hands.

32. Correctly label the specimen container and complete lab paperwork.

33. Help the client into a sitting position.

34. Assist the client to dress, as needed.

35. Ask the client if she has any questions.

36. Record the procedure in the client's chart immediately and process the urine specimen according to office policy.

Charting Example:

11/20/20xx   10:30 A.M.   Straight catheterization performed with #14 Fr. catheter as per doctor's order. Obtained 30 mL of cloudy, dark-yellow urine for specimen with 300 mL of residual urine drained. Urine specimen sent to lab for urinalysis and culture. Client instructed to call office for test results.

Shannon McGuire, S.M.A.

Shannon McGuire, S.M.A. (printed name)

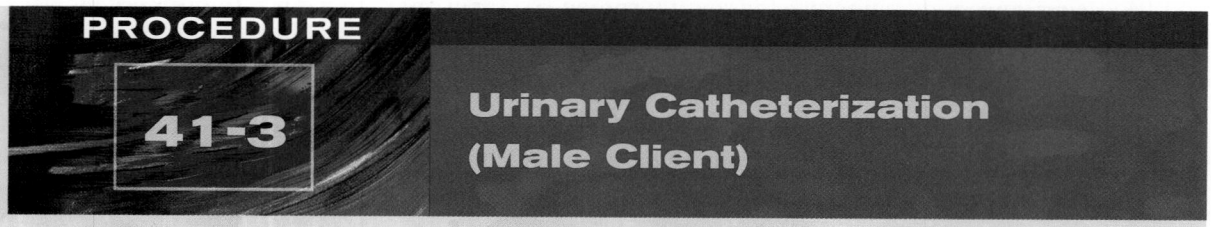

PROCEDURE 41-3 — Urinary Catheterization (Male Client)

Student Competency Objective: The medical assistant student will perform a urinary catheterization on a male client.

Items Needed: Catheter tray with #14 or #16 Fr. catheter, sterile gloves, antiseptic solution, urine specimen container, lubricant, biohazardous waste container, paper and pen

Steps:

1. Wash your hands.

2. Assemble equipment and supplies.

3. Introduce yourself to the client even if you have seen the client on previous visits to your office. The client may have forgotten your name. This also helps to establish a provider-client relationship, because it shows the client that you want him to know who you are.

(Continues)

PROCEDURE 41-3 (Continued)

4. Identify the client. Ask the client to state his name to establish that this is the right client, and then compare the name given to the name on the chart. Never enter a room and call out a client's name to determine if this person is the correct client. The client may not have heard you clearly and may just nod, smile, or answer yes. Clients almost never question if the medical assistant professional has the right client. It is up to the medical assistant to identify the right client before performing any procedure.

5. Tell the client, in everyday language, what you are going to do.

6. Ask if the client has any questions. If he does, give short and simple answers. Sometimes clients will start (and continue) talking because they are nervous about the procedure.

7. Ask the client to remove his clothing from the waist down.

8. Assist the client onto the examination table, as needed, and place him in supine position (on his back).

9. Ask the client to separate his legs a little (this helps to relax muscles).

10. Open the catheterization tray and place it to the client's side.

11. Put on sterile gloves.

12. Take out the sterile drape and place it under the client's penis.

13. Open the antiseptic wipes.

14. Open the lubricant and squeeze a sufficient amount on the catheter tip.

15. Using the nondominant hand, gently pick up the penis to expose the urinary meatus. If the male client is uncircumcised, gently pull back the foreskin. Hold the sides of the penis to prevent closing the urethra.

16. Using forceps, pick up an antiseptic wipe.

17. With the antiseptic wipe, cleanse the urinary meatus with a circular motion.

18. Discard the used wipe.

19. Pick up another antiseptic wipe and cleanse in a circular motion again.

20. Discard the used wipe.

21. Pick up a third antiseptic wipe and cleanse in a circular motion.

22. Discard the used wipe.

23. Using your sterile-gloved hand (that has not touched the penis), pick up the catheter.

24. Hold the penis at a 90-degree angle (perpendicular) to the client's body. Exert slight traction by pulling upward. (This straightens the urethra and aids in catheter insertion.)

25. Insert the lubricated tip of catheter into the urinary meatus about 6 inches.

26. When the urine begins to flow, hold the catheter in place with the nondominant hand (the hand that has been holding the penis).

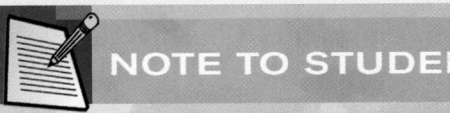

NOTE TO STUDENT:

If the catheter is hard to advance (meets resistance), place the penis at a 45-degree angle and ask the client to take a deep breath. If it is still difficult, gently remove the catheter and inform the doctor.

(Continues)

PROCEDURE 41-3 (Continued)

27. Place the sterile specimen container under the drainage tip of the catheter.

28. Fill the container with 30 mL of urine.

29. Allow the rest of the urine to drain into the collection tray.

30. Remove the catheter by pulling it out gently.

31. Note the amount of urine that drained into the collection tray.

32. Discard the extra urine, following standard precautions.

33. Take off your gloves and wash your hands.

34. Correctly label the specimen container and complete lab paperwork.

35. Help the client into a sitting position.

36. Assist the client to dress, as needed.

37. Ask the client if he has any questions.

38. Record the procedure in the client's chart immediately and process the urine specimen according to office policy.

Charting Example:

11/20/20xx   10:30 A.M.   Straight catheterization performed with #14 Fr. catheter as per doctor's order. Obtained 30 mL of clear, light-yellow urine for specimen with 700 mL of residual urine drained. Doctor informed of amount of residual urine. Urine specimen sent to lab for urinalysis and culture. Client instructed to call office for test results.

James Fox, S.M.A.

James Fox, S.M.A. (printed name)

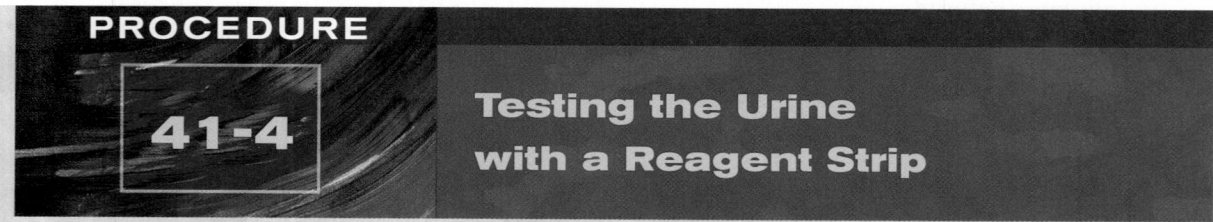

PROCEDURE 41-4

Testing the Urine with a Reagent Strip

Student Competency Objective: The medical assistant student will test urine using a reagent strip.

Items Needed: Reagent strips and chart, urine specimen container, urine specimen, watch with second hand, gloves, paper towel, biohazardous waste container

Steps:

1. Collect a urine specimen from the client.

2. Wash your hands.

3. Assemble equipment and supplies.

4. Check the expiration date on the reagent strip bottle.

5. Take one strip from the bottle.

(Continues)

PROCEDURE 41-4 (Continued)

6. Put the cap back on the bottle immediately.

7. Place the strip on a clean paper towel.

8. Put on gloves.

9. Dip the strip into the urine specimen so that all of the pads get immersed (Figure 41-7A).

10. Take the strip out immediately.

11. Gently rub the edge of the strip along the rim of the urine container to remove excess urine.

12. Hold the reagent strip next to, but not touching, the chart to match up the pads (Figure 41-7B).

13. Time the test using the second hand on your watch.

14. Read the results.

15. Write down the results.

16. Discard the urine and the reagent strip into the biohazardous waste container.

17. Clean the work area.

18. Take off your gloves.

19. Wash your hands.

20. Put the bottle of reagent strips away in the proper storage area.

21. Record the results of the urine test in the client's chart or lab slip, per the situation and office policy.

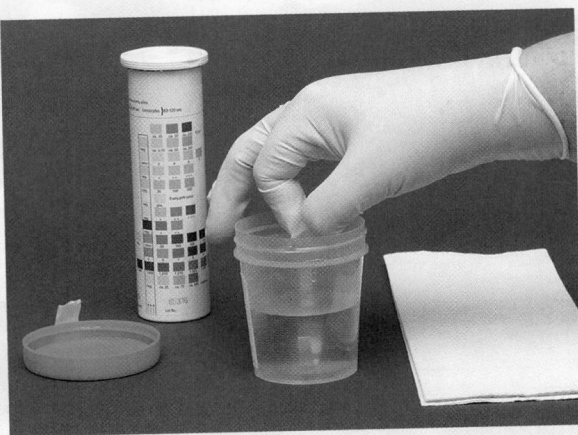

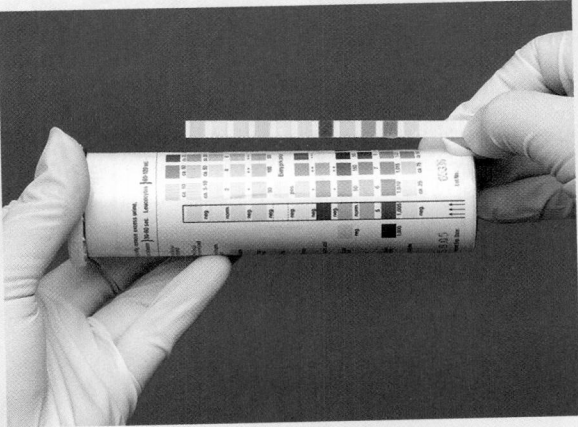

FIGURE 41-7A The medical assistant quickly and thoroughly immerses the strip in the urine specimen and removes the strip.

FIGURE 41-7B Compare the reagent strip with the color-coded chart or the chart on the bottle.

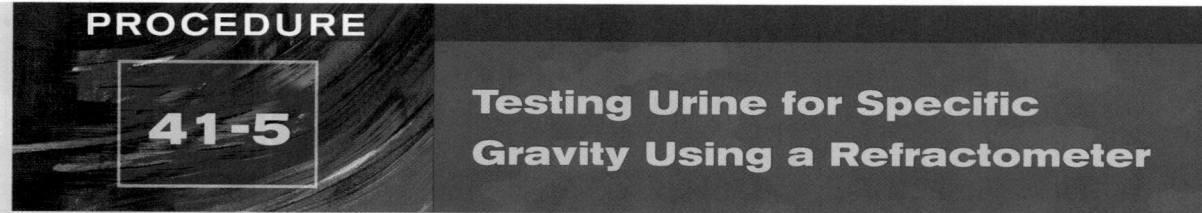

PROCEDURE

41-5

Testing Urine for Specific Gravity Using a Refractometer

Student Competency Objective: The medical assistant student will measure and record the specific gravity of a urine sample using a refractometer.

Items Needed: Refractometer, gloves, distilled water, urine specimen, pipettes, antiseptic cleaner, lint-free tissue or gauze, biohazardous waste container

Steps:

1. Wash your hands.
2. Put on gloves.
3. Assemble equipment and supplies.
4. Place a drop of distilled water on the prism and cover.
5. Dry the prism and cover with lint-free tissue or gauze.
6. Close the cover.
7. Using a pipette, place one drop of urine in the notched part of the cover. The urine should flow over the entire prism surface (Figure 41-8A).
8. Turn the refractometer so that it points to a strong light (Figure 41-8B).
9. Read the specific gravity line, which is the line that separates the light and dark areas.
10. Clean the cover and prism.
11. Dispose of used items, following standard precautions.
12. Clean the work area.
13. Remove your gloves.

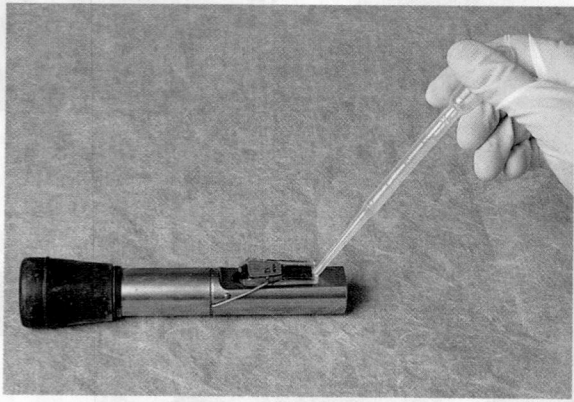

FIGURE 41-8A Fill the refractometer with one drop of urine using a pipette.

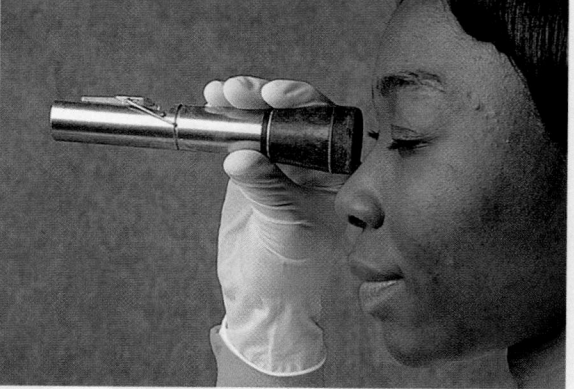

FIGURE 41-8B Turn the refractometer toward a light source to look through it.

(Continues)

PROCEDURE 41-5 (Continued)

14. Wash your hands.
15. Record the specific gravity measurement in the client's chart or on the laboratory requisition slip, depending on the situation and office policy.

NOTE TO STUDENT:

Quality control procedures must be done daily as stated by office policy. The procedure for the refractometer is the same, but distilled water is used. The specific gravity reading for the distilled water should be 1.000.

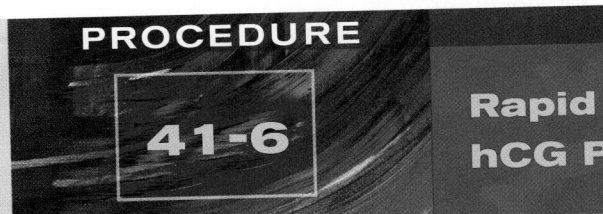

PROCEDURE 41-6

Rapid Test Procedure: hCG Pregnancy Test

Student Competency Objective: The medical assistant will perform a human chorionic gonadotropin (hCG) pregnancy test using a urine sample.

Items Needed: Gloves, urine collection cup with client's urine specimen (labeled), pregnancy kit, cassette urine dropper or pipette, clock or watch with second hand, biohazardous waste container

NOTE TO STUDENT:

Pregnancy kits vary, so it is important to read and follow exactly the manufacturer's directions for the kit you are using.

Steps:
1. Wash your hands.
2. Assemble equipment and supplies.
3. Put on gloves.
4. Compare the name on the urine specimen container to the name on the lab slip, to make sure they are the same.
5. Label the test cassette.
6. Using the urine dropper or pipette, draw up urine into the dropper or pipette.

(Continues)

PROCEDURE 41-6 (Continued)

7. Hold the urine dropper or pipette straight while pointing the tip down. Make sure the tip is high enough off the sample well that you can count drops.

8. Drop four drops into the well.

9. Wait 5 minutes. (Do not read or interpret after 10 minutes, as the results will be invalid.)

10. Read the results in the display window on the cassette. (Kits will vary as to color and/or number of lines indicating positive or negative.)

11. Record the results on the lab form or in the client's chart per office policy.

12. Notify the doctor of the results.

13. Dispose of the specimen and used supplies in the biohazardous waste container.

14. Remove your gloves.

15. Wash your hands.

Charting Example:

8/10/20xx   8:00 A.M.   Collected urine specimen. Performed hCG pregnancy test. Results positive. Results recorded in log and doctor notified.

Linda Rodden, S. M. A.

Linda Rodden, S.M.A. (printed name)

 BRIDGE TO CAAHEP

This chapter, which discusses urinalysis, provides information and content related to CAAHEP standards for Anatomy and Physiology, Medical Terminology, Medical Law and Ethics, Psychology, Communication, Medical Assisting Administrative Procedures, Medical Assisting Clinical Procedures, and Professional Components.

 ABHES LINKS

This chapter, which discusses urinalysis, links to ABHES course content for Anatomy and Physiology, Medical Terminology, Medical Law and Ethics, Psychology of Human Relations, Medical Office Clinical Procedures, and Medical Laboratory Procedures.

 AAMA AREAS OF COMPETENCE

This chapter, which discusses urinalysis, provides information or content within several areas listed in the Medical Assistant Role Delineation Study. These areas include: administrative, administrative procedures, clinical, fundamental principles, diagnostic orders, patient (client) care, general transdisciplinary, professionalism, communication skills, legal concepts, instruction, and operational functions.

 AMT PATHS

This chapter, which discusses urinalysis, provides a path to AMT competency in general medical assisting knowledge, anatomy and physiology, medical terminology, medical law, medical ethics, human relations, patient (client) education, clinical medical assisting, asepsis, sterilization, instruments, and laboratory procedures.

POINTS OF HIGHLIGHT

- Testing of urine is one of the tests most frequently performed in the medical office.
- Urine testing is done to screen for, diagnose, and monitor treatment or progress of disorders.
- Urinalysis consists of physical, chemical, and microscopic examinations.
- The physical examination of urine includes inspection of the color, clarity, odor, and specific gravity.
- Specific gravity can be measured by using a reagent strip, urinometer, or refractometer.
- Chemical examination of urine looks for the presence of specific chemicals or substances in the urine.
- Microscopic examination of urine often confirms the results of the physical and chemical examinations.
- Three major types of urine specimens for testing are random, timed, and eight-hour or first morning.
- Common methods of collecting urine are random and midstream or clean-catch.
- In urethral catheterization, a sterile tube is inserted into the urinary bladder to obtain a urine specimen.

STUDENT PORTFOLIO ACTIVITY

What would attract you to a particular health care setting? What factors would cause you to choose one over another? Write down what factors about a position are important to you. Is salary your only concern, or are benefits, flex time, support for continuing education, and other factors important? Note these things in order of their importance to you. Keeping this with your portfolio will help you ask questions during an interview. Employers will observe a prepared individual who understands the different aspects of employment. This ranking will also help you to make decisions about possible employers and places of employment.

APPLYING YOUR SKILLS

You are a newly hired, entry-level medical assistant in a medical office. You know that it is office policy to obtain a urine specimen when a client comes for a physical examination. However, today, as has happened several times in the past, the client cannot void because he urinated just before being called into the exam room. Because it would not give a true picture of the client's urinary system, you do not want to hand him a glass of water and ask for a sample before he leaves the office, as some of your colleagues have suggested. What can you do to avoid this situation in the future?

CRITICAL THINKING QUESTIONS

1. When performing the physical examination part of the urinalysis, you observe that the urine is cloudy and that it has an odor similar to ammonia. What are some possible reasons for this?

2. Describe possible reasons why urine specimens are very often collected, processed, and tested in the medical office.

3. What is meant by a timed test? How do these tests differ from random tests?

4. The doctor asks you to obtain a clean-catch urine specimen from a client. How do you explain this to the client in everyday language? List what you would say, step by step.

5. A urine sample has been left on the counter for more than two hours. How might this affect the pH reading? What might testing falsely indicate?

6. You test a freshly voided urine sample and find a high level of glucose in the urine. What is the most common cause of this? What other tests might be ordered based on these results?

7. A client questions why he must obtain a first morning urine sample. Why are first morning specimens often required? What do you say to this client?

8. Explain the importance of quality control measures in an office that performs urine testing.

9. Explain why the color of urine can vary but not indicate disease. What factors can cause differences in color?

10. How do you explain to a client the process of collecting a 24-hour urine specimen? (Put the discussion into everyday words that you would use with the client.)

11. Go back to the beginning of this chapter and review the Anticipatory Statements. Reread each statement and then indicate whether it is true or false. If the statement is false, rewrite it to make it a true statement.

CLIENT TEACHING PLAN

Midstream Urine Sample Collection

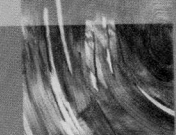

■ What Is to Be Taught:

- How to collect a midstream urine sample.

■ Objectives:

- Client will be able to collect a midstream urine sample at home and bring the specimen to the office.

■ Preparation Before Teaching:

- Review the midstream (clean-catch) urine collection procedure.
- Assemble teaching supplies: urine sample container; diagram of male and female perineal area, including urethral opening; gloves; soap and water, paper and pen.

■ Steps for the Medical Assistant:

1. Wash your hands.
2. Gather supplies needed.
3. Introduce yourself to the client.
4. Explain what you are going to teach and why.
5. Ask the client to wash his or her hands.
6. Using a diagram for illustration, instruct the client how to wash the area.
   Female: Use an antiseptic wipe or cloth and wipe once from front to back on one side of the labia. Using another wipe, repeat on the other side of the labia. Using a third wipe, wipe once from front to back down the center.
   Males: Wash in a circular motion around the penis using an antiseptic wipe or cloth. If uncircumcised, push back the foreskin and hold it while washing and thereafter.
7. Show the client the urine sample container. Demonstrate how to take off the lid and lay it upside down on a clean surface. Remind the client that the rim should not be put face down.
8. Tell the client to begin urinating in the toilet; then stop, put the container under the urethral opening, and resume voiding.

9. Instruct the client not to completely empty the bladder into the container. After the container is filled to the mark, remove it from the urine stream and finish urinating into the toilet.
10. Instruct the client to put the lid back on the container.
11. Remind the client to wash his or her hands.
12. Tell the client to bring the sample to the medical office within one hour. If this is not possible, have the client place the urine sample in the refrigerator until he or she can bring it to the office. A specimen must be brought in the same day it was collected.

■ Special Needs of the Client:

- Check the client's chart for any factors that might interfere with the client's ability to follow directions in collecting the urine sample and bringing it to the office.
- Ask the client if there is anything you should know that might affect the client's ability to carry out the procedure.

■ Evaluation:

- Client demonstrates correct handwashing.
- Client lists steps of procedure in correct order.
- Client is able to tell you when the sample should be collected and where it is to be brought.

■ Further Plans/Teaching:

- If the client is able to complete the procedure successfully, remark on that at the next office visit and ask if the client had any difficulties.
- If the client could not successfully complete any part of the procedure, evaluate and begin the process again. Ask the client what steps he or she took.

■ Follow-up:

- Call the client the next day to see if there are any questions.

(Continues)

CLIENT TEACHING PLAN (Continued)

- Check at the scheduled time to see if the client brought in the sample. If so, follow up with the lab report. If not, call the client and ask how you can help him or her.

Medical Assistant

Name: _____

Signature: _____

Date: _____

Client

Date: _____

Follow-up Date : _____

CHAPTER 42

Anticipatory Statements

People have different ideas about hematology and laboratory testing. Read and think about the following statements based upon what you believe now. Decide whether you agree or disagree. Write the word **agree** after the statement if you think the statement is true. Write the word **disagree** after the statement if you think the statement is false. Read the chapter to find out if your current beliefs can be supported.

1. Hematological tests examine the blood. _____

2. The medical assistant should always tell a client that getting blood drawn will not hurt. _____

3. Medical assistants can never draw blood. _____

4. Only a medical laboratory worker can test blood. _____

5. It is not necessary to wear gloves while drawing blood if it makes the client uncomfortable. _____

Hematology and Venipuncture

Learning Objectives

Upon completion of this chapter, the medical assistant student should be able to:

- Define hematology
- State the purpose of hematocrit testing
- Explain what is meant by a complete blood count
- List the steps in performing a venipuncture
- Identify the medical assistant's role in hematology testing

Key Terms

anemia Disorder in which there are either too few red blood cells, too little hemoglobin in the red blood cells, or low blood volume.

complete blood count (CBC) A series of tests that examines all three types of blood cells.

hematocrit In blood testing, the ratio of packed red blood cells to whole blood volume.

hemoglobin The oxygen-carrying part of the red blood cell.

leukocytes White blood cells.

platelet Part of the blood that is involved in blood clotting.

syringe method Method of obtaining a blood sample using a needle and a syringe; the blood from the syringe is then injected into a tube. Used most frequently on a person with small or fragile veins.

vacuum tube method Method of obtaining a blood sample using a needle and color-coded vacuum tube(s).

venipuncture Puncture of a vein for the purpose of removing blood for testing.

■ INTRODUCTION

Blood performs many functions vital to life itself. It carries oxygen and nutrients to the cells and carries away waste products through the circulatory system. Blood can help protect the body from infection and help regulate temperature. Blood can also spread disease, such as allowing cancer cells to move from one part of the body to another. *Hematology* is the study of blood, including the functions and diseases of the blood tissue. Specimens of blood are often collected for examination in a laboratory, whether for screening, diagnostic, or monitoring purposes. The medical assistant will prepare the client for these tests, as well as obtaining the blood samples and actually performing some of the tests. The type of test ordered, facility policy, and legal and regulatory guidelines will determine which tests the medical assistant is permitted to perform.

Blood cells can be grouped into three types: red blood cells, white blood cells, and platelets. The red blood cells carry oxygen to the cells and carry away carbon dioxide. The white blood cells fight infection. **Platelets** help the blood to maintain homeostasis (balance within the body). The blood must be thick enough not to bleed excessively when cut and not so thick that the blood cannot move or form clots.

To provide good client care, the medical assistant needs an understanding of the basic hematological tests. In addition to knowing the purpose of these tests, the medical assistant must be able to obtain specimens and either process the specimens or send them to the correct laboratory in the correct manner.

■ TESTING

Testing of blood can yield valuable information used in the diagnosis and treatment of many disorders. Blood samples are commonly obtained in the physician's office. Testing is done either in a physician's office laboratory (POL) or an outside laboratory facility.

Complete Blood Count

A **complete blood count (CBC)** is one of the most frequently ordered tests. It is actually a series of tests, the purpose of which is to examine all three types of blood cells. A CBC includes: hematocrit, hemoglobin, mean corpuscular volume, mean corpuscular hemoglobin, mean corpuscular hemoglobin concentration, platelet count, neutrophils, lymphocytes, monocytes, eosinophils, and basophils.

Hematocrit

A **hematocrit** blood test, which is abbreviated Hct, is commonly performed in the medical office (Figure 42-1). This test compares the amount of red blood cell mass to whole blood. The hematocrit level may indicate the presence of abnormal conditions. If the client has lost blood, either from visible external bleeding or hidden internal bleeding, the hematocrit reading will be low. A low hematocrit may also indicate that the client has **anemia.** The normal range for adult males is 40 to 54 percent. The normal hematocrit range for adult female is 37 to 47 percent.

Hemoglobin

The **hemoglobin** (Hgb or Hb) test or determination indirectly measures the oxygen-carrying capacity of the blood (Figure 42-2). (Remember, hemoglobin is a major part of the red blood cells,

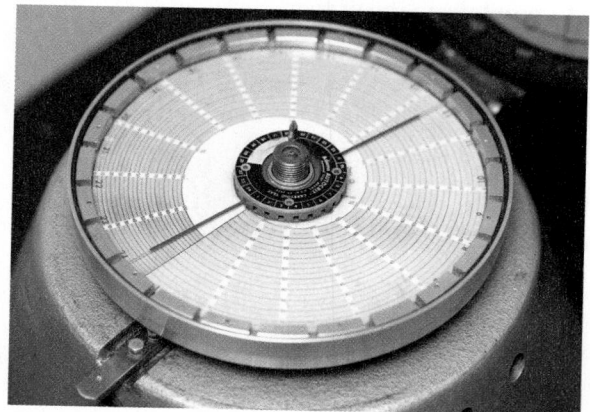

FIGURE 42–1 A microhematocrit centrifuge.

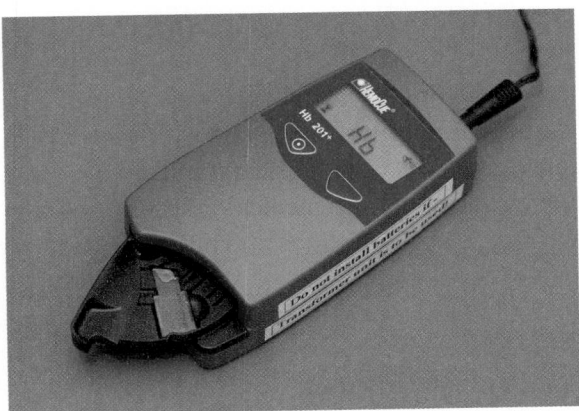

FIGURE 42-2 A HemoCue automated instrument, used for hemoglobin testing.

and is the substance that carries oxygen to the body's tissues.) The normal hemoglobin range for an adult male is 14 to 18 grams per 100 mL of blood. The normal hemoglobin range for an adult female is 12 to 16 grams per 100 mL of blood. An increase or decrease can indicate a disorder. An increase may point to congestive heart failure, chronic obstructive pulmonary disease, or polycythemia. Anemia, severe bleeding, cirrhosis of the liver, leukemia, and other disorders are associated with decreased hemoglobin levels. If the client has symptoms of anemia, a red blood cell count may be ordered. In adult females, the normal red blood cell count is 4 to 5 million per cubic millimeter of blood. In adult males, it is 4 to 6 million per cubic millimeter of blood.

Mean Corpuscular Volume, Mean Corpuscular Hemoglobin, and Mean Corpuscular Hemoglobin Concentration

The mean corpuscular volume, mean corpuscular hemoglobin, and mean corpuscular concentration are determined as part of a CBC. Knowing the values of these three components will assist the doctor in diagnosis, particularly with types of anemia.

The mean corpuscular volume (MCV) examines the size of the red blood cells. Is the cell smaller, larger, or the same as a normal red blood cell? The MCV refers to the volume of hemoglobin in the red blood cells. The normal range is 82 to 98 per cubic millimeter.

The mean corpuscular hemoglobin (MCH) is helpful in examining the blood of clients who have severe anemia. The MCH looks at the weight of the hemoglobin in the red blood cells. The normal range is 27 to 31 picograms per cell.

The mean corpuscular hemoglobin concentration (MCHC) looks at the average concentration of hemoglobin in the red blood cells. It is important to monitor this value during the treatment of anemia. The normal range is 32 to 36 grams per deciliter.

Platelet Count

Platelets are formed elements in the blood. They are critical to the body's ability to clot blood when necessary and in the amount necessary. The platelet count is used to monitor bleeding caused by organ disorders or cancers. The normal range is 150,000 to 400,000 platelets per cubic millimeter.

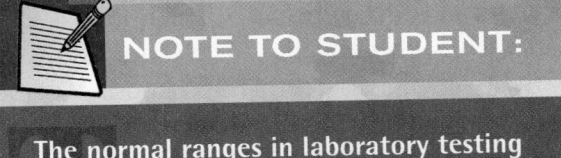

NOTE TO STUDENT: The normal ranges in laboratory testing can vary from laboratory to laboratory, depending on the instruments and the controls used. The medical assistant must look at the standard normal range listed on the laboratory reports from each facility.

White Blood Cell Count and Differential

The white blood cells help to fight infections. A white blood cell count is done when infection is suspected. In adults, the normal range for white blood cells (**leukocytes**) is 5,000 to 10,000 per cubic millimeter of blood. An increase in the number of white blood cells may indicate that the body is fighting an infection.

An increase often occurs because of an increase in only one type of white blood cells. It does not mean that all types have increased. A *differential white blood cell count* will identify the percentage of each kind of white blood cell. This includes neutrophils, eosinophils, basophils, lymphocytes, and monocytes. (See Chapter 13 for more information.) For this test, whole blood is usually used, and a blood smear or film is made to obtain a differential count. Laboratory technicians in specific laboratories normally perform this kind of test.

■ VENIPUNCTURE

Laboratory tests that use blood samples are a valuable part of the diagnosis and treatment of disorders. The client's blood is examined, which helps the doctor to screen, diagnose disorders, check the progress of the disorder and monitor the treatment prescribed. Blood samples are often obtained through **venipuncture** and the tests are frequently performed in a medical office setting.

Blood samples may be obtained as part of the client's routine physical examination. This promotes health by helping to identify risk factors for health problems or detecting the very early stages of a disorder. The prognosis of some disorders can be carefully watched through the periodic testing of blood. The prescribed treatment can also be monitored through observation of blood levels.

Client Preparation

The medical assistant's role includes client preparation, even if the blood sample is to be obtained by another health care provider. Many individuals are fearful about the drawing of blood. They may be anxious about the tightness of the tourniquet, pain from the needle, the amount of blood drawn, and the length of time needed to complete the procedure. Clients may even faint (experience syncope) during the procedure. Worry about what the doctor will discover from the blood test results also contributes to what is for many people an uncomfortable experience.

A calm, professional attitude with high skill competency is critical to successful procedure outcome and client satisfaction. The medical assistant must explain the procedure in terms that are easy to understand. After giving the explanation, the medical assistant needs to encourage any questions and allow the client to express fears and concerns. Answer all questions factually and clearly. Treat all client concerns with respect, and respond to client fears in a calm, nonjudgmental way. Never dismiss a client's concerns as minor. Venipuncture may be a common procedure in the everyday activities of a medical assistant, but it is not for the client.

Equipment and Supplies

Clients should either be sitting or in a supine position for venipuncture. Venipuncture (the puncturing or piercing of a vein to obtain a required amount of blood) requires specific equipment and supplies. Some medical settings have a special chair used for blood draws. The chair is sturdy, with a wide bar that can be opened and closed across the front of the client, similar to a lap tray. This bar supports and gives security. It also prevents the client from sliding out of the chair and being injured if the client faints. An examination table may be used instead of the chair.

A variety of vacuum tubes are required for different blood tests. These are color-coded (Figure 42-3). A *tourniquet,* which is a stretchy

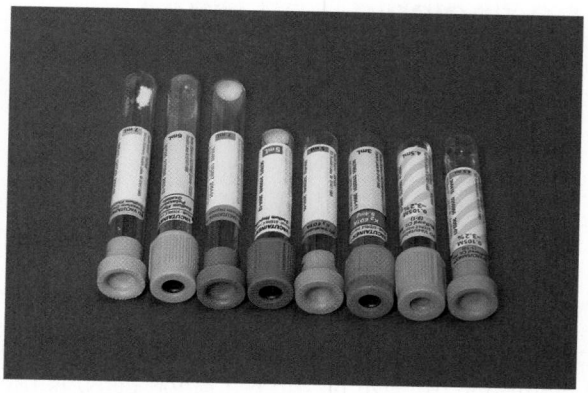

FIGURE 42-3 Vacuum tubes.

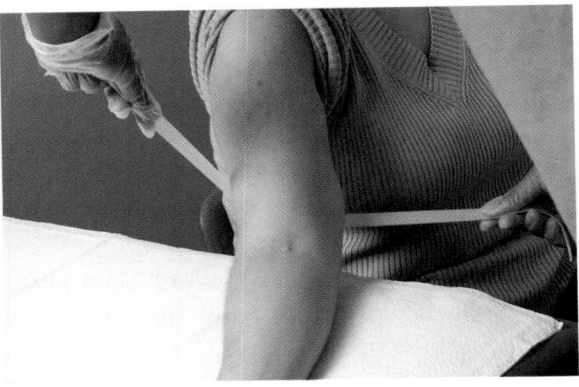

FIGURE 42-4A Wrap the tourniquet around the arm about 3 to 4 inches above the venipuncture site.

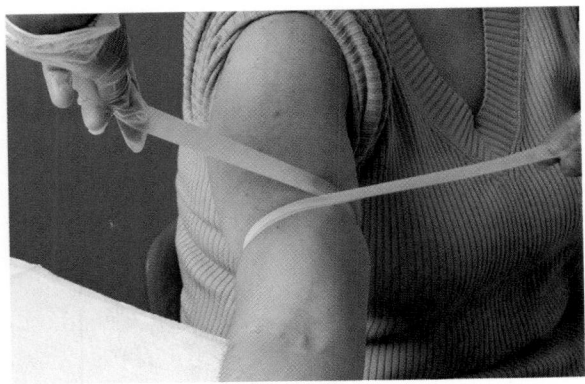

FIGURE 42-4B Stretch the tourniquet tightly and hold the ends across each other.

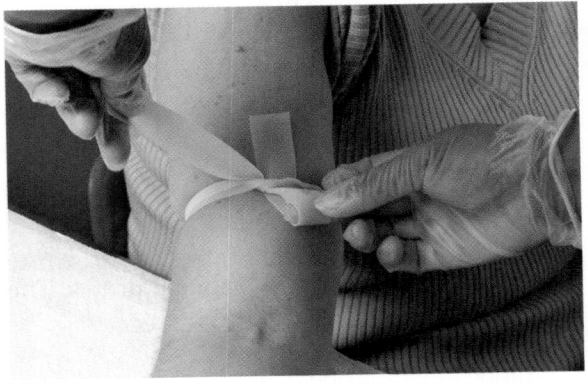

FIGURE 42-4C Tuck one of the ends under the other.

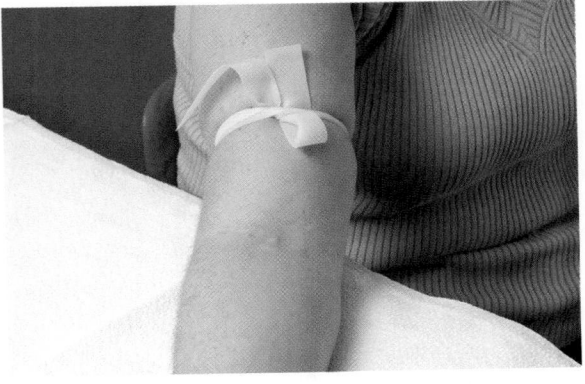

FIGURE 42-4D The ends of the tourniquet should be pointed away from the venipuncture site.

elastic band, is wrapped around the arm while the medical assistant selects and punctures the site (Figure 42-4A–D). Personal protective equipment such as gloves, gown, mask, and face shield must be available for use, according to OSHA regulations and standard precautions. Sterile needles, alcohol wipes, gauze, and various bandage sizes should be sorted and kept in a convenient container. A biohazardous waste container and a sharps container must also be nearby.

Site Selection

The **vacuum tube method** and the **syringe method** are common ways to obtain blood through venipuncture. The large veins in the antecubital area of the arms are usually selected (Figure 42-5). They are big, close to the skin surface, and easily accessed.

Both arms should be checked for appropriate veins. Use the following guidelines for site selection:

- The site should consist of unbroken skin.
- Skin should be free from scarring.
- No bruises should be visible at the site.
- Skin should not be inflamed or swollen.
- There should be no evidence of infection.
- Veins should feel springy when palpated.
- Veins are selected based on feel, not by sight. Veins that look good and are close to the surface may still collapse or roll once punctured.

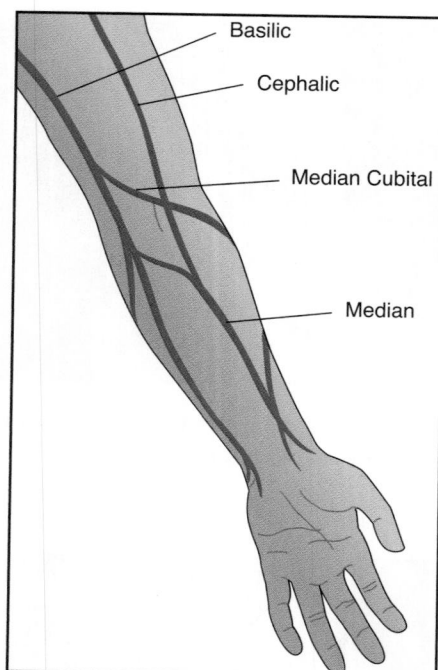

FIGURE 42–5 Superficial veins of the arm.

Points to Remember

While performing a venipuncture, the medical assistant can avoid problems by keeping in mind the following:

- Avoid probing; going back and forth once the needle is in the vein will cause a hematoma (bruise) and unnecessary pain.
- After two unsuccessful attempts to "hit" a vein, ask for the assistance of another health care provider in obtaining the blood sample.

- Avoid using the vacuum-tube method with a client who has small veins.
- Remove the tourniquet before you remove the needle from the vein.
- Apply pressure to the puncture site. Do not have the client bend the elbow; if she does, a hematoma may develop.
- If a vein that may "roll" must be used, apply firm pressure below the vein as you insert the needle.

Order of Draw

Frequently, more than one tube of blood is needed, depending on the doctor's order for tests. The order in which the various color-coded tubes are used to obtain blood samples does make a difference. Office policy determines the order in which the tubes are used; there are some variations among facilities. As of January 2005, the National Committee for Clinical Laboratory Standards (NCCLS), now known as the Clinical and Laboratory Standards Institute (CLSI), has established the following order of draw as a general rule.

1. Blood culture tube (yellow top or bottles)
2. Coagulation tube (light blue top)
3. Plain tube, nonadditive (red top)
4. Gel separator tube (speckled/tiger top)
5. Heparin tube
6. PST gel separator tube with heparin (green-gray top)
7. EDTA tube (lavender top)
8. Oxalate/fluoride tube (gray top)

PROCEDURE

42-1

Venipuncture (Vacuum-Tube Method)

Student Competency Objective: The medical assistant will obtain a blood sample using the vacuum-tube method.

Items Needed: Tubes specific to laboratory tests ordered; 20-, 21-, or 22-gauge needle made for vacuum-tube draws; gloves; mask or face shield if necessary; tourniquet; alcohol wipes; gauze; adhesive bandage; biohazardous waste container; sharps container; pen

Steps:

1. Read the doctor's orders for laboratory tests.
2. Wash your hands.
3. Assemble equipment and supplies. Check vacuum tubes for expiration date, make sure that additive in tubes is not adhering to the stopper or tube walls, and look for any flaws in tubes.
4. Twist the needle and take off the part that will puncture the top of the tube. Attach the needle to a holder.
5. Pick up the first collection tube (make sure you check the tests to be drawn for; there is an order for multiple-tube collection).
6. Place the tube into a holder. Do not push it in all the way (if punctured, it will lose the vacuum).
7. Introduce yourself to the client even if you have seen the client on previous visits to your office. The client may have forgotten your name. This also helps to establish a provider–client relationship, because it shows the client that you want her to know who you are.
8. Identify the client. Ask the client to state her name to establish that this is the right client, and then compare the name given to the name on the chart. Never enter a room and call out a client's name to determine if this person is the correct client. The client may not have heard you clearly and may just nod, smile, or answer yes. Clients almost never question if the medical assistant professional has the right client. It is up to the medical assistant to identify the right client before performing any procedure.
9. Tell the client, in everyday language, what you are going to do.
10. Ask if the client has any questions. If she does, give short and simple answers. Sometimes clients will start (and continue) talking because they are nervous about the procedure.
11. Help the client into a comfortable position. The client will either lie down with a pillow supporting the arm or sit in a laboratory chair with a bar or tray that crosses over in front of the client. This supports the arm in a stable position and helps to ensure the client's safety if she faints.
12. Line up the tubes in the order in which you will to use them.
13. Apply a tourniquet above desired venipuncture site on the client's arm.

(Continues)

14. Put on gloves, and a mask or face shield if needed.
15. Tell the client to close the hand into a fist, but do not pump the fist.
16. Find the vein (Figure 42-6A).
17. Wipe the site with an alcohol wipe (Figure 42-6B).
18. Let the site air-dry. Do not blow on the site; this will contaminate it.
19. Do not touch the venipuncture site after you clean it.
20. Place your thumb 1 to 2 inches below the site. Pull skin so that it is smooth and tight. This makes it easier for the needle to enter and keeps the vein from moving.
21. Line up the needle with the site. Keep the bevel of the needle pointed up.
22. Insert the needle into the vein (Figure 42-6C).
23. Take your thumb off the client's skin.
24. Grab the flange of the holder with your free hand.
25. Push the tube onto the needle inside of the holder (Figure 42-6D).
26. Allow blood to fill the tube.
27. When the blood flow stops, pull the tube off the needle and out of the holder with one hand (Figure 42-6E).
28. With the same hand, take the next tube in line and push it onto the needle in the holder. Let blood flow. Repeat this process until all test tubes are filled (Figure 42-6F).
29. Mix each tube that contains an additive by gently turning the tube upside down and back about five times. Do not shake or the blood cells will be damaged.
30. Ask the client to open the hand.
31. Take off the tourniquet with your free hand.
32. Place gauze just above the puncture site.
33. Take the needle out of the client's arm.
34. Apply pressure to the site for 3 minutes. If the client is able, ask her to hold gauze over the site while keeping the arm straight. Do not allow the client to bend the elbow; this can cause bruising.
35. Label all blood tubes before leaving the client's area (Figure 42-6G).
36. Check the venipuncture site and apply an adhesive bandage (Figure 42-6H).
37. Put the used needle into a sharps container (Figure 42-6I).
38. Take off your gloves (and mask or face shield, if used) and dispose of them in the biohazardous waste container.
39. Wash your hands.
40. Talk with the client and ask if she has any questions.
41. Record the procedure in the client's chart immediately.

(Continues)

PROCEDURE 42-1 (Continued)

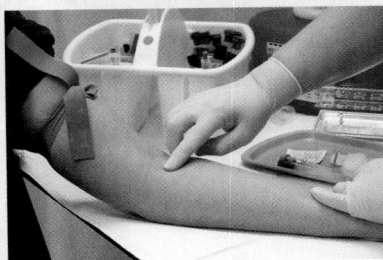

FIGURE 42-6A Palpate the client's arm to find the vein.

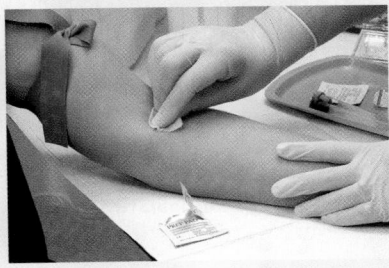

FIGURE 42-6B Cleanse the area with an alcohol wipe.

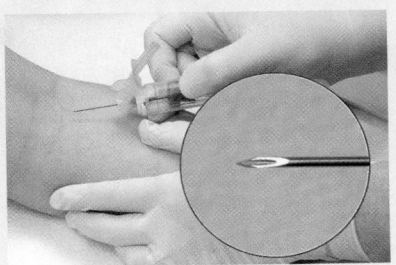

FIGURE 42-6C Insert the needle into the vein in a quick, smooth movement, holding the skin taut.

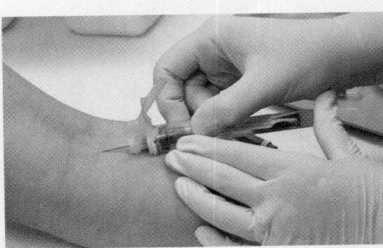

FIGURE 42-6D Push the tube forward until the needle has entered the tube.

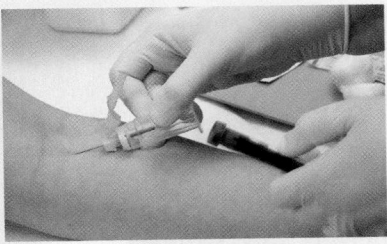

FIGURE 42-6E After it has stopped filling, take the tube out.

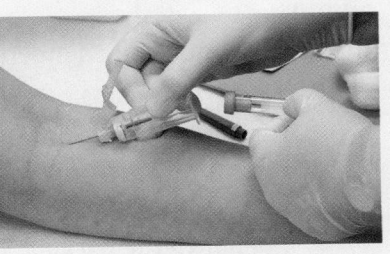

FIGURE 42-6F Place another tube onto the needle and let it fill.

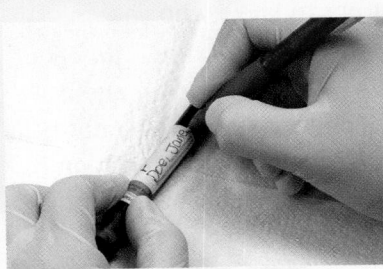

FIGURE 42-6G Label the tubes.

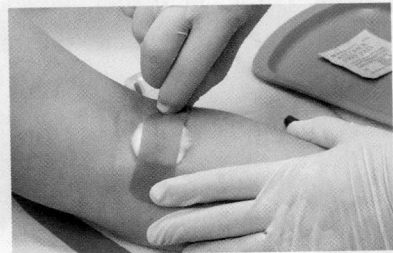

FIGURE 42-6H Apply an adhesive bandage to the client's arm.

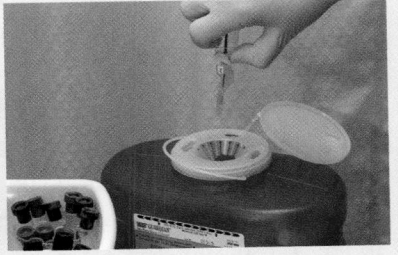

FIGURE 42-6I Properly dispose of the used needle in a sharps container.

Charting Example:

8/10/20xx   3:45 P.M.   Obtained multiple-tube blood sample from Mrs. Harting's right arm using vacuum-tube method. Adhesive bandage applied.

Catherine McDonald, S.M.A.

Catherine McDonald, S.M.A. (printed name)

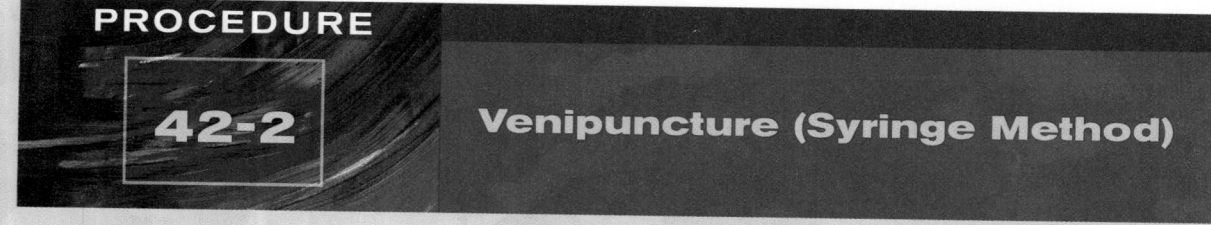

PROCEDURE

42-2

Venipuncture (Syringe Method)

Student Competency Objective: The medical assistant student will obtain a blood sample using the syringe method.

Items Needed: Tubes specific to laboratory test ordered, test tube rack, syringes, 21- or 22-gauge needle, gloves, mask or face shield if necessary, tourniquet, alcohol wipes, gauze, adhesive bandages, pen, biohazardous waste container, sharps container

Steps:

1. Read the doctor's orders for laboratory tests.
2. Wash your hands.
3. Assemble equipment and supplies. Choose the correct tubes for transfer of blood. Check expiration dates on the tubes. Make sure that additive is not adhering to the stopper and walls of the tube. Look for any flaws in tubes.
4. Open a sterile package of needles with syringes. Choose one and push the plunger up and down a few times to make sure that it will slide smoothly when drawing blood.
5. Introduce yourself to the client even if you have seen the client on previous visits to your office. The client may have forgotten your name. This also helps to establish a provider-client relationship, because it shows the client that you want her to know who you are.
6. Identify the client. Ask the client to state her name to establish that this is the right client, and then compare the name given to the name on the chart. Never enter a room and call out a client's name to determine if this person is the correct client. The client may not have heard you clearly and may just nod, smile, or answer yes. Clients almost never question if the medical assistant professional has the right client. It is up to the medical assistant to identify the right client before performing any procedure.
7. Tell the client, in everyday language, what you are going to do.
8. Ask if the client has any questions. If she does, give short and simple answers. Sometimes clients will start (and continue) talking because they are nervous about the procedure.
9. Help the client into a comfortable position. The client will either lie down with a pillow supporting the arm or sit in a laboratory chair with a bar or tray that crosses over in front of the client. This supports the arm in a stable position and helps to ensure the client's safety if she faints.
10. Line up the tubes in the order in which you will use them.
11. Apply a tourniquet above the desired venipuncture site.
12. Put on gloves, and a mask or face shield if needed.
13. Tell the client to close the hand into a fist, but do not pump the fist.
14. Find the vein.
15. Wipe the selected site with an alcohol wipe.
16. Let the site air-dry. Do not blow on the site; this will contaminate it.

(Continues)

PROCEDURE 42-2 (Continued)

17. Do not touch the venipuncture site after you clean it.

18. Place your thumb 1 to 2 inches below the site. Pull skin so that it is smooth and tight. This makes it easier for the needle to enter and keeps the vein from moving.

19. Line up the needle with the site. Keep the bevel of the needle pointed up (Figure 42-7A).

20. Insert the needle into the vein.

21. With the other hand, gently pull on the plunger of the syringe (Figure 42-7B).

22. Pull until the amount of blood needed has entered the syringe. Do not pull fast or the vein will collapse.

23. Tell the client to open the hand.

24. Using your free hand, take off the tourniquet.

25. Place gauze just above the injection site.

26. Take the needle and syringe out of the client's arm.

27. Apply pressure to the puncture area for 3 minutes. If the client is able, ask her to hold gauze over the site and keep the arm straight. Do not allow the client to bend the elbow; this can cause bruising (Figure 42-7C).

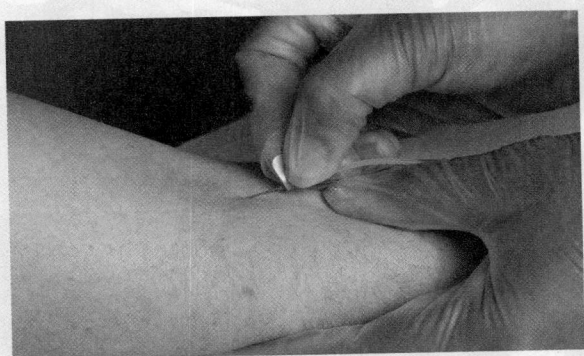

FIGURE 42-7A Line up the needle with the direction of the vein.

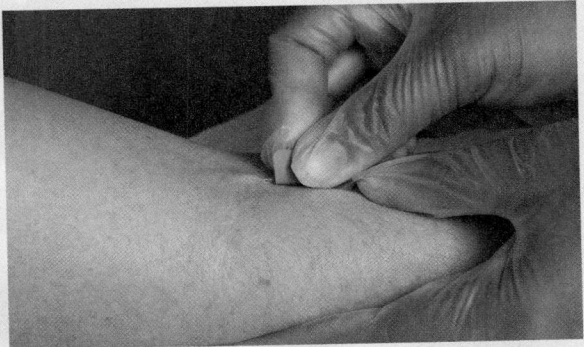

FIGURE 42-7B Insert the needle into the vein in a quick, smooth movement.

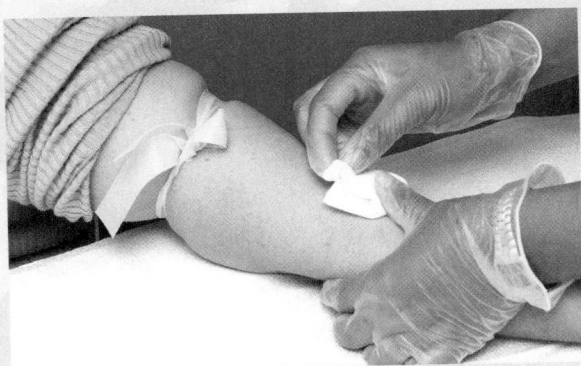

FIGURE 42-7C Remove the needle and apply pressure to the puncture area with sterile gauze.

(Continues)

PROCEDURE 42-2 (Continued)

28. Take the syringe to the test tube rack.
29. Push the needle into the stopper of the first tube.
30. Inject the required amount of blood into the tube.
31. Put the used syringe and needle into a sharps container.
32. Throw away the used gauze and alcohol wipes in a biohazardous waste container.
33. Label all blood tubes before you leave the client's area.
34. Check the injection site and apply an adhesive bandage.
35. Take off your gloves and dispose of them in the biohazardous waste container.
36. Wash your hands.
37. Talk with the client and ask if she has any questions.
38. Record the procedure in the client's chart immediately.

Charting Example:

2/17/20xx   10:30 A.M.   Obtained blood specimen from Mrs. Tate's left arm using the syringe method. Adhesive bandage applied.

Timothy Robinson, S.M.A.

Timothy Robinson, S.M.A. (printed name)

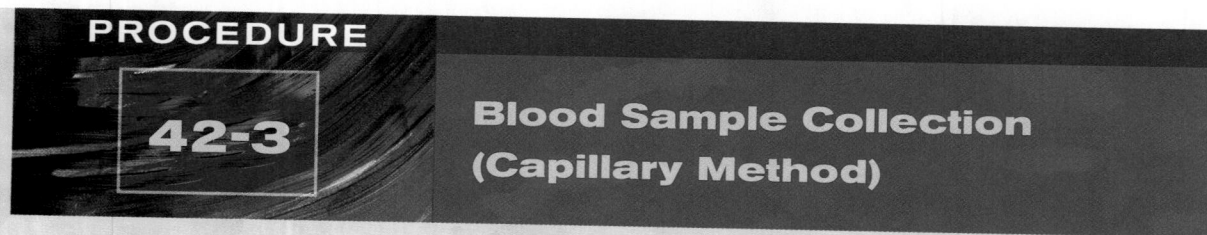

PROCEDURE

42-3

Blood Sample Collection (Capillary Method)

Student Competency Objective: The medical assistant student will collect a blood sample using the capillary method.

Items Needed: Gloves, sterile lancet, sterile gauze, alcohol wipes, sharps container, biohazardous waste container

Steps:

1. Check the doctor's order for the test.
2. Wash your hands.
3. Assemble equipment and supplies.
4. Introduce yourself to the client even if you have seen the client on previous visits to your office. The client may have forgotten your name. This also helps to establish a provider–client relationship, because it shows the client that you want her to know who you are.

(Continues)

PROCEDURE 42-3 (Continued)

5. Identify the client. Ask the client to state her name to establish that this is the right client, and then compare the name given to the name on the chart. Never enter a room and call out a client's name to determine if this person is the correct client. The client may not have heard you clearly and may just nod, smile, or answer yes. Clients almost never question if the medical assistant professional has the right client. It is up to the medical assistant to identify the right client before performing any procedure.

6. Tell the client, in everyday language, what you are going to do.

7. Ask if the client has any questions. If she does, give short and simple answers. Sometimes clients will start (and continue) talking because they are nervous about the procedure.

8. Look at possible sites. As with venipuncture, the area for capillary blood collection should be free of bruises, scars, or open skin.

9. Select a site. Common sites are on the ring finger, the middle finger, and the earlobes (Figure 42-8A). In infants, the heel may also be used. If a finger is selected, the site should be in the fleshy part of the fingertip to the side of the center.

10. Wash your hands.

11. Put on gloves.

12. Using an alcohol wipe, clean the area selected (Figure 42-8B).

13. Let the area air-dry; do not blow on it.

14. Open a sterile lancet package.

15. Using your nondominant hand, grasp the client's finger (selected site) firmly with your thumb and middle finger.

16. With your dominant hand, take the lancet and point it down.

17. Puncture the site with a clear, decisive down-and-up motion (do not slowly push the lancet in; this should be a darting movement) (Figure 42-8C).

18. Discard the first drop of blood by wiping it away with the sterile gauze (Figure 42-8D).

19. Continue to apply pressure on either side of the site until you obtain the desired amount of blood. Do not "milk" the site by squeezing hard.

20. Allow the blood to drop onto the collection device without touching the skin (Figure 42-8E).

21. Apply gentle pressure to the puncture site until bleeding stops.

22. Label collection containers in preparation for testing or processing.

23. Discard contaminated items in the biohazardous waste container and put the lancet in the sharps container.

24. Remove your gloves.

25. Wash your hands.

26. Record the procedure in the client's chart immediately.

(Continues)

PROCEDURE 42-3 (Continued)

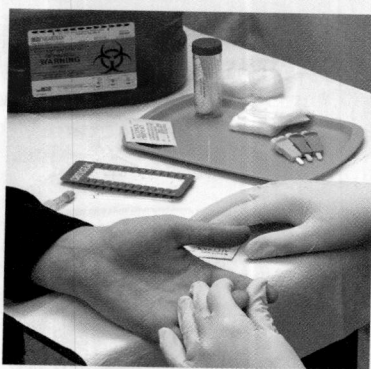

FIGURE 42-8A Assemble the items needed to collect a specimen into a capillary tube. Select a site that is free from bruises, scars, and open wounds.

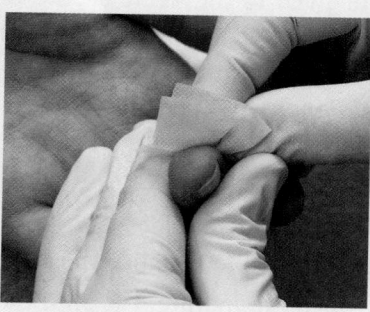

FIGURE 42-8B Cleanse the site with an alcohol wipe.

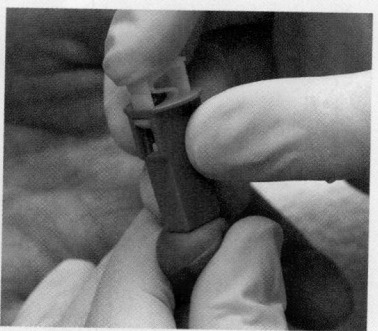

FIGURE 42-8C Perform the puncture.

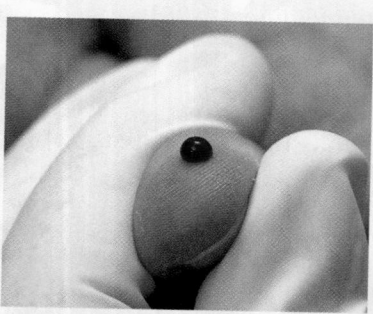

FIGURE 42-8D Wipe off the first drop of blood with sterile gauze.

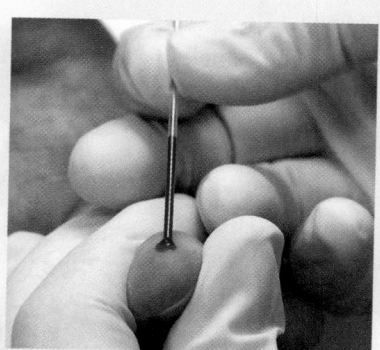

FIGURE 42-8E Allow the collection tube to fill, being careful not to touch the skin.

Charting Example:

06/17/20xx   10:15 A.M.   Blood sample collected from client using capillary method on client's ring finger left hand. Sample labeled and sent to lab.

Carrie Adams, S.M.A.

Carrie Adams, S.M.A. (printed name)

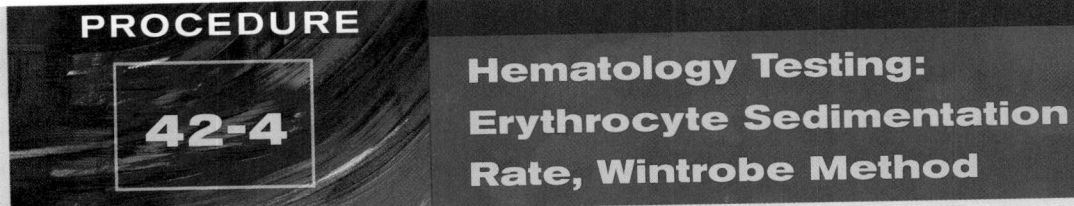

PROCEDURE

42-4

Hematology Testing: Erythrocyte Sedimentation Rate, Wintrobe Method

Student Competency Objective: The medical assistant student will perform an erythrocyte sedimentation rate (ESR) test using the Wintrobe method.

Items Needed: Gloves, PPE as appropriate, Wintrobe tube, pipette, lavender-top tube (anticoagulant), clock or watch with second hand, biohazardous waste container

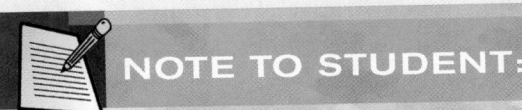

NOTE TO STUDENT:

The Westergreen method is more commonly used to test sedimentation rates. The basic difference between this and the Wintrobe method is the length of the pipette and the anticoagulant used.

Steps:

1. Wash your hands.
2. Assemble equipment and supplies.
3. Obtain a 5 mL blood sample using a lavender-top tube (anticoagulant) (see Procedure 42-1).
4. Gently invert the tube a number of times, but do not shake or agitate the contents.
5. Using a pipette, fill the Wintrobe tube to the 0 point. Be accurate.
6. Put the filled tube in a holder. The tube should be supported and straight up.
7. Leave undisturbed for 1 hour.
8. Read the level of the top of the red blood cells. (Normal ranges for adult males under the age of 50 = 0 to15 mm/hr; for adult females under the age of 50 = 0 to 20 mm/hr.)
9. Write results in a log.
10. Clean equipment.
11. Dispose of specimen and tubes and used supplies in biohazardous waste container.
12. Remove your gloves.
13. Wash your hands.
14. Record the procedure in the client's chart immediately.
15. Notify the doctor of the results.

Charting Example:

12/9/20xx   9:30 A.M.   Obtained blood sample from 40-year-old male. Performed ESR with Wintrobe method. Results: 50 mm/hr. Recorded in log and doctor notified of results.

Jerome Winters, S.M.A.

Jerome Winters, S.M.A. (printed name)

BRIDGE TO CAAHEP

This chapter, which discusses hematology and venipuncture, provides information and content related to CAAHEP standards for Anatomy and Physiology, Medical Terminology, Medical Law and Ethics, Psychology, Communication, Medical Assisting Administrative Procedures, Medical Assisting Clinical Procedures, and Professional Components.

AAMA AREAS OF COMPETENCE

This chapter, which discusses hematology and venipuncture, provides information or content within several areas listed in the Medical Assistant Role Delineation Study. These areas include: clinical, fundamental principles, diagnostic orders, patient (client) care, general transdisciplinary professionalism, communication, legal concepts, instruction, and operational functions.

ABHES LINKS

This chapter, which discusses hematology and venipuncture, links to ABHES course content for Anatomy and Physiology, Medical Terminology, Medical Law and Ethics, Psychology of Human Relations, Medical Office Clinical Procedures, and Medical Laboratory Procedures.

AMT PATHS

This chapter, which discusses hematology and venipuncture, provides a path to AMT competency in general medical assisting knowledge, anatomy and physiology, medical terminology, and patient (client) education.

POINTS OF HIGHLIGHT

- Hematology is the study of blood, including how it works and disorders of the blood.
- The medical assistant's role includes preparing the client for specialized blood tests.
- The medical assistant may obtain the blood samples for the ordered tests.
- Red blood cells, white blood cells, and platelets are the major types of blood cells.
- A complete blood count is one of the most frequently ordered tests.
- The hematocrit test examines the amount of red blood cell mass in relation to whole blood.
- Hemoglobin tests measure the oxygen-carrying capacity of the blood.
- An abnormal white blood cell count may indicate the presence of an infection.
- A differential white blood cell count will help to determine levels of specific subtypes of white blood cells.
- Blood draws, or venipuncture, can be done by either the vacuum-tube method or the syringe method.
- Certain blood tests only require a capillary puncture. The medical assistant needs to understand hematological tests and become skilled in obtaining the blood specimens used to perform these tests.

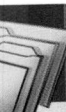

STUDENT PORTFOLIO ACTIVITY

Select a clinical laboratory in the region where you would like to work. Make an appointment with the manager for a tour and to observe. Write an observational report to share with your classroom instructor and peers. Make sure to ask the manager at the lab to sign a confirmation of your visit with times and dates.

APPLYING YOUR SKILLS

A laboratory report is faxed to the office. The hemoglobin level was tested, and is reported as 10 grams per 100 mL of blood. Is this within the normal range? As a medical assistant, what actions should you take, if any?

CRITICAL THINKING QUESTIONS

1. The doctor orders a CBC. As a medical assistant, you need to obtain the blood sample and send it to the lab. You must choose between venipuncture with vacuum tubes or venipuncture with a syringe. What are some factors that will help you decide which to use?

2. How can a laboratory chair make a venipuncture procedure safer?

3. What is the role of hemoglobin in the red blood cells?

4. What does it mean that platelets help the blood to maintain homeostasis?

5. How can blood affect the progression of cancer?

6. What could cause a low reading on a hematocrit blood test?

7. What might an increase in the white blood cell count indicate?

8. What conditions might cause an increase in the hemoglobin level?

9. How will medical assistants know which hematological tests they can perform?

10. Is the complete blood count one test? What is the purpose of the CBC?

11. Go back to the beginning of this chapter and review the Anticipatory Statements. Reread each statement and then indicate whether it is true or false. If the statement is false, rewrite it to make it a true statement.

CLIENT TEACHING PLAN

Applying Cold to an Area

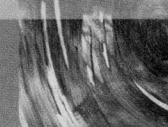

◼ What Is to Be Taught:

• Application of cold to a specific site, using either a commercial ice pack or a homemade ice compress.

◼ Objectives:

• Client will apply a cold treatment to an area of the body as prescribed by the doctor.

◼ Preparation Before Teaching:

• Check the doctor's orders for details of instruction.
• Review the purpose and benefits of cold treatment to an area of the body.
• Assemble items needed for teaching, such as ice, bag, towel, commercial ice pack, and paper and pen for written instructions.
• Make sure the area is free from distractions while you are teaching.

◼ Steps for the Medical Assistant:

1. Gather supplies needed.
2. Introduce yourself to the client.
3. Explain what you are going to teach and why.
4. Tell the client that the doctor has prescribed a cold treatment to help heal an injury.
5. Inform the client that you will apply the cold treatment and show her how to do the same thing at home.
6. Wash your hands.
7. Look at the area on the client where the cold treatment is to be applied.
8. Show the client how to fill a plastic bag with ice chips. Pick out small ice pieces. Small pieces, almost crushed, will mold to the client's body and cause less discomfort.
9. Tell the client not to completely fill the bag; some room is needed to close the bag and prevent leakage.
10. Place ice on the ordered area and place a towel over the ice bag.
11. Ask the client how it feels: Is there much discomfort?
12. Leave in the ice bag place for the amount of time ordered by the doctor (usually 20 to 30 minutes).
13. If the client will use a commercial ice pack at home, demonstrate correct use and include the following directions:
    a. Handle the pack with care so as not to puncture or damage it.
    b. Check the pack for leaks or damage. If present, do not use that pack.
    c. Read the directions on the cold pack. These items contain chemicals and should be handled with care.
14. Ask the client to tell you the steps that you just performed.
15. Repeat the instructions if the client cannot remember or is hesitant.
16. Write down instructions for the client to take home. Make sure to include the doctor's office telephone number.
17. Ask the client if she has any questions.
18. Remove the ice bag after the ordered amount of time.
19. Tell the client that if she has any questions, concerns, or problems when she does this at home, she should call the doctor.
20. Look at the area treated. See if there is any redness or unusual paleness.
21. Ask the client how the area feels.
22. Discard the used towel and ice chip bag.
23. Wash your hands.
24. Record the procedure and teaching in the client's chart immediately.

◼ Special Needs of the Client:

• If the client is elderly, use extra caution. The skin of older adults is more sensitive and intolerant of extreme temperatures.

(Continues)

CLIENT TEACHING PLAN (Continued)

- Look at the client's chart to see if there are any factors that might interfere with the client's ability to carry out this procedure at home.
- Ask the client, before and after the teaching and cold treatment application, if there is anything you should know that might affect her ability to apply cold treatments.

■ Evaluation:

- Client states the steps involved in applying cold treatments.
- Client is able to demonstrate the steps correctly, in the proper order.

■ Further Plans/Teaching:

- Ask the client if she thinks she can apply the cold treatments at home.
- Review the steps at the client's next office visit if needed.

■ Follow-up:

- Call the client at home to find out if she has any questions.

Medical Assistant

Name: _____

Signature: _____

Date: _____

Client

Date: _____

Follow-up Date: _____

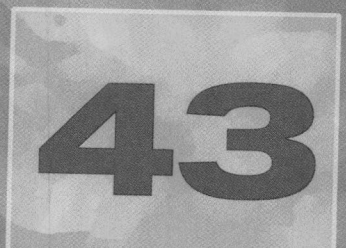
Anticipatory Statements

Read and think about the following statements based upon what you believe now. Decide whether you agree or disagree. Write the word **agree** after the statement if you think the statement is true. Write the word **disagree** after the statement if you think the statement is false. Read the chapter to find out if your current beliefs can be supported.

1. A medical assistant will often perform an ECG or EKG test in the office as part of clinical skills.

   _____

2. The medical assistant's role in cardiac stress testing is to provide client preparation and teaching.

   _____

3. An echocardiogram is performed by the clinical medical assistant.

   _____

4. Much client preparation is necessary before an ECG or EKG test.

   _____

5. A Holter monitor test is similar to an ECG or EKG test.

   _____

Learning Objectives

Upon completion of this chapter, the medical assistant student should be able to:

- State the purpose of cardiac diagnostic tests
- Define *electrocardiogram*
- Explain the medical assistant's role in the electrocardiogram test
- Perform an electrocardiogram test

Cardiac Diagnostic Laboratory

- Describe the use of a Holter monitor
- Explain the medical assistant's role in Holter monitor use
- Set up a Holter monitor test
- Define *stress test*
- Explain the medical assistant's role in a stress test
- Define *echocardiogram*
- Explain the medical assistant's role in the echocardiogram test
- Plan and carry out a client teaching plan for cardiac testing

Key Terms

artifacts In testing, something that shows up on a test (such as an ECG printout) that is not a valid result of the testing; for example, signals that are really caused by defective equipment or client movement during testing.

cardiac conduction system System that sends electrical impulses through the heart.

echocardiogram Graphic record of the structure and activity of the different parts of the heart.

electrocardiogram (ECG or EKG) Graphic record of the electrical impulses of the heart muscle.

electrode Consists of a wire connected to a patch that is applied to a client's skin; acts as a sensor to pick up and record electrical activity of the heart.

Holter monitor Similar to an electrocardiograph, but is portable, which allows recordings to be done as a client goes through daily activities.

leads The wires that go from the electrocardiograph machine to the client.

monitor Machine that watches and (usually) records.

transducer Piece of equipment that changes or adjusts power or a signal from one system to transfer the power or signal in a usable form to another system.

transesophageal echo (TEE) A type of echocardiogram.

ultrasound Sound waves used in echocardiography.

■ INTRODUCTION

Heart and cardiovascular problems affect many people in the United States. Cardiovascular events are the leading cause of death in this country. The number of problems is expected to grow as the population ages and the rate of obesity increases across all age groups. In an effort to prevent heart problems and to discover heart problems before great harm is done, diagnostic cardiac testing is often done in the doctor's office, diagnostic laboratory, or hospital. Medical assistants need to be aware of the basic cardiac diagnostic tests, the purpose of these tests, and the medical assistant's role in helping and caring for the client who is being tested. Cardiac tests include electrocardiograms, Holter monitoring, stress tests, and echocardiograms. The medical assistant prepares the client for the test, and may also perform or assist in conducting these tests.

■ ELECTROCARDIOGRAM

An **electrocardiogram (ECG** or sometimes **EKG)** is a common cardiac diagnostic test often performed in the doctor's office as part of a general physical examination, or to check specifically for heart problems. This test records the electrical impulses of the heart; the *electrocardiograph* is the tool that records these impulses. This is a noninvasive procedure, meaning that it is not necessary to pierce the skin or enter any body cavity to perform the test. The results of the test help the doctor to see if the **cardiac conduction system** is running smoothly (see Chapter 12). The ECG gives much information about the heart and can answer questions such as:

- Is the client experiencing arrhythmias (irregular or uneven heartbeats)?
- Are all parts of the heart receiving electrical impulses in the right amount, at the right time, and in the right order?
- Does the client have heart damage from a heart attack?
- Are any chambers or areas of the heart enlarged?

Client Preparation

The client need not do anything special before an ECG test. The medical assistant should explain to the client, in simple terms, what will be done, what will happen, and what to expect. A basic explanation states that the ECG records information about how the heart is working today, and that the doctor can use these facts to help the client. The medical assistant can stress that the client will not experience any pain or discomfort. Clients can become frightened when they see the electrocardiograph machine with its many cords (**leads**) that have to be attached directly to the skin of the client's chest, arms, and legs. When clients hear the word *electric*, they may fear getting a shock. The client may not openly say this to the medical assistant; therefore, the medical assistant should talk about common fears regarding ECGs. Ensure client privacy and comfort during the test. The client must lie on his back while remaining very still. Maintain a comfortable temperature in the room to prevent shivering, which causes error marks on the recording called **artifacts.** The ECG will have to be repeated after the cause of the artifacts is discovered and corrected.

Conducting the Test

For an ECG test, the client is positioned on his back, in supine position. The medical assistant finds the appropriate areas on the skin and attaches the correct leads for each area (Figure 43-1). The machine is turned on and the electrical impulses are recorded (Figure 43-2). When completed, the **electrodes** are removed. The entire test takes about 15 minutes. Afterward, the doctor will read the recordings and discuss the results with the client (see Procedure 43-1).

■ HOLTER MONITOR

A number of client problems may require use of a **Holter monitor** (Figure 43-3). Sometimes an electrocardiogram may not record any arrhythmias, yet the client still experiences strange

(A) Standard limb or bipolar leads

	Electrodes Connected
Lead I	LA and RA
Lead II*	LL and RA
Lead III	LL and LA

* Also used for rhythm strip

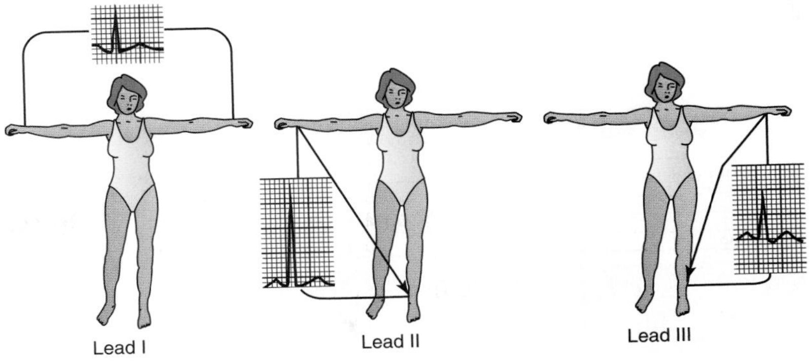

Lead I   Lead II   Lead III

(B) Augmented limb leads

aVR	RA and (LA-LL)
aVL	LA and (RA-LL)
aVF	LL and (RA-LA)

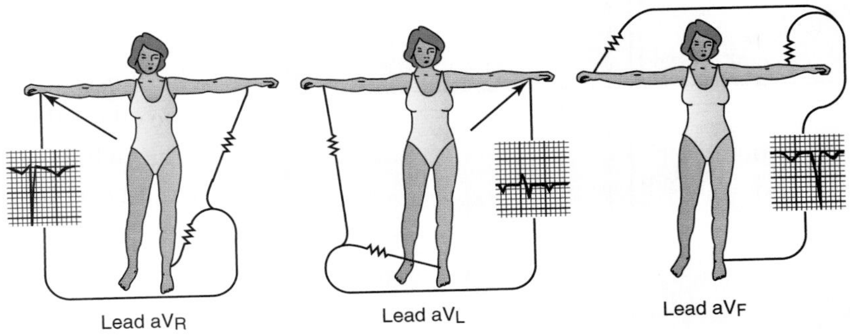

Lead aV$_R$ Lead aV$_L$ Lead aV$_F$

(C) Precordial or chest leads

	Electrodes connected	Placement
V$_1$	V$_1$ and (LA-RA-LL)	Fourth intercostal space at right margin of sternum
V$_2$	V$_2$ and (LA-RA-LL)	Fourth intercostal space at left margin of sternum
V$_4$	V$_4$ and (LA-RA-LL)	Fifth intercostal space at junction of left midclavicular line
V$_3$	V$_3$ and (LA-RA-LL)	Midway between position 2 and position 4
V$_5$	V$_5$ and (LA-RA-LL)	At horizontal level of position 4 at left anterior axillary line
V$_6$	V$_6$ and (LA-RA-LL)	At horizontal level of position 4 at left midaxillary line

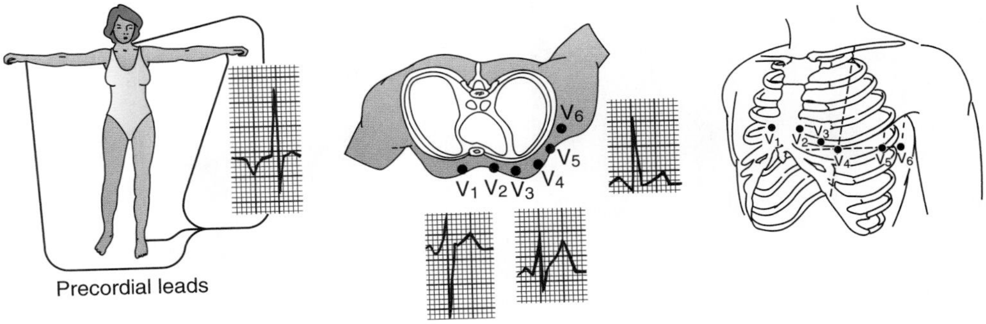

Precordial leads

V$_6$
V$_5$
V$_1$ V$_2$ V$_3$ V$_4$

FIGURE 43-1 Lead types, connections, and placement for electrocardiogram.

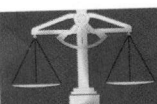

LEGAL/ETHICAL THOUGHTS

While working as a medical assistant, you may be asked to place telephone calls to a cardiac diagnostic laboratory. Office policy will help determine safety for outgoing calls. You need to make sure of the identity of the person receiving your call and that the person is the correct individual to speak to.

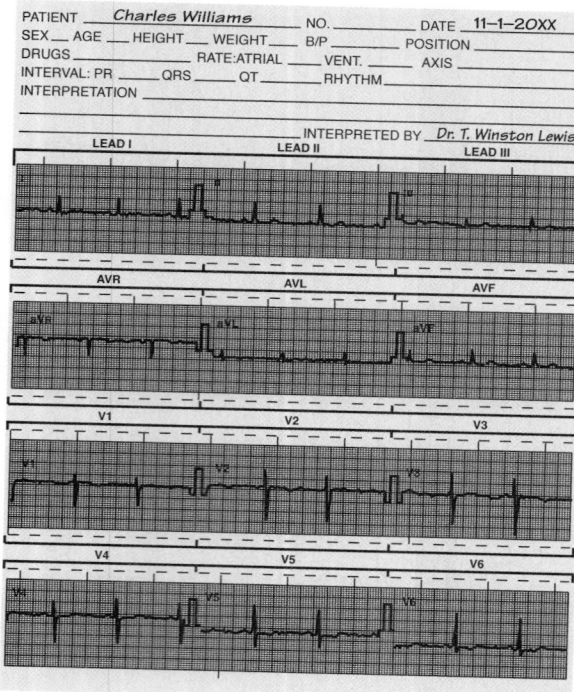

PATIENT ___Charles Williams___ NO. _____ DATE __11–1–20XX__
SEX __ AGE __ HEIGHT __ WEIGHT __ B/P _____ POSITION _____
DRUGS _____ RATE:ATRIAL __ VENT. __ AXIS _____
INTERVAL: PR _____ QRS _____ QT _____ RHYTHM _____
INTERPRETATION _____

INTERPRETED BY __Dr. T. Winston Lewis__

LEAD I   LEAD II   LEAD III

AVR   AVL   AVF

V1   V2   V3

V4   V5   V6

FIGURE 43–2 Single ECG recording.

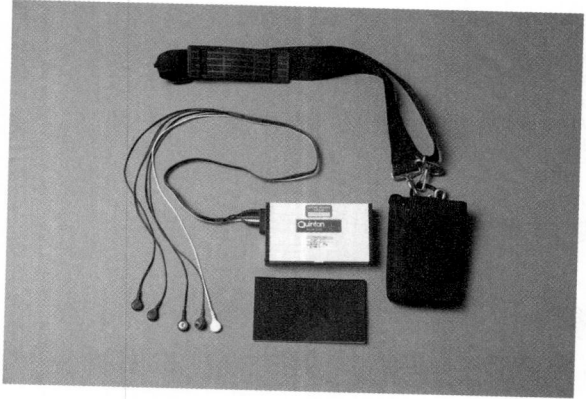

FIGURE 43–3 Holter monitor and supplies.

feelings in the chest. Also, an ECG may show some uneven heartbeats, and the doctor may want to investigate these further. A third reason to use a Holter monitor is to see how well a prescribed medicine is helping the client's heart. A Holter monitor test is similar to an electrocardiogram. This piece of equipment records the electrical impulses of the client's heart over a 24- to 48-hour time period while the client goes about his activities of daily living. The client should not, however, take a shower or bath, because the **monitor** and leads must not get wet.

Client Preparation

The client need not do anything special to prepare for a Holter monitor test. The client does need to be oriented and able to follow directions for a two-day period, including using hands to push the button on the monitor. If the client does not follow the directions, the test will be useless. When the client feels anything unusual with the heart (such as skipped beats, sense of a fast pulse, palpitations, or just an odd feeling in the chest), the client presses the monitor button. The client then writes in a booklet the date, the time, what he felt, and what he was doing or what was happening at that moment.

Conducting the Test

The medical assistant attaches the electrode leads to the chest and places the monitor in the shoulder strap or belt (Figure 43–4). Over the next 24 to 48 hours, the client pushes the button whenever he experiences strange feelings in the chest and writes in the record booklet what was going on at that moment. At the end of the testing period, the client returns the monitor and booklet to the doctor's office. If the client cannot remove the electrodes, the medical assistant can remove them when the client returns to the office (see Procedure 43–2).

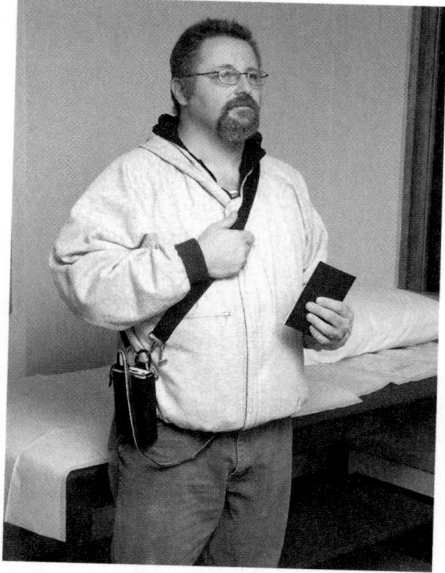

FIGURE 43–4 Correct placement of a Holter monitor on the client.

■ STRESS TEST

An ECG is also used with a third type of heart test: The *cardiac stress test* uses the ECG to monitor or watch the heart while it is being stressed during exercise (Figure 43-5). While hooked up to the ECG, the client exercises by walking on a treadmill. The purpose of the stress test is to see how well the heart works when the added strain of exercise is placed on it. The doctor may be looking for causes of chest pain or arrhythmias. A client who lives a sedentary lifestyle should have a stress test done before beginning an exercise program or sport. The cardiac stress test is done in a doctor's office or diagnostic laboratory. Emergency equipment must be available at the setting in case of life-threatening heart problems brought on by the stress of exercise.

Client Preparation

The medical assistant's role in cardiac stress testing is to provide client preparation and teaching. The client may not smoke, drink coffee (or other caffeine-containing beverages), or eat before the test. The number of hours of preparation depends on the doctor and the policy of the lab. The medical assistant will explain the purpose of the test to the client and tell him what to expect. Inform the client that a health care provider (usually the doctor) will be present during the exercise time. Answer questions to make the client comfortable.

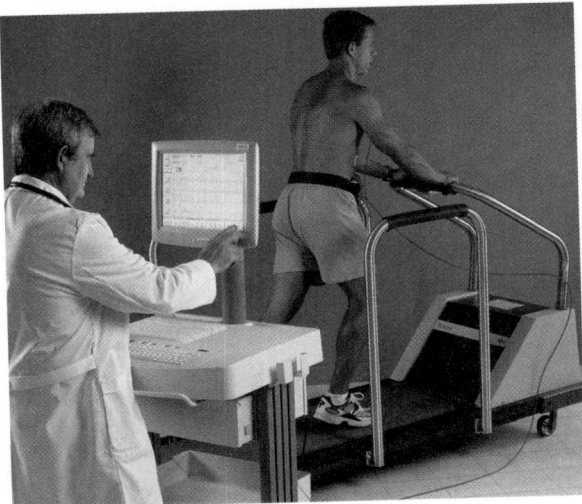

FIGURE 43-5 The Quest Exercise Stress System. (Courtesy of Quinton Cardiology, Inc.)

Conducting the Test

The medical assistant will attach the ECG leads to the client before the test begins. Sometimes the medical assistant will take the client's blood pressure, but often it is the doctor who obtains these readings. It depends on the scope of practice and the policy of the laboratory where the test is being conducted.

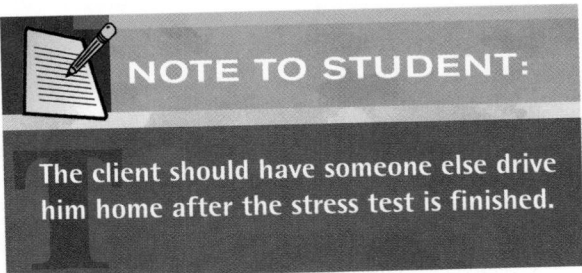

NOTE TO STUDENT:

The client should have someone else drive him home after the stress test is finished.

■ ECHOCARDIOGRAM

An **echocardiogram** is an **ultrasound** test that uses sound waves to look at the heart's structure and function. The size and position of the heart and valves, as well as the flow of blood, can be examined. This noninvasive test takes about 45 minutes to complete. There is a second type, called a **transesophageal echo (TEE)** test, in which a tube is passed down the client's throat so that an internal picture can be taken.

Client Preparation

The major role of the medical assistant is to provide client preparation and teaching. Most commonly, an echocardiogram technician holds a **transducer** (a piece of equipment that looks like a television remote control) and slides it across areas of the chest wall. With this method, no special client preparation is needed before the test. Reassure the client that there should be no pain or discomfort from the procedure.

Conducting the Test

The procedure will be performed by a trained echocardiogram technician. The technician will ask the client to lie on his side. Gel will be put on the client's chest. The technician will then move the transducer over the chest area.

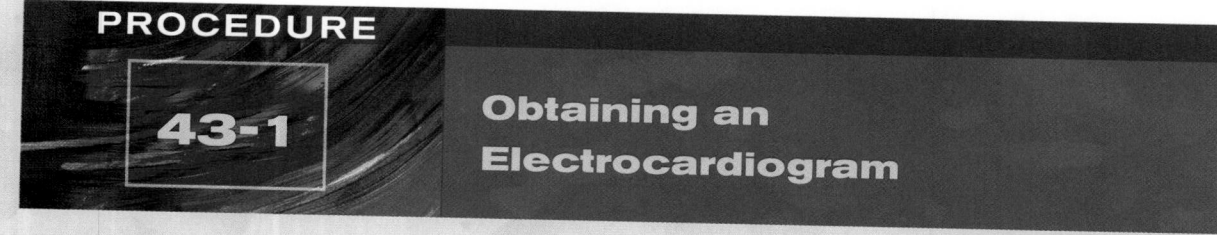

PROCEDURE

43-1

Obtaining an Electrocardiogram

Student Competency Objective: The medical assistant student will obtain a 12-lead electro-cardiogram using a computerized electrocardiograph.

Items Needed: Electrocardiograph with leads and cables, ECG paper, disposable electrodes with gel, gown, drape, pillow, disposable towels, alcohol wipes, pen, paper

Steps:

1. Wash your hands.
2. Assemble equipment and supplies.
3. Plug in the ECG machine.
4. Check all cable wires.
5. Look around the area to make sure nothing will create electrical interference.
6. Snap electrodes into pads.
7. Check the room to ensure that the atmosphere is quiet and comfortable and that the room is at a comfortable temperature.
8. Introduce yourself to the client even if you have seen the client on previous visits to your office. The client may have forgotten your name. This also helps to establish a provider-client relationship, because it shows the client that you want him to know who you are.
9. Identify the client. Ask the client to state his name to establish that this is the right client, and then compare the name given to the name on the chart. Never enter a room and call out a client's name to determine if this person is the correct client. The client may not have heard you clearly and may just nod, smile, or answer yes. Clients almost never question if the medical assistant professional has the right client. It is up to the medical assistant to identify the right client before performing any procedure.
10. Tell the client, in everyday language, what you are going to do.
11. Ask if the client has any questions. If he does, give short and simple answers. Sometimes clients will start (and continue) talking because they are nervous about the procedure.
12. Ask the client about any allergies.
13. Tell the client to remain still, as the machine will pick up any movement and thus distort the readings.
14. Remind the client that there is no pain from an ECG.
15. Hand the client a gown.
16. Tell the client to remove clothing from the waist up (female clients who are wearing tights or pantyhose must remove those also).
17. Help the client onto the examination table.
18. Ask the client to lie on his back (supine position).
19. Place a pillow under the client's head.

(Continues)

PROCEDURE 43-1 (Continued)

20. Drape the client for privacy.

21. Turn the ECG machine on.

22. Put in the client's name and other required data.

23. Wipe the sites for electrode placement with alcohol wipes (Figure 43-6A).

24. Place the arm electrodes on fleshy, muscular, outer area of upper arms (RA, LA) (Figure 43-6B).

25. Place the leg electrodes on the fleshy inner area of the calves of the lower legs (RL, LL).

26. Make sure the lead wires are not tangled.

27. Connect the lead wires to the electrodes and the ECG machine. Follow the color-coded markings.

28. Place chest electrodes (V_1–V_6) (Figure 43-6C).

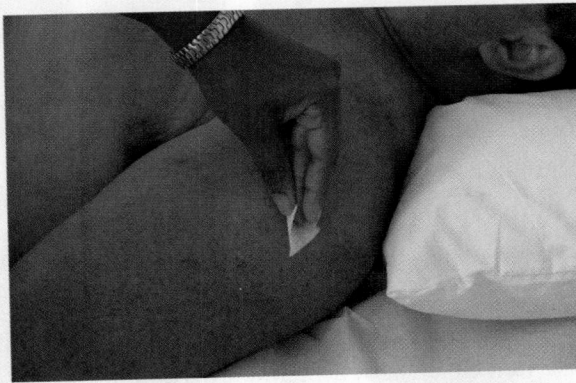

FIGURE 43-6A With the client lying supine, cleanse the sites for electrode placement with alcohol wipes.

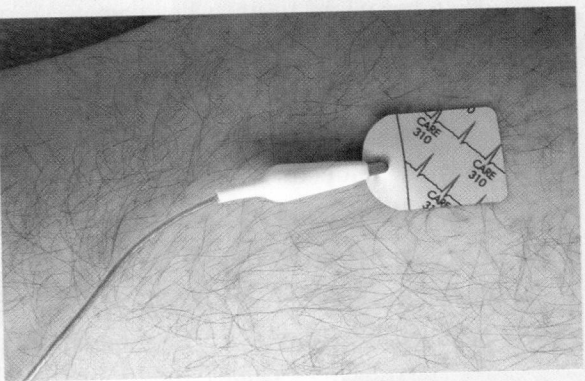

FIGURE 43-6B Attach the arm electrodes (RA, LA) on the client.

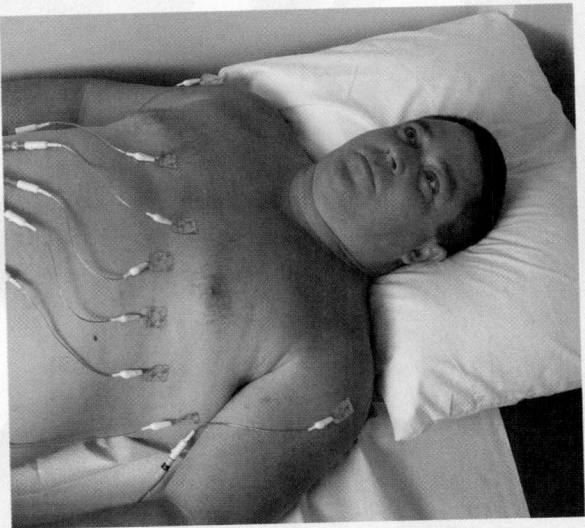

FIGURE 43-6C Place the chest electrodes (V_1–V_6) on the client.

(Continues)

PROCEDURE 43-1 (Continued)

29. Recheck electrode placement.
30. Press the "auto" button on the ECG machine.
31. Allow the 12-lead ECG to run through.
32. Remove the ECG printout from the machine.
33. Look at the printout for any artifacts.
34. If no artifacts are seen, turn the machine off.
35. Take the electrodes off the client.
36. Wipe the electrode placement sites dry, cleaning all the gel off.
37. Dispose of used towels and wipes in the appropriate waste container.
38. Help the client to a sitting position.
39. Assist the client to get off the table, as needed.
40. Help the client to dress as needed.
41. Discard used items such as the paper table cover and gown, according to office policy.
42. Wash your hands.
43. Record the procedure in the client's chart immediately.
44. Inform the doctor that the test has been completed.
45. Place the ECG printout in the client's chart or give it to the doctor, according to office policy.

Charting Example:

10/28/20xx   9:14 A.M.   Set up and obtained 12-lead ECG. Computerized printout placed in client's chart. Doctor informed. Assisted client with dressing. Instructions given to client on how to obtain ECG results.

Therese Towers, S.M.A.

Therese Towers, S.M.A. (printed name)

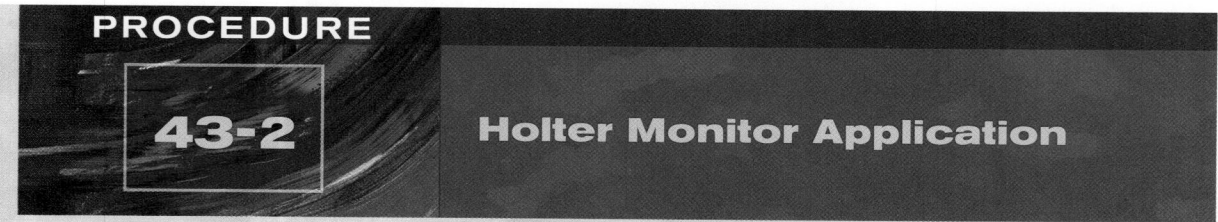

PROCEDURE

43-2   Holter Monitor Application

Student Competency Objective: The medical assistant student will apply a Holter monitor.

Items Needed: Holter monitor, gauze, cotton swabs, electrodes, cassette with case and strap, blank tape, batteries

Steps:

1. Wash your hands.
2. Gather equipment and supplies.

(Continues)

3. Introduce yourself to the client even if you have seen the client on previous visits to your office. The client may have forgotten your name. This also helps to establish a provider-client relationship, because it shows the client that you want him to know who you are.

4. Identify the client. Ask the client to state his name to establish that this is the right client, and then compare the name given to the name on the chart. Never enter a room and call out a client's name to determine if this person is the correct client. The client may not have heard you clearly and may just nod, smile, or answer yes. Clients almost never question if the medical assistant professional has the right client. It is up to the medical assistant to identify the right client before performing any procedure.

5. Tell the client, in everyday language, what you are going to do.

6. Ask if the client has any questions. If he does, give short and simple answers. Sometimes clients will start (and continue) talking because they are nervous about the procedure.

7. Tell the client, in simple terms, that the doctor needs to identify what is happening with the heartbeat and determine what the client can do to help his own heart health. Finding out what is going on will also help the doctor to prescribe the best treatment.

8. Show the client the monitor and all the parts, which are color-coded. Different manufacturers may use different colors. Follow the manufacturer's directions regarding where to place which color. The colored parts and the places they attach are not interchangeable.

9. Snap the white wire to an electrode or patch, snap the green electrode to an electrode or patch, and snap the black wire to an electrode or patch.

10. Ask the client to unbutton his shirt (he need not remove it completely).

11. Find an area on the client's chest that is one to two fingers' width below the clavicle (collarbone) on the right side of the chest. Clean the area with an alcohol wipe.

12. Remove the backing from the patch attached to the white wire and place it at the point located.

13. Find an area on the client's chest that is one to two fingers' width below the clavicle on the left side of the chest. Clean the area with an alcohol wipe.

14. Remove the backing from the patch attached to the green wire and place it at the point located.

15. Find an area under the left breast and move your hand to the side until it is below the client's underarm. Clean the area with an alcohol wipe.

16. Remove the backing from the patch attached to the black wire and place it at the point located.

17. Pick up the cassette. Put the battery into the cassette. Attach the plug at the end of each wire into the opening in the cassette.

18. Show client the "event" button, the "clear" button and the "low battery" button.

19. Perform a baseline recording.

20. Push and hold the "event" button down until it beeps.

21. Tell the client that when he feels any symptoms, he should push the "event" button.

22. Tell the client to write on a piece of paper (or log booklet) what he was doing when he felt the symptoms. Keep the written information to bring to the doctor.

(Continues)

PROCEDURE 43-2 (Continued)

Charting Example:

09/21/20xx   4:00 P.M.   Applied Holter monitor at 4:00 P.M. Client given written and verbal instructions regarding the event button, activities, and how to complete the diary. Client instructed to return to the medical office on 9/23/XX for removal of the monitor.

Krista Young, S.M.A.

Krista Young, S.M.A. (printed name)

BRIDGE TO CAAHEP

This chapter, which discusses cardiac diagnostic laboratory, provides information and content related to CAAHEP standards for Anatomy and Physiology, Medical Terminology, Psychology, Communications, Administrative Procedures, Medical Assisting Clinical Procedures, Diagnostic Testing, Patient (Client) Care, and Professional Components.

ABHES LINKS

This chapter, which discusses cardiac diagnostic laboratory, links to ABHES course content for Anatomy and Physiology, Medical Terminology, Medical Law and Ethics, Psychology of Human Relations, Medical Office Clinical Procedures, and Medical Laboratory Procedures.

AAMA AREAS OF COMPETENCE

This chapter, which discusses cardiac diagnostic laboratory, provides information or content within several areas listed in the Medical Assistant Role Delineation Study. These areas include: clinical, fundamental principles, diagnostic orders, patient (client) care, general transdisciplinary, professionalism, communication skills, instruction, and operational functions.

AMT PATHS

This chapter, which discusses cardiac diagnostic laboratory, provides a path to AMT competency in general medical assisting knowledge, anatomy and physiology, medical terminology, medical law, medical ethics, human relations, patient (client) education, clinical medical assisting, asepsis, instruments, and laboratory procedures.

POINTS OF HIGHLIGHT

- Tests to evaluate cardiac function are the electrocardiogram, Holter monitor, stress test, and echocardiogram.
- An electrocardiogram, commonly performed in the medical office, checks the heart's electrical impulse generation and conduction.
- A Holter monitor is similar to an electrocardiogram; it is portable and measures the electrical impulses of the heart over a 24- to 48-hour period.
- A cardiac stress test checks how well the heart works under the added stress of exercise or activity.
- An echocardiogram uses sound waves to examine the heart's structure and function.
- The medical assistant's role in cardiac testing will vary according to the scope of practice and office policy.

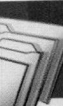

STUDENT PORTFOLIO ACTIVITY

Electrocardiograms and Holter monitoring are routinely done in many health care settings. Keep documentation that you are knowledgeable and competent regarding electrocardiograms and use of Holter monitors. This might include a test on which you earned a high grade or the signed competency form used in the laboratory practice part of the clinical course. You might choose a client preparation teaching plan for cardiac testing that you compiled.

APPLYING YOUR SKILLS

A doctor looks at the records for an ECG. He thinks that some of the records may actually be artifacts. What are artifacts? How might they have been prevented during the testing?

CRITICAL THINKING QUESTIONS

1. What does an ECG measure? What can it tell the doctor about a client's heart?

2. A doctor orders an ECG. The client tells you that he is afraid of the electricity going through him. As a medical assistant, how do you respond? What do you say to this client?

3. A client who complained of chest pain had an ECG done. There were no abnormal findings. However, the doctor ordered a Holter monitor test. Why would the doctor do this? What must the client do during this test?

4. Explain the role of the medical assistant in cardiac stress testing.

5. What does the echocardiogram use to examine the heart? What would you, as a medical assistant, tell the client to expect during an echocardiogram?

6. Explain how a Holter monitor is similar to an electrocardiograph.

7. Why are so many cardiac diagnostic tests performed?

8. How do you prepare and position a client for an ECG?

9. As a medical assistant, what precautions can you take to prevent artifacts during an ECG test?

10. Why is emergency equipment always available during cardiac stress testing?

11. Go back to the beginning of this chapter and review the Anticipatory Statements. Reread each statement and then indicate whether it is true or false. If the statement is false, rewrite it to make it a true statement.

CLIENT TEACHING PLAN

Cardiac Holter Event Monitor

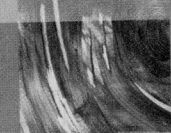

What Is to Be Taught:

- How to use a cardiac Holter event monitor.

Objectives:

- Client will be able to perform steps necessary to use a cardiac Holter event monitor for diagnostic testing at home.

Preparation Before Teaching:

- Review the cardiac heart cycle, including the pathways of the heart and especially the conduction of electrical impulses. Make sure to put technical medical terms into everyday language for teaching purposes.
- Look over the purposes of using an event monitor. (Irregular heartbeats are the most frequent reason for such a test.) Be prepared to be supportive of the client, who may have many worries and fears about heart problems.
- Assemble supplies and equipment, including the Holter event monitor, alcohol wipes, written or printed information about the working of the heart, and paper and pen.
- Make sure that the area is free from distractions while you are teaching.

Steps for the Medical Assistant:

1. Wash your hands.
2. Gather supplies needed.
3. Introduce yourself to the client.
4. Explain what you are going to teach and why.
5. Tell the client, in simple terms, about the need to identify what is happening with the heartbeat and what the client can do to help his own heart health. Inform him that finding out what is going on will also help the doctor to prescribe the best treatment.
6. Show the client the monitor and all the parts. *Different manufacturers may use different colors. Follow the manufacturer's directions regarding*

where to place which color. The colored parts and the places where they attach are not interchangeable.

7. Snap the white wire to an electrode or patch, snap the green electrode to an electrode or patch, and snap the black wire to an electrode or patch.
8. If possible, demonstrate the following steps on a teaching mannequin and then have the client repeat the steps on himself.
9. Ask the client to unbutton his shirt (he need not remove it completely).
10. Find an area on the client's chest that is one to two fingers' width below the clavicle on the right side of the chest. Clean the area with an alcohol wipe.
11. Remove the backing from the patch attached to the white wire and place it at the point located.
12. Find an area on the client's chest that is one to two fingers' width below the clavicle on the left side of the chest. Clean the area with an alcohol wipe.
13. Remove the backing from the patch attached to the green wire and place it at the point located.
14. Find an area under the client's left breast and move your hand to the side until it is below the client's underarm. Clean the area with an alcohol wipe.
15. Remove the backing from the patch attached to the black wire and place it at the point located.
16. Pick up the cassette. Put the battery into the cassette. Attach the plug at the end of each wire into the opening in the cassette.
17. Show client the "event" button, the "clear" button, and the "low battery" button. Ask the client to change the battery when the "low battery" indicator flashes. Give the client extra batteries in case replacements are needed.

(Continues)

CLIENT TEACHING PLAN (Continued)

18. Perform a baseline recording. This also demonstrates to the client how he is to perform a recording at home:
    a. Push and hold the "event" button down until it beeps.
    b. Release the button and sit still. Movement will interfere with the recording and give false information. The client will hear a low noise while the monitor is recording. Another beep will sound when the recording is complete. Additionally, a light will flash, indicating that the recording is complete.
    c. Call the laboratory where the recording is to be sent. The laboratory technician will inform the client how to transmit the recording.
19. Instruct the client to erase the baseline/demonstration recording. Push the "event" button; the cassette will beep when the recording is erased and the light will flash.
20. Tell the client that he should push the "event" button and begin the recording process whenever he feels any symptoms.
21. Tell the client to record (on a piece of paper or a log booklet) what he was doing when he felt the symptoms. Keep the written information to bring to the doctor.

■ Special Needs of the Client:

- Check the client's chart to see if there are any factors that might interfere with the client's ability to understand and follow all the steps necessary to use the cardiac Holter event monitor.
- Ask the client if there is anything you should know that might affect his ability to carry out the testing plan.

■ Evaluation:

- If a teaching mannequin is available, client is able to attach and place the electrodes correctly after your demonstration.
- If a mannequin is not available, client is able to state where each electrode should be placed.
- Client can describe the process for recording the heart-beat and sending the recording to diagnostic laboratory.

■ Further Plans/Teaching:

- Review information and correct any misunderstandings.
- Ask the client if he has any questions.

■ Follow-up:

- Call the client the next day at home to see if he has experienced any symptoms and (if so) whether he was able to record those symptoms and send the recording to the laboratory.
- Based on the client's response, review the information that was taught and answer any additional questions.

Medical Assistant

Name: _____

Signature: _____

Date: _____

Client

Date: _____

Follow-up Date: _____

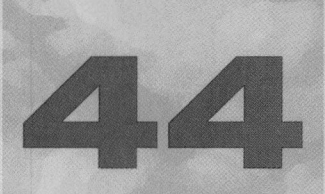

CHAPTER 44

Anticipatory Statements

People have different levels of knowledge about blood chemistry. Read and think about the following statements based upon what you believe now. Decide whether you agree or disagree. Write the word **agree** after the statement if you think the statement is true. Write the word **disagree** after the statement if you think the statement is false. Read the chapter to find out if your current beliefs can be supported.

1. There is "good" cholesterol and "bad" cholesterol in a person's body.   _____

2. Fats or lipids are not essential to life.   _____

3. Blood chemistry tests can look at the amount of carbohydrates, proteins, and fats in a client's blood.   _____

4. Hormones have no effect on the level of glucose in the body.   _____

5. There is an effort in public education to have people know their own cholesterol numbers.   _____

Blood Chemistry

Learning Objectives

Upon completion of this chapter, the medical assistant student should be able to:

- List common blood chemistry tests
- Explain the difference between hyperglycemia and hypoglycemia
- Identify the purpose of the glucose tolerance test
- Discuss what is meant by "good" cholesterol and "bad" cholesterol
- Define and explain BUN
- State the purpose of a creatinine blood chemistry test
- Explain the role of the medical assistant in blood chemistry testing

Key Terms

blood urea nitrogen (BUN) Test that measures the amount of urea nitrogen in the blood.

carbohydrates The major source of energy for the body.

glucose Sugar.

high-density lipoprotein (HDL) Also called "good" cholesterol; helps to protect against coronary artery disease.

hypercholesteremia Too much cholesterol in the blood.

hyperglycemia High blood sugar levels.

hypoglycemia Low blood sugar levels.

lipids Fats.

low-density lipoprotein (LDL) Also called "bad" cholesterol; travels through the bloodstream and then lodges in peripheral tissues.

triglycerides Also called *fat*; stored in adipose tissue.

INTRODUCTION

Carbohydrates, proteins, and fats or lipids are vital to life. The amounts, combination, and availability of these substances all have a direct effect on the functioning of body systems. Conversely, the functioning of body systems also directly affects the availability and use of these substances. Blood carries these substances to and from the body cells. The amount of carbohydrates, proteins, and lipids can be tested and analyzed using a small sample of blood. Questions such as, "How much glucose is present?," "Is this value within the normal range?," and "Is my cholesterol too high?" can all be answered. Blood chemistry tests can help the health care provider find out if a disorder in a body system is causing a problem in the body's use of carbohydrates, proteins, or fats.

CARBOHYDRATES

Carbohydrates provide the body with energy. Carbohydrates include sugars and starches, which are found abundantly in most people's diets. **Glucose,** or sugar, is in most foods, or as a product of metabolism of most foods. The amount of glucose and the speed with which it becomes available to body cells varies according to the type of food. If a person takes in more carbohydrates than are necessary at the moment, the body stores the glucose for future use. Some is stored in the liver as glycogen; some is stored in fat or adipose tissue as **triglycerides** (fat). The liver can also change glucose into the smaller components of protein. Chemical substances called *hormones* help to keep the body in balance. The hormones insulin, glucagon, epinephrine, and thyroxin all work to keep the glucose levels in balance with the energy needs of the body.

TESTS

The doctor may order tests to see if a client's blood glucose levels are within the normal range (Figure 44-1). The blood tested may point

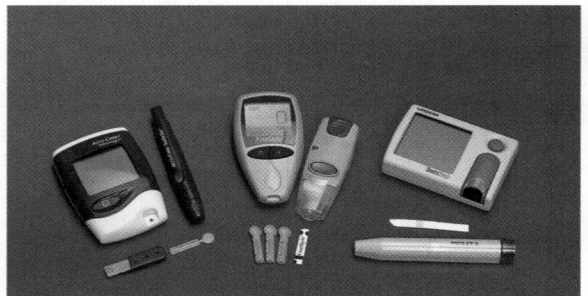

FIGURE 44–1 Handheld glucose analyzers for home and office use.

to **hyperglycemia,** a condition in which the level of glucose in the blood is higher than normal. Above 126 mg/dL in a fasting person is considered too high. The disorder that most commonly causes high blood glucose levels is diabetes mellitus. The blood test may also point to **hypoglycemia,** a condition in which the level of glucose in the blood is lower than normal. Below 70 mg/dL in a nonfasting person is considered too low. The most common cause is too much insulin taken as a medication by a person with diabetes mellitus. Tumors can also cause hypoglycemia.

Tests to Measure Blood Glucose

Tests that can measure blood glucose levels include the random blood glucose test, a fasting blood glucose test, a two-hour postprandial blood glucose test, and the standard glucose tolerance test. The tests vary as to when during the day the blood specimen is taken and the timing of glucose taken in by the client.

In a random blood glucose test, the blood is taken without any special client preparation, and may be taken at any time of the day. This helps to screen for high blood glucose levels under normal, everyday conditions.

Fasting blood glucose tests help to eliminate any false positives from a random blood glucose test. The client may not eat, drink (except water), or smoke for 12 hours before the blood is taken for this test.

The two-hour postprandial blood glucose test checks blood glucose levels after glucose intake. The client fasts, then is given liquid glucose to drink. Two hours later, blood and urine samples are obtained and tested.

The standard glucose tolerance test (GTT) measures how a person's blood glucose levels respond when she is given a large dose of glucose. The test is ordered when diabetes mellitus is suspected. It is also frequently ordered for a pregnant woman, to check for gestational diabetes.

In the standard GTT, the client fasts. At the end of the fast, blood and urine samples are obtained. The client then ingests a specific amount of glucose. Blood and urine samples are obtained at 30 minutes, 1 hour, 1½ hours, and finally at 2 hours. The doctor will decide how many samples are to be taken and how much time should elapse between sampling. This more complex test procedure shows how effectively the body metabolizes glucose and how long it takes the client's blood glucose levels to return to normal. The medical assistant will need to make sure the client understands the process and the preparation necessary, as much cooperation is needed from the client over a long period of time. A GTT can take as long as 6 hours.

■ LIPIDS

Lipids, also called *fats*, are highly concentrated sources of energy. A certain amount of lipids is necessary for life.

Cholesterol

Cholesterol (which is a lipid) is needed for cell membranes, digestion, and hormone production. Most of the cholesterol the body needs is produced by the liver. However, additional cholesterol is taken in from the foods that are eaten. Much of the dietary cholesterol is found in foods from animal sources, such as dairy products.

Although cholesterol is necessary, too much cholesterol (**hypercholesteremia**) can

lead to serious disease and even death. Thus, the medical assistant must understand the functions of and problems with cholesterol and serum triglycerides. High levels of cholesterol in the blood are linked to cardiovascular disorders, heart attacks, and stroke. It is important not to exceed certain levels. Blood is tested for total cholesterol, low-density lipoprotein, and high-density lipoprotein. **Low-density lipoprotein (LDL)** is thick, dense fat that can adhere to the walls of blood vessels and eventually clog up the vessels, preventing the free flow of blood. LDL is sometimes called the "bad" cholesterol. **High-density lipoprotein (HDL)** is composed of less fat and thus moves more freely with the blood; it does not accumulate the way LDL does. HDL is sometimes called the "good" cholesterol. HDL actually helps to carry off some of the LDL, thus keeping the blood vessels from clogging.

Total cholesterol for adults should be under 200 mg/dL. The LDL level should be less than 100 mg/dL, and the HDL level should be greater than 50 mg/dL. An HDL level of more than 60 mg/dL is beneficial to the heart. These targets and normal ranges reflect the relationship between good and bad cholesterol, and the fact that good cholesterol can keep bad cholesterol from harming the blood vessels. Therefore, the ratio of HDL to LDL, compared to the total cholesterol, is more important than the total cholesterol number by itself.

Public education efforts are being made to have people know their own cholesterol numbers. Information about cholesterol levels, and ways to reduce high cholesterol numbers, is made available through advertisements, media, and other public education campaign materials.

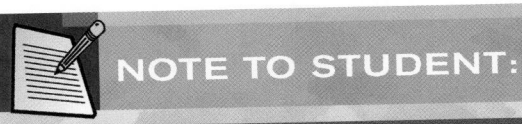

NOTE TO STUDENT:

The ratio of HDL to LDL is a more important indicator for risk of cardiovascular disease than the total cholesterol number.

Manufacturers of medicines used to treat high cholesterol advertise directly to the public about their products. Thus, clients may already know something about cholesterol when they come to the office, and may look to the medical assistant for more information or to clarify the information they already have. Cholesterol has a very direct link to many disorders. It is important for the medical assistant to teach clients healthy choices to keep cholesterol at a safe level.

Triglycerides

Triglycerides are composed of various fatty acids with glycerol. The normal level of triglycerides in the blood is 30 to 150 mg/dL. Higher levels are a risk factor for cardiovascular disorders. A family history can predispose a person to increased triglyceride levels. Heavy alcohol consumption and a diet of foods rich in fat are also a risk factors for high triglyceride levels. Blood tests for triglycerides are often done with cholesterol blood tests to give a more complete picture of the client's status.

Medical Assistant's Role

Testing for total cholesterol, HDL, LDL, and triglycerides is done as part of a *lipid profile test.* Medical assistants, in their clinical role, prepare clients for these tests. Medical assistants may also be asked to obtain blood specimens through venipuncture.

Client preparation includes fasting: the client must not eat or drink (except water) for a period of time before the blood sample is drawn. (The fasting time period is usually about 12 hours, depending on the doctor's orders and laboratory requirements.) The client should not drink alcohol for 24 hours before the test. If the medical assistant is obtaining the blood sample, it is critical to find out if the client has followed the preparation steps. Failure to follow the steps can affect the laboratory results and give a false impression of what is happening in the client's body.

NOTE TO STUDENT:

The client may be taking medication, either over-the-counter or prescription. You must check with the doctor to find out what, if any, of her usual medications the client should take during the time of fasting.

■ PROTEIN

Protein is made up of amino acids, which have been called the building blocks of life. Protein forms hormones, enzymes, and antibodies, as well as the blood that carries substances throughout the body. Most blood serum is *albumin;* the rest is mostly *globulin.* When testing for blood protein, the examiner generally looks first at total protein and then at albumin and globulins as a ratio (A/G) of the total protein.

■ OTHER CHEMISTRY TESTS

Chemistry tests can report on nitrogen substances that are not proteins. Ammonia, urea, uric acid, and creatinine are all examples.

When bacteria in the intestine break down foods, protein and then ammonia are formed. The liver changes ammonia to urea, so there should be very little ammonia in the blood. Abnormally high levels of ammonia in the blood may indicate a liver disorder. Abnormally low levels may indicate high blood pressure or kidney damage.

On a lab report, urea in the blood is labeled as **blood urea nitrogen** or **BUN.** This test measures ingestion of protein, whether the liver works well at using proteins, and whether the kidneys can get rid of the end products of protein metabolism efficiently. For adults, the normal BUN value is 5 to 20 mg/dL; for the elderly client, the normal value is 8 to 21mg/dL. The client's values should remain the same over time. These blood chemistry tests give an indication of how well the kidneys are working. High levels will occur if the body cannot get rid of urea; the most common cause of this problem is kidney failure. Disorders of the various systems can cause changes in the BUN. Bleeding in the digestive system or congestive heart failure can cause the BUN level to rise; dehydration and high-protein diets can also have this effect. Even some prescription medications, such as steroids (used over a long period) and some types of diuretics, can cause an increase in BUN. Other medications can cause a decrease in BUN. It is important for the medical assistant to be aware that an abnormal blood urea nitrogen level must be brought to the doctor's attention.

Uric acid in the blood also reflects the breakdown of protein. In a system that is functioning normally, the kidneys get rid of uric acid. The normal blood level in adult males is 2.0 to 8.5 mg/dL; for adult females, it is 2.0 to 8.0 mg/dL. The doctor may order this test for a client who has gout. During a gout flare-up, the client experiences painful joints. Urate crystals settle in the joints and other body tissues and cause painful symptoms similar to those of arthritis. Kidney failure and cancers, as well as gout, can all cause increased levels of uric acid in the blood.

Creatinine, which is the end product of a portion of metabolism, is picked up by the blood to be excreted by the kidneys. The blood level of creatinine and the amount excreted in the urine change very little in a healthy person. This test is used to determine kidney function: The creatinine blood level rises as the kidneys fail or stop working efficiently.

Medical Assistant's Role

The role of the medical assistant in blood chemistry testing varies according to scope of practice and office policy. Client preparation for blood chemistry testing is a major task for the medical assistant. Obtaining blood specimens

from clients, processing specimens, and sometimes doing the actual testing of blood samples may all be medical assistant clinical responsibilities (Figure 44-2A-C). If an outside laboratory

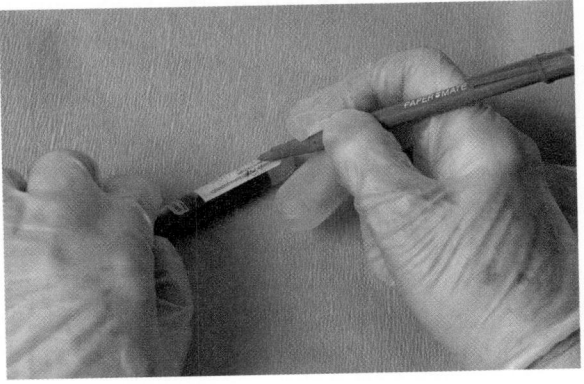

FIGURE 44–2A The medical assistant labels the tube.

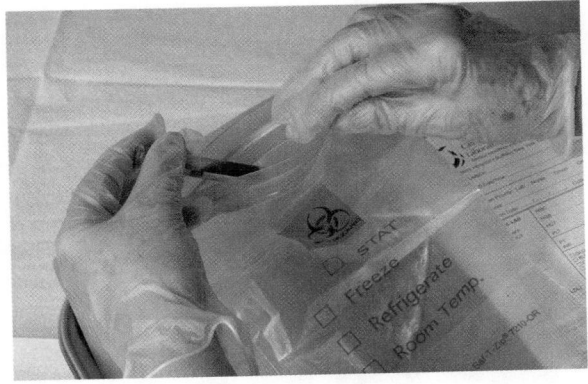

FIGURE 44–2B The medical assistant prepares the tube for transport.

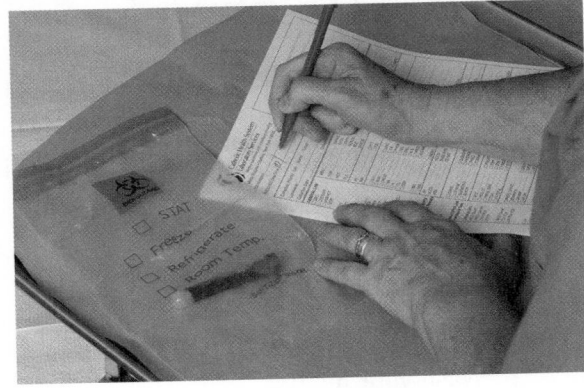

FIGURE 44–2C The medical assistant completes the requisition slip.

tests the sample; the medical assistant will probably be responsible for receiving the results and reporting the findings to the doctor. The steps involved will vary according to office policy. In some offices, lab reports are placed in clients files, flagged, and given to the physician to review. In other offices, the physician may want lab reports kept separately and not filed until she has reviewed them.

Clients may call the office asking for test results, not wanting to wait until the next appointment. Remember, a test may seem routine to those working in a medical office, but anxious clients may worry a lot as they wait for their results. The medical assistant must have a clear understanding of office policy regarding what information can be shared over the telephone, and with whom. If the client is also being cared for by another doctor, personnel from that office may call asking for results (by phone or fax). It is critical to know the procedures for and legal issues involved in sharing information!

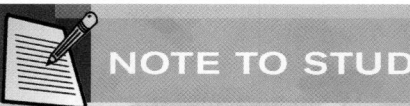

NOTE TO STUDENT:

Always make sure that you know who you are talking with, whether in person or on the telephone.

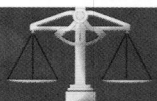

LEGAL/ETHICAL THOUGHTS

Callers to a physician's office laboratory may ask for protected health information. Office policy and regulations under the Health Insurance Portability and Accountability Act (HIPAA) determine what information can be released, and to whom. Positive identification is required before any information is shared, by any means of transmission.

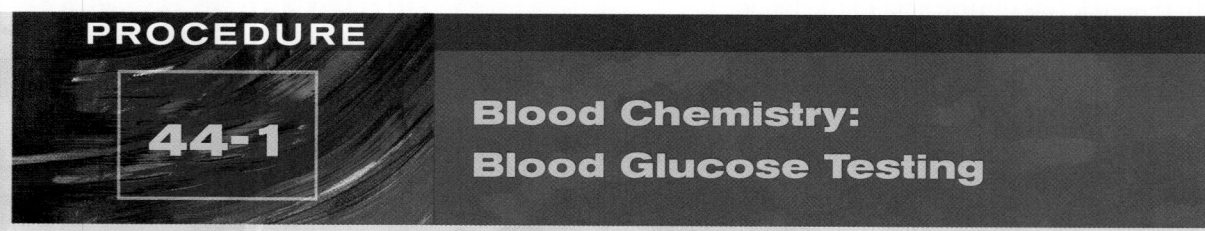

PROCEDURE

44-1

Blood Chemistry: Blood Glucose Testing

Student Competency Objective: The medical assistant student will obtain a blood sample and test the blood glucose level.

Items Needed: Sterile lancet, gloves, alcohol wipe, meter, test strips, blood sampler, protective cap, biohazardous waste container

Steps:

1. Wash your hands.
2. Gather equipment and supplies.

(Continues)

PROCEDURE 44-1 (Continued)

3. Introduce yourself to the client even if you have seen the client on previous visits to your office. The client may have forgotten your name. This also helps to establish a provider–client relationship, because it shows the client that you want her to know who you are.

4. Identify the client. Ask the client to state her name to establish that this is the right client, and then compare the name given to the name on the chart. Never enter a room and call out a client's name to determine if this person is the correct client. The client may not have heard you clearly and may just nod, smile, or answer yes. Clients almost never question if the medical assistant professional has the right client. It is up to the medical assistant to identify the right client before performing any procedure.

5. Tell the client, in everyday language, what you are going to do.

6. Ask if the client has any questions. If she does, give short and simple answers. Sometimes clients will start (and continue) talking because they are nervous about the procedure.

7. Put a test strip into the opening on the meter.

8. Look at the code number displayed as the meter turns on.

9. Compare this number with the code number on the test strip vial.

10. Put on gloves.

11. Firmly place a lancet into a lancet holder. Do not twist.

12. Choose the puncture depth using the adjustment knob or wheel.

13. Clean the side of the client's fingertip with an alcohol wipe. Allow the site to air-dry before puncturing.

14. Place the lancet against the selected site on the client's finger and push the release button.

15. Massage the puncture site gently to increase blood flow. Do not squeeze.

16. Hold the drop of blood on the test strip when the display symbol appears. The test strip will draw in the blood.

17. Wait for the meter to count down.

18. Read the blood glucose test results displayed in the meter window.

19. Write down the number displayed.

20. Remove the used test strip. This turns off the meter.

21. Ask the client if she has any questions.

22. Dispose of the used test strip and alcohol wipe in a biohazardous waste container.

23. Remove the cap from the lancet holder. With the lancet pointing down, eject the used lancet into a sharps container.

24. Remove your gloves.

25. Wash your hands.

26. Record the procedure and results in the client's chart immediately.

Charting Example:

1/11/20xx   3:35 P.M.   Tested blood glucose level in sample drawn from fingertip fourth finger left hand. Result 110 mg/dL. Answered client's questions. Informed doctor of test result.

Amy J. Clinton, S.M.A.

Amy J. Clinton, S.M.A. (printed name)

BRIDGE TO CAAHEP

This chapter, which discusses blood chemistry, provides information and content related to CAA-HEP standards for Anatomy and Physiology, Medical Terminology, Medical Law and Ethics, Psychology, Communication, Administrative Procedures, Medical Assisting Clinical Procedures, and Professional Components.

ABHES LINKS

This chapter, which discusses blood chemistry, links to ABHES course content for Anatomy and Physiology, Medical Terminology, Medical Law and Ethics, Psychology, Human Relations, Medical Office Clinical Procedures, and Medical Laboratory Procedures.

AAMA AREAS OF COMPETENCE

This chapter, which discusses blood chemistry, provides information or content within several areas listed in the Medical Assistant Role Delineation Study. These areas include: administrative, administrative procedures, clinical, fundamental principles, diagnostic orders, patient (client) care, general transdisciplinary, professionalism, communication skills, legal concepts, instruction, and operational functions.

AMT PATHS

This chapter, which discusses blood chemistry, provides a path to AMT competency in general medical assisting knowledge, anatomy and physiology, medical terminology, medical law, medical ethics, human relations, patient (client) education, clinical medical assisting, asepsis, sterilization, instruments, and laboratory procedures.

POINTS OF HIGHLIGHT

- Carbohydrates supply the body with energy.
- Hormones help to keep carbohydrate levels in balance with the energy needs of the body.
- The most common disorder with the symptom of hyperglycemia (high level of sugar in the blood) is diabetes mellitus.
- Blood chemistry tests examine the existence and amount of specific chemical substances in the blood.
- Many blood chemistry tests include dietary restrictions and fasting as part of client preparation before the test.
- Lipids or fats are concentrated sources of energy.
- Low-density lipoprotein is often called the "bad" cholesterol because it lines and clogs the blood vessels. High-density lipoprotein is often called the "good" cholesterol because it keeps moving in the blood vessels and helps to carry off LDL.
- High levels of triglycerides are a risk factor for cardiovascular disorders.
- A blood urea nitrogen test measures how well the liver is using the proteins ingested and how well the kidneys get rid of the end waste products of protein metabolism.
- A creatinine test is used to determine kidney function.
- Uric acid is produced by the breakdown of protein.

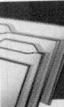

STUDENT PORTFOLIO ACTIVITY

Opportunities for client teaching regarding cholesterol levels, blood work, and dietary and exercise considerations should be observed by your supervisor. Ask the supervisor to evaluate your performance and write in your experience work log or journal. Use this to chart the development of your skills. This allows future employers to see how you are able to apply what you learned in the classroom to real-life situations.

APPLYING YOUR SKILLS

How can public education about cholesterol have a positive effect on health outcomes? In what ways can you as a medical assistant keep up to date with current information about cholesterol after you graduate? How will this help you and the clients you work with?

CRITICAL THINKING QUESTIONS

1. A client comes into the office asking about "good' and "bad" cholesterol. How would you, as a medical assistant, explain this to the client?

2. As a medical assistant, how would you explain the standard glucose tolerance test to a client? How can you tell if the client has understood the instructions for preparing for a GTT?

3. What is creatinine? What organs and systems does it give information about?

4. What is BUN, and what does a BUN test measure?

5. Explain the difference between hyperglycemia and hypoglycemia.

6. A male client's lab report states that his uric acid level is 9.5 mg/dL. Is this within the normal range? What might this level indicate about the client?

7. A client asks you to explain triglycerides. What would you tell her?

8. What is a common test to determine kidney function? In a healthy person, what do you expect to find in this laboratory value over time?

9. The doctor orders a fasting blood glucose test. The client wants to know why she can't have her blood drawn right away, as she is already at the office. How do you prepare the client for this test?

10. Why is it important for people to know and understand their cholesterol levels?

11. Go back to the beginning of this chapter and review the Anticipatory Statements. Reread each statement and then indicate whether it is true or false. If the statement is false, rewrite it to make it a true statement.

CLIENT TEACHING PLAN

Lowering Cholesterol

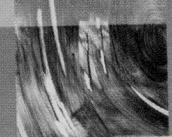

■ What Is to Be Taught:

• Client awareness of high cholesterol number (hypercholesteremia) and behaviors that can help to lower cholesterol levels.

■ Objectives:

• Client will be aware of own cholesterol blood levels and take steps to lower the cholesterol level.

■ Preparation Before Teaching:

• Review causes of increased blood cholesterol levels (hypercholesteremia).
• Translate a medical discussion of cholesterol levels into everyday language.
• Find and review the latest data on the desired range for cholesterol levels.
• Look over the possible complications caused by untreated high cholesterol levels.
• Gather any items needed for teaching, such as diagrams, pictures, paper and pen for note-taking and instructions.
• Make sure the area is free from distractions while you are teaching.

■ Steps for the Medical Assistant:

1. Wash your hands.
2. Gather supplies needed.
3. Introduce yourself to the client.
4. Explain what you are going to teach and why.
5. Tell the client that you want to work with her so that she will better understand the connection between cholesterol blood levels and her health.
6. Ask the client if she is willing to work together toward a goal of lowering her cholesterol.
7. Use a variety of methods (spoken, visual, written) to share the following information:
   a. Even if there is a family history of high cholesterol, there are actions the client can take to bring her cholesterol level down.
   b. Physical exercise is the most important factor in lowering the LDL "bad" cholesterol (even with improved diet, exercise is needed).
   c. Walking is the single best and cheapest form of exercise (you just need a pair of walking shoes that fit well). Ask others to walk with you. If they cannot, then walk alone. If the weather is too cold, hot, rainy, or snowy, consider mall walking or using a treadmill.
   d. Walking for a few minutes every day and slowly building up to about half an hour daily will be beneficial.
8. Share with the client the following tips on how to choose healthier foods:
   a. Choose chicken, turkey, or fish. As a general rule, stay away from red meat.
   b. Select only low-fat cheese. Although cheese is a good source of calcium, it adds too much fat to the diet unless a low-fat variety or type is eaten.
   c. Buy fresh fruits and vegetables.
   d. Read labels carefully. Makers of food products want people to buy their products, so some create labels that seem to promise health. Some foods that promise to "lower cholesterol" usually have a disclaimer on the label (e.g., "when used as part of a low-fat diet and exercise").
9. Share tips on food preparation and healthy eating with the client:
   a. The simple general rule is to bake or grill lean meat, rather than frying it. Avoid heavy cream sauces or fried-batter coatings.
   b. Watch portions (how much food is put on the plate). Check the serving size printed on the food label.
   c. Use smaller plates or dishes; this helps to make food portions appear larger and more appetizing.

(Continues)

CLIENT TEACHING PLAN (Continued)

d. Play enjoyable music during a meal, especially if eating alone.

e. Eat slowly and savor the food that you have taken the time to prepare.

■ Special Needs of the Client:

- Look at the client's chart to see if there are any factors that might interfere with the client's ability to remember and carry out these instructions.
- Ask the client if she or someone else does the food shopping and preparation in her home. If someone else does these activities, ask the client if that person could be included in the teaching session. Remember, it is up to the client to take responsibility for her own health.
- Ask the client if there is someone with whom she can exercise or walk.

■ Evaluation:

- Client knows and can state her most recent cholesterol blood levels.
- Client outlines steps in a plan to lower her cholesterol levels.

■ Further Plans/Teaching:

- At the next office visit, review the plan with the client.
- Ask for the client's input.
- Make changes as necessary, based on the client's input as well as results of blood cholesterol testing done since changes in the client's actions.

■ Follow-up:

- Call the client after one week. Ask if she has been able to start the plan and if she has any questions or concerns.

Medical Assistant

Name: _____

Signature: _____

Date: _____

Client

Date: _____

Follow-up Date: _____

CHAPTER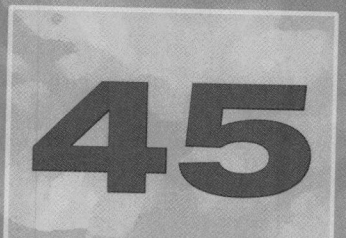

Anticipatory Statements

Read and think about the following statements based upon what you believe now. Decide whether you agree or disagree. Write the word **agree** after the statement if you think the statement is true. Write the word **disagree** after the statement if you think the statement is false. Read the chapter to find out if your current beliefs can be supported.

1. X-rays are used only for diagnostic purposes. _____

2. It is not necessary for workers who handle X-rays to take special precautions, because they are trained to work with X-rays. _____

3. Nuclear medicine uses radioactive substances to find diseases in the body. _____

4. Bone is radiopaque and will appear white on an X-ray film. _____

5. An MRI scan is never used to view problems in the neck or brain. _____

Learning Objectives

Upon completion of this chapter, the medical assistant student should be able to:
- Define *radiology*
- Tell the difference between radiopaque tissue and radiolucent tissue
- List the three groups within radiology
- Explain four safety concerns with X-rays
- Describe the purpose of contrast medium

Radiological Diagnostic Laboratory

- Explain the role of the medical assistant in X-ray studies
- Develop a teaching plan for a radiological procedure

Key Terms

angiography Procedure that visualizes the blood vessels of the body.

barium sulfate A substance used in some X-ray procedures to give contrast or distinguish internal structures from each other.

cholecystography X-ray procedure to view the gallbladder; this procedure is currently being replaced with ultrasound.

computerized tomography (CT scan) X-ray procedure that uses a small beam of radiation to produce a cross-sectional picture.

contrast medium Substance administered internally to client that helps distinguish between organs and surrounding structures during a radiological study.

cystography X-ray examination of the bladder.

diagnostic radiology The use of X-rays or radioactive substances to diagnose disorders.

fluoroscopy X-ray procedure done to observe movement and action inside the body.

intravenous pyelography (IVP) X-ray examination of the kidneys, ureters, and bladder.

iodine compound A substance used in some X-ray procedures as a contrast medium; helps distinguish internal structures from each other.

magnetic resonance imaging (MRI) Procedure that uses a strong magnetic field and radio waves to view internal structures; does not use X-rays.

mammogram X-ray of the breast.

nuclear medicine Branch of medicine that uses radioactive material to diagnose or treat disorders.

radiologist Physician who specializes in using X-rays and radioactive substances to diagnose and treat disease.

radiology Science that studies the use of X-rays and radioactive substances in diagnosis and treatment of disease.

radiolucent Lets X-rays pass through; on an X-ray film, a radiolucent structure looks black.

radiopaque Blocks X-rays; on an X-ray film, a radiopaque structure looks white.

therapeutic radiology The use of X-rays to treat diseases.

■ INTRODUCTION

X-rays are a valuable tool in diagnosis (**diagnostic radiology**) and treatment (**therapeutic radiology**) of disease. Clients can greatly benefit from the correct use of these powerful rays. However, steps must be taken by both the client and medical assistant to prevent these rays from becoming harmful to the body. The major role of a medical assistant in radiology is client preparation and teaching.

■ X-RAYS

Wilhelm Roentgen, a German physicist, discovered that certain rays could pass through solid objects (including the human body). He did not know exactly what kind of radiation he had found, so he did not know what to call the rays: hence the word *X-rays*. **Radiology** is the study of radioactive substances and ionizing substances and their effects on the human body. X-rays make it possible to see internal organs on a film or picture. An X-ray image is a negative image. Tissue that blocks X-rays is called **radiopaque** and will appear white on the film; for example, bone is radiopaque and thus appears white on an X-ray film. Tissue that allows more X-rays to pass through (such as the lungs) is called **radiolucent**, and will appear gray or black on the film.

Medical doctors who specialize in radiology are **radiologists.** The major role in radiology for the medical assistant is client teaching and preparation. An understanding of the basics of radiology is necessary if the medical assistant is to help clients know what is going to happen during a radiological study and how to prepare for the test.

In health care, radiological studies are used for both diagnostic and therapeutic purposes. Certain tests can help the doctor reach a diagnosis. For example, a small bone fracture or a tumor will show up on an X-ray. X-rays can also be used to treat diseases, in which case it is termed *therapeutic radiology*; radiation is used in the treatment of many cancers.

■ DIVISIONS OF RADIOLOGY

Radiology is a highly specialized area of medicine that is often divided into three groups: diagnostic radiology, therapeutic radiology, and nuclear medicine.

Diagnostic Radiology

X-ray studies are a very helpful tool in aiding the doctor to discover what is wrong with a client; that is, they help the doctor arrive at a diagnosis. Diagnostic tests are one part of a more complete examination. Diagnostic X-ray tests can be simple, needing no special client preparation before the test. They can also be complex, and require the client to follow a detailed diet and take medicine for days before the test. Most people will have diagnostic X-ray tests done at some time during their lives. Clients may have concerns about the amount of radiation ("I don't want too many X-rays.") or discomfort during the procedure ("Will it hurt?"); they may not, however, talk about these questions and fears. The medical assistant should actively approach the subject with the client to discover any fears or concerns. Often, telling the client in simple terms what to expect can ease fears and gain the client's cooperation with the diagnostic test.

Therapeutic Radiology

X-rays can be used in the treatment of certain diseases; for example, these waves are used to kill cancer cells. Different methods deliver therapeutic X-rays. The X-rays can be aimed at and sent to a site by an instrument similar to a laser gun. Radioactive isotopes (forms of chemical elements) may be put on or injected into the targeted area. This is done by implanting the isotopes (putting them inside the person) or inserting a tube to deliver the isotopes to a cancer site. The client who is undergoing X-ray treatment to kill cancer cells will require emotional support from the medical assistant. The client also needs to be made aware of the side effects of radiation therapy and how to deal with these effects.

Nuclear Medicine

Nuclear medicine uses radioactive substances to find diseases in the body. A small amount of a radioactive substance is injected or inhaled. The doctor tracks the radioactivity to find where the substance goes and how much settles in the specific area of interest. Nuclear medicine tests are designed to find cancers, heart or heart valve diseases, and gastrointestinal bleeding. They can also reveal how well the kidneys, thyroid, or other organs are working. Nuclear medicine bone scans can help visualize bone and skeletal abnormalities—some so small that they do not show up on plain X-rays. Depending on the test, the client may expect to have a needle inserted through a vein to deliver the substance.

■ SAFETY

X-rays are a valuable tool in finding and treating disease and helping the client to be healthy. They are, however, very powerful, and can harm a person who is overexposed, causing sickness and even death. By understanding the basics of radiology, the medical assistant can work safely to protect all the people involved in a procedure.

Exposure to radiation must be controlled to avoid problems. Four basic principles are:

1. Cover the place where the rays come from.
2. Shield both clients and health care providers.
3. Stay a safe distance from the source.
4. Limit the amount of time and frequency of exposure to X-rays.

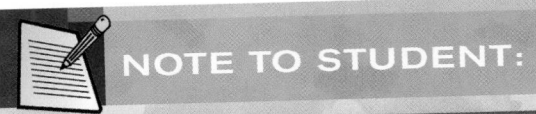

NOTE TO STUDENT:

All places that use or store radioactive materials display the universal radiation symbol. This warns people entering the area to take precautions.

Source

X-ray equipment is kept in a specific room. These rooms are lined with special material containing lead. The walls, floor, and even the doors are treated. This prevents the source from sending rays out to a wider area than is intended or desired.

Clients and Health Care Providers

Human tissue can be damaged by X-rays. In extreme cases, the reproductive organs and reproductive cells can be harmed. This damage may cause abnormalities in future children. Health care providers who conduct the studies and take the pictures (often radiological technicians) stand behind the special walls when the X-ray machine is turned on. Clients' reproductive organs are covered with a lead shield or apron during radiological testing.

NOTE TO STUDENT:

Ask every woman of childbearing years if there is any possibility that she is pregnant right now. Ask for the date of her last menstrual period (LMP). There will be signs in diagnostic facilities instructing women to inform the X-ray technician if there is any possibility of pregnancy. Most forms that have to be completed by the client ask this question, but do not rely on this. Ask every woman. X-rays can hurt a developing fetus.

Exposure

How much radiation the health care provider is exposed to, and the amount of time he is exposed to X-rays must be closely watched and limited. Every radiological worker wears a film badge that records his personal amount of radiation exposure. After a certain period of time, the badge is checked to see how much radiation the worker has received. This safety practice helps to protect the worker by limiting contact before he is exposed to a harmful amount of radiation.

■ SELECTED TESTS AND CLIENT PREPARATION

There are many radiological tests. Some of these tests are noninvasive (do not penetrate body cavities or skin) and cause very little, if any, discomfort to the client. Other tests may require the client to swallow substances or have a solution (contrast medium) injected into the body. These test procedures may be uncomfortable for the client.

The client may need very little preparation (except for client teaching) for some diagnostic tests, such as the plain chest X-ray. Several days of preparation may be necessary for some of the more complicated diagnostic tests. The medical assistant needs to understand the more common radiological diagnostic tests. This includes knowing the purpose of the test and what happens during the test, as well as understanding the required client preparation. Some of the tests that are often ordered in a primary care setting are presented in the following sections.

Plain X-Ray

Plain X-ray is the basic X-ray test done to aid in diagnosis. It is used to view broken bones, injured joints, and lung problems (Figure 45-1), among other things. It is an inexpensive test that requires little or no advance client prepara-

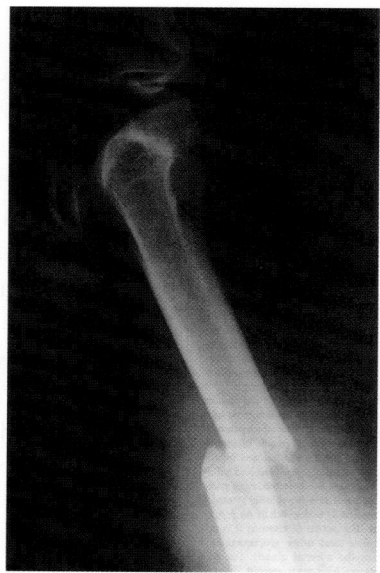

FIGURE 45-1 This X-ray shows a fractured bone in the leg.

tion. The results will show the doctor whether additional tests are needed.

Mammography

Mammography uses X-rays to look for abnormal growths or cancer in the breast (Figure 45-2). Used in conjunction with breast self-examination, this is a valuable tool to detect breast cancer in its early stages. It is recommended that women get a baseline **mammogram** at age 40 and periodically thereafter. If a client has a family history of breast cancer, she may have a mammogram done at an earlier age. This baseline (starting point) image is used for comparison with future mammograms.

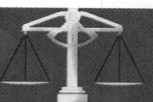

LEGAL/ETHICAL THOUGHTS

The physician's office frequently needs the results of radiological diagnostic testing quickly. Therefore, information may be faxed to the office. All faxes should contain a cover letter indicating who should receive the information and who sent it. The cover letter should contain instructions in case the fax accidentally reaches a person other than the intended recipient.

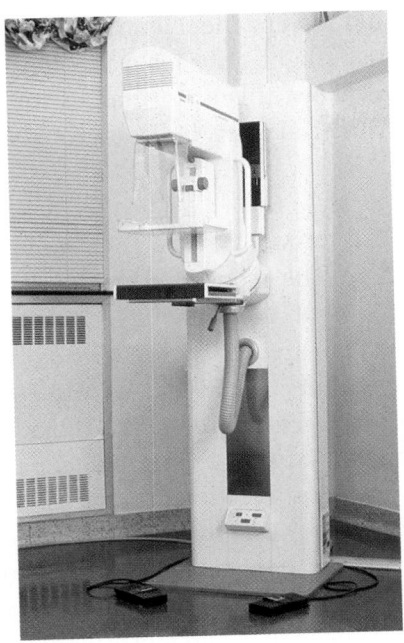

FIGURE 45-2 A mammographic unit.

At the time of testing, the client removes her clothing from the waist up. During the test, the breasts are compressed and the client holds her breath while the picture is taken (Figure 45-3). Each breast is tested separately. The client needs to know that she may feel some discomfort or pain during compression and may incur some slight bruising from the compression. However, the compression is necessary to get a clear,

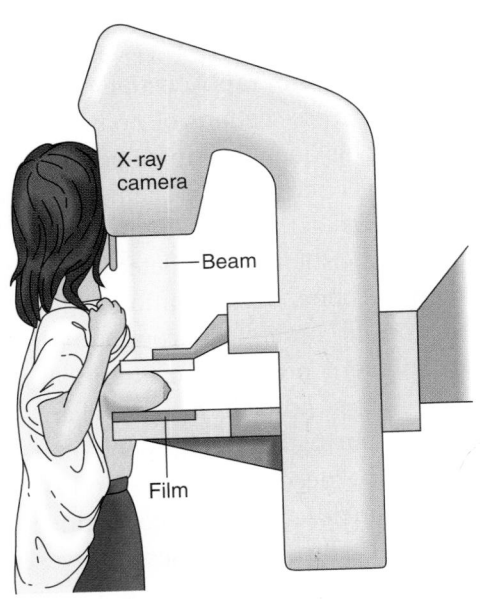

FIGURE 45-3 Client positioned for mammogram.

detailed picture that will let the doctor find any small abnormalities. There are no dietary restrictions before the tests. Lotions and deodorants can interfere with the imaging, so the client should not apply them on the day of the test.

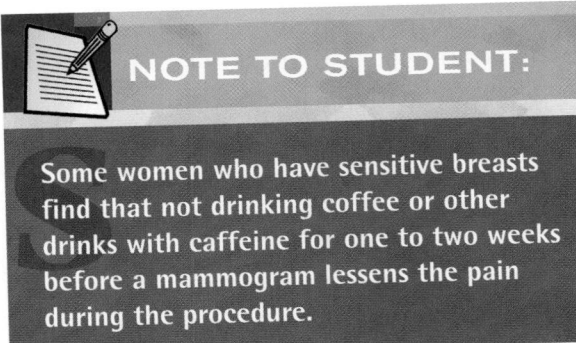

NOTE TO STUDENT:

Some women who have sensitive breasts find that not drinking coffee or other drinks with caffeine for one to two weeks before a mammogram lessens the pain during the procedure.

Tests with Contrast Medium

The value of X-rays depends on getting a clear contrast between tissues and organs. The image or picture is produced by the absorption or blocking of the rays. In some parts of the body, it is difficult to tell the various tissues apart, because of similar tissue density. In these instances, a contrast medium is given to the client. A **contrast medium** is a substance that helps highlight tissue, so that it can be distinguished from nearby tissues and structures. This is especially beneficial with hollow organs or blood vessels. The contrast medium can be injected, swallowed, or inserted rectally. Two common contrast media are barium sulfate and iodine compounds.

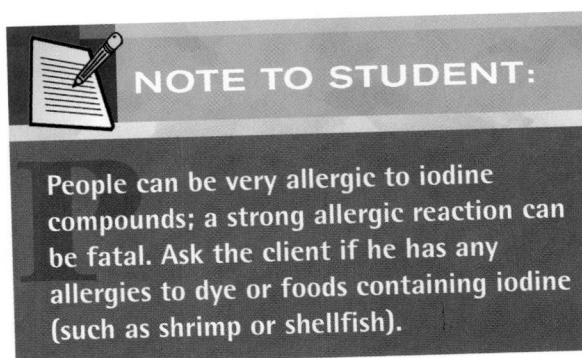

NOTE TO STUDENT:

People can be very allergic to iodine compounds; a strong allergic reaction can be fatal. Ask the client if he has any allergies to dye or foods containing iodine (such as shrimp or shellfish).

Tests with Barium Sulfate. Barium sulfate is used to help view gastrointestinal organs, such as the esophagus, stomach, small intestine, and large intestine. The *upper GI series* (*barium swallow*) and *lower GI series* (*barium enema*) use barium sulfate as the contrast medium (Figures 45-4A and 45-4B). These tests require client action before the X-ray test: the client must not eat or drink for eight hours before the test. Additional, specific dietary instructions will depend on the doctor and the laboratory that performs the test. For an upper GI series, the client actually swallows the barium sulfate. The medical assis-

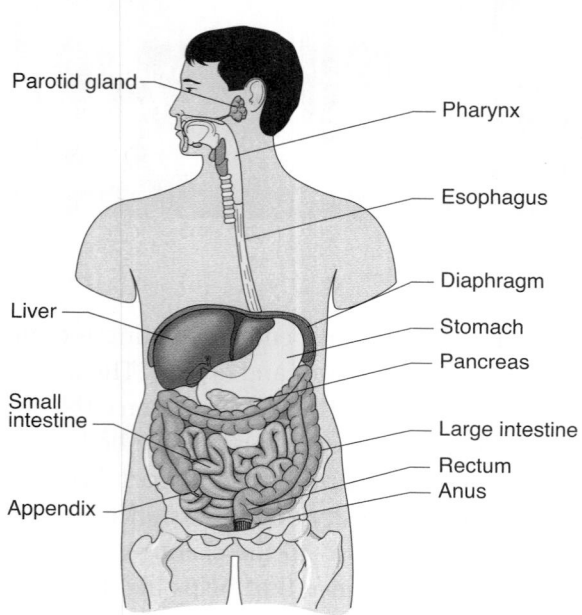

FIGURE 45–4A Upper GI series (light area).

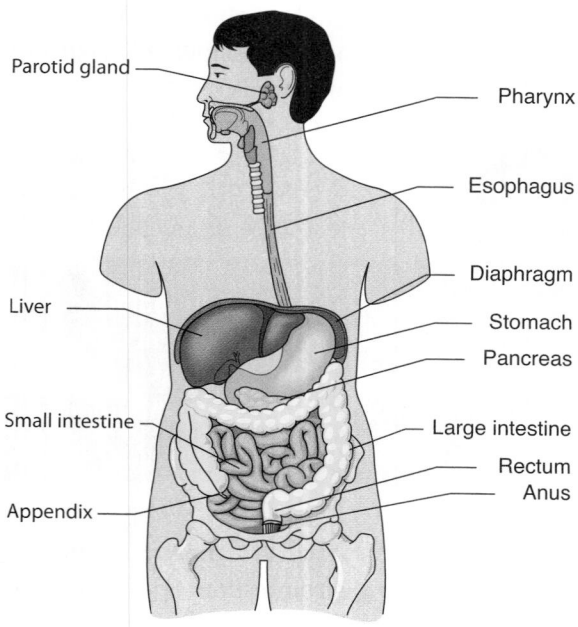

FIGURE 45–4B Lower GI series (light area).

tant should inform the client that the stool or feces may be light gray for a few days after a barium swallow; this is normal, as the barium contrast material is gradually excreted from the body.

Tests with Iodine Compounds. Iodine compounds are the contrast medium used in examinations of the kidneys, gallbladder, and thyroid. They are also used in **angiography**, which examines the insides of blood vessels. **Intravenous pyelography (IVP)** looks at how well the kidneys, ureter, and bladder function after intravenous injection of contrast medium. *Retrograde pyelography* looks at the kidneys and urinary tract. **Cystography** views the urinary bladder. **Cholecystography** uses contrast medium to check the gallbladder for blockage or stones. These tests are common, so the medical assistant should become familiar with them in order to prepare the client and answer questions.

Fluoroscopy. Radiological tests done with a contrast medium often use **fluoroscopy.** After the contrast medium is given, the doctor views its movement or flow through the organs being examined, with the aid of a fluoroscope. This type of test is becoming less common with the advent of newer technology for such imaging.

CT Scan

Computerized tomography, usually called a *CT scan*, looks at cross-sections of body tissue. The client lies on his back, in supine position, while X-ray emitters encircling the client obtain cross-sectional views of the body (Figure 45-5). This valuable diagnostic test can detect tumors, displacement of bone, accumulation of fluid, and other abnormal conditions throughout the body.

Good client preparation is critical to the success of this procedure. The client must remain still during the test. People can made nervous by the need for stillness and the relatively small, enclosed area of the scanner. Often it is helpful if the client closes his eyes while passing through the CT machine. Playing soft music during the test can also help. A contrast

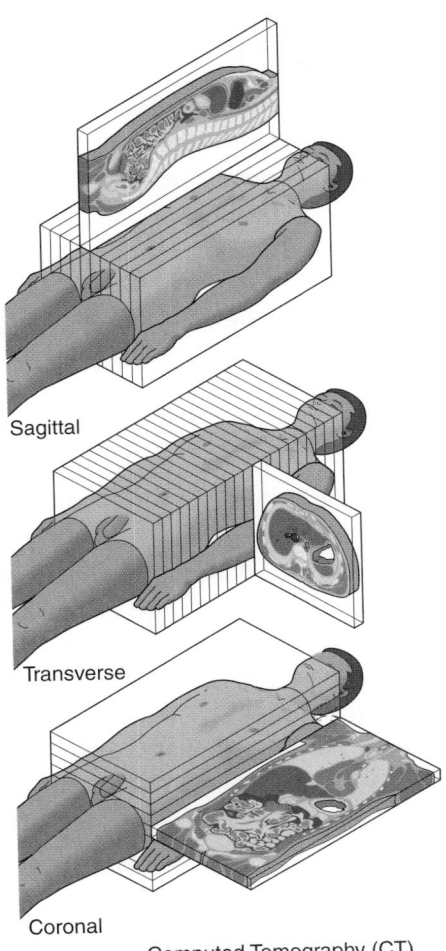

FIGURE 45-5 X-rays scan the cross-sections of a client's body during a CT scan.

medium is given intravenously. Before the test, the medical assistant must ask the client about any allergies to iodine or foods such as eggs or shellfish; allergies to contrast media can cause serious, life-threatening reactions.

MRI

Magnetic resonance imaging (MRI) takes pictures or images of body tissues using radio frequency waves. Because of its electromagnetic properties, tissues absorb and release energy, creating an image. An MRI does not use X-rays, and can show details that cannot be picked up by a CT scan. A contrast medium is sometimes used to make the MRI pictures even clearer.

This test can provide images from any body position. It is an excellent tool to view problems in the brain, head, and neck, such as tumors, multiple sclerosis, dementia, bleeding, or stroke. It is also used to look for spinal cord compression, herniated disks, and other problems with the spine. Heart disease and blood clots also show up.

The client will need specific information and teaching from the medical assistant. The client must remain still during an MRI, which is done while the client is lying on his back. Clients can feel claustrophobic during an MRI, because the person being tested is passed through a narrow opening into the machine. (This is similar to a CT scan, in that the client appears to be in a narrow tunnel.) Closing the eyes may help to lessen the fear of being trapped. The client will also hear loud knocking noises from the machine, as the magnetic coils change direction. To help ease fears and gain the client's cooperation, soft music is played. In addition, the client may speak to the technician, using a microphone in the machine, and the technician will talk with the client throughout the test. Some MRIs are equipped with mirrors so that the client can see outside while he is in the machine. The client cannot have any metal anywhere in or on the body during an MRI. Earrings, studs, rings, chains, and other body jewelry or piercing material must be removed. There can be no pacemaker or other medical metal (pins, rods, plates) surgically implanted in the body. Also ask if the client has ever worked with metal; very tiny pieces of metal may become embedded in the eye without the person being aware of them. A CT scan can be done to see if any metal is present before an MRI is done.

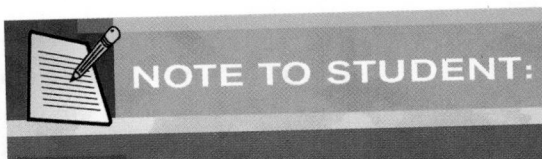

NOTE TO STUDENT:

There must not be any form of metal on or in the client. This could cause very serious harm to the client, because the force of the magnets will pull the metal right off or out of the body.

BRIDGE TO CAAHEP

This chapter, which discusses the radiological diagnostic laboratory, provides information and content related to CAAHEP standards for Medical Assisting Clinical Procedures, Principles of Radiology, Patient (Client) care, Anatomy and Physiology, Medical Terminology, Medical Law and Ethics, Psychology, Diagnostic/Treatment Modalities, Communication, Clinical Procedures, Professional Components, and Internship.

ABHES LINKS

This chapter, which discusses the radiological diagnostic laboratory, links to ABHES course content for Anatomy and Physiology, Medical Terminology, Medical Law and Ethics, Psychology of Human Relations, Medical Office Clinical Procedures, and Medical Laboratory Procedures.

AAMA AREAS OF COMPETENCE

This chapter, which discusses the radiological diagnostic laboratory, provides information or content within several areas listed in the Medical Assistant Role Delineation Study. These areas include: clinical, fundamental principles, diagnostic orders, patient (client) care, general transdisciplinary, professionalism, communication skills, instruction, and operational functions.

AMT PATHS

This chapter, which discusses the radiological diagnostic laboratory, provides a path to AMT competency in general medical assisting knowledge, anatomy and physiology, medical terminology, medical law, medical ethics, human relations, patient (client) education, clinical medical assisting, asepsis, clinical pharmacology, therapeutic modalities, and laboratory procedures.

POINTS OF HIGHLIGHT

- X-rays can be used to find disorders (diagnostic radiology) and to treat disorders (therapeutic radiology).
- The medical assistant's major role in radiology is client preparation.
- Nuclear medicine uses radioactive substances to find diseases in the body.
- Exposure to too much radiation can cause sickness or even death.
- X-ray equipment is kept in specially designed rooms that have lead shielding.
- Mammography, along with monthly self breast-examination, is valuable in detecting breast cancer in the early stages.
- The value of X-rays depends on the clarity of the images. Client preparation and cooperation are essential for useful, successful radiological studies.
- A contrast medium may be used to more clearly distinguish between tissues. Barium sulfate and iodine compounds are two commonly used contrast media.
- Computerized tomography scanning takes pictures or images that are cross-sections of body tissues.
- Magnetic resonance imaging provides details about body tissues using radio frequency waves rather than X-rays.

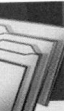

STUDENT PORTFOLIO ACTIVITY

Keep a separate list of radiological procedures that you observed or for which you gave client preparation and instruction. Explain the purpose of each test. Write down how the sample instructions you selected relate to the skills of either the certified medical assistant or the registered medical assistant. In your reflection, tell why you chose this example to illustrate your skill. (Hint: Make sure to include communication skills for a medical assistant.)

APPLYING YOUR SKILLS

The doctor has ordered a CT scan for a client. You need to complete the client preparation for the scan. The client appears nervous and tells you that he has heard "horror stories" about CT machines and testing. How do you respond? How can you best prepare this client for the CT scan?

CRITICAL THINKING QUESTIONS

1. List the three groups or divisions in radiology.

2. State the purpose of diagnostic radiology.

3. Discuss the role of the medical assistant in diagnostic radiology.

4. What is a critical question to ask any client before any test using an iodine contrast medium? What should you do if the client's answer is yes?

5. What group of diseases can be treated with X-rays? How are therapeutic X-rays given to the client?

6. Explain how an MRI saves a client from exposure to X-rays.

7. What steps can a medical assistant take to prevent and avoid harm from X-rays, both for the medical assistant and for the client?

8. A client tells you that she does not need a mammogram because she does monthly breast self-examinations. As a medical assistant, what do you tell her?

9. Your instructor tells you that in addition to the question on the medical form, you must always ask a female client if there is any possibility that she is pregnant. Why must you ask a female client the date of her last menstrual period?

10. If radiological procedures are performed by radiological technology professionals, why do medical assistants need to learn about these tests and procedures?

11. Go back to the beginning of this chapter and review the Anticipatory Statements. Reread each statement and then indicate whether it is true or false. If the statement is false, rewrite it to make it a true statement.

CLIENT TEACHING PLAN

Preparation for Mammogram

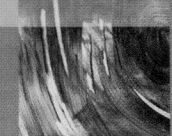

■ What Is to Be Taught:

- Client preparation before a mammographic radiological procedure.

■ Objectives:

- Client will understand the purpose of the diagnostic mammogram.

■ Preparation Before Teaching:

- Review the mammogram procedure and the reasons for the procedure. Make sure to put any technical medical terms into everyday language.
- Gather any printed educational pamphlets available, and paper and pen for note-taking and instructions.

■ Steps for the Medical Assistant:

1. Wash your hands.
2. Gather supplies needed.
3. Introduce yourself to the client.
4. Explain what you are going to teach and why.
5. Tell the client that having a mammogram is one of the three important steps a woman can take to detect breast cancer and other breast disorders. A mammogram is the most valuable method the doctor can use to detect breast cancer.
6. Show the client pictures and diagrams of the breast and positioning of the client during the procedure. Show drawings of the typical size of lumps found without mammography compared with those found during regular mammograms.
7. Suggest to the client that she not schedule the mammogram right before her menstrual period; the breasts can be tender during this time and may make the examination more uncomfortable.
8. Inform the client that if she experiences tender breasts, it might be helpful not to have any caffeine for one to two weeks before the procedure. Caffeine is found in coffee, tea, many colas and soft drinks, and chocolate.
9. Instruct the client not to use deodorant under the arms or any creams or lotions on the breasts the day of the mammogram.
10. Inform the client that no other preparatory steps are needed.
11. Tell the client what to expect during the test.
12. Tell the client that she will be asked to remove her clothing from the waist up and to put on a gown. The technician will place the breast on a flat surface of the machine. The breast will be compressed to obtain the X-ray image. The client may experience some discomfort or pain during the procedure. It is important to compress the breasts to get a clear picture to detect any problems.
13. Ask the client if she has any questions about the preparation or the mammogram procedure.

■ Special Needs of the Client:

- Check the client's chart to see if there are any factors that might interfere with the client's ability to follow through with your instructions.
- Ask the client if there is anything you should know that might affect her ability to prepare for or undertake the mammography procedure.

■ Evaluation:

- Client is able to state the steps to take before a mammogram.
- Client is able to explain what to expect during a mammogram.

■ Further Plans/Teaching:

- Give the client appropriate printed material to use as a reference at home.
- If no printed material or instructions are available, write the information down and give it to the client.

CLIENT TEACHING PLAN (Continued)

Follow-up:

- Call the client at home and inquire if the mammogram has been scheduled.
- Ask the client if she has any questions or if she would like you to repeat any information about preparation or what to expect during the X-ray.

Medical Assistant

Name: _____

Signature: _____

Date: _____

Client

Date: _____

Follow-up Date: _____

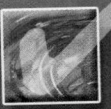

Name _____   Course _____

PROCEDURE

3-1

Handwashing for Medical Asepsis

	1st Observation	2nd Observation	Mastery
1. Takes off watch and any rings.	_____	_____	_____
2. Makes sure sleeves are above elbows.	_____	_____	_____
3. Stands close to the sink without touching it.	_____	_____	_____
4. Turns on faucet with paper towel, unless faucet is operated with foot or knee control or is motion-activated.	_____	_____	_____
5. Adjusts water temperature.	_____	_____	_____
6. Rinses hands under warm running water.	_____	_____	_____
7. Keeps hands lower than forearms.	_____	_____	_____
8. Lets soap from soap dispenser squirt into palm of hand.	_____	_____	_____
9. Rubs hands together, working soap into a lather.	_____	_____	_____
10. Rubs soap over palms, backs of hands, and between fingers, using a circular motion.	_____	_____	_____
11. Puts fingertips of right hand into palm of left hand and scrubs.	_____	_____	_____
12. Puts fingertips of left hand into palm of right hand and scrubs.	_____	_____	_____
13. Takes orange stick and cleans under fingernails of both hands. If using nail brush, brushes under each nail and around cuticles.	_____	_____	_____
14. Rinses well, making sure to get off all soap. Does not touch the inside of the sink with hands.	_____	_____	_____
15. If hands have come into contact with blood, drainage, pus, or body fluids, repeats the handwashing.	_____	_____	_____
16. Dries hands gently and thoroughly with paper towels.	_____	_____	_____
17. Discards used paper towels and orange stick or nail brush.	_____	_____	_____
18. Using a paper towel, turns off faucet (unless automatic or knee-controlled).	_____	_____	_____
19. Discards paper towel.	_____	_____	_____
20. Puts on watch and rings.	_____	_____	_____

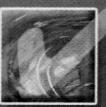

Competency Skill Checklist (Continued)

Documentation

```

```

1st Observation

Date: _____ Evaluator Signature and Printed Name: _____

Comments:

2nd Observation

Date: _____ Evaluator Signature and Printed Name: _____

Comments:

Mastery

Date: _____ Evaluator Signature and Printed Name: _____

Comments:

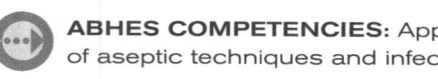 **ABHES COMPETENCIES:** Apply principles of aseptic techniques and infection control.

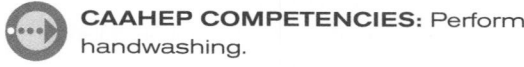 **CAAHEP COMPETENCIES:** Perform handwashing.

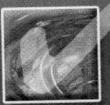
Name _____ Course _____

PROCEDURE 3-2

Handwashing for Surgical Asepsis

	1st Observation	2nd Observation	Mastery
1. Takes off watch and any rings.	_____	_____	_____
2. Makes sure sleeves are above elbows.	_____	_____	_____
3. Stands close to sink without touching it.	_____	_____	_____
4. Turns on faucet with paper towel, unless faucet is operated with foot or knee control or is motion-activated.	_____	_____	_____
5. Adjusts water temperature.	_____	_____	_____
6. Holds hands under faucet above waist level.	_____	_____	_____
7. Rinses hands under warm running water.	_____	_____	_____
8. Keeps hands lower than forearms.	_____	_____	_____
9. Lets soap from soap dispenser squirt into palm of hand.	_____	_____	_____
10. Rubs hands together, working soap into a lather.	_____	_____	_____
11. Rubs soap over palms, backs of hands, and between fingers, using a circular motion.	_____	_____	_____
12. Puts fingertips of right hand into palm of left hand and scrubs.	_____	_____	_____
13. Puts fingertips of left hand into palm of right hand and scrubs.	_____		
14. Takes orange stick and cleans under fingernails of both hands.	_____	_____	_____
15. Picks up nail brush and scrubs palms and backs of hands, nails, wrists, and forearms.	_____	_____	_____
16. Starts rinsing from tips of fingers to forearms.	_____	_____	_____
17. Rinses well, making sure to get off all soap. Does not touch inside of sink with hands.	_____	_____	_____
18. Continues to keep hands higher than elbows.	_____	_____	_____
19. Picks up sterile towel.	_____	_____	_____
20. Dries hands gently and thoroughly with sterile towel, starting with fingers and hands and working up forearms.	_____	_____	_____
21. Discards used sterile towel, orange stick, and nail brush.	_____	_____	_____
22. Takes dry sterile towel and turns off faucet, or turns it off with elbow (unless faucet is automatic or knee-controlled).	_____	_____	_____
23. Discards used sterile towel.	_____	_____	_____

Competency Skill Checklist (Continued)

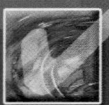

Documentation

1st Observation
Date: _____ Evaluator Signature and Printed Name: _____
Comments:

2nd Observation
Date: _____ Evaluator Signature and Printed Name: _____
Comments:

Mastery
Date: _____ Evaluator Signature and Printed Name: _____
Comments:

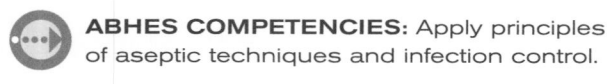 **ABHES COMPETENCIES:** Apply principles of aseptic techniques and infection control.

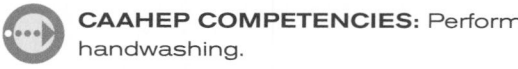 **CAAHEP COMPETENCIES:** Perform handwashing.

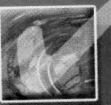

Competency Skill Checklist

Name _____ Course _____

PROCEDURE 3-3

Application of Sterile Gloves

	1st Observation	2nd Observation	Mastery
1. Removes rings from hands.	_____	_____	_____
2. Washes hands.	_____	_____	_____
3. Selects correct glove size.	_____	_____	_____
4. Reads package label.	_____	_____	_____
5. Places glove package on clean surface with left glove in front of left hand and right glove in front of right hand.	_____	_____	_____
6. Breaks seal on package for left glove.	_____	_____	_____
7. Opens flap and folds it away from self.	_____	_____	_____
8. Makes sure that cuff of glove is closest to self.	_____	_____	_____
9. Breaks seal on package for right glove.	_____	_____	_____
10. Opens flap and folds it away from self.	_____	_____	_____
11. Makes sure that cuff of glove is closest to self.	_____	_____	_____
12. Using thumb and forefinger of nondominant hand, grabs cuff of glove for dominant hand.	_____	_____	_____
13. Fits dominant hand into glove, being careful not to let ungloved hand touch any other area of glove.	_____	_____	_____
14. Using sterile-gloved dominant hand, slips four fingers under cuff of other sterile glove. Does not let thumb touch other glove.	_____	_____	_____
15. Fits nondominant hand into glove.	_____	_____	_____
16. Does not touch anything that is not sterile.	_____	_____	_____
17. While waiting to assist doctor or undertake a procedure, interlaces fingers.	_____	_____	_____
18. Keeps sterile-gloved hands above waist.	_____	_____	_____

Documentation

_____

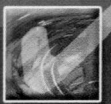
1st Observation

Date: _____ Evaluator Signature and Printed Name: _____

Comments:

2nd Observation

Date: _____ Evaluator Signature and Printed Name: _____

Comments:

Mastery

Date: _____ Evaluator Signature and Printed Name: _____

Comments:

 ABHES COMPETENCIES: Apply principles of aseptic techniques and infection control.

Prepare patient for and assist physician with routine and specialty examinations and treatments and minor office surgeries.

 CAAHEP COMPETENCIES: Prepare patient for and assist with procedures, treatments, and minor office surgeries.

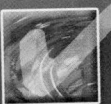

Name _____   Course _____

PROCEDURE
3-4

Removal of Contaminated Gloves

	1st Observation	2nd Observation	Mastery
1. With nondominant hand, grabs outside of sterile glove on dominant hand at palm.	_____	_____	_____
2. Pulls that glove off and holds it in sterile-gloved nondominant hand.	_____	_____	_____
3. Slips fingers of dominant hand (ungloved) under cuff of sterile glove on nondominant hand.	_____	_____	_____
4. Pulls glove off nondominant hand inside out, inverting it over the first glove.	_____	_____	_____
5. Disposes of contaminated gloves in biohazardous waste container.	_____	_____	_____
6. Washes hands.	_____	_____	_____

Documentation

_____

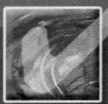

Competency Skill Checklist (Continued)

1st Observation

Date: _____ Evaluator Signature and Printed Name: _____

Comments:

2nd Observation

Date: _____ Evaluator Signature and Printed Name: _____

Comments:

Mastery

Date: _____ Evaluator Signature and Printed Name: _____

Comments:

 ABHES COMPETENCIES: Apply principles of aseptic techniques and infection control.

Dispose of biohazardous materials.

Practice standard precautions.

 CAAHEP COMPETENCIES: Practice standard precautions.

Dispose of biohazardous materials.

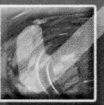
Name _____ Course _____

PROCEDURE

3-5

Cleanup after a Spill of a Biohazardous Substance

	1st Observation	2nd Observation	Mastery
1. Gathers items needed for cleanup.	_____	_____	_____
2. Puts on gloves.	_____	_____	_____
3. Puts on other personal protective equipment (as needed).	_____	_____	_____
4. Wipes with disposable towels any spill that can be seen.	_____	_____	_____
5. Disposes of used towels in biohazardous waste container.	_____	_____	_____
6. Sprays or pours germicide solution or bleach onto surface to decontaminate it; is careful not to splash outside contaminated area.	_____	_____	_____
7. Wipes surface with disposable towels.	_____	_____	_____
8. Disposes of used towels in biohazardous waste container.	_____	_____	_____
9. Puts away unused supplies.	_____	_____	_____
10. Takes off personal protective equipment.	_____	_____	_____
11. Takes off gloves.	_____	_____	_____
12. Washes hands.	_____	_____	_____

Documentation

737

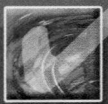

1st Observation

Date: _____ Evaluator Signature and Printed Name: _____

Comments:

2nd Observation

Date: _____ Evaluator Signature and Printed Name: _____

Comments:

Mastery

Date: _____ Evaluator Signature and Printed Name: _____

Comments:

 ABHES COMPETENCIES: Apply principles of aseptic techniques and infection control.

Dispose of biohazardous materials.

Practice standard precautions.

 CAAHEP COMPETENCIES: Practice standard precautions.

Dispose of biohazardous materials.

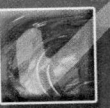

Competency Skill Checklist

Name _____ Course _____

PROCEDURE

4-1

Radial Pulse: Rate, Rhythm, and Volume

	1st Observation	2nd Observation	Mastery
1. Washes hands.	_____	_____	_____
2. Gathers equipment and supplies.	_____	_____	_____
3. Introduces self to client.	_____	_____	_____
4. Identifies client.	_____	_____	_____
5. Tells client, in everyday language, what medical assistant is going to do.	_____	_____	_____
6. Asks if client has any questions.	_____	_____	_____
7. If client is sitting, asks client to rest arm comfortably on table or other supportive surface that will keep wrist at heart level.	_____	_____	_____
8. If client is lying down, places client's arm across client's chest.	_____	_____	_____
9. Places pads of first two fingers on radial site.	_____	_____	_____
10. Applies steady, gentle pressure.	_____	_____	_____
11. Counts each tap or pulsation felt for 30 seconds and multiplies by 2.	_____	_____	_____
12. While counting pulse beats, notes if beats are regular and equally spaced.	_____	_____	_____
13. Notes volume or force while counting.	_____	_____	_____
14. Records procedure correctly in client's chart.	_____	_____	_____

Documentation

```



```

739

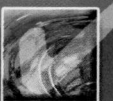

Competency Skill Checklist (Continued)

1st Observation

Date: _____ Evaluator Signature and Printed Name: _____

Comments:

2nd Observation

Date: _____ Evaluator Signature and Printed Name: _____

Comments:

Mastery

Date: _____ Evaluator Signature and Printed Name: _____

Comments:

 ABHES COMPETENCIES: Take vital signs.

 CAAHEP COMPETENCIES: Obtain vital signs.

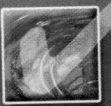

Name _____ Course _____

PROCEDURE

4-2

Respirations

	1st Observation	2nd Observation	Mastery
1. Washes hands.	_____	_____	_____
2. Gathers equipment and supplies.	_____	_____	_____
3. Introduces self to client.	_____	_____	_____
4. Identifies client.	_____	_____	_____
5. Tells client, in everyday language, what medical assistant is going to do.	_____	_____	_____
6. Asks if client has any questions. If client does, gives short and simple answers.	_____	_____	_____
7. If client is sitting, asks client to rest arm on surface that will comfortably support the arm.	_____	_____	_____
8. If client is lying down, rests client's arm across client's chest.	_____	_____	_____
9. Places pads of first two fingers of hand on radial site.	_____	_____	_____
10. Watches rise and fall of client's chest and counts number of respirations for 30 seconds. Does not stare at client's chest.	_____	_____	_____
11. Multiplies number of respirations counted by 2 and records that number.	_____	_____	_____
12. Records rhythm.	_____	_____	_____
13. Records depth.	_____	_____	_____
14. Records procedure correctly in client's chart.	_____	_____	_____

Documentation

```



```

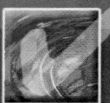

1st Observation

Date: _____ Evaluator Signature and Printed Name: _____

Comments:

2nd Observation

Date: _____ Evaluator Signature and Printed Name: _____

Comments:

Mastery

Date: _____ Evaluator Signature and Printed Name: _____

Comments:

 ABHES COMPETENCIES: Take vital signs.

 CAAHEP COMPETENCIES: Obtain vital signs.

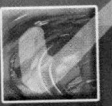

Name _____ Course _____

PROCEDURE

4-3 Oral Temperature: Electronic Thermometer

	1st Observation	2nd Observation	Mastery
1. Washes hands.	_____	_____	_____
2. Gathers equipment and supplies.	_____	_____	_____
3. Introduces self to client.	_____	_____	_____
4. Identifies client.	_____	_____	_____
5. Tells client, in everyday language, what medical assistant is going to do.	_____	_____	_____
6. Asks if client has any questions. If client does, gives short and simple answers.	_____	_____	_____
7. If there is probe connector for electronic thermometer, puts it in the unit base holder.	_____	_____	_____
8. Holding probe by collar, takes probe from holder.	_____	_____	_____
9. Pushes probe into probe cover.	_____	_____	_____
10. Asks client to open mouth; then places probe in client's mouth.	_____	_____	_____
11. Tells client to keep lips closed.	_____	_____	_____
12. Holds thermometer probe cover to keep it steady while probe is in client's mouth.	_____	_____	_____
13. Holds probe steady for approximately 10 seconds until unit indicates that measurement is complete.	_____	_____	_____
14. Removes probe from client's mouth without touching probe cover.	_____	_____	_____
15. Reads and writes down temperature number showing on thermometer's screen.	_____	_____	_____
16. Pushes button to eject probe cover directly into biohazardous waste container.	_____	_____	_____
17. Puts probe back into its unit.	_____	_____	_____
18. Washes hands.	_____	_____	_____
19. Records procedure correctly in client's chart.	_____	_____	_____

Documentation

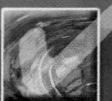

1st Observation

Date: _____ Evaluator Signature and Printed Name: _____

Comments:

2nd Observation

Date: _____ Evaluator Signature and Printed Name: _____

Comments:

Mastery

Date: _____ Evaluator Signature and Printed Name: _____

Comments:

 ABHES COMPETENCIES: Take vital signs.

 CAAHEP COMPETENCIES: Obtain vital signs.

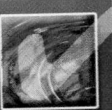

Name _____   Course _____

PROCEDURE

4-4

Oral Temperature: Dot-Matrix Thermometer

	1st Observation	2nd Observation	Mastery
1. Washes hands.	_____	_____	_____
2. Gathers equipment and supplies.	_____	_____	_____
3. Introduces self to client.	_____	_____	_____
4. Identifies client.	_____	_____	_____
5. Tells client, in everyday language, what medical assistant is going to do.	_____	_____	_____
6. Asks if client has any questions. If client does, gives short and simple answers.	_____	_____	_____
7. Asks client to open mouth. Puts thermometer under client's tongue toward back.	_____	_____	_____
8. Asks client to keep tongue down on thermometer and keep thermometer in mouth for 60 seconds.	_____	_____	_____
9. After 60 seconds, removes thermometer.	_____	_____	_____
10. Reads and writes down number at last colored dot.	_____	_____	_____
11. Disposes of used thermometer in biohazardous waste container.	_____	_____	_____
12. Washes hands.	_____	_____	_____
13. Records procedure correctly in client's chart.	_____	_____	_____

Documentation

745

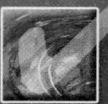

1st Observation

Date: _____ Evaluator Signature and Printed Name: _____

Comments:

2nd Observation

Date: _____ Evaluator Signature and Printed Name: _____

Comments:

Mastery

Date: _____ Evaluator Signature and Printed Name: _____

Comments:

 ABHES COMPETENCIES: Take vital signs.

 CAAHEP COMPETENCIES: Obtain vital signs.

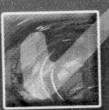

Name _____ Course _____

PROCEDURE

4-5

Oral Temperature: Digital Thermometer

	1st Observation	2nd Observation	Mastery
1. Washes hands.	_____	_____	_____
2. Gathers equipment and supplies.	_____	_____	_____
3. Familiarizes self with parts of digital thermometer.	_____	_____	_____
4. Introduces self to client.	_____	_____	_____
5. Identifies client.	_____	_____	_____
6. Tells client, in everyday language, what medical assistant is going to do.	_____	_____	_____
7. Asks if client has any questions. If client does, gives short and simple answers.	_____	_____	_____
8. Pushes on-off button on thermometer.	_____	_____	_____
9. Checks display window.	_____	_____	_____
10. Switches measurement scale if necessary.	_____	_____	_____
11. Asks client to open mouth. Puts thermometer under client's tongue, toward back.	_____	_____	_____
12. Asks client to keep tongue down on thermometer and keep it in mouth.	_____	_____	_____
13. After the number has stopped flashing, removes thermometer from client's mouth.	_____	_____	_____
14. Reads and writes down number from display window.	_____	_____	_____
15. Discards probe cover directly into biohazardous waste container.	_____	_____	_____
16. Pushes on-off button.	_____	_____	_____
17. Cleans thermometer tip with alcohol wipe.	_____	_____	_____
18. Stores thermometer in protective case.	_____	_____	_____
19. Washes hands.	_____	_____	_____
20. Records procedure correctly in client's chart.	_____	_____	_____

Documentation

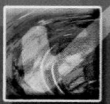

1st Observation

Date: _____ Evaluator Signature and Printed Name: _____

Comments:

2nd Observation

Date: _____ Evaluator Signature and Printed Name: _____

Comments:

Mastery

Date: _____ Evaluator Signature and Printed Name: _____

Comments:

 ABHES COMPETENCIES: Take vital signs.

 CAAHEP COMPETENCIES: Obtain vital signs.

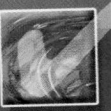

Name _____   Course _____

	1st Observation	2nd Observation	Mastery
1. Washes hands.	_____	_____	_____
2. Gathers equipment and supplies.	_____	_____	_____
3. Introduces self to client.	_____	_____	_____
4. Identifies client.	_____	_____	_____
5. Tells client, in everyday language, what medical assistant is going to do.	_____	_____	_____
6. Asks if client has any questions. If client does, gives short and simple answers.	_____	_____	_____
7. Puts on gloves.	_____	_____	_____
8. If there is a probe connector for electronic thermometer, puts it in unit base holder.	_____	_____	_____
9. Holding probe by collar, takes probe from holder.	_____	_____	_____
10. Pushes probe into probe cover.	_____	_____	_____
11. Assists client to lie on side.	_____	_____	_____
12. Drapes client to ensure privacy.	_____	_____	_____
13. Makes sure probe is lubricated.	_____	_____	_____
14. With one gloved hand, lifts client's buttock to expose anus.	_____	_____	_____
15. With other gloved hand, gently inserts probe into client's anus.	_____	_____	_____
16. Holds probe in place until thermometer indicates that temperature measurement is complete.	_____	_____	_____
17. Removes probe from client without touching probe cover.	_____	_____	_____
18. Covers client's buttock with the drape.	_____	_____	_____
19. Reads temperature number shown on thermometer's screen.	_____	_____	_____
20. Pushes button to eject probe cover directly into biohazardous waste container.	_____	_____	_____
21. Removes gloves and disposes of them in waste container.	_____	_____	_____
22. Puts probe back into unit.	_____	_____	_____
23. Assists client as needed to adjust clothing and sit up.	_____	_____	_____
24. Washes hands.	_____	_____	_____
25. Records procedure correctly in client's chart.	_____	_____	_____

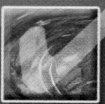
Documentation

1st Observation

Date: _____ Evaluator Signature and Printed Name: _____

Comments:

2nd Observation

Date: _____ Evaluator Signature and Printed Name: _____

Comments:

Mastery

Date: _____ Evaluator Signature and Printed Name: _____

Comments:

 ABHES COMPETENCIES: Take vital signs.

 CAAHEP COMPETENCIES: Obtain vital signs.

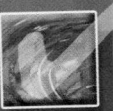

Competency Skill Checklist

Name _____ Course _____

	1st Observation	2nd Observation	Mastery
1. Washes hands.	_____	_____	_____
2. Gathers equipment and supplies.	_____	_____	_____
3. Introduces self to client.	_____	_____	_____
4. Identifies client.	_____	_____	_____
5. Tells client, in everyday language, what medical assistant is going to do.	_____	_____	_____
6. Asks if client has any questions. If client does, gives short and simple answers.	_____	_____	_____
7. Puts probe cover on ear-probe part of thermometer. Checks to see if screen flashes "READY."	_____	_____	_____
8. Pulls gently on client's ear to straighten ear canal.	_____	_____	_____
9. Puts covered probe into client's ear canal securely and gently.	_____	_____	_____
10. Presses scan button.	_____	_____	_____
11. Waits for thermometer sound.	_____	_____	_____
12. Takes probe out of client's ear.	_____	_____	_____
13. Reads temperature number shown on screen.	_____	_____	_____
14. Presses release button to dispose of probe cover directly into waste container.	_____	_____	_____
15. Places thermometer unit back on its base.	_____	_____	_____
16. Washes hands.	_____	_____	_____
17. Records procedure correctly in client's chart.	_____	_____	_____

Documentation

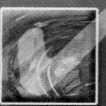

1st Observation

Date: _____ Evaluator Signature and Printed Name: _____

Comments:

2nd Observation

Date: _____ Evaluator Signature and Printed Name: _____

Comments:

Mastery

Date: _____ Evaluator Signature and Printed Name: _____

Comments:

 ABHES COMPETENCIES: Take vital signs.

 CAAHEP COMPETENCIES: Obtain vital signs.

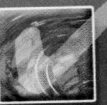
Name _____ Course _____

PROCEDURE

4-8

Axillary Temperature: Dot-Matrix Thermometer

	1st Observation	2nd Observation	Mastery
1. Washes hands.	_____	_____	_____
2. Gathers equipment and supplies.	_____	_____	_____
3. Introduces self to client.	_____	_____	_____
4. Identifies client.	_____	_____	_____
5. Tells client, in everyday language, what medical assistant is going to do.	_____	_____	_____
6. Asks if client has any questions. If client does, gives short and simple answers.	_____	_____	_____
7. Asks client to lift arm.	_____	_____	_____
8. Places thermometer high up in armpit, vertically.	_____	_____	_____
9. Places dots on thermometer against client's torso.	_____	_____	_____
10. Moves client's arm down to hold thermometer in place.	_____	_____	_____
11. Checks watch to note time.	_____	_____	_____
12. After 3 minutes, asks client to lift arm; removes thermometer.	_____	_____	_____
13. Reads and writes down number at last colored dot on thermometer.	_____	_____	_____
14. Disposes of used thermometer in waste container.	_____	_____	_____
15. Washes hands.	_____	_____	_____
16. Records procedure correctly in client's chart.	_____	_____	_____

Documentation

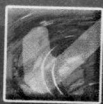
1st Observation

Date: _____ Evaluator Signature and Printed Name: _____

Comments:

2nd Observation

Date: _____ Evaluator Signature and Printed Name: _____

Comments:

Mastery

Date: _____ Evaluator Signature and Printed Name: _____

Comments:

 ABHES COMPETENCIES: Take vital signs.

 CAAHEP COMPETENCIES: Obtain vital signs.

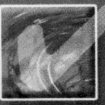

Name _____ Course _____

PROCEDURE

4-9 Apical Pulse

	1st Observation	2nd Observation	Mastery
1. Washes hands.	_____	_____	_____
2. Gathers equipment and supplies.	_____	_____	_____
3. Introduces self to client.	_____	_____	_____
4. Identifies client.	_____	_____	_____
5. Tells client, in everyday language, what medical assistant is going to do.	_____	_____	_____
6. Asks if client has any questions. If client does, gives short and simple answers.	_____	_____	_____
7. Removes clothing from left side of client's chest; provides gown, if needed.	_____	_____	_____
8. Has client either sit or lie down.	_____	_____	_____
9. Puts stethoscope earpiece in ear.	_____	_____	_____
10. Finds apical pulse site by starting at midclavicular line and counting intercostal spaces on left side of chest. Stops at fifth intercostal space.	_____	_____	_____
11. Puts chestpiece of stethoscope directly on client's skin at this spot.	_____	_____	_____
12. Listens for the heartbeat.	_____	_____	_____
13. Counts number of beats for one full minute.	_____	_____	_____
14. While counting, pays attention to pulse rhythm.	_____	_____	_____
15. Notes volume or quality of apical pulse.	_____	_____	_____
16. Removes stethoscope earpieces from ears.	_____	_____	_____
17. Records findings. Notes that this measurement is an apical pulse.	_____	_____	_____
18. Asks client if client needs help to dress; assists as needed.	_____	_____	_____
19. Cleans stethoscope earpieces and chestpiece with disinfectant wipes.	_____	_____	_____
20. Washes hands.	_____	_____	_____
21. Records procedure correctly in client's chart.	_____	_____	_____

Documentation

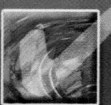

1st Observation

Date: _____ Evaluator Signature and Printed Name: _____

Comments:

2nd Observation

Date: _____ Evaluator Signature and Printed Name: _____

Comments:

Mastery

Date: _____ Evaluator Signature and Printed Name: _____

Comments:

 ABHES COMPETENCIES: Take vital signs.

 CAAHEP COMPETENCIES: Obtain vital signs.

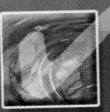

Name _____ Course _____

PROCEDURE

4-10   Blood Pressure

	1st Observation	2nd Observation	Mastery
1. Washes hands.	_____	_____	_____
2. Gathers equipment and supplies.	_____	_____	_____
3. Introduces self to client.	_____	_____	_____
4. Identifies client.	_____	_____	_____
5. Tells client, in everyday language, what medical assistant is going to do.	_____	_____	_____
6. Asks if client has any questions. If client does, gives short and simple answers.	_____	_____	_____
7. Wipes earpieces and chestpiece of stethoscope with alcohol wipes.	_____	_____	_____
8. Has client either sit or lie down. If sitting, arm is extended at heart level with palm of hand facing up.	_____	_____	_____
9. Removes any clothing from client's arm.	_____	_____	_____
10. Turns valve on bulb of cuff counterclockwise to open valve and completely empty air from blood pressure cuff.	_____	_____	_____
11. Wraps blood pressure cuff snugly around client's arm, approximately 2 inches above elbow.	_____	_____	_____
12. Checks fit of cuff with two fingers.	_____	_____	_____
13. If using aneroid sphygmomanometer, makes sure dial is placed so numbers are clearly visible. If using mercury sphygmomanometer, makes sure it is placed on flat surface where numbers are easily visible.	_____	_____	_____
14. With pads of first two fingers, finds client's radial pulse.	_____	_____	_____
15. With other hand, turns valve on bulb clockwise to close it.	_____	_____	_____
16. Pumps bulb to inflate cuff to 30 mm Hg above where no longer feels radial pulse.	_____	_____	_____
17. Turns valve counterclockwise to deflate cuff until feels radial pulse.	_____	_____	_____
18. Notes number where radial pulse felt (*palpatory systolic pressure*).	_____	_____	_____
19. Quickly finishes turning valve to release rest of air.	_____	_____	_____
20. Places earpieces of stethoscope in ears.	_____	_____	_____
21. Finds brachial artery.	_____	_____	_____

757

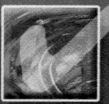
22. Puts stethoscope chestpiece at this site. _____ _____ _____

23. Turns valve clockwise to close it. Quickly inflates cuff 30 mm Hg above palpatory systolic pressure. _____ _____ _____

24. Turns valve counterclockwise to open valve and slowly keeps turning to release 2 to 3 mm Hg per second. _____ _____ _____

25. Reads number at which first hears sound (*systolic pressure*). _____ _____ _____

26. Keeps turning valve until sound changes. Keeps turning valve slowly and steadily until no longer hears any sound (*diastolic pressure*). _____ _____ _____

27. Quickly releases rest of air. _____ _____ _____

28. Takes cuff off client. _____ _____ _____

29. Writes down blood pressure measurement as systolic over diastolic. _____ _____ _____

30. Using alcohol wipes, cleans stethoscope chestpiece and earpieces. _____ _____ _____

31. Folds cuff and puts it away with sphygmomanometer and stethoscope. _____ _____ _____

32. Washes hands. _____ _____ _____

33. Records procedure correctly in client's chart. _____ _____ _____

Documentation

```
[ blank box ]
```

1st Observation

Date: _____ Evaluator Signature and Printed Name: _____

Comments:

2nd Observation

Date: _____ Evaluator Signature and Printed Name: _____

Comments:

Mastery

Date: _____ Evaluator Signature and Printed Name: _____

Comments:

 ABHES COMPETENCIES: Take vital signs.

 CAAHEP COMPETENCIES: Obtain vital signs.

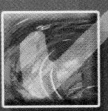

Name _____   Course _____

	1st Observation	2nd Observation	Mastery
1. Washes hands.	_____	_____	_____
2. Gathers equipment and supplies.	_____	_____	_____
3. Reviews forms before entering room with client.	_____	_____	_____
4. Introduces self to client.	_____	_____	_____
5. Identifies client.	_____	_____	_____
6. Tells client, in everyday language, what medical assistant is going to do.	_____	_____	_____
7. Asks if client has any questions. If client does, gives short and simple answers.	_____	_____	_____
8. Asks client to sit in chair rather than on examination table.	_____	_____	_____
9. Sits in chair opposite or next to client.	_____	_____	_____
10. Speaks clearly. When asking questions, looks at client and not down at clipboard.	_____	_____	_____
11. Gives client time to answer questions.	_____	_____	_____
12. Repeats question and uses words that client can understand if client hesitates.	_____	_____	_____
13. When medical/health history form is completed, asks again if client has any questions. If client does, gives short and simple answers.	_____	_____	_____
14. Thanks client and informs client what will happen next.	_____	_____	_____
15. Washes hands.	_____	_____	_____
16. Signs form and records information in client's chart according to office policy.	_____	_____	_____

Documentation

_____
| |
| |
| |
| |
|_____|

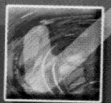

1st Observation

Date: _____ Evaluator Signature and Printed Name: _____

Comments:

2nd Observation

Date: _____ Evaluator Signature and Printed Name: _____

Comments:

Mastery

Date: _____ Evaluator Signature and Printed Name: _____

Comments:

 ABHES COMPETENCIES: Interview and record patient history.

Perform telephone and in-person screening.

 CAAHEP COMPETENCIES: Obtain and record patient history.

Perform telephone and in-person screening.

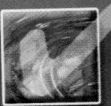

Name _____   Course _____

PROCEDURE

5-2

Height

	1st Observation	2nd Observation	Mastery
1. Washes hands.	_____	_____	_____
2. Gathers equipment and supplies.	_____	_____	_____
3. Introduces self to client.	_____	_____	_____
4. Identifies client.	_____	_____	_____
5. Tells client, in everyday language, what medical assistant is going to do.	_____	_____	_____
6. Asks if client has any questions. If client does, gives short and simple answers.	_____	_____	_____
7. Asks client to remove shoes.	_____	_____	_____
8. Places paper towel on base of balance-beam scale.	_____	_____	_____
9. With one hand, raises vertical bar. Keeps extension against vertical bar and raises bar several inches above client's head.	_____	_____	_____
10. Helps client to step up onto scale.	_____	_____	_____
11. Stands close enough to client to help if client becomes unsteady.	_____	_____	_____
12. Opens extension from vertical bar. While holding it open, pushes bar down until it rests gently on client's head.	_____	_____	_____
13. Helps client off scale as needed.	_____	_____	_____
14. Offers to help client put on shoes.			
15. Reads and records number shown at line on vertical bar.	_____	_____	_____
16. Changes number into feet and inches.	_____	_____	_____
17. Disposes of paper towel in waste container.	_____	_____	_____
18. Washes hands.	_____	_____	_____
19. Records procedure correctly in client's chart.	_____	_____	_____

Documentation

_____

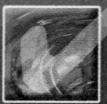

Competency Skill Checklist (Continued)

1st Observation

Date: _____ Evaluator Signature and Printed Name: _____

Comments:

2nd Observation

Date: _____ Evaluator Signature and Printed Name: _____

Comments:

Mastery

Date: _____ Evaluator Signature and Printed Name: _____

Comments:

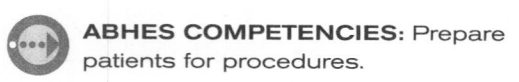 **ABHES COMPETENCIES:** Prepare patients for procedures.

 CAAHEP COMPETENCIES: Prepare patient for and assist with procedures, treatments, and minor office surgeries.

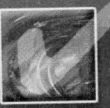

Name _____   Course _____

PROCEDURE

5-3   Weight

	1st Observation	2nd Observation	Mastery
1. Washes hands.	_____	_____	_____
2. Gathers equipment and supplies.	_____	_____	_____
3. Introduces self to client.	_____	_____	_____
4. Identifies client.	_____	_____	_____
5. Tells client, in everyday language, what medical assistant is going to do.	_____	_____	_____
6. Asks if client has any questions. If client does, gives short and simple answers.	_____	_____	_____
7. Asks client to remove shoes.	_____	_____	_____
8. Places paper towel on base of balance-beam scale.	_____	_____	_____
9. Helps client to step up onto scale with client's face to scale and back to medical assistant.	_____	_____	_____
10. Stands close enough to client to help if client becomes unsteady while standing.	_____	_____	_____
11. Moves large poise along long horizontal bar.	_____	_____	_____
12. Moves small poise along upper measuring bar.	_____	_____	_____
13. When pointed end of balance beam remains in middle between top and bottom, stops moving poises.	_____	_____	_____
14. Reads number at large poise.	_____	_____	_____
15. Reads number at small poise.	_____	_____	_____
16. Adds numbers from large and small poises.	_____	_____	_____
17. Helps client off scale.	_____	_____	_____
18. Offers to help client put on shoes.	_____	_____	_____
19. Reads and records weight measurement.	_____	_____	_____
20. Pushes poises back to left.	_____	_____	_____
21. Disposes of paper towel in waste container.	_____	_____	_____
22. Washes hands.	_____	_____	_____
23. Records procedure correctly in client's chart.	_____	_____	_____

Documentation

_____

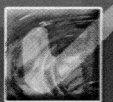

1st Observation

Date: _____ Evaluator Signature and Printed Name: _____

Comments:

2nd Observation

Date: _____ Evaluator Signature and Printed Name: _____

Comments:

Mastery

Date: _____ Evaluator Signature and Printed Name: _____

Comments:

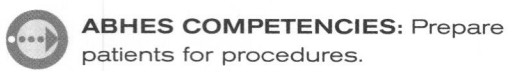 **ABHES COMPETENCIES:** Prepare patients for procedures.

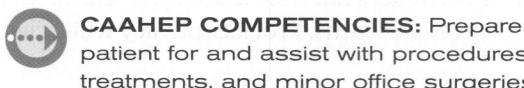 **CAAHEP COMPETENCIES:** Prepare patient for and assist with procedures, treatments, and minor office surgeries.

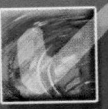

Name _____ Course _____

PROCEDURE

5-4

Semi-Fowler's and Fowler's Positions

	1st Observation	2nd Observation	Mastery
1. Washes hands.	_____	_____	_____
2. Gathers equipment and supplies.	_____	_____	_____
3. Introduces self to client.	_____	_____	_____
4. Identifies client.	_____	_____	_____
5. Tells client, in everyday language, what medical assistant is going to do.	_____	_____	_____
6. Asks if client has any questions. If client does, gives short and simple answers.	_____	_____	_____
7. Asks client if client needs help undressing and putting on gown. Assists as needed.	_____	_____	_____
8. If client does not need assistance, tells client which way gown opens. Provides privacy while client changes.	_____	_____	_____
9. Moves footstool to side of examination table.	_____	_____	_____
10. Standing close to client, in position ready to help as needed, asks client to step up backward onto footstool.	_____	_____	_____
11. Asks client to sit back comfortably on side of examination table.	_____	_____	_____
12. Raises head of examination table to 45 degrees for semi-Fowler's position or to 90 degrees for Fowler's position.	_____	_____	_____
13. Asks client to rest back on support.	_____	_____	_____
14. Drapes client as needed.	_____	_____	_____
15. Stays with client and assists doctor during examination or procedure, as needed.	_____	_____	_____
16. Informs client before head of table is lowered. Has client lean forward before moving head of table.	_____	_____	_____
17. Supports head of table as needed while lowering.	_____	_____	_____
18. After examination or procedure is completed, asks client to sit with legs over table edge, before getting off table. Assists as needed, then helps client to get off table.	_____	_____	_____
19. If necessary, assists clients to take off gown and get dressed.	_____	_____	_____
20. Disposes of paper table covering, paper covering for pillow, and gown (if paper) in appropriate waste container.	_____	_____	_____

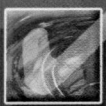

21. Cleans table and room according to office policy.   _____   _____   _____

22. Records procedure correctly in client's chart.   _____   _____   _____

Documentation

1st Observation

Date: _____ Evaluator Signature and Printed Name: _____

Comments:

2nd Observation

Date: _____ Evaluator Signature and Printed Name: _____

Comments:

Mastery

Date: _____ Evaluator Signature and Printed Name: _____

Comments:

 ABHES COMPETENCIES: Prepare patient for and assist physician with routine and specialty examinations and treatments and minor office surgeries.

Prepare patients for procedures.

 CAAHEP COMPETENCIES: Prepare patient for and assist with routine and specialty examinations.

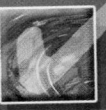

Name _____ Course _____

PROCEDURE

5-5   Prone Position

		1st Observation	2nd Observation	Mastery
1.	Washes hands.	_____	_____	_____
2.	Gathers equipment and supplies.	_____	_____	_____
3.	Introduces self to client.	_____	_____	_____
4.	Identifies client.	_____	_____	_____
5.	Tells client, in everyday language, what medical assistant is going to do.	_____	_____	_____
6.	Asks if client has any questions. If client does, gives short and simple answers.	_____	_____	_____
7.	Asks client if client needs help undressing and putting on gown. Assists as needed.	_____	_____	_____
8.	If client does not need assistance, tells client which way gown opens. Provides privacy while client changes.	_____	_____	_____
9.	Moves footstool to side of examination table.	_____		
10.	Standing close to client, and in position ready to help as needed for balance, asks client to step up backward onto footstool.	_____	_____	_____
11.	Asks client to sit back comfortably on side of examination table.	_____	_____	_____
12.	Pulls out foot extension of table, if needed.	_____	_____	_____
13.	Asks client to lie on back.	_____	_____	_____
14.	Covers client with drape.	_____	_____	_____
15.	Standing at side of table, asks client to turn toward the medical assistant so that client is lying on stomach. Tells client to turn slowly.	_____	_____	_____
16.	Has client turn head to side.	_____	_____	_____
17.	Asks client to bend arms at elbow and place hands near head.	_____	_____	_____
18.	Makes sure client is covered for privacy and modesty.	_____	_____	_____
19.	Stays with client and assists doctor with examination or procedure, as needed.	_____	_____	_____
20.	After examination is completed, asks client to turn on back. Remains with client during this movement.	_____	_____	_____
21.	Asks client to sit, with legs over table edge, before getting off table. Assists as needed, then helps client to get off table.	_____	_____	_____

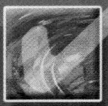

22. If necessary, assists client to take off gown and get dressed. _____ _____ _____

23. Disposes of paper table covering and paper gown in appropriate waste container. _____ _____ _____

24. Cleans table and room according to office policy. _____ _____ _____

25. Records procedure correctly in client's chart. _____ _____ _____

Documentation

```
```

1st Observation

Date: _____ Evaluator Signature and Printed Name: _____

Comments:

2nd Observation

Date: _____ Evaluator Signature and Printed Name: _____

Comments:

Mastery

Date: _____ Evaluator Signature and Printed Name: _____

Comments:

 ABHES COMPETENCIES: Prepare patient for and assist physician with routine and specialty examinations and treatments and minor office surgeries.

Prepare patients for procedures.

 CAAHEP COMPETENCIES: Prepare patient for and assist with routine and specialty examinations.

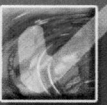
Name _____ Course _____

PROCEDURE

5-6 Supine Position

	1st Observation	2nd Observation	Mastery
1. Washes hands.	_____	_____	_____
2. Gathers equipment and supplies.	_____	_____	_____
3. Introduces self to client.	_____	_____	_____
4. Identifies client.	_____	_____	_____
5. Tells client, in everyday language, what medical assistant is going to do.	_____	_____	_____
6. Asks if client has any questions. If client does, gives short and simple answers.	_____	_____	_____
7. Asks client if client needs help undressing and putting on gown. Assists as needed.	_____	_____	_____
8. If client does not need assistance, tells client which way gown opens. Provides privacy while client changes.	_____	_____	_____
9. Moves footstool to side of examination table.	_____	_____	_____
10. Standing close to client, and in position ready to help as needed for balance, asks client to step up backward onto footstool.	_____	_____	_____
11. Asks client to sit back comfortably on side of examination table.	_____	_____	_____
12. Pulls out foot extension of table, if needed.	_____	_____	_____
13. Asks client to lie on back.	_____	_____	_____
14. Covers client with drape.	_____	_____	_____
15. Places small pillow under client's head.	_____	_____	_____
16. Stays with client and assists doctor during examination or procedure, as needed.	_____	_____	_____
17. After examination or procedure is completed, asks client to sit, with legs over table edge, before getting off table. Assists as needed, then helps client to get off table.	_____	_____	_____
18. If necessary, assists client to take off gown and get dressed.	_____	_____	_____
19. Disposes of paper table covering, paper covering for pillow, and paper gown in appropriate waste container.	_____	_____	_____
20. Cleans table and room according to office policy.	_____	_____	_____
21. Records procedure correctly in client's chart.	_____	_____	_____

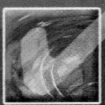

Documentation

1st Observation

Date: _____ Evaluator Signature and Printed Name: _____

Comments:

2nd Observation

Date: _____ Evaluator Signature and Printed Name: _____

Comments:

Mastery

Date: _____ Evaluator Signature and Printed Name: _____

Comments:

 ABHES COMPETENCIES: Prepare patient for and assist physician with routine and specialty examinations and treatments and minor office surgeries.

Prepare patients for procedures.

 CAAHEP COMPETENCIES: Prepare patient for and assist with routine and specialty examinations.

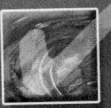

Competency Skill Checklist

Name _____ Course _____

PROCEDURE 5-7 — Dorsal Recumbent Position

	1st Observation	2nd Observation	Mastery
1. Washes hands.	_____	_____	_____
2. Gathers equipment and supplies.	_____	_____	_____
3. Introduces self to client.	_____	_____	_____
4. Identifies client.	_____	_____	_____
5. Tells client, in everyday language, what medical assistant is going to do.	_____	_____	_____
6. Asks if client has any questions. If client does, gives short and simple answers.	_____	_____	_____
7. Asks client if client needs help undressing and putting on gown. Assists as needed.	_____	_____	_____
8. If client does not need assistance, tells client which way gown opens. Provides privacy while client changes.	_____	_____	_____
9. Moves footstool to side of examination table.	_____	_____	_____
10. Standing close to client, and in position ready to help as needed for balance, asks client to step up backward onto footstool.	_____	_____	_____
11. Asks client to sit back comfortably on side of examination table.	_____	_____	_____
12. Pulls out foot extension of table, if needed.	_____	_____	_____
13. Asks client to bend knees and put feet flat on table.	_____	_____	_____
14. Drapes client.	_____	_____	_____
15. Places small pillow under client's head for comfort.	_____	_____	_____
16. Stays with client and assists doctor during examination or procedure, as needed.	_____	_____	_____
17. After examination or procedure is completed, asks client to sit, with legs over table edge, before getting off table. Assists as needed, then helps client to get off table.	_____	_____	_____
18. If necessary, assists client to take off gown and get dressed.	_____	_____	_____
19. Disposes of paper table covering, paper covering for pillow, and paper gown in appropriate waste container.	_____	_____	_____
20. Cleans table and room according to office policy.	_____	_____	_____
21. Records procedure correctly in client's chart.	_____	_____	_____

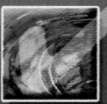

Documentation

[ ]

1st Observation

Date: _____ Evaluator Signature and Printed Name: _____

Comments:

2nd Observation

Date: _____ Evaluator Signature and Printed Name: _____

Comments:

Mastery

Date: _____ Evaluator Signature and Printed Name: _____

Comments:

 ABHES COMPETENCIES: Prepare patient for and assist physician with routine and specialty examinations and treatments and minor office surgeries.

Prepare patients for procedures.

 CAAHEP COMPETENCIES: Prepare patient for and assist with routine and specialty examinations.

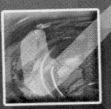

Name _____   Course _____

PROCEDURE

5-8   Lithotomy Position

	1st Observation	2nd Observation	Mastery
1. Washes hands.	_____	_____	_____
2. Gathers equipment and supplies.	_____	_____	_____
3. Introduces self to client.	_____	_____	_____
4. Identifies client.	_____		
5. Tells client, in everyday language, what medical assistant is going to do.	_____	_____	_____
6. Asks if client has any questions. If client does, gives short and simple answers.	_____	_____	_____
7. Asks client if client needs help undressing and putting on gown. Assists as needed.	_____	_____	_____
8. If client does not need assistance, tells client which way gown opens. Provides privacy while client changes.	_____	_____	_____
9. Moves footstool to side of examination table.	_____		
10. Standing close to client, and in position ready to help as needed for balance, asks client to step up backward onto footstool.	_____	_____	_____
11. Asks client to sit back comfortably on side of examination table.	_____	_____	_____
12. Pulls out foot extension of table, if needed.	_____	_____	_____
13. Asks client to lie on back.	_____	_____	_____
14. Drapes client.	_____		
15. Turns stirrups away from table and adjusts height as needed for client comfort.	_____	_____	_____
16. Asks client to slide down toward end of table. Places client's feet into stirrups.	_____	_____	_____
17. Pushes in foot extension of table.	_____	_____	_____
18. Ensures that footstool and light are placed correctly for examiner.	_____	_____	_____
19. Stays with client and assists doctor during examination or procedure, as needed.	_____	_____	_____
20. After examination or procedure is completed, helps client to lift feet out of stirrups.	_____	_____	_____
21. Asks client to sit, with legs over table edge, before getting off table. Assists as needed, then helps client to get off table.	_____	_____	_____

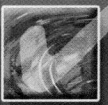

22. If necessary, assists client to take off gown and get dressed. _____ _____ _____

23. Disposes of paper table covering, paper covering for pillow, and paper gown in appropriate waste container. _____ _____ _____

24. Cleans table and room according to office policy. _____ _____ _____

25. Records procedure correctly in client's chart. _____ _____ _____

Documentation

```
┌─────────────────────────────────────────────────┐
│                                                   │
│                                                   │
│                                                   │
│                                                   │
└─────────────────────────────────────────────────┘
```

1st Observation

Date: _____ Evaluator Signature and Printed Name: _____

Comments:

2nd Observation

Date: _____ Evaluator Signature and Printed Name: _____

Comments:

Mastery

Date: _____ Evaluator Signature and Printed Name: _____

Comments:

 ABHES COMPETENCIES: Prepare patient for and assist physician with routine and specialty examinations and treatments and minor office surgeries.

Prepare patients for procedures.

 CAAHEP COMPETENCIES: Prepare patient for and assist with routine and specialty examinations.

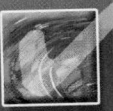

Name _____ Course _____

PROCEDURE

5-9 Sims' Position

	1st Observation	2nd Observation	Mastery
1. Washes hands.	_____	_____	_____
2. Gathers equipment and supplies.	_____	_____	_____
3. Introduces self to client.	_____	_____	_____
4. Identifies client.	_____	_____	_____
5. Tells client, in everyday language, what medical assistant is going to do.	_____	_____	_____
6. Asks if client has any questions. If client does, gives short and simple answers.	_____	_____	_____
7. Asks client if client needs help undressing and putting on gown. Assists as needed.	_____	_____	_____
8. If client does not need assistance, tells client which way gown opens. Provides privacy while client changes.	_____	_____	_____
9. Moves footstool to side of examination table.	_____	_____	_____
10. Standing close to client, and in position ready to help as needed for balance, asks client to step up backward onto footstool.	_____	_____	_____
11. Asks client to sit back comfortably on side of examination table.	_____	_____	_____
12. Pulls out foot extension of table, if needed.	_____	_____	_____
13. Tells client to lie on left side.	_____	_____	_____
14. Tells client to bend right arm at elbow, placing hand near head.	_____	_____	_____
15. Has client flex left leg slightly and flex right leg sharply.	_____	_____	_____
16. Places drape over client.	_____	_____	_____
17. Stays with client and assists doctor during examination or procedure, as needed.	_____	_____	_____
18. Tells client to turn onto back. Stands by table to prevent client from falling off examination table while turning.	_____	_____	_____
19. After examination or procedure is completed, asks client to sit, with legs over table edge, before getting off table. Assists as needed, then helps client to get off table.	_____	_____	_____
20. If necessary, assists client to take off gown and get dressed.	_____	_____	_____

775

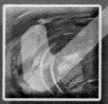

21. Disposes of paper table covering, paper covering for pillow, and paper gown in appropriate waste container.   _____   _____   _____
22. Cleans table and room according to office policy.   _____   _____   _____
23. Records procedure correctly in client's chart.   _____   _____   _____

Documentation

```


```

1st Observation
Date: _____   Evaluator Signature and Printed Name: _____
Comments:

2nd Observation
Date: _____   Evaluator Signature and Printed Name: _____
Comments:

Mastery
Date: _____   Evaluator Signature and Printed Name: _____
Comments:

 ABHES COMPETENCIES: Prepare patient for and assist physician with routine and specialty examinations and treatments and minor office surgeries.

Prepare patients for procedures.

 CAAHEP COMPETENCIES: Prepare patient for and assist with routine and specialty examinations.

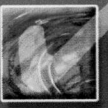

Competency Skill Checklist

Name _____ Course _____

PROCEDURE 5-10 — Knee-Chest Position

	1st Observation	2nd Observation	Mastery
1. Washes hands.	_____	_____	_____
2. Gathers equipment and supplies.	_____	_____	_____
3. Introduces self to client.	_____	_____	_____
4. Identifies client.	_____	_____	_____
5. Tells client, in everyday language, what medical assistant is going to do.	_____	_____	_____
6. Asks if client has any questions. If client does, gives short and simple answers.	_____	_____	_____
7. Asks client if client needs help undressing and putting on gown. Assists as needed.	_____	_____	_____
8. If client does not need assistance, tells client which way gown opens. Provides privacy while client changes.	_____	_____	_____
9. Moves footstool to side of examination table.	_____	_____	_____
10. Standing close to client, and in position ready to help as needed for balance, asks client to step up backward onto footstool.	_____	_____	_____
11. Instructs client to lie prone on exam table.	_____	_____	_____
12. Asks client to rest on knees and chest.	_____	_____	_____
13. Tells client to turn head to side.	_____	_____	_____
14. Places small pillow under client's chest for comfort.	_____	_____	_____
15. Drapes client's back, buttocks, and legs.	_____	_____	_____
16. Tells client to place arm above head or down at side, whichever is more comfortable for client.	_____	_____	_____
17. Stays with client and assists doctor during examination or procedure, as needed.	_____	_____	_____
18. After examination or procedure is completed, asks client to sit, with legs over table edge, before getting off table. Assists as needed, then helps client to get off table.	_____	_____	_____
19. If necessary, assists client to take off gown and get dressed.	_____	_____	_____
20. Disposes of paper table covering, paper covering for pillow, and paper gown in appropriate waste container.	_____	_____	_____
21. Cleans table and room according to office policy.	_____	_____	_____
22. Records procedure correctly in client's chart.	_____	_____	_____

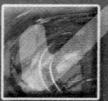
Documentation

1st Observation

Date: _____ Evaluator Signature and Printed Name: _____

Comments:

2nd Observation

Date: _____ Evaluator Signature and Printed Name: _____

Comments:

Mastery

Date: _____ Evaluator Signature and Printed Name: _____

Comments:

 ABHES COMPETENCIES: Prepare patient for and assist physician with routine and specialty examinations and treatments and minor office surgeries.

Prepare patients for procedures.

 CAAHEP COMPETENCIES: Prepare patient for and assist with routine and specialty examinations.

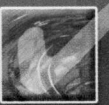

Name _____   Course _____

PROCEDURE

5-11   Modified Standing Position

	1st Observation	2nd Observation	Mastery
1. Washes hands.	_____	_____	_____
2. Gathers equipment and supplies.	_____	_____	_____
3. Introduces self to client.	_____	_____	_____
4. Identifies client.	_____	_____	_____
5. Tells client, in everyday language, what medical assistant is going to do.	_____	_____	_____
6. Asks if client has any questions. If client does, gives short and simple answers.	_____	_____	_____
7. Asks client if client needs help undressing and putting on gown. Assists as needed.	_____	_____	_____
8. If client does not need assistance, tells which way gown opens. Provides privacy while client changes.	_____	_____	_____
9. Asks client to stand facing end of examination table.	_____	_____	_____
10. Covers client with drape.	_____	_____	_____
11. Instructs client to bend forward from waist or hips.	_____	_____	_____
12. Tells client to rest head, chest, and arms on exam table.	_____	_____	_____
13. Places small pillow under client's head for comfort.	_____	_____	_____
14. Stays with client and assists doctor during examination or procedure, as needed.	_____	_____	_____
15. After examination or procedure is completed, assists client to take off gown and get dressed, as needed.	_____	_____	_____
16. Disposes of paper table covering, paper covering for pillow, and paper gown in appropriate waste container.	_____	_____	_____
17. Cleans table and room according to office policy.	_____	_____	_____
18. Records procedure correctly in client's chart.	_____	_____	_____

Documentation

```



```

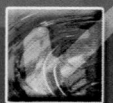

1st Observation

Date: _____ Evaluator Signature and Printed Name: _____

Comments:

2nd Observation

Date: _____ Evaluator Signature and Printed Name: _____

Comments:

Mastery

Date: _____ Evaluator Signature and Printed Name: _____

Comments:

 ABHES COMPETENCIES: Prepare patient for and assist physician with routine and specialty examinations and treatments and minor office surgeries.

Prepare patients for procedures.

 CAAHEP COMPETENCIES: Prepare patient for and assist with routine and specialty examinations.

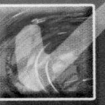

Name _____ Course _____

PROCEDURE

5-12

Vision Acuity: Measuring with Snellen Chart

	1st Observation	2nd Observation	Mastery
1. Washes hands.	_____	_____	_____
2. Gathers equipment and supplies.	_____	_____	_____
3. Introduces self to client.	_____	_____	_____
4. Identifies client.	_____	_____	_____
5. Tells client, in everyday language, what medical assistant is going to do.	_____	_____	_____
6. Asks if client has any questions. If client does, gives short and simple answers.	_____	_____	_____
7. Has client stand or sit 20 feet from Snellen chart. Makes sure that chart is at client's eye level.	_____	_____	_____
8. Identifies line on chart by pointing to it.	_____	_____	_____
9. Asks client to read that line with both eyes. Has client keep glasses on for this part of examination.	_____	_____	_____
10. Tells client to cover left eye with eye occluder. If client wears glasses, procedure is done first with glasses on, then without corrective lenses.	_____	_____	_____
11. Asks client to keep both eyes open, even though one eye is covered.	_____	_____	_____
12. Observes and records if client leans forward, squints, or turns head in effort to read lines.	_____	_____	_____
13. Records whether each line was read with corrective lenses or without corrective lenses.	_____	_____	_____
14. Writes down number by smallest line that client can read with right eye without mistakes.	_____	_____	_____
15. Tells client to cover right eye with occluder. Tests left eye.	_____	_____	_____
16. Writes down number by smallest line that client can read with left eye without mistake.	_____	_____	_____
17. Records vision acuity for distance as fraction.	_____	_____	_____
18. Washes hands.	_____	_____	_____
19. Records procedure correctly in client's chart.	_____	_____	_____

Documentation

_____

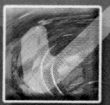

1st Observation

Date: _____ Evaluator Signature and Printed Name: _____

Comments:

2nd Observation

Date: _____ Evaluator Signature and Printed Name: _____

Comments:

Mastery

Date: _____ Evaluator Signature and Printed Name: _____

Comments:

 ABHES COMPETENCIES: Prepare patient for and assist physician with routine and specialty examinations and treatments and minor office surgeries.

 CAAHEP COMPETENCIES: Prepare patient for and assist with routine and specialty examinations.

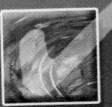

Name _____   Course _____

PROCEDURE

5-13   Near Visual Acuity Assessment

	1st Observation	2nd Observation	Mastery
1. Washes hands.	_____	_____	_____
2. Gathers equipment and supplies.	_____	_____	_____
3. Introduces self to client.	_____	_____	_____
4. Identifies client.	_____	_____	_____
5. Tells client, in everyday language, what medical assistant is going to do.	_____	_____	_____
6. Asks if client has any questions. If client does, gives short and simple answers.	_____	_____	_____
7. Asks client to sit comfortably.	_____	_____	_____
8. Reminds client to keep both eyes open.	_____	_____	_____
9. Holds Jaeger card about 15 to 16 inches from client's face.	_____	_____	_____
10. Positions card at comfortable reading level for client.	_____	_____	_____
11. Points to a line and instructs client to begin reading aloud.	_____	_____	_____
12. Notes number by smallest printed line that client reads without mistake.	_____	_____	_____
13. Wipes card off with small gauze pad.	_____	_____	_____
14. Discards gauze pad in appropriate waste container.	_____	_____	_____
15. Washes hands.	_____	_____	_____
16. Records procedure correctly in client's chart.	_____	_____	_____

Documentation

_____
_____
_____
_____

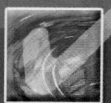

1st Observation

Date: _____ Evaluator Signature and Printed Name: _____

Comments:

2nd Observation

Date: _____ Evaluator Signature and Printed Name: _____

Comments:

Mastery

Date: _____ Evaluator Signature and Printed Name: _____

Comments:

 ABHES COMPETENCIES: Prepare patient for and assist physician with routine and specialty examinations and treatments and minor office surgeries.

 CAAHEP COMPETENCIES: Prepare patient for and assist with routine and specialty examinations.

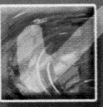

Name _____ Course _____

PROCEDURE

5-14   Color Acuity Assessment

	1st Observation	2nd Observation	Mastery
1. Washes hands.	_____	_____	_____
2. Gathers equipment and supplies.	_____	_____	_____
3. Introduces self to client.	_____	_____	_____
4. Identifies client.	_____	_____	_____
5. Tells client, in everyday language, what medical assistant is going to do.	_____	_____	_____
6. Asks if client has any questions. If client does, gives short and simple answers.	_____	_____	_____
7. Makes sure room has adequate lighting.	_____	_____	_____
8. Explains procedure to client and performs sample session with practice card.	_____	_____	_____
9. Positions plate or chart at right angles to client's vision.	_____	_____	_____
10. Holds chart about 30 inches from client's face.	_____	_____	_____
11. Instructs client to keep both eyes open.	_____	_____	_____
12. Asks client to look at colored dots and state what number or symbol is seen in dots.	_____	_____	_____
13. After practice plate, holds up plate #1 and asks client to read number seen.	_____	_____	_____
14. Notes if client read number correctly.	_____	_____	_____
15. Continues until all plates or charts have been completed.	_____	_____	_____
16. Cleans plates with small gauze pad if charts are laminated.	_____	_____	_____
17. Stores plates properly, away from light.	_____	_____	_____
18. Washes hands.	_____	_____	_____
19. Records procedure correctly in client's chart.	_____	_____	_____

Documentation

_____
_____
_____
_____
_____

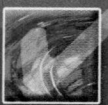

1st Observation

Date: _____ Evaluator Signature and Printed Name: _____

Comments:

2nd Observation

Date: _____ Evaluator Signature and Printed Name: _____

Comments:

Mastery

Date: _____ Evaluator Signature and Printed Name: _____

Comments:

 ABHES COMPETENCIES: Prepare patient for and assist physician with routine and specialty examinations and treatments and minor office surgeries.

 CAAHEP COMPETENCIES: Prepare patient for and assist with routine and specialty examinations.

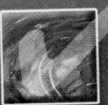

Name _____ Course _____

	1st Observation	2nd Observation	Mastery
1. Washes hands.	_____	_____	_____
2. Gathers equipment and supplies.	_____	_____	_____
3. Introduces self to client.	_____	_____	_____
4. Identifies client.	_____	_____	
5. Tells client, in everyday language, what medical assistant is going to do.	_____	_____	_____
6. Asks if client has any questions. If client does, gives short and simple answers.	_____	_____	_____
7. Asks client to lie on his back on examination table.	_____	_____	_____
8. Drapes absorbent towel over client's shoulder.	_____	_____	_____
9. Asks client to turn head toward affected eye.	_____		
10. Using moist gauze pad, gently wipes from inner canthus of eye to outer canthus.	_____	_____	_____
11. Places basin snugly against side of client's face.	_____	_____	_____
12. Fills bulb of syringe with ordered solution. Compares ophthalmic solution with doctor's order.	_____	_____	_____
13. Using thumb and index finger, gently exposes lower conjunctiva and holds open client's upper eyelid.	_____	_____	_____
14. Starting at inner canthus of eye, holds syringe 1 inch above eye and points flow of solution toward lower conjunctiva. Does not let tip of syringe touch eye.	_____	_____	_____
15. When flow from syringe is completed, blots excess moisture from client's eye with sterile gauze or cotton.	_____	_____	_____
16. Observes returned solution in basin.	_____	_____	_____
17. Removes basin, towel, and supplies. Disposes of these items according to office policy.	_____	_____	_____
18. Helps client to upright sitting position.	_____	_____	_____
19. Removes gloves and disposes of them properly.	_____	_____	_____
20. Washes hands.	_____	_____	_____
21. Records procedure correctly in client's chart.	_____	_____	_____

Documentation

_____

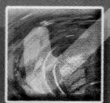
1st Observation

Date: _____ Evaluator Signature and Printed Name: _____

Comments:

2nd Observation

Date: _____ Evaluator Signature and Printed Name: _____

Comments:

Mastery

Date: _____ Evaluator Signature and Printed Name: _____

Comments:

 ABHES COMPETENCIES: Prepare patient for and assist physician with routine and specialty examinations and treatments and minor office surgeries.

 CAAHEP COMPETENCIES: Prepare patient for and assist with routine and specialty examinations.

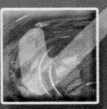

Competency Skill Checklist

Name _____ Course _____

PROCEDURE

5-16   Ear Irrigation

	1st Observation	2nd Observation	Mastery
1. Washes hands.	_____	_____	_____
2. Gathers equipment and supplies.	_____	_____	_____
3. Warms irrigation solution to approximately 100° F.	_____	_____	_____
4. Introduces self to client.	_____	_____	_____
5. Identifies client.	_____	_____	_____
6. Tells client, in everyday language, what medical assistant is going to do.	_____	_____	_____
7. Asks if client has any questions. If client does, gives short and simple answers.	_____	_____	_____
8. Positions client in comfortable sitting position.	_____	_____	_____
9. Asks client to bend head slightly toward affected ear.	_____	_____	_____
10. Places absorbent towel on client's shoulder.	_____	_____	_____
11. Puts on gloves.	_____	_____	_____
12. Wipes client's outer ear with moist gauze.	_____	_____	_____
13. Asks client to hold basin against ear. If client is unable, asks for help.	_____	_____	_____
14. Draws up ordered solution into syringe.	_____	_____	_____
15. Gently pulls outer ear up and back for adult client. (In infants and small children, pulls auricle down and back.)	_____	_____	_____
16. Places tip of syringe into client's ear canal and points flow of solution upward toward roof of ear canal.	_____	_____	_____
17. Refills syringe and irrigates again.	_____	_____	_____
18. Wipes excess moisture from outer part of ear with gauze.	_____	_____	_____
19. Observes returned solution in basin.	_____	_____	_____
20. Removes basin and towel and disposes of them according to office policy.	_____	_____	_____
21. Allows client to sit for a few minutes.	_____	_____	_____
22. Assists client to get off exam table or out of chair.	_____	_____	_____
23. Removes gloves and disposes of them properly.	_____	_____	_____
24. Washes hands.	_____	_____	_____
25. Records procedure correctly in client's chart.	_____	_____	_____

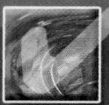

Documentation

___

1st Observation

Date: _____ Evaluator Signature and Printed Name: _____

Comments:

2nd Observation

Date: _____ Evaluator Signature and Printed Name: _____

Comments:

Mastery

Date: _____ Evaluator Signature and Printed Name: _____

Comments:

 ABHES COMPETENCIES: Prepare patient for and assist physician with routine and specialty examinations and treatments and minor office surgeries.

 CAAHEP COMPETENCIES: Prepare patient for and assist with routine and specialty examinations.

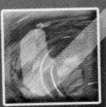

Name _____   Course _____

	1st Observation	2nd Observation	Mastery
1. Washes hands.	_____	_____	_____
2. Gathers equipment and supplies.	_____	_____	_____
3. Introduces self to client.	_____	_____	_____
4. Identifies client.	_____	_____	_____
5. Tells client, in everyday language, what medical assistant is going to do. Inform client that he will be asked to repeat the breathing step three times.	_____	_____	_____
6. Asks if client has any questions. If client does, gives short and simple answers.	_____	_____	_____
7. Puts in client information on chart.	_____		
8. Asks client to stand or sit and put on nose clip. Notes in chart whether client stands or sits during procedure.	_____	_____	_____
9. Makes sure correct test is being done.	_____	_____	_____
10. Puts on gloves.	_____	_____	_____
11. Instructs client to put disposable mouthpiece in mouth.	_____	_____	_____
12. Tells client to take deep breath and blow hard into mouthpiece. Observe while client is breathing into mouthpiece.	_____	_____	_____
13. Encourages client to keep blowing until machine indicates to stop.	_____	_____	_____
14. Instructs client to remove mouthpiece and relax.	_____	_____	_____
15. Encourages client and instructs client on how to improve blowing out of air.	_____	_____	_____
16. Tells client again to take deep breath and blow hard into mouthpiece.	_____	_____	_____
17. After third attempt, tells client to remove mouthpiece and nose clip.	_____	_____	_____
18. Disposes of mouthpiece in biohazardous waste container.	_____	_____	_____
19. Removes gloves and disposes of them in appropriate waste container.	_____	_____	_____
20. Washes hands.	_____	_____	_____
21. Asks client if client is experiencing any discomforts or has any questions.	_____	_____	_____
22. Prints results of procedure.	_____	_____	_____

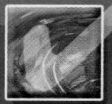

23. Notifies doctor of completion of testing or adds results to chart per office policy.

_____   _____   _____

Documentation

```



```

1st Observation

Date: _____ Evaluator Signature and Printed Name: _____

Comments:

2nd Observation

Date: _____ Evaluator Signature and Printed Name: _____

Comments:

Mastery

Date: _____ Evaluator Signature and Printed Name: _____

Comments:

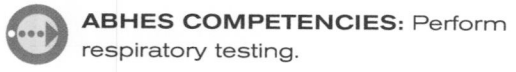 **ABHES COMPETENCIES:** Perform respiratory testing.

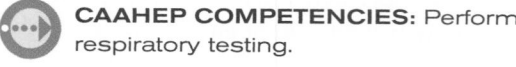 **CAAHEP COMPETENCIES:** Perform respiratory testing.

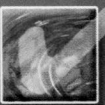
Name _____ Course _____

PROCEDURE

32-1 — Breast Examination Assistance

	1st Observation	2nd Observation	Mastery
1. Washes hands.	_____	_____	_____
2. Gathers equipment and supplies.	_____	_____	_____
3. Introduces self to client.	_____	_____	_____
4. Identifies client.	_____	_____	_____
5. Tells client, in everyday language, what medical assistant is going to do.	_____	_____	_____
6. Asks if client has any questions. If client does, gives short and simple answers.	_____	_____	_____
7. Asks client to remove clothing from waist up.	_____	_____	_____
8. Asks client to put on gown with opening in front.	_____	_____	_____
9. Helps client with undressing as needed.	_____	_____	_____
10. Asks client to sit at end of examination table.	_____	_____	_____
11. When doctor has completed examining breasts with client sitting, positions client supine on table.	_____	_____	_____
12. Drapes client as needed.	_____	_____	_____
13. When examination is finished, helps client into sitting position.	_____	_____	_____
14. Asks client if client has any questions. Teaches or reviews steps for breast self-examination with client.	_____	_____	_____
15. Asks client to dress and helps as needed.	_____	_____	_____
16. Washes hands.	_____	_____	_____
17. Records procedure correctly in client's chart.	_____	_____	_____

Documentation

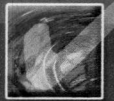

1st Observation

Date: _____ Evaluator Signature and Printed Name: _____

Comments:

2nd Observation

Date: _____ Evaluator Signature and Printed Name: _____

Comments:

Mastery

Date: _____ Evaluator Signature and Printed Name: _____

Comments:

 ABHES COMPETENCIES: Prepare patient for and assist physician with routine and specialty examinations and treatments and minor office surgeries.

Instruct patients with special needs.

 CAAHEP COMPETENCIES: Prepare patient for and assist with routine and specialty examinations.

Instruct individuals according to their needs.

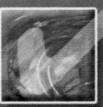
Name _____ Course _____

PROCEDURE

32-2 Pelvic Examination with Pap Test Assistance

	1st Observation	2nd Observation	Mastery
1. Sets up examination room according to office policy.	_____	_____	_____
2. Washes hands.	_____	_____	_____
3. Gathers equipment and supplies.	_____	_____	_____
4. Introduces self to client.	_____	_____	_____
5. Identifies client.	_____	_____	_____
6. Tells client, in everyday language, what medical assistant is going to do.	_____	_____	_____
7. Asks if client has any questions. If client does, gives short and simple answers.	_____	_____	_____
8. Asks client to empty bladder and collect urine specimen if needed.	_____	_____	_____
9. Hands client a drape and instructs client to remove all clothing from waist down.	_____	_____	_____
10. Assists client to sit at end of examination table.	_____	_____	_____
11. Adjusts drape on client.	_____	_____	_____
12. Talks with client to reassure.	_____	_____	_____
13. When doctor is ready, positions client in lithotomy position, with buttocks at edge of table and feet in stirrups.	_____	_____	_____
14. Passes instruments to doctor in correct order.	_____	_____	_____
15. Helps with Pap smear by covering slide with fixative and labeling slide.	_____	_____	_____
16. Tells client when doctor is going to take out speculum and do a manual exam.	_____	_____	_____
17. Holds basin for used speculum.	_____	_____	_____
18. Squeezes water-soluble lubricant on doctor's gloved fingers.	_____	_____	_____
19. Instructs client to breathe deeply and slowly.	_____	_____	_____
20. Takes client's feet out of stirrups when doctor is finished.	_____	_____	_____
21. Assists client to sitting position.	_____	_____	_____
22. Gives client wipes to remove any excess lubricant; assists as needed.	_____	_____	_____
23. Asks client if client has any questions.	_____	_____	_____
24. Helps client to get off examination table; assists with dressing as needed.	_____	_____	_____

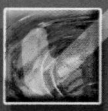

25. Completes processing for transportation of specimens to lab.

_____ _____ _____

26. Cleans, disinfects, or discards equipment and supplies as required.

_____ _____ _____

27. Cleans exam room.

_____ _____ _____

28. Removes gloves.

_____ _____ _____

29. Washes hands.

_____ _____ _____

30. Records procedure correctly in client's chart.

_____ _____ _____

Documentation

1st Observation

Date: _____ Evaluator Signature and Printed Name: _____

Comments:

2nd Observation

Date: _____ Evaluator Signature and Printed Name: _____

Comments:

Mastery

Date: _____ Evaluator Signature and Printed Name: _____

Comments:

 ABHES COMPETENCIES: Prepare patient for and assist physician with routine and specialty examinations and treatments and minor office surgeries.

 CAAHEP COMPETENCIES: Prepare patient for and assist with routine and specialty examinations.

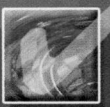

Competency Skill Checklist

Name _____ Course _____

PROCEDURE

33-1   Measurement for Axillary Crutches

	1st Observation	2nd Observation	Mastery
1. Washes hands.	_____	_____	_____
2. Gathers equipment and supplies.	_____	_____	_____
3. Introduces self to client.	_____	_____	_____
4. Identifies client.	_____	_____	_____
5. Tells client, in everyday language, what medical assistant is going to do.	_____	_____	_____
6. Asks if client has any questions. If client does, gives short and simple answers.	_____	_____	_____
7. Asks client to stand straight. Assists client as needed for support.	_____	_____	_____
8. Places tips of crutches 2 inches in front of client and 4 to 6 inches to side of client.	_____	_____	_____
9. Adjusts length of crutches by removing bolts and wing nuts and sliding central support up or down at bottom until shoulder rests or axillary bar is two fingers' breadth below client's axilla. Replaces bolts and wing nuts and fastens them securely.	_____	_____	_____
10. Asks client to stand with crutches supporting client's weight.	_____	_____	_____
11. Moves handgrips to level so that client's elbows are flexed at 30-degree angle.	_____	_____	_____
12. Makes sure that shoulder rests or axilla bars and handgrips are sufficiently padded for client's comfort.	_____	_____	_____
13. Checks fit of crutches.	_____	_____	_____
14. Gives instructions as ordered.	_____	_____	_____
15. Asks client if client has any questions or concerns.	_____	_____	_____
16. Washes hands.	_____	_____	_____
17. Records procedure correctly in client's chart.	_____	_____	_____

Documentation

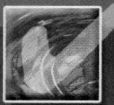

1st Observation

Date: _____ Evaluator Signature and Printed Name: _____

Comments:

2nd Observation

Date: _____ Evaluator Signature and Printed Name: _____

Comments:

Mastery

Date: _____ Evaluator Signature and Printed Name: _____

Comments:

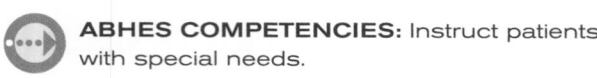 **ABHES COMPETENCIES:** Instruct patients with special needs.

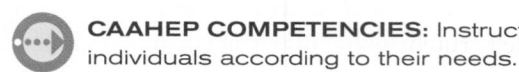 **CAAHEP COMPETENCIES:** Instruct individuals according to their needs.

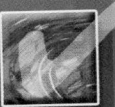
Name _____   Course _____

PROCEDURE

33-2   Crutch Walking: Four-Point Gait

	1st Observation	2nd Observation	Mastery
1. Washes hands.	_____	_____	_____
2. Gathers equipment and supplies.	_____	_____	_____
3. Introduces self to client.	_____	_____	_____
4. Identifies client.	_____	_____	_____
5. Tells client, in everyday language, what medical assistant is going to do.	_____	_____	_____
6. Asks if client has any questions. If client does, gives short and simple answers.	_____	_____	_____
7. Stands straight with crutches in tripod position.	_____	_____	_____
8. Moves right crutch forward about 6 inches.	_____	_____	_____
9. Moves left foot forward to just slightly ahead of left crutch.	_____	_____	_____
10. Moves left crutch forward.	_____	_____	_____
11. Moves right foot forward to just slightly ahead of right crutch.	_____	_____	_____
12. Moves right crutch forward and repeats steps.	_____	_____	_____

Documentation

_____
| |
| |
| |
| |
|_____|

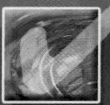

1st Observation

Date: _____ Evaluator Signature and Printed Name: _____

Comments:

2nd Observation

Date: _____ Evaluator Signature and Printed Name: _____

Comments:

Mastery

Date: _____ Evaluator Signature and Printed Name: _____

Comments:

 ABHES COMPETENCIES: Instruct patients with special needs.

 CAAHEP COMPETENCIES: Instruct individuals according to their needs.

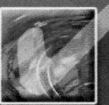
Name _____ Course _____

	1st Observation	2nd Observation	Mastery
1. Washes hands.	_____	_____	_____
2. Gathers equipment and supplies.	_____	_____	_____
3. Introduces self to client.	_____	_____	_____
4. Identifies client.	_____	_____	_____
5. Tells client, in everyday language, what medical assistant is going to do.	_____	_____	_____
6. Asks if client has any questions. If client does, gives short and simple answers.	_____	_____	_____
7. Stands straight with crutches in tripod position.	_____	_____	_____
8. Moves both crutches and affected leg forward.	_____	_____	_____
9. Balances weight on both crutches while moving unaffected leg forward.	_____	_____	_____
10. Moves both crutches and affected leg forward and repeats steps.	_____	_____	_____

Documentation

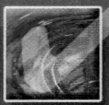

1st Observation

Date: _____ Evaluator Signature and Printed Name: _____

Comments:

2nd Observation

Date: _____ Evaluator Signature and Printed Name: _____

Comments:

Mastery

Date: _____ Evaluator Signature and Printed Name: _____

Comments:

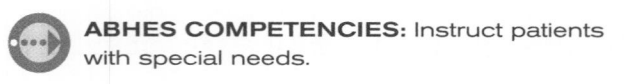 **ABHES COMPETENCIES:** Instruct patients with special needs.

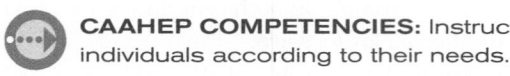 **CAAHEP COMPETENCIES:** Instruct individuals according to their needs.

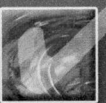

Name _____ Course _____

33-4   Crutch Walking: Two-Point Gait

	1st Observation	2nd Observation	Mastery
1. Washes hands.	_____	_____	_____
2. Gathers equipment and supplies.	_____	_____	_____
3. Introduces self to client.	_____	_____	_____
4. Identifies client.	_____	_____	_____
5. Tells client, in everyday language, what medical assistant is going to do.	_____	_____	_____
6. Asks if client has any questions. If client does, gives short and simple answers.	_____	_____	_____
7. Stands straight with crutches in tripod position.	_____	_____	_____
8. At same time, moves left crutch and right foot forward.	_____	_____	_____
9. Moves right crutch and left foot forward together.	_____	_____	_____
10. Repeats steps.	_____	_____	_____

Documentation

```


```

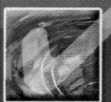

1st Observation

Date: _____ Evaluator Signature and Printed Name: _____

Comments:

2nd Observation

Date: _____ Evaluator Signature and Printed Name: _____

Comments:

Mastery

Date: _____ Evaluator Signature and Printed Name: _____

Comments:

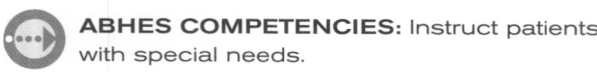 **ABHES COMPETENCIES:** Instruct patients with special needs.

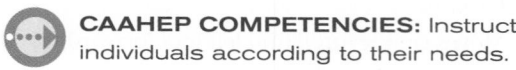 **CAAHEP COMPETENCIES:** Instruct individuals according to their needs.

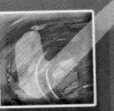
Name _____   Course _____

	1st Observation	2nd Observation	Mastery
Swing-to:			
1. Washes hands.	_____	_____	_____
2. Gathers equipment and supplies.	_____	_____	_____
3. Introduces self to client.	_____	_____	_____
4. Identifies client.	_____	_____	_____
5. Tells client, in everyday language, what medical assistant is going to do.	_____	_____	_____
6. Asks if client has any questions. If client does, gives short and simple answers.	_____	_____	_____
7. Stands straight with crutches in tripod position.	_____	_____	_____
8. Moves both crutches forward.	_____	_____	_____
9. Bears weight on hands.	_____	_____	_____
10. Swings body to bring both feet to level of crutches.	_____	_____	_____
11. Repeats steps.	_____	_____	_____
Swing-through:			
7. Stands straight with crutches in tripod position.	_____	_____	_____
8. Moves both crutches forward.	_____	_____	_____
9. Bears weight on hands.	_____	_____	_____
10. Swings body to bring both feet through to spot ahead of crutches.	_____	_____	_____
11. Repeats steps.	_____	_____	_____

Documentation

```



```

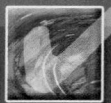

Competency Skill Checklist (Continued)

1st Observation

Date: _____ Evaluator Signature and Printed Name: _____

Comments:

2nd Observation

Date: _____ Evaluator Signature and Printed Name: _____

Comments:

Mastery

Date: _____ Evaluator Signature and Printed Name: _____

Comments:

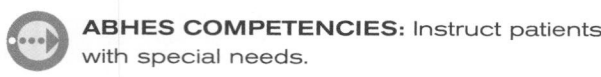 **ABHES COMPETENCIES:** Instruct patients with special needs.

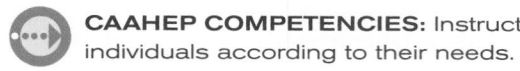 **CAAHEP COMPETENCIES:** Instruct individuals according to their needs.

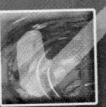

Competency Skill Checklist

Name _____   Course _____

PROCEDURE

33-6 Cast Application Assistance

	1st Observation	2nd Observation	Mastery
1. Washes hands.	____	____	____
2. Gathers equipment and supplies.	____	____	____
3. Introduces self to client.	____	____	____
4. Identifies client.	____	____	____
5. Tells client, in everyday language, what medical assistant is going to do.	____	____	____
6. Asks if client has any questions. If client does, gives short and simple answers.	____	____	____
7. Assists as doctor inspects area and places stockinette and padding on site.	____	____	____
8. Fills bucket with room-temperature water.	____	____	____
9. Waits for doctor's instructions; then puts on gloves and places casting material in water bucket.	____	____	____
10. Waits for bubbles to stop rising from water.	____	____	____
11. Takes roll out and gently squeezes it.	____	____	____
12. Hands roll to doctor to wrap limb.	____	____	____
13. Places knife in doctor's hand when wrapping is complete.	____	____	____
14. Wipes away any loose pieces of cast material from client's skin with warm, damp cloth.	____	____	____
15. Helps client to dress as necessary. Does not cover cast while it is still wet. Does not apply pressure or handle cast with fingertips.	____	____	____
16. Teaches cast care to client, making sure to include any special instructions from doctor.	____	____	____
17. Asks client if client has any questions.	____	____	____
18. Cleans, disinfects, or discards supplies and equipment according to regulations and office policy.	____	____	____
19. Washes hands.	____	____	____
20. Records procedure correctly in client's chart.	____	____	____

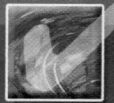

Documentation

```



```

1st Observation

Date: _____ Evaluator Signature and Printed Name: _____

Comments:

2nd Observation

Date: _____ Evaluator Signature and Printed Name: _____

Comments:

Mastery

Date: _____ Evaluator Signature and Printed Name: _____

Comments:

 ABHES COMPETENCIES: Instruct patients with special needs.

 CAAHEP COMPETENCIES: Instruct individuals according to their needs.

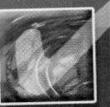

Name _____ Course _____

PROCEDURE

33-7

Arm Sling Application

	1st Observation	2nd Observation	Mastery
1. Washes hands.	⎯⎯	⎯⎯	⎯⎯
2. Gathers equipment and supplies.	⎯⎯	⎯⎯	⎯⎯
3. Introduces self to client.	⎯⎯	⎯⎯	⎯⎯
4. Identifies client.	⎯⎯	⎯⎯	⎯⎯
5. Tells client, in everyday language, what medical assistant is going to do.	⎯⎯	⎯⎯	⎯⎯
6. Asks if client has any questions. If client does, gives short and simple answers.	⎯⎯	⎯⎯	⎯⎯
7. Asks client to sit.	⎯⎯	⎯⎯	⎯⎯
8. Places affected arm across client's chest with thumb pointing up.	⎯⎯	⎯⎯	⎯⎯
9. Gently places arm in sling so that client's elbow fits snugly into corner of sling.	⎯⎯	⎯⎯	⎯⎯
10. Takes strap attached to sling, brings it around back of client's neck, and pulls it through metal hoops.	⎯⎯	⎯⎯	⎯⎯
11. Carefully pulls on strap until sling is at a right angle to body.	⎯⎯	⎯⎯	⎯⎯
12. Checks position of elbow and wrist.	⎯⎯	⎯⎯	⎯⎯
13. Asks client if client is comfortable. Checks neck area and applies padding if needed to ease pressure.	⎯⎯	⎯⎯	⎯⎯
14. Gives client information and written instructions as ordered by doctor.	⎯⎯	⎯⎯	⎯⎯
15. Asks client if client has any questions.	⎯⎯	⎯⎯	⎯⎯
16. Washes hands.	⎯⎯	⎯⎯	⎯⎯
17. Records procedure correctly in client's chart.	⎯⎯	⎯⎯	⎯⎯

Documentation

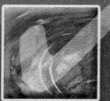

1st Observation

Date: _____ Evaluator Signature and Printed Name: _____

Comments:

2nd Observation

Date: _____ Evaluator Signature and Printed Name: _____

Comments:

Mastery

Date: _____ Evaluator Signature and Printed Name: _____

Comments:

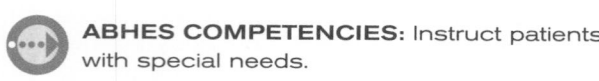 **ABHES COMPETENCIES:** Instruct patients with special needs.

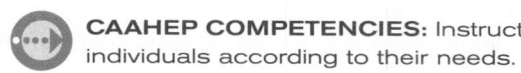 **CAAHEP COMPETENCIES:** Instruct individuals according to their needs.

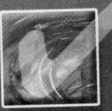

Name _____   Course _____

PROCEDURE

33-8   Triangular Sling Application

	1st Observation	2nd Observation	Mastery
1. Washes hands.	_____	_____	_____
2. Gathers equipment and supplies.	_____	_____	_____
3. Introduces self to client.	_____	_____	_____
4. Identifies client.	_____	_____	_____
5. Tells client, in everyday language, what medical assistant is going to do.	_____	_____	_____
6. Asks if client has any questions. If client does, gives short and simple answers.	_____	_____	_____
7. Asks client to sit.			
8. Bends client's elbow with hand at a little less than 90 degrees.	_____	_____	_____
9. Places one corner of triangular cloth over unaffected shoulder.	_____	_____	_____
10. Extends cloth down client's chest.	_____	_____	_____
11. Slides cloth under affected arm.	_____	_____	_____
12. Makes sure that middle point of cloth is at elbow.	_____	_____	_____
13. Takes lowest point of triangular cloth over affected arm, with point ending at side of neck.	_____	_____	_____
14. Ties or pins sling points at side of neck.	_____	_____	_____
15. Takes loose folds of material at elbow, folds neatly, and fastens with pin.	_____	_____	_____
16. Gives client information and written instructions as ordered by doctor.	_____	_____	_____
17. Asks client if client has any questions.	_____	_____	_____
18. Washes hands.	_____	_____	_____
19. Records procedure correctly in client's chart.	_____	_____	_____

Documentation

_____

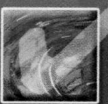

1st Observation

Date: _____ Evaluator Signature and Printed Name: _____

Comments:

2nd Observation

Date: _____ Evaluator Signature and Printed Name: _____

Comments:

Mastery

Date: _____ Evaluator Signature and Printed Name: _____

Comments:

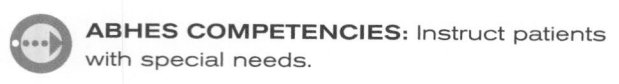 **ABHES COMPETENCIES:** Instruct patients with special needs.

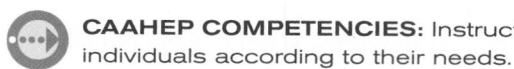 **CAAHEP COMPETENCIES:** Instruct individuals according to their needs.

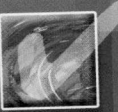

Name _____ Course _____

PROCEDURE

35-1

Measuring Infant Chest Circumference

	1st Observation	2nd Observation	Mastery
1. Washes hands.	___	___	___
2. Gathers equipment and supplies.	___	___	___
3. Introduces self to client's parent.	___	___	___
4. Identifies infant client.	___	___	___
5. Smiles at infant and talks in soothing, calm voice.	___	___	___
6. Lays infant on back on examination table.	___	___	___
7. Asks parent to help by talking to infant and gently holding head.	___	___	___
8. Tells parent what medical assistant is going to do.	___	___	___
9. Places end marking of tape measure at center of infant's chest, in line with infant's nipples. Holds it in place with finger. Slips tape measure under infant's body and brings it around to meet other end of tape at center of chest.	___	___	___
10. Reads number where tape measure ends meet (to nearest 0.01 cm or nearest half-inch).	___	___	___
11. Makes sure that parent is holding infant before turns to write number in infant's chart.	___	___	___
12. Records procedure correctly in client's chart.	___	___	___
13. Washes hands.	___	___	___

Documentation

```



```

813

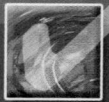
1st Observation

Date: _____ Evaluator Signature and Printed Name: _____

Comments:

2nd Observation

Date: _____ Evaluator Signature and Printed Name: _____

Comments:

Mastery

Date: _____ Evaluator Signature and Printed Name: _____

Comments:

 ABHES COMPETENCIES: Prepare patient for and assist physician with routine and specialty examinations and treatments and minor office surgeries.

 CAAHEP COMPETENCIES: Prepare patient for and assist with routine and specialty examinations.

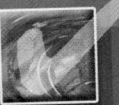
Name _____   Course _____

PROCEDURE

35-2   Infant Head Circumference

	1st Observation	2nd Observation	Mastery
1. Washes hands.	_____	_____	_____
2. Gathers equipment and supplies.	_____	_____	_____
3. Introduces self to client's parent.	_____	_____	_____
4. Identifies infant client.	_____	_____	_____
5. Smiles at infant and talks in soothing, calm voice.	_____	_____	_____
6. Lays infant on back on examination table.	_____		
7. Asks parent to help by talking to infant and gently holding head.	_____	_____	_____
8. Tells parent what medical assistant is going to do.	_____	_____	_____
9. Wraps tape measure around largest part of infant's head. Makes sure tape measure meets at middle of forehead. Does not pull too tightly or stretch tape measure.	_____	_____	_____
10. Reads number where tape measure ends meet (to nearest 0.01 cm or nearest half-inch).	_____		
11. Makes sure that parent is holding infant before turns to write number in infant's chart.	_____	_____	_____
12. Records procedure correctly in client's chart.	_____	_____	_____
13. Washes hands.	_____	_____	_____
14. If head and chest circumference are both being taken, continues without giving child to parent. Gives infant to parent and records both numbers when both measurements have been completed.	_____	_____	_____

Documentation

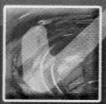
1st Observation

Date: _____ Evaluator Signature and Printed Name: _____

Comments:

2nd Observation

Date: _____ Evaluator Signature and Printed Name: _____

Comments:

Mastery

Date: _____ Evaluator Signature and Printed Name: _____

Comments:

 ABHES COMPETENCIES: Prepare patient for and assist physician with routine and specialty examinations and treatments and minor office surgeries.

 CAAHEP COMPETENCIES: Prepare patient for and assist with routine and specialty examinations.

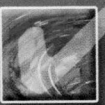

Name _____ Course _____

PROCEDURE

35-3 Infant Weight

	1st Observation	2nd Observation	Mastery
1. Washes hands.	_____	_____	_____
2. Gathers equipment and supplies.	_____	_____	_____
3. Introduces self to client's parent.	_____	_____	_____
4. Identifies infant client.	_____	_____	_____
5. Smiles at infant and talks in soothing, calm voice.	_____	_____	_____
6. Asks parent to help by talking to infant.	_____	_____	_____
7. Tells parent what medical assistant is going to do.	_____	_____	_____
8. Removes client's diaper (per office policy).	_____	_____	_____
9. Lays infant on back on infant scale.	_____	_____	_____
10. Places one hand very close to but not touching infant.	_____	_____	_____
11. With other hand, moves slide on scale bar marked pounds.	_____	_____	_____
12. Moves slide on scale bar marked ounces until beam balances or bounces in middle.	_____	_____	_____
13. Reads number marked on pound bar.	_____	_____	_____
14. Reads number marked on ounce bar.	_____	_____	_____
15. Takes infant out of scale and makes sure that parent is holding client before turning away to record weight in infant's chart.	_____	_____	_____
16. Asks parent if parent has any questions.	_____	_____	_____
17. Cleans scale.	_____	_____	_____
18. Washes hands.	_____	_____	_____

Documentation

_____

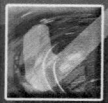

Competency Skill Checklist (Continued)

1st Observation

Date: _____ Evaluator Signature and Printed Name: _____

Comments:

2nd Observation

Date: _____ Evaluator Signature and Printed Name: _____

Comments:

Mastery

Date: _____ Evaluator Signature and Printed Name: _____

Comments:

 ABHES COMPETENCIES: Prepare patient for and assist physician with routine and specialty examinations and treatments and minor office surgeries.

 CAAHEP COMPETENCIES: Prepare patient for and assist with routine and specialty examinations.

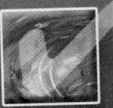

Name _____   Course _____

PROCEDURE

35-4

Infant Length

	1st Observation	2nd Observation	Mastery
1. Washes hands.	____	____	____
2. Gathers equipment and supplies.	____	____	____
3. Introduces self to client's parent.	____	____	____
4. Identifies infant client.	____	____	____
5. Smiles at infant and talks in soothing, calm voice.	____	____	____
6. Tells parent what medical assistant is going to do.	____	____	____
7. Lays infant on back on examination table. Places infant so that head lines up at beginning of markings on side of scale.	____	____	____
8. Asks parent to help by talking to infant and gently holding head.	____	____	____
9. Extends infant's leg until foot touches footboard. If scale does not have a footboard, uses hand as footboard.	____	____	____
10. Reads number on ruler to which infant's feet extend.	____	____	____
11. Makes sure that parent is holding infant before turns to record number in infant's chart.	____	____	____
12. Asks parent if parent has any questions.	____	____	____
13. Records procedure correctly in client's chart.	____	____	____
14. Washes hands.	____	____	____

Documentation

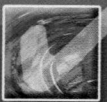

1st Observation

Date: _____ Evaluator Signature and Printed Name: _____

Comments:

2nd Observation

Date: _____ Evaluator Signature and Printed Name: _____

Comments:

Mastery

Date: _____ Evaluator Signature and Printed Name: _____

Comments:

 ABHES COMPETENCIES: Prepare patient for and assist physician with routine and specialty examinations and treatments and minor office surgeries.

 CAAHEP COMPETENCIES: Prepare patient for and assist with routine and specialty examinations.

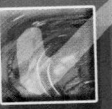

Name _____   Course _____

PROCEDURE

35-5

Pediatric Urine Specimen Collection

	1st Observation	2nd Observation	Mastery
1. Washes hands.	_____	_____	_____
2. Gathers equipment and supplies. Puts items needed within reach of examination table.	_____	_____	_____
3. Introduces self to client's parent.	_____	_____	_____
4. Identifies infant client.	_____	_____	_____
5. Smiles at infant and talks in soothing, calm voice.	_____	_____	_____
6. Asks parent to help by talking to infant and standing near infant.	_____	_____	_____
7. Puts on gloves.	_____	_____	_____
8. Removes infant's diaper.	_____	_____	_____
9. Washes infant's perineum with soap and water. Dries gently.	_____	_____	_____
10. Following directions on urine collection bag, places bag over infant's perineum. For male infants, center of bag is placed over penis and scrotum. For female infants, urine bag is centered over labia.	_____	_____	_____
11. Once bag is in place, gently presses adhesive on bag so that it adheres to skin.	_____	_____	_____
12. Carefully places diaper over bag.	_____	_____	_____
13. Hands infant to parent.	_____	_____	_____
14. Checks bag in 5 minutes and periodically thereafter until urine is present in bag.	_____	_____	_____
15. When enough urine is in bag, removes bag carefully.	_____	_____	_____
16. Makes sure that parent is holding infant securely before proceeds to next step.	_____	_____	_____
17. Places urine specimen in container, per office procedure.	_____	_____	_____
18. Labels specimen container.	_____	_____	_____
19. Discards collection bag in biohazardous waste container.	_____	_____	_____
20. Removes gloves.	_____	_____	_____
21. Asks parent if parent has any questions.	_____	_____	_____
22. Records amount of urine collected in client's chart.	_____	_____	_____
23. Washes hands.	_____	_____	_____
24. Records procedure correctly in client's chart.	_____	_____	_____

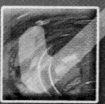

Documentation

1st Observation

Date: _____ Evaluator Signature and Printed Name: _____

Comments:

2nd Observation

Date: _____ Evaluator Signature and Printed Name: _____

Comments:

Mastery

Date: _____ Evaluator Signature and Printed Name: _____

Comments:

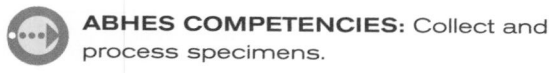 **ABHES COMPETENCIES:** Collect and process specimens.

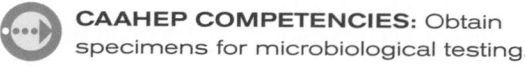 **CAAHEP COMPETENCIES:** Obtain specimens for microbiological testing.

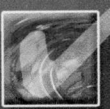

Name _____ Course _____

PROCEDURE

35-6

Body Mass Index for Children (BMI for Age)

	1st Observation	2nd Observation	Mastery
1. Washes hands.	_____	_____	_____
2. Gathers equipment and supplies.	_____	_____	_____
3. Introduces self to client's parent.	_____	_____	_____
4. Identifies child client.	_____	_____	_____
5. Obtains child's height and weight, if not known.	_____	_____	_____
6. If measurements are in pounds and inches, writes down child's weight in pounds (per office policy).	_____	_____	_____
7. Writes down child's height in inches.	_____	_____	_____
8. Inserts these numbers in correct places in BMI formula.	_____	_____	_____
9. Works through formula: Divides weight in pounds by height in inches and multiplies result by height in inches. Takes that number and multiplies it by 703.	_____	_____	_____
10. If measurements are in kilograms and meters, writes down child's weight in kilograms (per office policy).	_____	_____	_____
11. Writes down child's height in meters.	_____	_____	_____
12. Inserts these numbers in correct places in BMI formula,	_____	_____	_____
13. Works through formula: Divides weight in kilograms by height in meters and multiplies result by height in meters. Takes that number and multiplies it by 703.	_____	_____	_____
14. Records result as BMI in child's chart.	_____	_____	_____

Documentation

```



```

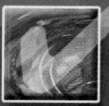

Competency Skill Checklist (Continued)

1st Observation

Date: _____ Evaluator Signature and Printed Name: _____

Comments:

2nd Observation

Date: _____ Evaluator Signature and Printed Name: _____

Comments:

Mastery

Date: _____ Evaluator Signature and Printed Name: _____

Comments:

 ABHES COMPETENCIES: Prepare patient for and assist physician with routine and specialty examinations and treatments and minor office surgeries.

 CAAHEP COMPETENCIES: Prepare patient for and assist with routine and specialty examinations.

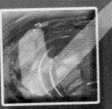

Name _____ Course _____

	1st Observation	2nd Observation	Mastery
1. Reads doctor's order for medication.	_____	_____	
2. Goes to cupboard in supply room where medication is kept.	_____	_____	_____
3. Washes hands.	_____	_____	_____
4. Places disposable medication cup on medicine tray.	_____	_____	_____
5. Finds ordered medication.	_____	_____	_____
6. Checks expiration date.			
7. Reads label on medication and compares it to doctor's orders.	_____	_____	
8. Opens lid of medicine container and puts lid upside down on clean surface. Does not let rim of lid touch any surface.	_____	_____	_____
9. Puts ordered number of tablets or capsules into lid.	_____	_____	
10. Puts contents of lid into medicine cup on medicine tray.	_____	_____	_____
11. Replaces lid on container and closes it tightly.	_____	_____	_____
12. Compares medicine container label with doctor's order as puts medicine container back on shelf.	_____	_____	_____
13. Goes to client's examination room.	_____	_____	_____
14. Introduces self to client.	_____	_____	
15. Identifies client.			
16. Tells client, in everyday language, what medical assistant is going to do.	_____	_____	_____
17. Asks if client has any questions. If client does, gives short and simple answers.	_____	_____	_____
18. Tells client that medical assistant is going to give client medicine doctor ordered.	_____	_____	_____
19. Hands disposable cup with tablet(s) or capsule(s) in it to client. Hands client glass of water.	_____	_____	_____
20. Makes sure that client is able to swallow tablet(s) or capsule(s). Offers more water as needed.	_____	_____	_____
21. Washes hands.	_____		_____
22. Charts medication given in client's medical record. Includes date, time medication was given, amount of medication, route, and any client reactions.	_____	_____	_____

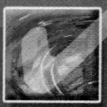

Documentation

1st Observation

Date: _____ Evaluator Signature and Printed Name: _____

Comments:

2nd Observation

Date: _____ Evaluator Signature and Printed Name: _____

Comments:

Mastery

Date: _____ Evaluator Signature and Printed Name: _____

Comments:

 ABHES COMPETENCIES: Prepare and administer oral and parenteral medications as ordered by physician.

Maintain medication and immunization records.

 CAAHEP COMPETENCIES: Apply pharmacology principles to prepare and administer oral and parenteral (excluding IV) medications.

Maintain medication and immunization records.

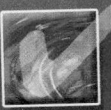

Name _____   Course _____

	1st Observation	2nd Observation	Mastery
1. Reads doctor's order for medication.	_____	_____	_____
2. Goes to cupboard in supply room where medication is kept.			
3. Washes hands.	_____	_____	_____
4. Finds ordered medicine.	_____	_____	_____
5. Checks expiration date.	_____	_____	_____
6. Reads label on medicine container and compares it to doctor's order.	_____		
7. Opens lid of medicine container and puts lid upside down on clean surface. Does not let rim of lid touch any surface.	_____	_____	_____
8. Pours ordered amount of liquid into measured plastic cup. Holds bottle and cup at eye level while pouring.	_____	_____	_____
9. Places lid back on container and closes it tightly.	_____	_____	_____
10. Compares medicine container label with doctor's order as puts medicine container back on shelf.	_____	_____	_____
11. Goes to client's examination room.	_____	_____	_____
12. Introduces self to client.	_____	_____	_____
13. Identifies client.	_____		
14. Tells client, in everyday language, what medical assistant is going to do.	_____	_____	_____
15. Asks if client has any questions. If client does, gives short and simple answers.	_____	_____	_____
16. Tells client that medical assistant is going to give client medication doctor ordered.	_____	_____	_____
17. Hands plastic measured medicine cup, with ordered amount of liquid medicine in it, to client.	_____	_____	_____
18. Makes sure that client is able to swallow medicine. Checks medication order to see if client can have water immediately.	_____	_____	_____
19. Washes hands.	_____	_____	_____
20. Charts medication given in client's medical record. Includes date, time medication was given, amount of medication, route, and any client reactions.	_____	_____	_____

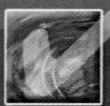

Documentation

1st Observation

Date: _____ Evaluator Signature and Printed Name: _____

Comments:

2nd Observation

Date: _____ Evaluator Signature and Printed Name: _____

Comments:

Mastery

Date: _____ Evaluator Signature and Printed Name: _____

Comments:

 ABHES COMPETENCIES: Prepare and administer oral and parenteral medications as ordered by physician.

Maintain medication and immunization records.

 CAAHEP COMPETENCIES: Apply pharmacology principles to prepare and administer oral and parenteral (excluding IV) medications.

Maintain medication and immunization records.

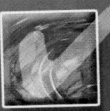
Name _____   Course _____

PROCEDURE

36-3

Draw Up Medication from an Ampule

	1st Observation	2nd Observation	Mastery
1. Reads doctor's order for medication.	_____	_____	_____
2. Goes to cupboard in supply room where medication is kept.	_____	_____	_____
3. Washes hands.	_____	_____	_____
4. Finds ordered medication.	_____	_____	_____
5. Reads label on ampule and compares it to doctor's order.	_____	_____	_____
6. Checks expiration date.	_____	_____	_____
7. Selects correct size needle and syringe, filter needle, and alcohol wipe.	_____	_____	_____
8. Puts on gloves.	_____	_____	_____
9. Picks up ampule and holds it upright. Flicks index finger against stem of ampule.	_____	_____	_____
10. Grabs stem of ampule with alcohol wipe.	_____	_____	_____
11. Pointing ampule away from face, snaps off neck of ampule.	_____	_____	_____
12. Picks up syringe and needle.	_____	_____	_____
13. Uncaps needle and puts needle into solution in ampule.	_____		
14. Pulls back on plunger and draws up ordered amount of solution.	_____	_____	_____
15. Takes syringe and needle out of solution.	_____	_____	_____
16. Points needle straight up into air.	_____	_____	_____
17. Allows air to float to top of barrel of syringe.	_____	_____	_____
18. Pushes plunger of syringe in to get rid of any remaining air.	_____	_____	_____
19. Checks amount of medication in syringe.	_____	_____	_____
20. Changes needle if needed, or puts safety sheath over it.	_____	_____	_____
21. Puts used ampule in sharps container.	_____	_____	_____
22. Washes hands.	_____	_____	_____

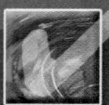

Documentation

1st Observation

Date: _____ Evaluator Signature and Printed Name: _____

Comments:

2nd Observation

Date: _____ Evaluator Signature and Printed Name: _____

Comments:

Mastery

Date: _____ Evaluator Signature and Printed Name: _____

Comments:

 ABHES COMPETENCIES: Prepare and administer oral and parenteral medications as ordered by physician.

Maintain medication and immunization records.

 CAAHEP COMPETENCIES: Apply pharmacology principles to prepare and administer oral and parenteral (excluding IV) medications.

Maintain medication and immunization records.

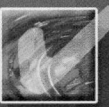

Name _____ Course _____

PROCEDURE 36-4   Draw Up Medication from a Vial

	1st Observation	2nd Observation	Mastery
1. Reads doctor's order for medication.	_____	_____	_____
2. Washes hands.	_____	_____	_____
3. Goes to cupboard in supply room where medication is kept.	_____	_____	_____
4. Finds ordered medication.	_____	_____	_____
5. Reads label on medication container and compares it to doctor's order.	_____	_____	_____
6. Checks expiration date.	_____	_____	_____
7. Puts on gloves.	_____	_____	_____
8. Places vial on flat surface.	_____	_____	_____
9. If vial is new, takes off plastic lid.	_____	_____	_____
10. Rubs alcohol wipe over rubber port.	_____	_____	_____
11. Picks up syringe and needle. Pulls back plunger and draws in air until plunger is at mark for amount of medication ordered. Uses filter needle if required.	_____	_____	_____
12. Inserts needle and injects air into vial through rubber covering.	_____	_____	_____
13. Keeps needle above solution level.	_____	_____	_____
14. With nondominant hand, holds vial and needle in vial and inverts them.	_____	_____	_____
15. Keeps vial at eye level.	_____	_____	_____
16. Pushes needle into solution.	_____	_____	_____
17. Pulls back on plunger with nondominant hand until solution reaches ordered line on syringe.	_____	_____	_____
18. Pulls needle and syringe out of vial.	_____	_____	_____
19. Holds syringe with needle pointing straight up.	_____	_____	_____
20. Flicks barrel of syringe with index finger. Pushes in plunger to expel any air.	_____	_____	_____
21. Checks amount of solution. If not enough medication is left in syringe, inserts needle into vial and repeat steps 13–19.	_____	_____	_____
22. Changes needle if needed, or puts safety sheath over it.	_____	_____	_____
23. Stores multiple-dose vial according to office policy. Discards single-dose vial according to office policy.	_____	_____	_____
24. Puts syringe and needle into sharps container.	_____	_____	_____
25. Washes hands.	_____	_____	_____

831

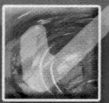

Documentation

```



```

1st Observation

Date: _____ Evaluator Signature and Printed Name: _____

Comments:

2nd Observation

Date: _____ Evaluator Signature and Printed Name: _____

Comments:

Mastery

Date: _____ Evaluator Signature and Printed Name: _____

Comments:

 ABHES COMPETENCIES: Prepare and administer oral and parenteral medications as ordered by physician.

Maintain medication and immunization records.

 CAAHEP COMPETENCIES: Apply pharmacology principles to prepare and administer oral and parenteral (excluding IV) medications.

Maintain medication and immunization records.

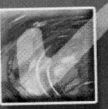

Competency Skill Checklist

Name _____ Course _____

PROCEDURE

36-5   Subcutaneous Injection

	1st Observation	2nd Observation	Mastery
1. Reads doctor's order for medication.	_____	_____	_____
2. Washes hands.	_____	_____	_____
3. Goes to cupboard in supply room where medication is kept.	_____	_____	_____
4. Finds ordered medication.	_____	_____	_____
5. Reads label on medication container and compares it to doctor's order.	_____	_____	_____
6. Checks expiration date.	_____	_____	_____
7. Draws up medication in syringe following Procedure 36-3 or Procedure 36-4.	_____	_____	_____
8. Checks medication label against doctor's order again and then puts medication back into cupboard, or discards single-dose container.	_____	_____	_____
9. Gathers equipment and supplies.	_____	_____	_____
10. Goes to client's examination room.	_____	_____	_____
11. Introduces self to client.	_____	_____	_____
12. Identifies client.	_____	_____	_____
13. Tells client, in everyday language, what medical assistant is going to do.	_____	_____	_____
14. Asks if client has any questions. If client does, gives short and simple answers.	_____	_____	_____
15. Puts on gloves.	_____	_____	_____
16. Helps client into comfortable position, depending on body site selected for injection. Uses anatomical landmarks.	_____	_____	_____
17. Starts at center of injection site and wipes with alcohol wipe in circular movement.	_____	_____	_____
18. Lets area dry. Does not blow on area.	_____	_____	_____
19. Takes cap off needle or pulls back safety sheath.	_____	_____	_____
20. With one hand, gently grabs up skin and tissue or spreads it flat for injection.	_____	_____	_____
21. With other hand, holds syringe by barrel. Does not put thumb on plunger yet.	_____	_____	_____
22. Inserts needle at 45-degree angle (according to office policy).	_____	_____	_____
23. Lets go of skin.	_____	_____	_____

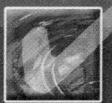
24. Pulls back plunger to see if any blood comes into needle. If it does, takes out needle and syringe and starts over after drawing up new medication in new needle and syringe. _____ _____ _____

25. If no blood enters syringe, pushes plunger in steadily. Does not push fast. _____ _____ _____

26. Takes out needle at same angle as inserted. _____ _____ _____

27. Wipes area gently with alcohol wipe. _____ _____ _____

28. Pulls safety sheath over needle. Does not recap needle. Disposes of needle and syringe in sharps container. _____ _____ _____

29. Talks with client while observing client's response to injection. _____ _____ _____

30. Takes off gloves. _____ _____ _____

31. Washes hands. _____ _____ _____

32. Records procedure correctly in client's chart. _____ _____ _____

Documentation

```


```

1st Observation

Date: _____ Evaluator Signature and Printed Name: _____

Comments:

2nd Observation

Date: _____ Evaluator Signature and Printed Name: _____

Comments:

Mastery

Date: _____ Evaluator Signature and Printed Name: _____

Comments:

 ABHES COMPETENCIES: Prepare and administer oral and parenteral medications as ordered by physician.

Maintain medication and immunization records.

 CAAHEP COMPETENCIES: Apply pharmacology principles to prepare and administer oral and parenteral (excluding IV) medications.

Maintain medication and immunization records.

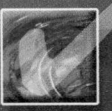

Competency Skill Checklist

Name _____ Course _____

PROCEDURE

36-6 Intramuscular Injection

	1st Observation	2nd Observation	Mastery
1. Reads doctor's order for medication.	_____	_____	_____
2. Washes hands.	_____	_____	_____
3. Goes to cupboard in supply room where medication is kept.	_____	_____	_____
4. Finds ordered medication.	_____	_____	_____
5. Reads label on medication container and compares it to doctor's order.	_____	_____	_____
6. Checks expiration date.	_____	_____	_____
7. Draws up medication in syringe following Procedure 36-3 or Procedure 36-4.	_____	_____	_____
8. Checks medication label against doctor's order again and puts medication container back into cupboard, or discards single-dose package.	_____	_____	_____
9. Gathers equipment and supplies.	_____	_____	_____
10. Goes to client's examination room.	_____	_____	_____
11. Introduces self to client.	_____	_____	_____
12. Identifies client.	_____	_____	_____
13. Tells client, in everyday language, what medical assistant is going to do.	_____	_____	_____
14. Asks if client has any questions. If client does, gives short and simple answers.	_____	_____	_____
15. Puts on gloves.	_____	_____	_____
16. Helps client into comfortable position, depending on body site selected for injection. Uses anatomical landmarks.	_____	_____	_____
17. Starts at center of injection site and wipes in circular movement with alcohol wipe.	_____	_____	_____
18. Lets area dry. Does not blow on area.	_____	_____	_____
19. Takes cap off needle or pulls back safety sheath.	_____	_____	_____
20. Spreads skin at injection site.	_____	_____	_____
21. With other hand, holds syringe by barrel. Does not put thumb on plunger yet.	_____	_____	_____
22. Inserts needle at 90-degree angle.	_____	_____	_____
23. Lets go of skin.	_____	_____	_____

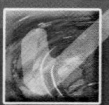
24. Pulls back plunger to see if any blood comes into syringe. If it does, takes out needle and starts over, drawing up new medication into new needle and syringe.   _____   _____   _____

25. If no blood enters syringe, pushes plunger in steadily. Does not push fast.   _____   _____   _____

26. Takes out needle and syringe at same angle as inserted.   _____   _____   _____

27. Wipes area gently with alcohol wipe.   _____   _____   _____

28. Pulls safety sheath over needle; does not recap needle. Disposes of needle and syringe in sharps container.   _____   _____   _____

29. Talks with client while observing client's response to injection.   _____   _____   _____

30. Takes off gloves.   _____   _____   _____

31. Washes hands.   _____   _____   _____

32. Records procedure correctly in client's chart.   _____   _____   _____

Documentation

1st Observation

Date: _____ Evaluator Signature and Printed Name: _____

Comments:

2nd Observation

Date: _____ Evaluator Signature and Printed Name: _____

Comments:

Mastery

Date: _____ Evaluator Signature and Printed Name: _____

Comments:

 ABHES COMPETENCIES: Prepare and administer oral and parenteral medications as ordered by physician.

Maintain medication and immunization records.

 CAAHEP COMPETENCIES: Apply pharmacology principles to prepare and administer oral and parenteral (excluding IV) medications.

Maintain medication and immunization records.

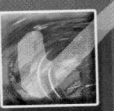

Competency Skill Checklist

Name _____ Course _____

PROCEDURE

36-7

Intramuscular Injection— Z-Track Method

	1st Observation	2nd Observation	Mastery
1. Reads doctor's order for medication.	_____	_____	_____
2. Goes to cupboard in supply room where medication is kept.	_____	_____	_____
3. Washes hands.	_____	_____	_____
4. Finds ordered medication.	_____	_____	_____
5. Reads label on medication container and compares it to doctor's order.	_____	_____	_____
6. Checks expiration date.	_____	_____	_____
7. Draws up medication in syringe following Procedure 36-3 or Procedure 36-4.	_____	_____	_____
8. Checks medication label against doctor's order again and puts medication back into cupboard, or discards single-dose container.	_____	_____	_____
9. Gathers equipment and supplies.	_____	_____	_____
10. Goes to client's examination room.	_____	_____	_____
11. Introduces self to client.	_____	_____	_____
12. Identifies client.	_____	_____	_____
13. Tells client, in everyday language, what medical assistant is going to do.	_____	_____	_____
14. Asks if client has any questions. If client does, gives short and simple answers.	_____	_____	_____
15. Puts on gloves.	_____	_____	_____
16. Helps client into comfortable position, depending on body site selected for injection. Uses anatomical landmarks.	_____	_____	_____
17. Starts at center of injection site and wipes site in circular movement with alcohol wipe.	_____	_____	_____
18. Lets area dry. Does not blow on area.	_____	_____	_____
19. Takes cap off needle or pulls back safety sheath.	_____	_____	_____
20. Pulls skin to side of injection site.	_____	_____	_____
21. Pulls skin, subcutaneous layer, and fat into a Z form.	_____	_____	_____
22. Holds syringe by barrel. Does not put thumb on plunger yet.	_____	_____	_____
23. Spreads skin taut at injection site.	_____	_____	_____
24. Inserts needle at 90-degree angle.	_____	_____	_____

837

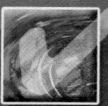

25. Pulls back plunger to see if any blood comes into syringe. If it does, takes out needle and syringe and starts over, drawing up new medication using new needle and syringe.

26. If no blood enters syringe, pushes plunger in steadily. Does not push fast.

27. Waits a few seconds before taking out needle and syringe, while still holding skin taut to side.

28. Takes out needle and syringe and lets skin return to its normal position.

29. Does not rub injection site.

30. Pulls safety sheath over needle; does not recap needle. Disposes of needle and syringe in sharps container.

31. Talks with client while observing client's response to injection.

32. Takes off gloves.

33. Washes hands.

34. Records procedure correctly in client's chart.

Documentation

1st Observation

Date: _____ Evaluator Signature and Printed Name: _____

Comments:

2nd Observation

Date: _____ Evaluator Signature and Printed Name: _____

Comments:

Mastery

Date: _____ Evaluator Signature and Printed Name: _____

Comments:

 ABHES COMPETENCIES: Prepare and administer oral and parenteral medications as ordered by physician.

Maintain medication and immunization records.

 CAAHEP COMPETENCIES: Apply pharmacology principles to prepare and administer oral and parenteral (excluding IV) medications.

Maintain medication and immunization records.

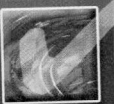
Name _____   Course _____

PROCEDURE

36-8   Intradermal Injection

	1st Observation	2nd Observation	Mastery
1. Reads doctor's order for medication.	_____	_____	_____
2. Washes hands.	_____		
3. Goes to cupboard in supply room where medication is kept.	_____	_____	_____
4. Finds ordered medication.	_____	_____	_____
5. Reads label on medication container and compares it to doctor's order.	_____	_____	_____
6. Checks expiration date.	_____	_____	_____
7. Draws up medication in syringe following Procedure 36-3 or Procedure 36-4.	_____		
8. Checks medication label against doctor's order again and puts medication back into cupboard, or discards single-dose container.	_____	_____	_____
9. Gathers equipment and supplies.	_____		
10. Goes to client's examination room.	_____		
11. Introduces self to client.	_____		
12. Identifies client.	_____		
13. Tells client, in everyday language, what medical assistant is going to do.	_____	_____	_____
14. Asks if client has any questions. If client does, gives short and simple answers.	_____	_____	_____
15. Puts on gloves.	_____	_____	_____
16. Helps client into comfortable position, depending on body site selected for injection. Uses anatomical landmarks.	_____	_____	_____
17. Picks area on inner side of either forearm.	_____	_____	_____
18. Starts at center of injection site and wipes site in circular motion with alcohol wipe.	_____	_____	_____
19. Lets area dry. Does not blow on area.	_____	_____	_____
20. Takes cap off needle or pulls back safety sheath.	_____	_____	_____
21. Holds skin tight and smooth.	_____	_____	_____
22. Holds needle and syringe at right angles to skin site.	_____	_____	_____
23. Moves tip of needle to 15-degree angle with bevel pointing up.	_____	_____	_____
24. Inserts needle just under top layer of skin.	_____	_____	_____
25. Pushes plunger and injects medication slowly.	_____	_____	_____
26. Takes out needle at same angle.	_____	_____	_____

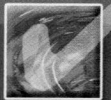

27. Does not rub area.
28. Tells client not to rub or scratch area.
29. Pulls safety sheath over needle; does not recap needle.
30. Disposes of needle and syringe in sharps container.
31. Talks with client while observing client's response to injection.
32. Reminds client not to rub or scratch area.
33. Takes off gloves.
34. Washes hands.
35. Records procedure correctly in client's chart.

Documentation

1st Observation

Date: _____ Evaluator Signature and Printed Name: _____

Comments:

2nd Observation

Date: _____ Evaluator Signature and Printed Name: _____

Comments:

Mastery

Date: _____ Evaluator Signature and Printed Name: _____

Comments:

 ABHES COMPETENCIES: Prepare and administer oral and parenteral medications as ordered by physician.

Maintain medication and immunization records.

 CAAHEP COMPETENCIES: Apply pharmacology principles to prepare and administer oral and parenteral (excluding IV) medications.

Maintain medication and immunization records.

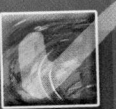

Competency Skill Checklist

Name _____ Course _____

PROCEDURE

36-9   Nasal Medication

	1st Observation	2nd Observation	Mastery
1. Washes hands.	___	___	___
2. Gathers equipment and supplies.	___	___	___
3. Checks medication three times, comparing it to doctor's order.	___	___	___
4. Introduces self to client.	___	___	___
5. Identifies client.	___	___	___
6. Tells client, in everyday language, what medical assistant is going to do.	___	___	___
7. Asks if client has any questions. If client does, gives short and simple answers.	___	___	___
8. Asks client to lie back on examination table.	___	___	___
9. Places pillow under client's shoulder.	___	___	___
10. Supports client's neck.	___	___	___
11. Puts on gloves.	___	___	___
12. Holds medication straight up above nostril (does not touch nostril with dropper tip). Administers one drop at a time, up to ordered numbered of drops.	___	___	___
13. Repeats step 12 with other nostril.	___	___	___
14. Instructs client to remain lying down for a few minutes.	___	___	___
15. Wipes any excess moisture away from skin or around nose.	___	___	___
16. Assists client to sitting position.	___	___	___
17. Asks if client has any questions.	___	___	___
18. Helps client get off exam table.	___	___	___
19. Takes off gloves.	___	___	___
20. Washes hands.	___	___	___
21. Records procedure correctly in client's chart.	___	___	___

Documentation

841

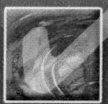

1st Observation

1st Observation

Date: _____ Evaluator Signature and Printed Name: _____

Comments:

2nd Observation

Date: _____ Evaluator Signature and Printed Name: _____

Comments:

Mastery

Date: _____ Evaluator Signature and Printed Name: _____

Comments:

 ABHES COMPETENCIES: Prepare patient for and assist physician with routine and specialty examinations and treatments and minor office surgeries.

 CAAHEP COMPETENCIES: Prepare patient for and assist with routine and specialty examinations.

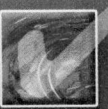

Competency Skill Checklist

Name _____ Course _____

PROCEDURE

36-10   Instillation of Eye Medication

	1st Observation	2nd Observation	Mastery
1. Reads doctor's order.	_____	_____	_____
2. Goes to medication cupboard.	_____	_____	_____
3. Washes hands.	_____	_____	_____
4. Finds correct medication.	_____	_____	_____
5. Checks expiration date.	_____	_____	_____
6. Compares label on medication container with doctor's order.	_____	_____	_____
7. Gathers equipment and supplies.	_____	_____	_____
8. Introduces self to client.	_____	_____	_____
9. Identifies client.	_____	_____	_____
10. Tells client, in everyday language, what medical assistant is going to do.	_____	_____	_____
11. Asks if client has any questions. If client does, gives short and simple answers.	_____	_____	_____
12. Opens eye medication container.	_____	_____	_____
13. Holds medication in hand to avoid contamination.	_____	_____	_____
14. Has client sit or lie down.	_____	_____	_____
15. Asks client to look up.	_____	_____	_____
16. Gently pulls down on lower lid of eye into which drops are to be instilled.	_____	_____	_____
17. Lines up eyedrop container at middle of lower lid.	_____	_____	_____
18. Gently squeezes container and directs liquid drops into lower-lid conjunctival area.	_____	_____	_____
19. Instructs client to close eye gently to allow medication to be absorbed. Makes sure client does not squeeze eyelids together tightly.	_____	_____	_____
20. Replaces lid on medication container.	_____	_____	_____
21. Hands client a dry cotton ball to remove extra moisture.	_____	_____	_____
22. Washes hands.	_____	_____	_____
23. Records procedure correctly in client's chart.	_____	_____	_____

Documentation

_____

843

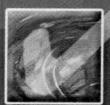

Competency Skill Checklist (Continued)

1st Observation

Date: _____ Evaluator Signature and Printed Name: _____

Comments:

2nd Observation

Date: _____ Evaluator Signature and Printed Name: _____

Comments:

Mastery

Date: _____ Evaluator Signature and Printed Name: _____

Comments:

 ABHES COMPETENCIES: Prepare patient for and assist physician with routine and specialty examinations and treatments and minor office surgeries.

 CAAHEP COMPETENCIES: Prepare patient for and assist with routine and specialty examinations.

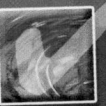

Name _____   Course _____

	1st Observation	2nd Observation	Mastery
1. Reads doctor's order.	_____	_____	_____
2. Goes to medication cupboard.	_____	_____	_____
3. Washes hands.	_____	_____	_____
4. Finds correct medication.	_____	_____	_____
5. Compares label on medication container with doctor's order.	_____	_____	_____
6. Checks expiration date.	_____	_____	_____
7. Gathers equipment and supplies.	_____	_____	_____
8. Introduces self to client.	_____	_____	_____
9. Identifies client.	_____	_____	_____
10. Tells client, in everyday language, what medical assistant is going to do.	_____	_____	_____
11. Asks if client has any questions. If client does, gives short and simple answers.	_____	_____	_____
12. Asks client to sit with head tilted toward unaffected ear.	_____	_____	_____
13. Straightens ear canal of affected ear.	_____	_____	_____
14. Places tip of otic medication container in ear canal without touching ear canal.	_____	_____	_____
15. Gently squeezes correct number of drops along side of ear canal without touching ear canal.	_____	_____	_____
16. Tells client to remain in this position for 2 to 3 minutes.	_____	_____	_____
17. Loosely places cotton ball into external ear of affected ear.	_____	_____	_____
18. Washes hands.	_____	_____	_____
19. Records procedure correctly in client's chart.	_____	_____	_____

Documentation

_____

845

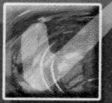

1st Observation

Date: _____ Evaluator Signature and Printed Name: _____

Comments:

2nd Observation

Date: _____ Evaluator Signature and Printed Name: _____

Comments:

Mastery

Date: _____ Evaluator Signature and Printed Name: _____

Comments:

 ABHES COMPETENCIES: Prepare patient for and assist physician with routine and specialty examinations and treatments and minor office surgeries.

 CAAHEP COMPETENCIES: Prepare patient for and assist with routine and specialty examinations.

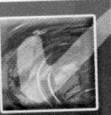

Name _____   Course _____

PROCEDURE

36-12

Preparing and Administering a Sublingual Medication

	1st Observation	2nd Observation	Mastery
1. Reads doctor's order.	_____	_____	_____
2. Goes to medication cupboard.	_____	_____	_____
3. Washes hands.	_____	_____	_____
4. Finds correct medication.	_____	_____	_____
5. Compares label on medication container with doctor's order.	_____	_____	_____
6. Checks expiration date.	_____	_____	_____
7. Gathers equipment and supplies.	_____	_____	_____
8. Introduces self to client.	_____	_____	_____
9. Identifies client.	_____	_____	_____
10. Tells client, in everyday language, what medical assistant is going to do.	_____	_____	_____
11. Asks if client has any questions. If client does, gives short and simple answers.	_____	_____	_____
12. Instructs client not to swallow medication, but allow it to dissolve under tongue.	_____	_____	_____
13. Hands client sublingual medication in disposable cup.	_____	_____	_____
14. Tells client to place medication under tongue.	_____	_____	_____
15. Stays with client until medication has dissolved completely.	_____	_____	_____
16. Washes hands.	_____	_____	_____
17. Records procedure correctly in client's chart.	_____	_____	_____

Documentation

```
[blank box]
```

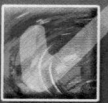
1st Observation

Date: _____ Evaluator Signature and Printed Name: _____

Comments:

2nd Observation

Date: _____ Evaluator Signature and Printed Name: _____

Comments:

Mastery

Date: _____ Evaluator Signature and Printed Name: _____

Comments:

 ABHES COMPETENCIES: Prepare patient for and assist physician with routine and specialty examinations and treatments and minor office surgeries.

 CAAHEP COMPETENCIES: Prepare patient for and assist with routine and specialty examinations.

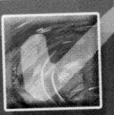
Name _____ Course _____

Preparing and Administering Topical Medication

	1st Observation	2nd Observation	Mastery
1. Reads doctor's order.	_____	_____	_____
2. Goes to medication cupboard.	_____	_____	_____
3. Washes hands.	_____	_____	_____
4. Finds correct medication.	_____	_____	_____
5. Compares label on medication container with doctor's order.	_____	_____	_____
6. Checks expiration date.	_____	_____	_____
7. Gathers equipment and supplies.	_____	_____	_____
8. Introduces self to client.	_____	_____	_____
9. Identifies client.	_____	_____	_____
10. Tells client, in everyday language, what medical assistant is going to do.	_____	_____	_____
11. Asks if client has any questions. If client does, gives short and simple answers.	_____	_____	_____
12. Puts on gloves.	_____	_____	_____
13. Checks skin area where medication will be applied.	_____	_____	_____
14. Squeezes medication onto large cotton swab or tongue blade.	_____	_____	_____
15. Starts applying topical medication from center of selected area and works outward in a circle.	_____	_____	_____
16. Leaves application area open to air unless doctor orders differently.	_____	_____	_____
17. Removes gloves.	_____	_____	_____
18. Washes hands.	_____	_____	_____
19. Records procedure correctly in client's chart.	_____	_____	_____

Documentation

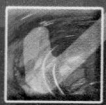

1st Observation

Date: _____ Evaluator Signature and Printed Name: _____

Comments:

2nd Observation

Date: _____ Evaluator Signature and Printed Name: _____

Comments:

Mastery

Date: _____ Evaluator Signature and Printed Name: _____

Comments:

 ABHES COMPETENCIES: Prepare patient for and assist physician with routine and specialty examinations and treatments and minor office surgeries.

 CAAHEP COMPETENCIES: Prepare patient for and assist with routine and specialty examinations.

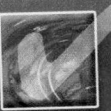

Competency Skill Checklist

Name _____   Course _____

PROCEDURE

36-14

Preparing and Administering Transdermal Medication

	1st Observation	2nd Observation	Mastery
1. Reads doctor's order.	_____	_____	_____
2. Goes to medication cupboard.	_____	_____	_____
3. Washes hands.	_____	_____	_____
4. Finds correct medication.	_____	_____	_____
5. Compares label on medication container with doctor's order.	_____	_____	_____
6. Checks expiration date.	_____	_____	_____
7. Gathers equipment and supplies.	_____	_____	_____
8. Introduces self to client.	_____	_____	_____
9. Identifies client.	_____	_____	_____
10. Tells client, in everyday language, what medical assistant is going to do.	_____	_____	_____
11. Asks if client has any questions. If client does, gives short and simple answers.	_____	_____	_____
12. Chooses area to place medicated patch.	_____	_____	_____
13. Puts on gloves.	_____	_____	_____
14. If old patch is still on client, removes it. Does not place new patch at same spot.	_____	_____	_____
15. Opens package by peeling it apart according to manufacturer's instructions.	_____	_____	_____
16. Does not touch medicated part of patch.	_____	_____	_____
17. Places transdermal patch at selected site. Gently but firmly presses edges down, starting at center.	_____	_____	_____
18. Removes gloves.	_____	_____	_____
19. Washes hands.	_____	_____	_____
20. Records procedure correctly in client's chart.	_____	_____	_____

Documentation

```
+--------------------------------------------------------------+
|                                                              |
|                                                              |
|                                                              |
|                                                              |
|                                                              |
+--------------------------------------------------------------+
```

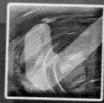

1st Observation

Date: _____ Evaluator Signature and Printed Name: _____

Comments:

2nd Observation

Date: _____ Evaluator Signature and Printed Name: _____

Comments:

Mastery

Date: _____ Evaluator Signature and Printed Name: _____

Comments:

 ABHES COMPETENCIES: Prepare patient for and assist physician with routine and specialty examinations and treatments and minor office surgeries.

 CAAHEP COMPETENCIES: Prepare patient for and assist with routine and specialty examinations.

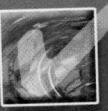

Name _____   Course _____

	1st Observation	2nd Observation	Mastery
1. Washes hands.	_____	_____	_____
2. Gathers equipment and supplies.	_____	_____	_____
3. Introduces self to client.	_____	_____	_____
4. Identifies client.	_____	_____	_____
5. Tells client, in everyday language, what medical assistant is going to do.	_____	_____	_____
6. Asks if client has any questions. If client does, gives short and simple answers.	_____		
7. Asks client to remove clothing as necessary to expose area to be prepped. Helps as needed and maintains privacy.	_____	_____	_____
8. Helps client into correct position on examination table.	_____	_____	_____
9. Places drapes around area.	_____	_____	_____
10. Puts on gloves.	_____	_____	_____
11. Dips gauze pad into soapy solution.	_____		
12. Wipes client's skin only once with each gauze pad and then disposes of pad into basin.	_____	_____	_____
13. Looks at area to be shaved. If needed, cuts it before shaving area.	_____	_____	_____
14. Cuts hair carefully so as not to cut or nick skin.	_____	_____	_____
15. Shaves area with safety razor. Shaves in direction in which hair grows. Pulls on skin below area being shaved.	_____		
16. Rinses soap and any remaining hair off with sterile gauze pad and sterile water.	_____	_____	_____
17. Dries area with sterile gauze.	_____	_____	_____
18. Using sterile forceps, dips gauze into antiseptic solution.	_____	_____	_____
19. Begins at center of area being prepped.	_____	_____	_____
20. Moves antiseptic-soaked gauze in circle, working from center of area into bigger circles. Does not go back and forth or change direction.	_____	_____	_____
21. Places a sterile drape over prepped area.	_____	_____	_____
22. Tells client not to touch area.	_____	_____	_____
23. Discards disposable items in biohazardous waste container.	_____	_____	_____

853

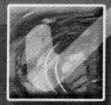

24. Places other items and instruments in appropriate place to be sanitized and sterilized.   _____   _____   _____

25. Remains in room with client. Talks with client to reassure, comfort, and distract as appropriate.   _____   _____   _____

26. Assists doctor as needed.   _____   _____   _____

Documentation

```
┌──────────────────────────────────────────────────────────┐
│                                                          │
│                                                          │
│                                                          │
│                                                          │
│                                                          │
└──────────────────────────────────────────────────────────┘
```

1st Observation

Date: _____ Evaluator Signature and Printed Name: _____

Comments:

2nd Observation

Date: _____ Evaluator Signature and Printed Name: _____

Comments:

Mastery

Date: _____ Evaluator Signature and Printed Name: _____

Comments:

 ABHES COMPETENCIES: Prepare patient for and assist physician with routine and specialty examinations and treatments and minor office surgeries.

 CAAHEP COMPETENCIES: Prepare patient for and assist with routine and specialty examinations.

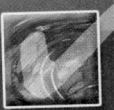

Name _____   Course _____

PROCEDURE

38-2   Pouring a Sterile Solution

	1st Observation	2nd Observation	Mastery
1. Washes hands.	_____	_____	_____
2. Gathers equipment and supplies.	_____	_____	_____
3. Reads label on bottle.	_____	_____	_____
4. Checks expiration date on bottle.	_____	_____	_____
5. Picks up solution and palms label.	_____	_____	_____
6. Takes cap off solution bottle with other hand; does not touch inside of cap.	_____	_____	_____
7. Places cap on flat surface with open side up, or holds cap right side up in hand. Does not touch inside of cap.	_____	_____	_____
8. Pours small amount of solution into separate container.	_____	_____	_____
9. Approaches sterile field.	_____	_____	_____
10. Pours correct amount of solution into sterile container; does not let rim of solution bottle touch sterile container.	_____	_____	_____
11. Does not reach over or touch any part of sterile field.	_____	_____	_____
12. Puts cap back on sterile solution bottle, using sterile technique.	_____	_____	_____

Documentation

_____

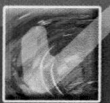

1st Observation

Date: _____ Evaluator Signature and Printed Name: _____

Comments:

2nd Observation

Date: _____ Evaluator Signature and Printed Name: _____

Comments:

Mastery

Date: _____ Evaluator Signature and Printed Name: _____

Comments:

 ABHES COMPETENCIES: Prepare patient for and assist physician with routine and specialty examinations and treatments and minor office surgeries.

 CAAHEP COMPETENCIES: Prepare patient for and assist with routine and specialty examinations.

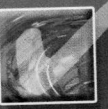
Name _____ Course _____

PROCEDURE

38-3   Sterile Dressing Application

	1st Observation	2nd Observation	Mastery
1. Washes hands.	_____	_____	_____
2. Gathers equipment and supplies.	_____	_____	_____
3. Introduces self to client.	_____	_____	_____
4. Identifies client.	_____	_____	_____
5. Tells client, in everyday language, what medical assistant is going to do.	_____	_____	_____
6. Asks if client has any questions. If client does, gives short and simple answers.	_____	_____	_____
7. Asks client about any allergies to tapes or adhesives.	_____	_____	_____
8. Reassures client and instructs client not to move during procedure.	_____		
9. Sets up sterile field.	_____		
10. Places waterproof bag away from sterile field, but within easy reach.	_____	_____	_____
11. Puts on sterile gloves.	_____	_____	_____
12. Looks at client's wound.	_____	_____	_____
13. Looks for any signs of infection. Notes type and amount of any drainage observed.	_____	_____	_____
14. Using forceps, picks up sterile dressing.	_____	_____	_____
15. Puts sterile dressing over area, using forceps or other sterile-gloved hand.	_____	_____	_____
16. Takes off sterile gloves.	_____	_____	_____
17. Using tape or elastic bandage, secures gauze to client's skin. Makes sure tape strips are even and smooth. If using elastic bandage, makes sure it is smooth and does not twist or bind.	_____	_____	_____
18. Teaches client proper care of gauze dressing. Includes other instructions from doctor. Tells client to call doctor if there is any swelling, pain, or discharge through gauze dressing.	_____	_____	_____
19. Asks client if client has any questions.	_____	_____	_____
20. Helps client to get off examination table.	_____	_____	_____
21. Cleans area according to regulations and office policy.	_____	_____	_____
22. Washes hands.	_____	_____	_____
23. Records procedure correctly in client's chart.	_____	_____	_____

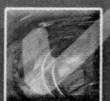

Documentation

1st Observation

Date: _____ Evaluator Signature and Printed Name: _____

Comments:

2nd Observation

Date: _____ Evaluator Signature and Printed Name: _____

Comments:

Mastery

Date: _____ Evaluator Signature and Printed Name: _____

Comments:

 ABHES COMPETENCIES: Prepare patient for and assist physician with routine and specialty examinations and treatments and minor office surgeries.

 CAAHEP COMPETENCIES: Prepare patient for and assist with routine and specialty examinations..

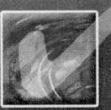
Name _____ Course _____

	1st Observation	2nd Observation	Mastery
1. Washes hands.	_____	_____	_____
2. Gathers equipment and supplies.	_____	_____	_____
3. Introduces self to client.	_____	_____	_____
4. Identifies client.	_____	_____	_____
5. Tells client, in everyday language, what medical assistant is going to do.	_____	_____	_____
6. Asks if client has any questions. If client does, gives short and simple answers.	_____	_____	_____
7. Sets up sterile field.	_____	_____	_____
8. Pours sterile solution.	_____	_____	_____
9. Places waterproof bag away from sterile field, but within easy reach.	_____	_____	_____
10. Reassures client and instructs client not to move during procedure.	_____	_____	_____
11. Puts on disposable examination gloves.	_____	_____	_____
12. Removes old dressing gently.	_____	_____	_____
13. Places soiled dressing in biohazardous waste container without touching sides of container.	_____	_____	_____
14. Does not pass old dressing over sterile field.	_____	_____	_____
15. Looks at wound.	_____	_____	_____
16. Looks for any signs of infection. Notes type and amount of any drainage observed.	_____	_____	_____
17. Takes off contaminated gloves.	_____	_____	_____
18. Washes hands.	_____	_____	_____
19. Puts on sterile gloves.	_____	_____	_____
20. Using forceps, picks up gauze or cotton balls moistened with sterile antiseptic solution.	_____	_____	_____
21. Cleans wound area, starting at center and working outward.	_____	_____	_____
22. Puts used gauze into waste bag.	_____	_____	_____
23. Puts sterile gauze over area, using forceps or sterile-gloved hand.	_____	_____	_____
24. Takes off sterile gloves.	_____	_____	_____
25. Using tape or elastic bandage, secures gauze to skin. Makes sure tape strips are even and smooth. If using elastic bandage, makes sure that it is smooth and does not twist or bind.	_____	_____	_____

859

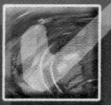

26. Teaches client proper care of gauze dressing.
    Includes other instructions from doctor. Tells client
    to call doctor if there is any swelling, pain, or
    discharge through gauze dressing.   _____   _____   _____
27. Asks client if client has any questions.   _____   _____   _____
28. Helps client to get off examination table.   _____   _____   _____
29. Disposes of contaminated items in biohazardous
    waste bag.   _____   _____   _____
30. Cleans room according to regulations and office policy. _____ _____ _____
31. Washes hands.   _____   _____   _____
32. Records procedure correctly in client's chart.   _____   _____   _____

Documentation

_____

1st Observation

Date: _____ Evaluator Signature and Printed Name: _____

Comments:

2nd Observation

Date: _____ Evaluator Signature and Printed Name: _____

Comments:

Mastery

Date: _____ Evaluator Signature and Printed Name: _____

Comments:

 ABHES COMPETENCIES: Prepare patient for and assist physician with routine and specialty examinations and treatments and minor office surgeries.

 CAAHEP COMPETENCIES: Prepare patient for and assist with routine and specialty examinations.

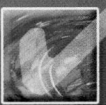

Competency Skill Checklist

Name _____ Course _____

PROCEDURE

38-5 Sanitizing Instruments

	1st Observation	2nd Observation	Mastery
1. Washes hands.	_____	_____	_____
2. Gathers equipment and supplies.	_____	_____	_____
3. Puts on gloves.	_____	_____	_____
4. Rinses instruments, then uses cleaning solution.	_____	_____	_____
5. Looks closely at instruments for any defect.	_____	_____	_____
6. Opens hinged instruments.	_____	_____	_____
7. Uses soft brush or gauze to clean grooves, joints, hinges, ratchets, and any uneven surfaces.	_____	_____	_____
8. Rinses instruments again thoroughly.	_____	_____	_____
9. Leaves all instruments in open positions.	_____	_____	_____
10. Dries thoroughly.	_____	_____	_____
11. Removes gown, mask, and gloves.	_____	_____	_____
12. Washes hands.	_____	_____	_____

Documentation

_____

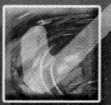

1st Observation

Date: _____ Evaluator Signature and Printed Name: _____

Comments:

2nd Observation

Date: _____ Evaluator Signature and Printed Name: _____

Comments:

Mastery

Date: _____ Evaluator Signature and Printed Name: _____

Comments:

 ABHES COMPETENCIES: Prepare patient for and assist physician with routine and specialty examinations and treatments and minor office surgeries.

 CAAHEP COMPETENCIES: Prepare patient for and assist with routine and specialty examinations.

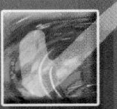

Competency Skill Checklist

Name _____ Course _____

PROCEDURE

38-6

Preparing Sanitized Instruments for Sterilization

	1st Observation	2nd Observation	Mastery
1. Washes hands.	_____	_____	_____
2. Gathers equipment and supplies.	_____	_____	_____
3. Opens all instruments to allow complete penetration of steam.	_____	_____	_____
4. Lays cloth on bottom of tray; lays larger items down first.	_____	_____	_____
5. Places items in order of use for specific pack.	_____	_____	_____
6. Puts gauze or cotton ball between tips of any sharp hinged instruments.	_____	_____	_____
7. Takes bottom edge of wrapper and folds it over article.	_____	_____	_____
8. Folds back this corner.	_____	_____	_____
9. Takes right side of wrapper and folds it over.	_____	_____	_____
10. Folds back this corner.	_____	_____	_____
11. Takes left side of wrapper and folds it over.	_____	_____	_____
12. Folds back this corner.	_____	_____	_____
13. Takes last corner of wrapper and folds it over.	_____	_____	_____
14. Tapes last corner with autoclave tape or tucks edge under other corners before taping, depending on office policy.	_____	_____	_____
15. Seals package with sterilization tape.	_____	_____	_____
16. Writes items included on tape.	_____	_____	_____
17. Writes date and initials on tape.	_____	_____	_____

Documentation

_____

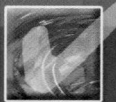

1st Observation

Date: _____ Evaluator Signature and Printed Name: _____

Comments:

2nd Observation

Date: _____ Evaluator Signature and Printed Name: _____

Comments:

Mastery

Date: _____ Evaluator Signature and Printed Name: _____

Comments:

 ABHES COMPETENCIES: Wrap items for autoclaving.

 CAAHEP COMPETENCIES: Wrap items for autoclaving.

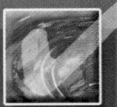

Competency Skill Checklist

Name _____ Course _____

PROCEDURE

38-7 Sterilization with Autoclave

	1st Observation	2nd Observation	Mastery
1. Washes hands.	_____	_____	_____
2. Gathers equipment and supplies.	_____	_____	_____
3. Reads manual for machine to be used.	_____	_____	_____
4. Looks at water level indicator, making sure water is at "fill" line.	_____	_____	_____
5. Places small packs in autoclave, keeping packs and articles separate from each other and away from sides of machine.	_____	_____	_____
6. Lays containers on their sides, with lids ajar or removed.	_____	_____	_____
7. Puts indicator in middle of items to be sterilized.	_____	_____	_____
8. Closes autoclave door securely.	_____	_____	_____
9. Turns on machine.	_____	_____	_____
10. Sets timer when temperature gauge reaches required temperature.	_____	_____	_____
11. Vents chamber when cycle is complete.	_____	_____	_____
12. Allows items to dry.	_____	_____	_____
13. Removes items when cooled.	_____	_____	_____
14. Checks sterilizer indicator.	_____	_____	_____
15. Places items in clean, dry area.	_____	_____	_____
16. Cleans and services autoclave according to manufacturer's directions.	_____	_____	_____

Documentation

```



```

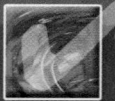

Competency Skill Checklist (Continued)

1st Observation

Date: _____ Evaluator Signature and Printed Name: _____

Comments:

2nd Observation

Date: _____ Evaluator Signature and Printed Name: _____

Comments:

Mastery

Date: _____ Evaluator Signature and Printed Name: _____

Comments:

 ABHES COMPETENCIES: Perform sterilization techniques.

Operate and maintain facilities and perform routine maintenance of administrative and clinical equipment safely.

 CAAHEP COMPETENCIES: Perform sterilization techniques.

Perform routine maintenance of administrative and clinical equipment.

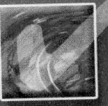

Name _____   Course _____

PROCEDURE

39-1

Cardiopulmonary Resuscitation— Two-Person Rescue

	1st Observation	2nd Observation	Mastery
1. Shakes client and shouts, "Are you okay?"	_____	_____	_____
2. If no response, one rescuer activates emergency medical services system.	_____	_____	_____
3. Places client on floor or other hard, flat surface.	_____	_____	_____
4. Rescuer One kneels at client's side.	_____	_____	_____
5. Rescuer Two kneels by side of client's head. Rescuer Two stays at client's head.	_____	_____	_____
6. Opens client's airway using head-tilt, chin-lift maneuver or jaw-thrust method.	_____	_____	_____
7. Looks, listens, and feels for breath and breathing.	_____	_____	_____
8. If client is not breathing, keeps head in head-tilt or jaw-thrust position.	_____	_____	_____
9. Pinches client's nostrils closed.	_____	_____	_____
10. Rescuer Two puts mouth over client's mouth.	_____	_____	_____
11. Gives two slow breaths (each two seconds long). Takes a breath in between two slow breaths.	_____	_____	_____
12. Observes client for chest rise.	_____	_____	_____
13. Turns head to side to listen and feel for return of air while looking for chest to rise.	_____	_____	_____
14. Checks for carotid pulse with index and middle finger. At same time, watches for signs of circulation, breathing, coughing, or movement.	_____	_____	_____
15. If circulation signs are observed but no breathing, gives rescue breathing (1 breath every 5 seconds, or 10 to 12 breaths per minute).	_____	_____	_____
16. If there is no sign of circulation (pulse), Rescuer One starts chest compressions. Finds correct position for hand placement by starting at lower edge of client's rib cage and following it with finger to notch or V at center of chest. Puts two fingers above notch. Places heel of hand that is closest to client's head over other hand and interlaces and locks fingers. Holds fingers off client's chest.	_____	_____	_____
17. Rescuer One positions himself on knees, with shoulders directly over hands, which are on client's sternum.	_____	_____	_____
18. Keeps arms straight and presses down on client's chest (1½ to 2 inches) and then releases.	_____	_____	_____

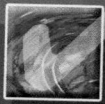

19. Repeats chest compression 15 times (at rate of 100 compressions per minute). _____ _____ _____

20. Rescuer Two gives client 2 slow breaths after each cycle of 15 compressions. _____ _____ _____

21. Repeats cycle of 15 compressions and 2 slow breaths (15:2) four times. _____ _____ _____

22. Rescuer Two rechecks carotid pulse and looks for signs of circulation and breathing. _____ _____ _____

23. If no signs of circulation are present, resumes cycle, beginning with chest compressions by Rescuer One. _____ _____ _____

24. If circulation is observed but no signs of breathing, Rescuer Two gives rescue breathing (1 breath every 5 seconds, or 10 to 12 per minute). Once CPR has been started, rescuers continue until client recovers or instructor says to stop. _____ _____ _____

25. Cleans mannequin thoroughly with alcohol wipes. Follows directions for mannequins with disposable parts. _____ _____ _____

26. Washes hands. _____ _____ _____

27. Records procedure immediately. _____ _____ _____

Documentation

```
┌─────────────────────────────────────────────────────────────┐
│                                                               │
│                                                               │
│                                                               │
│                                                               │
└─────────────────────────────────────────────────────────────┘
```

1st Observation

Date: _____ Evaluator Signature and Printed Name: _____

Comments:

2nd Observation

Date: _____ Evaluator Signature and Printed Name: _____

Comments:

Mastery

Date: _____ Evaluator Signature and Printed Name: _____

Comments:

 ABHES COMPETENCIES: Recognition and response to verbal and non-verbal communication.

Recognize emergencies.

Perform first aid and CPR.

 CAAHEP COMPETENCIES: Recognize and respond to nonverbal communications.

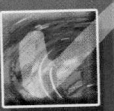

Name _____ Course _____

	1st Observation	2nd Observation	Mastery
1. Shakes client and shouts, "Are you okay?"	___	___	___
2. If there is no response, activates EMS system.	___	___	___
3. Places client on floor or other flat, hard surface.	___	___	___
4. Kneels at side of client's head.	___	___	___
5. Opens client's airway, using head-tilt, chin-lift maneuver or jaw-thrust method.	___	___	___
6. Looks, listens, and feels for breath and breathing.	___	___	___
7. If client is not breathing, keeps head in head-tilt or jaw-thrust position.	___	___	___
8. Pinches client's nostrils closed.	___	___	___
9. Puts mouth over client's mouth (or uses barrier respiration device).	___	___	___
10. Gives two slow breaths (each two seconds long). Takes a breath in between two slow breaths.	___	___	___
11. Observes client for chest rise.	___	___	___
12. Turns head to side to listen and feel for return of air while looking for chest to rise.	___		
13. Checks for carotid pulse with index and middle finger. At same time, watches for signs of circulation, breathing, coughing, or movement.	___	___	___
14. If circulation signs are observed, but no breathing, gives rescue breathing (1 breath every 5 seconds, or 10 to 12 breaths per minute).	___	___	___
15. If no sign of circulation present, begins chest compressions. Finds correct position for hand placement by starting at lower edge of client's rib cage and following it with finger to notch or V at center of chest. Puts two fingers above notch. Places heel of hand that is closest to client's head over other hand and interlaces and locks fingers. Holds fingers off client's chest.	___	___	___
16. Kneels with shoulders over hands, which are over client's sternum.	___	___	___
17. Keeps arms straight and tight.	___	___	___
18. Presses down on client's chest (1½ to 2 inches) and releases.	___	___	___
19. Repeats compression 15 times (at a rate of 100 compressions per minute).	___	___	___

869

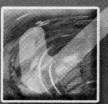
20. Gives client 2 slow breaths after each cycle of 15 compressions. _____ _____ _____

21. Does not move from position by client's side. _____ _____ _____

22. Repeats cycle of 15 compressions and 2 slow breaths (15:2) four times. _____ _____ _____

23. Rechecks carotid pulse and observes for signs of circulation and breathing. _____ _____ _____

24. If no signs of circulation, resumes cycle, beginning with chest compressions. _____ _____ _____

25. If circulation is observed but no signs of breathing, gives rescue breathing (1 breath every 5 seconds, or 10 to 12 per minute). Once CPR has been started, continues until client recovers or instructor says to stop. _____ _____ _____

26. Cleans mannequin thoroughly with alcohol wipes. Follows directions for mannequins with disposable parts. _____ _____ _____

27. Washes hands. _____ _____ _____

28. Records procedure immediately. _____ _____ _____

Documentation

```



```

1st Observation

Date: _____ Evaluator Signature and Printed Name: _____

Comments:

2nd Observation

Date: _____ Evaluator Signature and Printed Name: _____

Comments:

Mastery

Date: _____ Evaluator Signature and Printed Name: _____

Comments:

 ABHES COMPETENCIES: Recognition and response to verbal and non-verbal communication.

Recognize emergencies.

Perform first aid and CPR.

 CAAHEP COMPETENCIES: Recognize and respond to nonverbal communications.

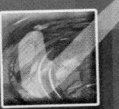
Name _____   Course _____

PROCEDURE

39-3   Recovery Position

	1st Observation	2nd Observation	Mastery
1. Kneels next to client.	_____	_____	_____
2. Straightens client's legs.	_____	_____	_____
3. Using nearest arm, bends client's arm at elbow.	_____	_____	_____
4. Places forearm of that arm near client's head, with palm facing up.	_____	_____	_____
5. Puts client's other arm across client's chest.	_____	_____	_____
6. Places hand on back of client's leg that is farthest away, about 2 to 3 inches above knee.	_____	_____	_____
7. Pulls thigh up toward client's body.	_____	_____	_____
8. Grabs client's shoulder that is farthest away with other hand.	_____	_____	_____
9. In smooth motion, rolls client onto side toward student.	_____	_____	_____
10. Makes sure that hip and knee of client's uppermost leg are flexed and at right angles. If not, adjusts them.	_____	_____	_____
11. Tilts client's head back to keep airway open.	_____	_____	_____
12. Takes client's uppermost hand and places it under cheek (with back of hand against cheek).	_____	_____	_____
13. Looks, listens, and feels for breathing and circulation.	_____	_____	_____
14. If breathing or circulation stops, begins CPR.	_____	_____	_____

Documentation

_____

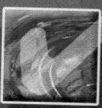
1st Observation

Date: _____ Evaluator Signature and Printed Name: _____

Comments:

2nd Observation

Date: _____ Evaluator Signature and Printed Name: _____

Comments:

Mastery

Date: _____ Evaluator Signature and Printed Name: _____

Comments:

 ABHES COMPETENCIES: Recognition and response to verbal and non-verbal communication.

Recognize emergencies.

 CAAHEP COMPETENCIES: Recognize and respond to nonverbal communications.

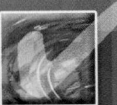

Name _____ Course _____

PROCEDURE

39-4

Care During a Seizure

	1st Observation	2nd Observation	Mastery
1. Gently assists client to floor, if not already seizing on floor.	_____	_____	_____
2. Moves objects away from client.	_____	_____	_____
3. Checks watch to note time.	_____	_____	_____
4. Removes bystanders and provides privacy.	_____	_____	_____
5. Calls physician.	_____	_____	_____
6. Observes characteristics of seizure.	_____	_____	_____
7. After seizure is over, positions client on side in recovery position.	_____	_____	_____

Documentation

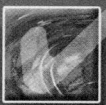

1st Observation

Date: _____ Evaluator Signature and Printed Name: _____

Comments:

2nd Observation

Date: _____ Evaluator Signature and Printed Name: _____

Comments:

Mastery

Date: _____ Evaluator Signature and Printed Name: _____

Comments:

 ABHES COMPETENCIES: Recognition and response to verbal and non-verbal communication.

Recognize emergencies.

 CAAHEP COMPETENCIES: Recognize and respond to nonverbal communications.

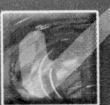
Name _____ Course _____

	1st Observation	2nd Observation	Mastery
1. Asks person, "Are you choking?" "Can you speak?" (If person does not or cannot respond, continues steps of this procedure.)	_____	_____	_____
2. Tells person that student will help and that student will stand behind client.	_____	_____	_____
3. Stands behind choking person.	_____	_____	_____
4. Places one foot between person's feet.	_____	_____	_____
5. Places arms around client's abdomen, locking one hand over other fist on upper abdomen (stays away from lower sternum or xiphoid).	_____	_____	_____
6. Pulls inward and upward sharply to give an abdominal thrust. Repeats abdominal thrusts until object is expelled or person becomes unresponsive. If client stops breathing and shows no signs of circulation, starts CPR.	_____	_____	_____

Documentation

```



```

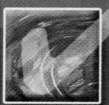

1st Observation

Date: _____ Evaluator Signature and Printed Name: _____

Comments:

2nd Observation

Date: _____ Evaluator Signature and Printed Name: _____

Comments:

Mastery

Date: _____ Evaluator Signature and Printed Name: _____

Comments:

 ABHES COMPETENCIES: Recognize emergencies.

Perform first aid and CPR.

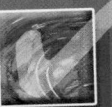

Competency Skill Checklist

Name _____ Course _____

PROCEDURE 39-6

Abdominal Thrusts (Unconscious Adult)

	1st Observation	2nd Observation	Mastery
1. Activates emergency response system.	_____	_____	_____
2. Opens client's airway with tongue-jaw lift.	_____	_____	_____
3. Sweeps finger through client's mouth to remove any foreign objects.	_____	_____	_____
4. Opens client's airway and tries to ventilate (gives rescue breaths). If client's chest does not go up, does steps 5 through 8.	_____	_____	_____
5. Reopens client's airway and tries again.	_____	_____	_____
6. If client's chest still does not rise, gives five abdominal thrusts. Makes sure to avoid lower sternum.	_____	_____	_____
7. Repeats until rescue breathing is effective.	_____	_____	_____
8. When airway has been successfully cleared, and client has signs of circulation and breathing, puts client in recovery position.	_____	_____	_____

Documentation

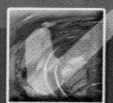

1st Observation

Date: _____ Evaluator Signature and Printed Name: _____

Comments:

2nd Observation

Date: _____ Evaluator Signature and Printed Name: _____

Comments:

Mastery

Date: _____ Evaluator Signature and Printed Name: _____

Comments:

ABHES COMPETENCIES: Recognize emergencies.

Perform first aid and CPR.

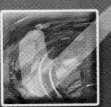
Name _____   Course _____

PROCEDURE

39-7

Clearing Foreign Body Airway Obstruction in a Responsive Infant

	1st Observation	2nd Observation	Mastery
1. Looks at infant for difficulty in breathing, weak cough, and weak or no cry.	_____	_____	_____
2. Picks up infant. Supports infant's head and abdomen on palm of hand and forearm.	_____	_____	_____
3. Gives five back blows with heel of hand.	_____	_____	_____
4. Turns child over and gives five chest thrusts. Uses only two fingers on chest.	_____	_____	_____
5. Repeats steps 3 and 4 until foreign body is expelled or infant becomes unresponsive.	_____	_____	_____
6. If unresponsive, initiates Procedure 39-8.	_____	_____	_____

Documentation

```
┌─────────────────────────────────────────────────────────────┐
│                                                               │
│                                                               │
│                                                               │
│                                                               │
└─────────────────────────────────────────────────────────────┘
```

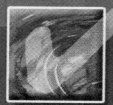

Competency Skill Checklist (Continued)

1st Observation

Date: _____ Evaluator Signature and Printed Name: _____

Comments:

2nd Observation

Date: _____ Evaluator Signature and Printed Name: _____

Comments:

Mastery

Date: _____ Evaluator Signature and Printed Name: _____

Comments:

ABHES COMPETENCIES: Recognize emergencies.

Perform first aid and CPR.

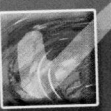

Competency Skill Checklist

Name _____   Course _____

PROCEDURE 39-8
Clearing a Foreign Body Airway Obstruction in an Unresponsive Infant

	1st Observation	2nd Observation	Mastery
1. Establishes unresponsiveness.	_____	_____	_____
2. If another person is available, sends that person to activate emergency response system.	_____	_____	_____
3. Opens client's airway and checks for breathing.	_____	_____	_____
4. Gives rescue breaths. If client's chest does not rise, reopens airway and gives another rescue breath.	_____	_____	_____
5. If unsuccessful (client is still not breathing), gives five back blows with heel of hand and then five chest thrusts. Uses only two fingers for chest thrusts.	_____	_____	_____
6. Opens airway with tongue-jaw lift. Removes foreign body if seen. Does not do blind finger sweep on infant.	_____	_____	_____
7. Repeats steps 3–6 until rescue breathing is effective. Continues CPR as needed.	_____	_____	_____
8. If alone and unable to remove airway obstruction within one minute, carries infant and activates emergency response system.	_____	_____	_____

Documentation

<!-- empty documentation box -->

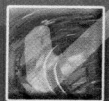

1st Observation

Date: _____ Evaluator Signature and Printed Name: _____

Comments:

2nd Observation

Date: _____ Evaluator Signature and Printed Name: _____

Comments:

Mastery

Date: _____ Evaluator Signature and Printed Name: _____

Comments:

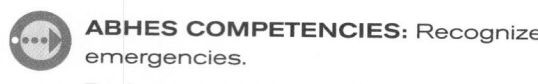 **ABHES COMPETENCIES:** Recognize emergencies.

Perform first aid and CPR.

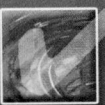

Competency Skill Checklist

Name _____ Course _____

PROCEDURE

40-1

Opening Physician's Office Laboratory

	1st Observation	2nd Observation	Mastery
1. Unlocks door and turns on lights.	_____	_____	_____
2. Washes hands.	_____	_____	_____
3. Reviews messages on answering machine.	_____	_____	_____
4. Sees if there are any fax messages.	_____	_____	_____
5. Looks over activities on day's schedule.	_____	_____	_____
6. Shuts off special ultraviolet lights.	_____	_____	_____
7. Walks area and switches machines on.	_____	_____	_____
8. Makes sure to switch machines from standby or energy-save mode to ready.	_____	_____	_____
9. Takes from refrigerator any supplies that must be at room temperature for use.	_____	_____	_____
10. Records on appropriate forms temperature readings on any equipment that must be at a certain temperature to work.	_____	_____	_____
11. Puts on gloves, gown, and mask (PPE) according to protocol.	_____	_____	_____
12. Goes through daily control checks and records results according to laboratory's quality assurance policy.	_____	_____	_____
13. Checks labels of disinfectants for expiration dates.	_____	_____	_____
14. Makes sure containers are filled and ready for use that day.	_____	_____	_____
15. Makes sure work surfaces that will be used that day are clean.	_____	_____	_____
16. Checks supplies and discards any outdated supplies according to safety standard precautions.	_____	_____	_____
17. Reorders supplies as needed.	_____	_____	_____
18. Arranges supplies on shelves with newest items at back.	_____	_____	_____
19. Signs name, date, and time in appropriate record when finished with these tasks.	_____	_____	_____
20. Looks over tests scheduled for day.	_____	_____	_____
21. Assembles items that will be needed for these tests.	_____	_____	_____
22. Reviews any requests or results that came in since closing day before.	_____	_____	_____
23. Informs doctor of any new requests or results.	_____	_____	_____
24. Writes test results in charts per laboratory/office policy.	_____	_____	_____

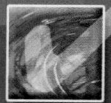
25. Checks sheet that lists weekly tasks.   _____ _____ _____
26. Compares weekly list to today's day/date.   _____ _____ _____
27. Completes tasks as required.   _____ _____ _____
28. Signs name, date, and time on laboratory sheet. _____ _____ _____
29. Begins day's client testing and procedures.   _____ _____ _____

Documentation

_____

1st Observation

Date: _____ Evaluator Signature and Printed Name: _____

Comments:

2nd Observation

Date: _____ Evaluator Signature and Printed Name: _____

Comments:

Mastery

Date: _____ Evaluator Signature and Printed Name: _____

Comments:

 ABHES COMPETENCIES: Maintain physical plant.

Operate and maintain facilities and perform routine maintenance of administrative and clinical equipment safely.

Inventory equipment and supplies.

 CAAHEP COMPETENCIES: Perform an inventory of equipment and supplies.

Perform routine maintenance of administrative and clinical equipment.

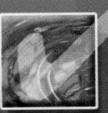

Competency Skill Checklist

Name _____ Course _____

	1st Observation	2nd Observation	Mastery
1. Using correct form, lists activities that should be done next day after opening POL.	_____	_____	_____
2. Sends out any samples that must go to more specialized laboratories.	_____	_____	_____
3. Stores properly any samples that will be tested following day.	_____	_____	_____
4. Gets authorization or "all clear" from doctor before shutting off machines or switching to standby.	_____	_____	_____
5. Puts away supplies.	_____	_____	_____
6. Checks supplies received or opened that day and makes sure these supplies are dated and signed.	_____	_____	_____
7. Picks up and straightens up lab area.	_____	_____	_____
8. Discards waste according to safety standard precautions.	_____	_____	_____
9. Cleans and sterilizes equipment and supplies as necessary.	_____	_____	_____
10. Cleans and disinfects surfaces where lab tests are done.	_____	_____	_____
11. Puts medical waste into biohazardous waste containers.	_____	_____	_____
12. Discards biohazardous waste container according to regulations.	_____	_____	_____
13. Shuts off machines or changes them to power save or standby.	_____	_____	_____
14. Replaces items that are in low supply.	_____	_____	_____
15. Checks fax communications and any last messages.	_____	_____	_____
16. Turns on answering machine.	_____	_____	_____
17. Washes hands.	_____	_____	_____
18. Puts on special ultraviolet lights.	_____	_____	_____
19. Turns off any other lights.	_____	_____	_____
20. Closes and locks doors and access to laboratory equipment.	_____	_____	_____

Documentation

_____

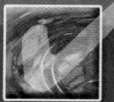
Competency Skill Checklist (Continued)

1st Observation

Date: _____ Evaluator Signature and Printed Name: _____

Comments:

2nd Observation

Date: _____ Evaluator Signature and Printed Name: _____

Comments:

Mastery

Date: _____ Evaluator Signature and Printed Name: _____

Comments:

 ABHES COMPETENCIES: Maintain physical plant.

Operate and maintain facilities and perform routine maintenance of administrative and clinical equipment safely.

Inventory equipment and supplies.

 CAAHEP COMPETENCIES: Perform an inventory of equipment and supplies.

Perform routine maintenance of administrative and clinical equipment.

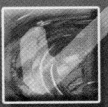

Name _____ Course _____

PROCEDURE

40-3

Throat Specimen Collection for Culture

	1st Observation	2nd Observation	Mastery
1. Washes hands.	_____	_____	_____
2. Gathers equipment and supplies.	_____	_____	_____
3. Introduces self to client.	_____	_____	_____
4. Identifies client.	_____	_____	_____
5. Tells client, in everyday language, what medical assistant is going to do.	_____	_____	_____
6. Asks if client has any questions. If client does, gives short and simple answers.	_____	_____	_____
7. Asks client to sit on examination table.	_____	_____	_____
8. Adjusts light if using examination light.	_____	_____	_____
9. Puts on gloves and a face mask.	_____	_____	_____
10. Takes sterile swab out of sterile container.	_____	_____	_____
11. Asks client to open mouth and say, "Ahhh."			
12. Presses on middle of client's tongue with tongue blade.	_____	_____	_____
13. Gently places swab at back of client's throat. Firmly touches with swab any red, inflamed, or white areas. Turns swab constantly while obtaining specimen.	_____	_____	_____
14. Keeps client's tongue down with tongue blade.	_____	_____	_____
15. Takes swab out of client's mouth. Keeps tongue depressed to avoid getting saliva on throat specimen.	_____	_____	_____
16. Puts swab into sterile container immediately. (Follows directions on container.).	_____	_____	_____
17. Labels specimen container with requested or required information.	_____	_____	_____
18. Asks client if client has any questions.	_____	_____	_____
19. Disposes of equipment and supplies according to office policy.	_____	_____	_____
20. Removes gloves and face mask.	_____	_____	_____
21. Washes hands.	_____	_____	_____
22. Records procedure correctly in client's chart.	_____	_____	_____
23. Stores and sends specimen to laboratory for testing.	_____	_____	_____

Documentation

```



```

887

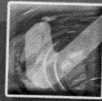

Competency Skill Checklist (Continued)

1st Observation

Date: _____ Evaluator Signature and Printed Name: _____

Comments:

2nd Observation

Date: _____ Evaluator Signature and Printed Name: _____

Comments:

Mastery

Date: _____ Evaluator Signature and Printed Name: _____

Comments:

 ABHES COMPETENCIES: Obtain throat specimen for microbiological testing. Perform microbiology testing.

 CAAHEP COMPETENCIES: Obtain specimens for microbiological testing. Perform microbiology testing.

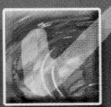

Name _____ Course _____

PROCEDURE

40-4

Sputum Specimen Collection

	1st Observation	2nd Observation	Mastery
1. Washes hands.	_____	_____	_____
2. Gathers equipment and supplies.	_____	_____	_____
3. Introduces self to client.	_____	_____	_____
4. Identifies client.	_____	_____	_____
5. Tells client, in everyday language, what medical assistant is going to do.	_____	_____	_____
6. Asks if client has any questions. If client does, gives short and simple answers.	_____	_____	_____
7. Asks client to rinse mouth well.	_____	_____	_____
8. Puts on gloves, gown, and face mask or face shield.	_____	_____	_____
9. Instructs client to breathe deeply and cough deeply.	_____	_____	_____
10. Tells client to use abdominal muscles to help cough up secretions from lower lungs.	_____	_____	_____
11. Tells client to expectorate sputum directly into specimen container.	_____	_____	_____
12. Instructs client not to touch inside of container.	_____	_____	_____
13. Asks client to avoid getting sputum on side of container.	_____	_____	_____
14. Immediately takes container from client, observing standard precautions.	_____	_____	_____
15. Puts lid on container.	_____	_____	_____
16. Completes label and lab request form.	_____	_____	_____
17. Instructs client to rinse mouth.	_____	_____	_____
18. Asks client if client has any questions.	_____	_____	_____
19. Disposes of used items according to office policy.	_____	_____	_____
20. Removes gloves, gown, and face mask or shield.	_____	_____	_____
21. Washes hands.	_____	_____	_____
22. Sends specimen to laboratory for testing.	_____	_____	_____
23. Records procedure correctly in client's chart.	_____	_____	_____

Documentation

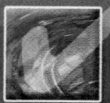

Competency Skill Checklist (Continued)

1st Observation

Date: _____ Evaluator Signature and Printed Name: _____

Comments:

2nd Observation

Date: _____ Evaluator Signature and Printed Name: _____

Comments:

Mastery

Date: _____ Evaluator Signature and Printed Name: _____

Comments:

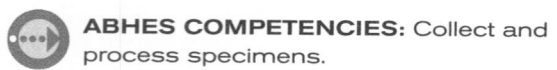 **ABHES COMPETENCIES:** Collect and process specimens.

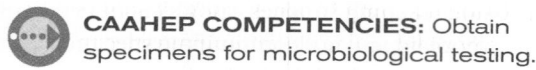 **CAAHEP COMPETENCIES:** Obtain specimens for microbiological testing.

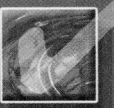

Name _____ Course _____

PROCEDURE

40-5

Client Instruction for Sputum Specimen Collection

	1st Observation	2nd Observation	Mastery
1. Washes hands.	_____	_____	_____
2. Gathers equipment and supplies.	_____	_____	_____
3. Introduces self to client.	_____	_____	_____
4. Identifies client.	_____	_____	_____
5. Tells client, in everyday language, what medical assistant is going to do.	_____	_____	_____
6. Asks if client has any questions. If client does, gives short and simple answers.	_____	_____	_____
7. Tells client that first morning, productive cough sputum is best.	_____	_____	_____
8. Using teaching supplies, shows client how to remove lid and not contaminate specimen. Reminds client not to touch inside of container and not to get sputum on sides of container.	_____	_____	_____
9. Tells client not to let saliva get into container.	_____	_____	_____
10. Instructs client to breathe deeply, cough deeply, and expectorate sputum from lower lungs into container.	_____	_____	_____
11. Tells client to put lid on container immediately after expectorating.	_____	_____	_____
12. Reminds client to wash hands after obtaining sputum specimen.	_____	_____	_____
13. Tells client to fill in information on label of container and lab request form.	_____	_____	_____
14. Instructs client to take sputum specimen to office or lab as directed by doctor.	_____	_____	_____
15. Gives written, step-by-step instructions to client.	_____	_____	_____
16. Asks client if client has any questions.	_____	_____	_____
17. Washes hands.	_____	_____	_____
18. Records procedure correctly in client's chart.	_____	_____	_____

Documentation

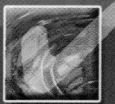

Competency Skill Checklist (Continued)

1st Observation

Date: _____ Evaluator Signature and Printed Name: _____

Comments:

2nd Observation

Date: _____ Evaluator Signature and Printed Name: _____

Comments:

Mastery

Date: _____ Evaluator Signature and Printed Name: _____

Comments:

 ABHES COMPETENCIES: Instruct patients with special needs.

 CAAHEP COMPETENCIES: Instruct individuals according to their needs.

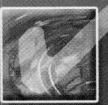

Name _____ Course _____

	1st Observation	2nd Observation	Mastery
1. Washes hands.	_____	_____	_____
2. Gathers equipment and supplies.	_____	_____	_____
3. Introduces self to client.	_____	_____	_____
4. Identifies client.	_____	_____	_____
5. Tells client, in everyday language, what medical assistant is going to do.	_____	_____	_____
6. Asks if client has any questions. If client does, gives short and simple answers.	_____	_____	_____
7. Instructs client to obtain stool or feces from next bowel movement.	_____	_____	_____
8. Informs client to urinate first; no urine should be mixed with stool specimen.	_____	_____	_____
9. Shows client how to use kit or how to use tongue depressor and specimen container to obtain stool specimen.	_____	_____	_____
10. Tells client that nothing but stool or feces should be in container. This includes toilet paper.	_____	_____	_____
11. Instructs client to put lid on container immediately after putting specimen in container.	_____	_____	_____
12. Reminds client to wash hands after obtaining specimen.	_____	_____	_____
13. Fills out label with client's name; has client fill in date and time specimen was collected.	_____	_____	_____
14. Completes laboratory request form with required information.	_____	_____	_____
15. Tells client to bring specimen container to office or lab as directed by doctor within two hours after obtaining specimen (if this is not possible, specimen must be refrigerated).	_____	_____	_____
16. Gives client written instructions for reference at home.	_____	_____	_____
17. Asks client if client has any questions.	_____	_____	_____
18. Records procedure correctly in client's chart.	_____	_____	_____

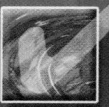

Documentation

┌───┐
│   │
│   │
│   │
│   │
└───┘

1st Observation

Date: _____ Evaluator Signature and Printed Name: _____

Comments:

2nd Observation

Date: _____ Evaluator Signature and Printed Name: _____

Comments:

Mastery

Date: _____ Evaluator Signature and Printed Name: _____

Comments:

 ABHES COMPETENCIES: Instruct patient in the collection of fecal specimen.

 CAAHEP COMPETENCIES: Instruct patients in the collection of fecal specimen.

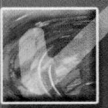

Name _____ Course _____

PROCEDURE

40-7

Wound Culture Collection for Microbiological Testing

	1st Observation	2nd Observation	Mastery
1. Washes hands.	_____	_____	_____
2. Gathers equipment and supplies.	_____	_____	_____
3. Introduces self to client.	_____	_____	_____
4. Identifies client.	_____	_____	_____
5. Tells client, in everyday language, what medical assistant is going to do.	_____	_____	_____
6. Asks if client has any questions. If client does, gives short and simple answers.	_____	_____	_____
7. Reassures client and instructs her not to move during procedure.	_____	_____	_____
8. Puts on gloves and other PPE as needed.	_____	_____	_____
9. Looks at wound and notes size, color, and smell (if any).	_____	_____	_____
10. Using sterile saline solution, rinses wound if pus or other drainage noted.	_____	_____	_____
11. Using sterile gauze, gently dries area.	_____	_____	_____
12. Disposes of used gauze in biohazardous waste container.	_____	_____	_____
13. Removes contaminated gloves, washes hands, and puts on clean gloves.	_____	_____	_____
14. Picks up sterile swab.	_____	_____	_____
15. With one gloved hand, holds wound area. With other gloved hand, rotates swab over wound, being careful not to wipe edges of wound.	_____	_____	_____
16. Puts swab in culture tube.	_____	_____	_____
17. Labels tube and fills out other lab forms.	_____	_____	_____
18. Asks client if client has any questions.	_____	_____	_____
19. Sends wound culture specimen to lab.	_____	_____	_____
20. Cleans area. Removes PPE and washes hands.	_____	_____	_____
21. Records procedure correctly in client's chart.	_____	_____	_____

Documentation

```
[blank documentation box]
```

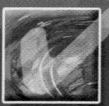

1st Observation

Date: _____ Evaluator Signature and Printed Name: _____

Comments:

2nd Observation

Date: _____ Evaluator Signature and Printed Name: _____

Comments:

Mastery

Date: _____ Evaluator Signature and Printed Name: _____

Comments:

 ABHES COMPETENCIES: Perform wound collection procedure for microbiological testing.

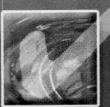

Name _____ Course _____

PROCEDURE

41-1

Obtaining a Clean-Catch Urine Specimen

	1st Observation	2nd Observation	Mastery
1. Washes hands.	_____	_____	_____
2. Reads doctor's order.	_____	_____	_____
3. Gathers equipment and supplies.	_____	_____	_____
4. Introduces self to client.	_____	_____	_____
5. Identifies client.	_____	_____	_____
6. Tells client, in everyday language, what medical assistant is going to do.	_____	_____	_____
7. Asks if client has any questions. If client does, gives short and simple answers.	_____	_____	_____

If client is female, gives her needed items and tells her to do steps 8 through 21:

	1st Observation	2nd Observation	Mastery
8. Wash hands.	_____	_____	_____
9. Spread labia apart with one hand.	_____	_____	_____
10. Take cotton ball with antiseptic solution, or antiseptic wipe, and wipe down on one side of meatus from front to back, using only a single stroke.	_____	_____	_____
11. Throw away used cotton ball or wipe.	_____	_____	_____
12. Take another cotton ball or wipe and wipe down other side of meatus from front to back, again using only a single stroke.	_____	_____	_____
13. Throw away used cotton ball or wipe.	_____	_____	_____
14. Take a third cotton ball or wipe and wipe down middle of meatus, from front to back.	_____	_____	_____
15. Throw away used cotton ball or wipe.	_____	_____	_____
16. Rinse area with sterile cotton balls.	_____	_____	_____
17. Throw away used cotton balls.	_____	_____	_____
18. Hold labia apart and void a small amount of urine into toilet.	_____	_____	_____
19. Take sterile container and bring it into urine stream while continuing to urinate.	_____	_____	_____
20. Void last small amount of urine into toilet.	_____	_____	_____
21. Put cap on sterile container when finished.	_____	_____	_____

If client is male, gives him needed items and tells him to do steps 22 through 34:

	1st Observation	2nd Observation	Mastery
22. Wash hands and remove underpants.	_____	_____	_____
23. Retract foreskin of penis.	_____	_____	_____
24. Take cotton ball with antiseptic solution or antiseptic wipe and wipe in a circular motion away from urinary meatus.	_____	_____	_____

897

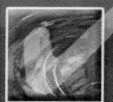

25. Throw away used cotton ball or wipe. _____ _____ _____

26. Take another cotton ball or wipe and wipe again in a circular motion. _____ _____ _____

27. Throw away used cotton ball or wipe. _____ _____ _____

28. Take a third cotton ball or wipe and wipe again in a circular motion. _____ _____ _____

29. Throw away used cotton ball or wipe. _____ _____ _____

30. Keep foreskin retracted. _____ _____ _____

31. Void a small amount into toilet. _____ _____ _____

32. Take sterile container and bring it into urine stream while continuing to urinate. _____ _____ _____

33. Void last small amount of urine into toilet. _____ _____ _____

34. Put cap on sterile container when finished. _____ _____ _____

Medical assistant then completes steps 35 to 39:

35. Labels and tests or processes urine specimen as directed by office policy. _____ _____ _____

36. Cleans area, following standard precautions. _____ _____ _____

37. Removes gloves. _____ _____ _____

38. Washes hands. _____ _____ _____

39. Records procedure correctly in client's chart. _____ _____ _____

Documentation

```



```

1st Observation

Date: _____ Evaluator Signature and Printed Name: _____

Comments:

2nd Observation

Date: _____ Evaluator Signature and Printed Name: _____

Comments:

Mastery

Date: _____ Evaluator Signature and Printed Name: _____

Comments:

 ABHES COMPETENCIES: Instruct patients in the collection of a clean-catch mid-stream urine specimen.

Collect and process specimens.

 CAAHEP COMPETENCIES: Instruct patients in the collection of a clean-catch mid-stream urine specimen.

Obtain specimens for microbiological testing.

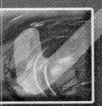

Name _____ Course _____

PROCEDURE 41-2

Urinary Catheterization (Female Client)

	1st Observation	2nd Observation	Mastery
1. Washes hands.	_____	_____	_____
2. Gathers equipment and supplies.	_____	_____	_____
3. Introduces self to client.	_____	_____	_____
4. Identifies client.	_____	_____	_____
5. Tells client, in everyday language, what medical assistant is going to do.	_____	_____	_____
6. Asks if client has any questions. If client does, gives short and simple answers.	_____	_____	_____
7. Asks client to remove clothing from waist down.	_____	_____	_____
8. Assists client onto examination table as needed.	_____	_____	_____
9. Positions client in dorsal recumbent position.	_____	_____	_____
10. Opens catheter tray and places it between client's legs.	_____	_____	_____
11. Puts on sterile gloves.	_____	_____	_____
12. Takes sterile drape from catheter tray and places it under client's buttocks. Does not contaminate gloves while doing this.	_____	_____	_____
13. Opens antiseptic wipes and lubricant. Squeezes lubricant onto tip of catheter.	_____	_____	_____
14. Using nondominant hand, gently spreads labia apart to expose urinary meatus.	_____	_____	_____
15. Picks up forceps and grabs antiseptic wipe.	_____	_____	_____
16. Starting at one side of urinary meatus, wipes from top to bottom in one stroke. Wipes once and discards used wipe.	_____	_____	_____
17. Picks up another antiseptic wipe with forceps.	_____	_____	_____
18. Goes to other side of urinary meatus and wipes from top to bottom. Wipes once and discards used wipe.	_____	_____	_____
19. Picks up another antiseptic wipe with forceps.	_____	_____	_____
20. Wipes from top to bottom down center of urinary meatus.	_____	_____	_____
21. Using sterile gloved hand, picks up catheter. Keeps labia separated at all times.	_____	_____	_____
22. Gently inserts catheter tip 2 or 3 inches into urinary meatus.	_____	_____	_____
23. When urine begins to flow, holds catheter in place with hand that had been keeping labia open.	_____	_____	_____

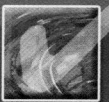

24. Places sterile specimen container under drainage tip of catheter.

25. Fills container with 30 mL of urine. _____ _____ _____

26. Allows rest of urine to drain into collection tray. _____ _____ _____

27. Removes catheter by pulling it out gently. _____ _____ _____

28. Removes collection tray from between client's legs and tells her she can relax her position. _____ _____ _____

29. Notes amount of urine that drained into collection tray. _____ _____ _____

30. Discards extra urine, following standard precautions. _____ _____ _____

31. Takes off gloves and washes hands. _____ _____ _____

32. Correctly labels specimen container and completes lab paperwork. _____ _____ _____

33. Helps client into a sitting position. _____ _____ _____

34. Assists client to dress, as needed. _____ _____ _____

35. Asks client if she has any questions. _____ _____ _____

36. Records procedure in client's chart immediately and processes urine specimen according to office policy. _____ _____ _____

Documentation

[ ]

1st Observation

Date: _____ Evaluator Signature and Printed Name: _____

Comments:

2nd Observation

Date: _____ Evaluator Signature and Printed Name: _____

Comments:

Mastery

Date: _____ Evaluator Signature and Printed Name: _____

Comments:

 ABHES COMPETENCIES: Prepare patient for and assist physician with routine and specialty examinations and treatments and minor office surgeries.

Collect and process specimens.

 CAAHEP COMPETENCIES: Prepare patient for and assist with routine and specialty examinations.

Obtain specimens for microbiological testing.

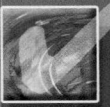

Name _____ Course _____

PROCEDURE

41-3

Urinary Catheterization (Male Client)

	1st Observation	2nd Observation	Mastery
1. Washes hands.	_____	_____	_____
2. Gathers equipment and supplies.	_____	_____	_____
3. Introduces self to client.	_____	_____	_____
4. Identifies client.	_____	_____	_____
5. Tells client, in everyday language, what medical assistant is going to do.	_____	_____	_____
6. Asks if client has any questions. If client does, gives short and simple answers.	_____	_____	_____
7. Asks client to remove clothing from waist down.	_____	_____	_____
8. Assists client onto examination table, as needed, and places him in supine position.	_____	_____	_____
9. Asks client to separate legs a little.	_____	_____	_____
10. Opens catheterization tray and places it to client's side.	_____	_____	_____
11. Puts on sterile gloves.	_____	_____	_____
12. Takes out sterile drape and places it under client's penis.	_____	_____	_____
13. Opens antiseptic wipes.	_____	_____	_____
14. Opens lubricant and squeezes sufficient amount on catheter tip.	_____	_____	_____
15. Using nondominant hand, gently picks up penis to expose urinary meatus. If male client is uncircumcised, gently pulls back foreskin. Holds sides of penis to prevent closing urethra.	_____	_____	_____
16. Using forceps, picks up antiseptic wipe.	_____	_____	_____
17. With antiseptic wipe, cleanses urinary meatus with a circular motion.	_____	_____	_____
18. Discards used wipe.	_____	_____	_____
19. Picks up another antiseptic wipe and cleanses in a circular motion again.	_____	_____	_____
20. Discards used wipe.	_____	_____	_____
21. Picks up third antiseptic wipe and cleanses in a circular motion.	_____	_____	_____
22. Discards used wipe.	_____	_____	_____
23. Using sterile-gloved hand, picks up catheter.	_____	_____	_____
24. Holds penis at 90-degree angle to client's body. Exerts slight traction by pulling upward.	_____	_____	_____
25. Inserts lubricated tip of catheter into urinary meatus about 6 inches.	_____	_____	_____

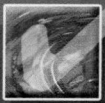

26. When urine begins to flow, holds catheter in place with nondominant hand. _____ _____ _____

27. Places sterile specimen container under drainage tip of catheter. _____ _____ _____

28. Fills container with 30 mL of urine. _____ _____ _____

29. Allows rest of urine to drain into collection tray. _____ _____ _____

30. Removes catheter by pulling it out gently. _____ _____ _____

31. Notes amount of urine that drained into collection tray. _____ _____ _____

32. Discards extra urine, following standard precautions. _____ _____ _____

33. Takes off gloves and washes hands. _____ _____ _____

34. Correctly labels specimen container and completes lab paperwork. _____ _____ _____

35. Helps client into sitting position. _____ _____ _____

36. Assists client to dress, as needed. _____ _____ _____

37. Ask client if he has any questions. _____ _____ _____

38. Records procedure in client's chart immediately and processes urine specimen according to office policy. _____ _____ _____

Documentation

1st Observation

Date: _____ Evaluator Signature and Printed Name: _____

Comments:

2nd Observation

Date: _____ Evaluator Signature and Printed Name: _____

Comments:

Mastery

Date: _____ Evaluator Signature and Printed Name: _____

Comments:

 ABHES COMPETENCIES: Prepare patient for and assist physician with routine and specialty examinations and treatments and minor office surgeries.

Collect and process specimens.

 CAAHEP COMPETENCIES: Prepare patient for and assist with routine and specialty examinations.

Obtain specimens for microbiological testing.

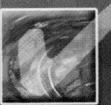

Competency Skill Checklist

Name _____   Course _____

PROCEDURE 41-4

Testing Urine with a Reagent Strip

	1st Observation	2nd Observation	Mastery
1. Collects urine specimen from client.	_____	_____	_____
2. Washes hands.	_____	_____	_____
3. Gathers equipment and supplies.	_____	_____	_____
4. Checks expiration date on reagent strip bottle.	_____	_____	_____
5. Takes one strip from bottle.	_____	_____	_____
6. Puts cap back on bottle immediately.	_____	_____	_____
7. Places strip on clean paper towel.	_____	_____	_____
8. Puts on gloves.	_____	_____	_____
9. Dips strip into urine specimen so that all pads get immersed.	_____	_____	_____
10. Takes strip out immediately.	_____	_____	_____
11. Gently rubs edge of strip along rim of urine container to remove excess urine.	_____	_____	_____
12. Holds reagent strip next to, but not touching, chart to match up pads.	_____	_____	_____
13. Times test using second hand on watch.	_____	_____	_____
14. Reads results.	_____	_____	_____
15. Writes down results.	_____	_____	_____
16. Discards urine and reagent strip into biohazardous waste container.	_____	_____	_____
17. Cleans work area.	_____	_____	_____
18. Takes off gloves.	_____	_____	_____
19. Washes hands.	_____	_____	_____
20. Puts bottle of reagent strips away in proper storage area.	_____	_____	_____
21. Records results of urine test in client's chart or lab slip, per situation and office policy.	_____	_____	_____

Documentation

903

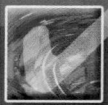

1st Observation

Date: _____ Evaluator Signature and Printed Name: _____

Comments:

2nd Observation

Date: _____ Evaluator Signature and Printed Name: _____

Comments:

Mastery

Date: _____ Evaluator Signature and Printed Name: _____

Comments:

 ABHES COMPETENCIES: Perform selected CLIA-waived tests (i.e., kit tests such as pregnancy, quick strep, dip sticks) that assist with diagnosis and treatment.

Perform urinalysis.

 CAAHEP COMPETENCIES: Perform urinalysis.

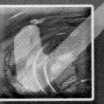

Name _____   Course _____

PROCEDURE

41-5 Testing Urine for Specific Gravity Using a Refractometer

	1st Observation	2nd Observation	Mastery
1. Washes hands.	_____	_____	_____
2. Puts on gloves.	_____	_____	_____
3. Gathers equipment and supplies.	_____	_____	_____
4. Places drop of distilled water on prism and cover.	_____	_____	_____
5. Dries prism and covers with lint-free tissue or gauze.	_____	_____	_____
6. Closes cover.	_____	_____	_____
7. Using a pipette, places one drop of urine in notched part of cover.	_____	_____	_____
8. Turns refractometer so that it points to a strong light.	_____	_____	_____
9. Reads specific gravity line.	_____	_____	_____
10. Cleans cover and prism.	_____	_____	_____
11. Disposes of used items, following standard precautions.	_____	_____	_____
12. Cleans work area.	_____	_____	_____
13. Removes gloves.	_____	_____	_____
14. Washes hands.	_____	_____	_____
15. Records specific gravity measurement in client's chart or on laboratory requisition slip, depending on situation and office policy.	_____	_____	_____

Documentation

_____

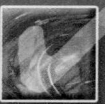

1st Observation

Date: _____ Evaluator Signature and Printed Name: _____

Comments:

2nd Observation

Date: _____ Evaluator Signature and Printed Name: _____

Comments:

Mastery

Date: _____ Evaluator Signature and Printed Name: _____

Comments:

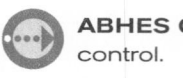 **ABHES COMPETENCIES:** Use quality control.

Perform urinalysis.

 CAAHEP COMPETENCIES: Use methods of quality control.

Perform urinalysis.

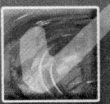

Name _____   Course _____

PROCEDURE

41-6   Rapid Test Procedure: hCG Pregnancy Test

	1st Observation	2nd Observation	Mastery
1. Washes hands.	_____	_____	_____
2. Gathers equipment and supplies.	_____	_____	_____
3. Puts on gloves.	_____	_____	_____
4. Compares name on urine specimen container to name on lab slip.	_____	_____	_____
5. Labels test cassette.	_____	_____	_____
6. Using urine dropper or pipette, draws up urine into dropper or pipette.	_____	_____	_____
7. Holds urine dropper or pipette straight while pointing tip down. Makes sure tip is high enough off sample well to count drops.	_____	_____	_____
8. Drops four drops into well.	_____	_____	_____
9. Waits 5 minutes.	_____	_____	_____
10. Reads results in display window on cassette.	_____	_____	_____
11. Records results on lab form or in client's chart per office policy.	_____	_____	_____
12. Notifies doctor of results.	_____	_____	_____
13. Disposes of specimen and used supplies in biohazardous waste container.	_____	_____	_____
14. Removes gloves.	_____	_____	_____
15. Washes hands.	_____	_____	_____

Documentation

_____

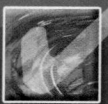

1st Observation

Date: _____ Evaluator Signature and Printed Name: _____

Comments:

2nd Observation

Date: _____ Evaluator Signature and Printed Name: _____

Comments:

Mastery

Date: _____ Evaluator Signature and Printed Name: _____

Comments:

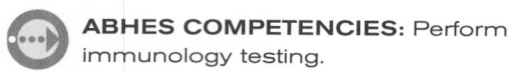 **ABHES COMPETENCIES:** Perform immunology testing.

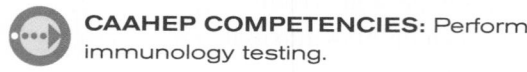 **CAAHEP COMPETENCIES:** Perform immunology testing.

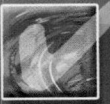

Name _____ Course _____

PROCEDURE

42-1 Venipuncture (Vacuum-Tube Method)

	1st Observation	2nd Observation	Mastery
1. Reads doctor's orders for laboratory tests.	_____	_____	_____
2. Washes hands.	_____	_____	_____
3. Gathers equipment and supplies. Checks vacuum tubes for expiration date, makes sure that additive in tubes is not adhering to stopper or tube walls, and looks for any flaws in tubes.	_____	_____	_____
4. Twists needle and takes off part that will puncture top of tube. Attaches needle to holder.	_____	_____	_____
5. Picks up first collection tube (checks test for order of collection).	_____	_____	_____
6. Places tube into holder. Does not push it in all the way.	_____	_____	_____
7. Introduces self to client.	_____	_____	_____
8. Identifies client.	_____	_____	_____
9. Tells client, in everyday language, what medical assistant is going to do.	_____	_____	_____
10. Asks if client has any questions. If client does, gives short and simple answers.	_____	_____	_____
11. Helps client into comfortable position.	_____	_____	_____
12. Lines up tubes in order of use.	_____	_____	_____
13. Applies tourniquet above desired venipuncture site on client's arm.	_____	_____	_____
14. Puts on gloves, and mask or face shield if needed.	_____	_____	_____
15. Tells client to close hand into a fist, but do not pump fist.	_____	_____	_____
16. Finds vein.	_____	_____	_____
17. Wipes site with alcohol wipe.	_____	_____	_____
18. Lets site air-dry. Does not blow on site.	_____	_____	_____
19. Does not touch venipuncture site after cleaning it.	_____	_____	_____
20. Places thumb 1 to 2 inches below site. Pulls skin smooth and tight.	_____	_____	_____
21. Lines up needle with site. Keeps bevel of needle pointed up.	_____	_____	_____
22. Inserts needle into vein.	_____	_____	_____
23. Takes thumb off client's skin.	_____	_____	_____
24. Grabs flange of holder with free hand.	_____	_____	_____
25. Pushes tube onto needle inside of holder.	_____	_____	_____
26. Allows blood to fill tube.	_____	_____	_____

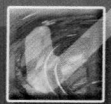
27. When blood flow stops, pulls tube off needle and out of holder with one hand.   _____   _____   _____

28. With same hand, takes next tube in line and pushes it onto needle in holder. Lets blood flow. Repeats this process until all test tubes are filled.   _____   _____   _____

29. Mixes each tube that contains additive by gently turning tube upside down and back about five times. Does not shake.   _____   _____   _____

30. Asks client to open hand.   _____   _____   _____

31. Takes off tourniquet with free hand.   _____   _____   _____

32. Places gauze just above puncture site.   _____   _____   _____

33. Takes needle out of client's arm.   _____   _____   _____

34. Applies pressure to site for 3 minutes. If client is able, asks client to hold gauze over site while keeping arm straight. Does not allow client to bend elbow.   _____   _____   _____

35. Labels all blood tubes before leaving client's area.   _____   _____   _____

36. Checks venipuncture site and applies adhesive bandage.   _____   _____   _____

37. Puts used needle into sharps container.   _____   _____   _____

38. Takes off gloves (and mask or face shield, if used) and disposes of them in biohazardous waste container.   _____   _____   _____

39. Washes hands.   _____   _____   _____

40. Talks with client and asks if client has any questions.   _____   _____   _____

41. Records procedure correctly in client's chart.   _____   _____   _____

Documentation

```
[                                                                    ]
```

1st Observation

Date: _____   Evaluator Signature and Printed Name: _____

Comments:

2nd Observation

Date: _____   Evaluator Signature and Printed Name: _____

Comments:

Mastery

Date: _____   Evaluator Signature and Printed Name: _____

Comments:

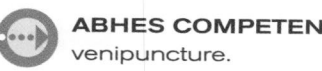

ABHES COMPETENCIES: Perform venipuncture.

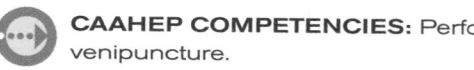

CAAHEP COMPETENCIES: Perform venipuncture.

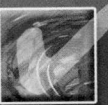

Name _____   Course _____

PROCEDURE

42-2

Venipuncture (Syringe Method)

	1st Observation	2nd Observation	Mastery
1. Reads doctor's orders for laboratory tests.	_____	_____	_____
2. Washes hands.	_____	_____	_____
3. Gathers equipment and supplies. Chooses correct tubes for transfer of blood. Checks expiration dates on tubes. Makes sure that additive is not adhering to stopper and walls of tube. Looks for any flaws in tubes.	_____	_____	_____
4. Opens sterile package of needles with syringes. Chooses one and pushes plunger up and down a few times to make sure it will slide smoothly when drawing blood.	_____	_____	_____
5. Introduces self to client.	_____	_____	_____
6. Identifies client.	_____	_____	_____
7. Tells client, in everyday language, what medical assistant is going to do.	_____	_____	_____
8. Asks if client has any questions. If client does, gives short and simple answers.	_____	_____	_____
9. Helps client into comfortable position.	_____	_____	_____
10. Lines up tubes in test rack in order of use.	_____	_____	_____
11. Applies tourniquet above desired venipuncture site.	_____	_____	_____
12. Puts on gloves, and mask or face shield if needed.	_____	_____	_____
13. Tells client to close hand into a fist, but do not pump fist.	_____	_____	_____
14. Finds vein.	_____	_____	_____
15. Wipes selected site with alcohol wipe.	_____	_____	_____
16. Lets site air-dry. Does not blow on site.	_____	_____	_____
17. Does not touch venipuncture site after cleaning it.	_____	_____	_____
18. Places thumb 1 to 2 inches below site. Pulls skin smooth and tight.	_____	_____	_____
19. Lines up needle with site. Keeps bevel of needle pointed up.	_____	_____	_____
20. Inserts needle into vein.	_____	_____	_____
21. With other hand, gently pulls on plunger of syringe.	_____	_____	_____
22. Pulls until amount of blood needed has entered syringe. Does not pull fast.	_____	_____	_____
23. Tells client to open hand.	_____	_____	_____
24. Using free hand, takes off tourniquet.	_____	_____	_____
25. Places gauze just above injection site.	_____	_____	_____
26. Takes needle and syringe out of client's arm.	_____	_____	_____

911

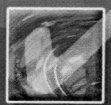
27. Applies pressure to puncture area for 3 minutes. If client is able, asks client to hold gauze over site and keep arm straight. Does not allow client to bend elbow. _____ _____ _____
28. Takes syringe to test tube rack. _____ _____ _____
29. Pushes needle into stopper of first tube. _____ _____ _____
30. Injects required amount of blood into tube. _____ _____ _____
31. Puts used syringe and needle into sharps container. _____ _____ _____
32. Throws away used gauze and alcohol wipes in biohazardous waste container. _____ _____ _____
33. Labels all blood tubes before leaving client's area. _____ _____ _____
34. Checks injection site and applies adhesive bandage. _____ _____ _____
35. Takes off gloves and disposes of them in biohazardous waste container. _____ _____ _____
36. Washes hands. _____ _____ _____
37. Talks with client and asks if client has any questions. _____ _____ _____
38. Records procedure correctly in client's chart. _____ _____ _____

Documentation

```



```

1st Observation

Date: _____ Evaluator Signature and Printed Name: _____

Comments:

2nd Observation

Date: _____ Evaluator Signature and Printed Name: _____

Comments:

Mastery

Date: _____ Evaluator Signature and Printed Name: _____

Comments:

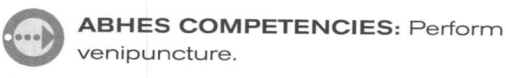

ABHES COMPETENCIES: Perform venipuncture.

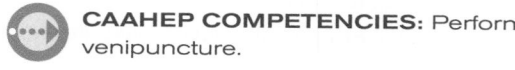

CAAHEP COMPETENCIES: Perform venipuncture.

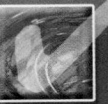

Name _____   Course _____

	1st Observation	2nd Observation	Mastery
1. Checks doctor's order for test.	_____	_____	_____
2. Washes hands.	_____	_____	_____
3. Gathers equipment and supplies.	_____	_____	_____
4. Introduces self to client.	_____	_____	_____
5. Identifies client.	_____	_____	_____
6. Tells client, in everyday language, what medical assistant is going to do.			
7. Asks if client has any questions. If client does, gives short and simple answers.	_____	_____	_____
8. Looks at possible sites. Makes sure area for capillary blood collection is free of bruises, scars, or open skin.	_____	_____	_____
9. Selects a site.	_____	_____	_____
10. Washes hands.	_____	_____	_____
11. Puts on gloves.	_____	_____	_____
12. Using alcohol wipe, cleans area selected.	_____	_____	_____
13. Lets area air-dry; does not blow on it.	_____	_____	_____
14. Opens sterile lancet package.	_____	_____	_____
15. Using nondominant hand, grasps client's finger (selected side) firmly with thumb and middle finger.	_____	_____	_____
16. With dominant hand, takes lancet and points it down.	_____	_____	_____
17. Punctures site with clear, decisive, down-and-up motion.	_____	_____	_____
18. Discards first drop of blood by wiping it away with sterile gauze.	_____	_____	_____
19. Continues to apply pressure on either side of site until obtains desired amount of blood. Does not "milk" site.	_____	_____	_____
20. Allows blood to drop onto collection device without touching skin.	_____	_____	_____
21. Applies gentle pressure to puncture site until bleeding stops.	_____	_____	_____
22. Labels collection containers in preparation for testing or processing.	_____	_____	_____
23. Discards contaminated items in biohazardous waste container and puts lancet in sharps container.	_____	_____	_____
24. Removes gloves.	_____	_____	_____
25. Washes hands.	_____	_____	_____
26. Records procedure correctly in client's chart.	_____	_____	_____

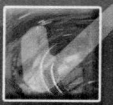

Competency Skill Checklist (Continued)

Documentation

1st Observation

Date: _____ Evaluator Signature and Printed Name: _____

Comments:

2nd Observation

Date: _____ Evaluator Signature and Printed Name: _____

Comments:

Mastery

Date: _____ Evaluator Signature and Printed Name: _____

Comments:

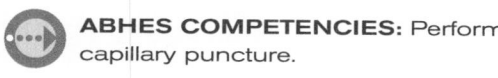 **ABHES COMPETENCIES:** Perform capillary puncture.

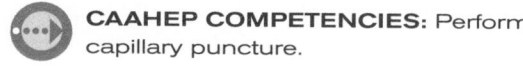 **CAAHEP COMPETENCIES:** Perform capillary puncture.

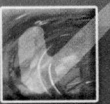

Name _____ Course _____

PROCEDURE

42-4

Hematology Testing: Erythrocyte Sedimentation Rate, Wintrobe Method

	1st Observation	2nd Observation	Mastery
1. Washes hands.	_____	_____	_____
2. Gathers equipment and supplies.	_____	_____	_____
3. Obtains 5 mL blood sample using lavender-top tube (anticoagulant).	_____	_____	_____
4. Gently inverts tube a number of times, but does not shake or agitate contents.	_____	_____	_____
5. Using a pipette, accurately fills Wintrobe tube to 0 point.	_____	_____	_____
6. Puts filled tube in holder. Tube is supported and straight up.	_____	_____	_____
7. Leaves undisturbed for 1 hour.	_____	_____	_____
8. Reads level of top of red blood cells.	_____	_____	_____
9. Writes results in log.	_____	_____	_____
10. Cleans equipment.	_____	_____	_____
11. Disposes of specimen and tubes and used supplies in biohazardous waste container.	_____	_____	_____
12. Removes gloves.	_____	_____	_____
13. Washes hands.	_____	_____	_____
14. Records procedure correctly in client's chart.	_____	_____	_____
15. Notifies doctor of results.	_____	_____	_____

Documentation

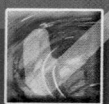

1st Observation

Date: _____ Evaluator Signature and Printed Name: _____

Comments:

2nd Observation

Date: _____ Evaluator Signature and Printed Name: _____

Comments:

Mastery

Date: _____ Evaluator Signature and Printed Name: _____

Comments:

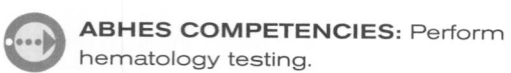 **ABHES COMPETENCIES:** Perform hematology testing.

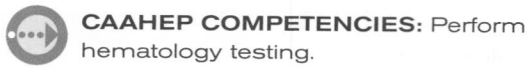 **CAAHEP COMPETENCIES:** Perform hematology testing.

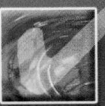

Name _____ Course _____

PROCEDURE

43-1

Obtaining an Electrocardiogram

	1st Observation	2nd Observation	Mastery
1. Washes hands.	_____	_____	_____
2. Gathers equipment and supplies.	_____	_____	_____
3. Plugs in ECG machine.	_____	_____	_____
4. Checks all cable wires.	_____	_____	_____
5. Looks around area to make sure nothing will create electrical interference.	_____	_____	_____
6. Snaps electrodes into pads.	_____	_____	_____
7. Checks room to ensure that atmosphere is quiet and comfortable and that room is at comfortable temperature.	_____	_____	_____
8. Introduces self to client.	_____	_____	_____
9. Identifies client.	_____	_____	_____
10. Tells client, in everyday language, what medical assistant is going to do.	_____	_____	_____
11. Asks if client has any questions. If client does, gives short and simple answers.	_____	_____	_____
12. Asks client about any allergies.	_____	_____	_____
13. Tells client to remain still, as machine will pick up any movement and thus distort readings.	_____	_____	_____
14. Reminds client that there is no pain from an ECG.	_____	_____	_____
15. Hands client a gown.	_____	_____	_____
16. Tells client to remove clothing from waist up.	_____	_____	_____
17. Helps client onto examination table.	_____	_____	_____
18. Asks client to lie on back.	_____	_____	_____
19. Places pillow under client's head.	_____	_____	_____
20. Drapes client for privacy.	_____	_____	_____
21. Turns ECG machine on.	_____	_____	_____
22. Puts in client's name and other required data.	_____	_____	_____
23. Wipes sites for electrode placement with alcohol wipes.	_____	_____	_____
24. Places arm electrodes on fleshy, muscular, outer area of upper arms (RA, LA).	_____	_____	_____
25. Places leg electrodes on fleshy inner area of calves of lower legs (RL, LL).	_____	_____	_____
26. Makes sure lead wires are not tangled.	_____	_____	_____
27. Connects lead wires to electrodes and ECG machine. Follows color-coded markings.	_____	_____	_____
28. Places chest electrodes (V1–V6).	_____	_____	_____

917

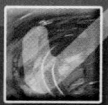

29. Rechecks electrode placement. _____ _____ _____
30. Presses "auto" button on ECG machine. _____ _____ _____
31. Allows 12-lead ECG to run through. _____ _____ _____
32. Removes ECG printout from machine. _____ _____ _____
33. Looks at printout for any artifacts. _____ _____ _____
34. If no artifacts are seen, turns machine off. _____ _____ _____
35. Takes electrodes off client. _____ _____ _____
36. Wipes electrode placement sites dry, cleaning all gel off. _____ _____ _____
37. Disposes of used towels and wipes in appropriate waste container. _____ _____ _____
38. Helps client to sitting position. _____ _____ _____
39. Assists client to get off table, as needed. _____ _____ _____
40. Helps client to dress, as needed. _____ _____ _____
41. Discards used items such as paper table cover and gown, according to office policy. _____ _____ _____
42. Washes hands. _____ _____ _____
43. Records procedure correctly in client's chart. _____ _____ _____
44. Informs doctor that test has been completed. _____ _____ _____
45. Places ECG printout in client's chart or gives it to doctor, according to office policy. _____ _____ _____

Documentation

```



```

1st Observation

Date: _____ Evaluator Signature and Printed Name: _____

Comments:

2nd Observation

Date: _____ Evaluator Signature and Printed Name: _____

Comments:

Mastery

Date: _____ Evaluator Signature and Printed Name: _____

Comments:

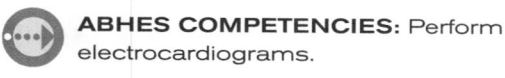
ABHES COMPETENCIES: Perform electrocardiograms.

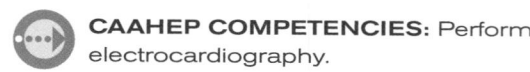
CAAHEP COMPETENCIES: Perform electrocardiography.

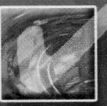
Name _____ Course _____

PROCEDURE

43-2   Holter Monitor Application

	1st Observation	2nd Observation	Mastery
1. Washes hands.	_____	_____	_____
2. Gathers equipment and supplies.	_____	_____	_____
3. Introduces self to client.	_____	_____	_____
4. Identifies client.	_____	_____	_____
5. Tells client, in everyday language, what medical assistant is going to do.	_____	_____	_____
6. Asks if client has any questions. If client does, gives short and simple answers.	_____	_____	_____
7. Tells client, in simple terms, that doctor needs to identify what is happening with heartbeat and determine what client can do to help his own heart health. Finding out what is going on will also help doctor to prescribe best treatment.	_____	_____	_____
8. Shows client monitor and all parts.	_____	_____	_____
9. Snaps white wire to electrode or patch; snaps green electrode to electrode or patch; snaps black wire to electrode or patch.	_____	_____	_____
10. Asks client to unbutton shirt (need not remove it completely).	_____	_____	_____
11. Finds area on client's chest that is one to two fingers' width below clavicle on right side of chest. Cleans area with alcohol wipe.	_____	_____	_____
12. Removes backing from patch attached to white wire and places it at point located.	_____	_____	_____
13. Finds area on client's chest that is one to two fingers' width below clavicle on left side of chest. Cleans area with alcohol wipe.	_____	_____	_____
14. Removes backing from patch attached to green wire and places it at point located.	_____	_____	_____
15. Finds area under left breast and moves hand to side until it is below client's underarm. Cleans area with alcohol wipe.	_____	_____	_____
16. Removes backing from patch attached to black wire and places it at point located.	_____	_____	_____
17. Picks up cassette. Puts battery into cassette. Attaches plug at end of each wire into opening in cassette.	_____	_____	_____

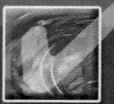
18. Shows client "event" button, "clear" button, and "low battery" button.
19. Performs a baseline recording.
20. Pushes and holds "event" button down until it beeps.
21. Tells client that when client feels any symptoms, client should push "event" button.
22. Tells client to write on a piece of paper (or log booklet) what client was doing when client felt symptoms. Keep written information to bring to doctor.

Documentation

1st Observation

Date: _____ Evaluator Signature and Printed Name: _____

Comments:

2nd Observation

Date: _____ Evaluator Signature and Printed Name: _____

Comments:

Mastery

Date: _____ Evaluator Signature and Printed Name: _____

Comments:

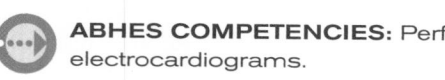 **ABHES COMPETENCIES:** Perform electrocardiograms.

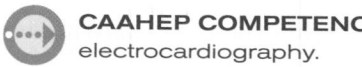 **CAAHEP COMPETENCIES:** Perform electrocardiography.

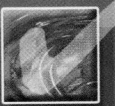

Name _____ Course _____

PROCEDURE

44-1

Blood Chemistry: Blood Glucose Testing

	1st Observation	2nd Observation	Mastery
1. Washes hands.	_____	_____	_____
2. Gathers equipment and supplies.	_____	_____	_____
3. Introduces self to client.	_____	_____	_____
4. Identifies client.	_____	_____	_____
5. Tells client, in everyday language, what medical assistant is going to do.	_____	_____	_____
6. Asks if client has any questions. If client does, gives short and simple answers.	_____	_____	_____
7. Puts test strip into opening on meter.	_____	_____	_____
8. Looks at code number displayed as meter turns on.	_____	_____	_____
9. Compares this number with code number on test strip vial.	_____	_____	_____
10. Puts on gloves.	_____	_____	_____
11. Firmly places lancet into lancet holder. Does not twist.	_____	_____	_____
12. Chooses puncture depth using adjustment knob or wheel.	_____	_____	_____
13. Cleans side of client's fingertip with alcohol wipe. Allows site to air-dry before puncturing.	_____	_____	_____
14. Places lancet against selected site on client's finger and pushes release button.	_____	_____	_____
15. Massages puncture site gently to increase blood flow. Does not squeeze.	_____	_____	_____
16. Holds drop of blood on test strip when display symbol appears.	_____	_____	_____
17. Waits for meter to count down.	_____	_____	_____
18. Reads blood glucose test results displayed in meter window.	_____	_____	_____
19. Writes down number displayed.	_____	_____	_____
20. Removes used test strip.	_____	_____	_____
21. Asks client if client has any questions.	_____	_____	_____
22. Disposes of used test strip and alcohol wipe in biohazardous waste container.	_____	_____	_____
23. Removes cap from lancet holder. With lancet pointing down, ejects used lancet into sharps container.	_____	_____	_____
24. Removes gloves.	_____	_____	_____

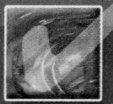
25. Washes hands. _____   _____   _____
26. Records procedure correctly in client's chart. _____   _____   _____

Documentation

```



```

1st Observation

Date: _____ Evaluator Signature and Printed Name: _____

Comments:

2nd Observation

Date: _____ Evaluator Signature and Printed Name: _____

Comments:

Mastery

Date: _____ Evaluator Signature and Printed Name: _____

Comments:

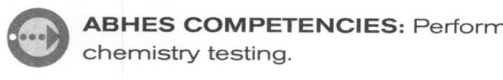
ABHES COMPETENCIES: Perform chemistry testing.

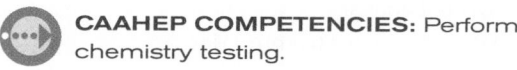
CAAHEP COMPETENCIES: Perform chemistry testing.

Glossary

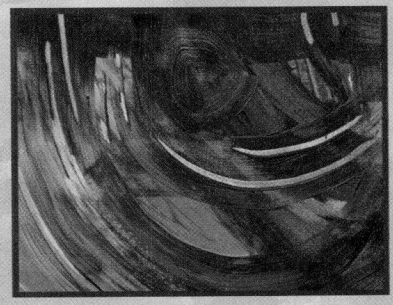

A

abdominal thrusts Procedure to aid in the removal of a foreign body airway obstruction (FBAO) in adults and children over one year of age; also called the *Heimlich maneuver* or *subdiaphragmatic abdominal thrusts.*

abscess Specific area or localized site that contains pus made up of dead bacteria, blood, and tissue.

absorption Process by which a substance is taken in and used; the taking up of a substance, such as medication, into or within the body.

accredited Standing awarded to a school program that meets the standards of an accrediting organization.

Accrediting Bureau of Health Education Schools (ABHES) A national organization that grants accreditation to medical assisting programs.

acquired immunodeficiency syndrome (AIDS) Disorder that causes the immune system to be suppressed; a serious, life-threatening disorder.

acromegaly Condition in which the bones of the face, hands, and feet become larger as a result of overproduction of growth hormone during adulthood.

activities of daily living (ADLs) Tasks that a person performs in everyday life, such as walking, eating, and toileting.

acupressure Use of fingers and hands to press on certain body points to ease pain and decrease harmful stress.

acupuncture Therapy that uses needles, inserted at specific body points, for relief of pain.

acute coryza Respiratory viral infection; also called the common cold.

Addison's disease Disorder in which the adrenal glands do not make enough corticosteroids.

adipose tissue Fat tissue.

administrative Skills and tasks regarding the business aspects of the office setting.

adrenal cortex Outer part of the adrenal gland; these glands are located above the kidneys.

adrenal medulla Inner part of the adrenal gland; these glands are located above the kidneys.

agglutination Clumping of red blood cells.

agranular White blood cells that do not have granules in the cytoplasm.

albumin The smallest of the plasma proteins.

allergen A protein or substance that sets off an allergic response in a person.

alveoli Small sacs at the end of the bronchial tree. Alveoli look like a bunch of grapes.

ambulatory Describes health care settings where a client who is not hospitalized receives care; the client ambulates (walks) into these settings.

American Academy of Pediatrics National organization that sets guidelines for the practice of pediatricians and the care of children.

American Association of Medical Assistants (AAMA) A national professional organization of medical assistants. The AAMA is a three-level group with local, state, and national divisions. It certifies medical assistants and maintains professional standards.

American Medical Technologists (AMT) A national professional organization that certifies medical assistants and other health professionals.

anatomical Position of the body when standing straight, facing forward, arms down at side with the palms of the hands forward.

anemia Disorder in which too little oxygen is delivered to the cells, either because there are too few red blood cells, the red blood cells lack hemoglobin, or there is low blood volume.

angina pectoris Condition in which the vessels to the heart are narrowed, causing pain upon physical activity or stress.

angiography Procedure that visualizes the blood vessels of the body.

anorexia nervosa Eating disorder in which a person starves herself or himself because of a distorted self-image of obesity.

antibodies Produced by the body to fight off foreign proteins and other substances.

anticipatory guidance Explanation of what to expect from a child at a specific age; given for the purpose of encouraging parents to respond in a helpful way.

antidiuretic hormone (ADH) Released by the pituitary gland; tells the kidneys to conserve water.

antigen Protein or foreign substance, the entry of which into the body causes the body to respond by producing antibodies.

antioxidant effects Change free radicals from harmful substances, which can change DNA and increase a person's cancer risk, into nonharmful substances.

aorta The largest artery in the body.

appendicitis Inflammation of the appendix.

appendicular skeleton Bones of arms and legs.

aromatherapy Use of scents or odors from herbs or flowers to promote wellness or relief from stress and pain.

arteries Thick-walled blood vessels that carry blood away from the heart.

arteriosclerosis Coronary artery disorder in which the coronary arteries narrow and harden.

arthritis Inflammation of the joints.

artifacts In testing, something that shows up on a test (such as an ECG printout) that is not a valid result of the testing; for example, signals that are really caused by defective equipment or client movement during testing.

asepsis A state of being free from pathogenic microorganisms.

asthma Reactive airway disorder in which the tubes of the bronchial tree become narrowed; often caused by allergies or infection; client experiences difficulty in breathing during an acute episode.

astigmatism Abnormal curve or shape of the cornea (lens of the eye); causes blurry vision.

atelectasis Collapsed lung.

atherosclerosis Condition in which the walls of the arteries harden and collect fatty deposits.

atopic dermatitis Inflammation of skin caused by an allergic-type reaction.

atrophy Shrinking or decrease in size of tissue.

audiometer Instrument used to measure sharpness (acuity) of hearing.

auscultation Listening to sounds in the body.

autoclave Machine used to sterilize instruments and medical items.

autoimmune Describes a response in which the body mistakes its own tissue as foreign and begins to attack itself.

automated method Method of testing specimens by means of instruments that both perform tests and complete mathematical calculations to yield results.

autonomic nervous system The part of the nervous system that controls involuntary muscles and actions.

axial skeleton Bones of the trunk of the body.

axon The part of a neuron that carries impulses away from the cell body.

B

barium sulfate A substance used in some X-ray procedures to give contrast or distinguish internal structures from each other.

basal cell carcinoma Common type of skin cancer.

baseline Starting point or beginning set of measurements or observations that are used as a basis of comparison with future data.

basophil A type of white blood cell; sends out histamine and heparin to initiate and promote inflammation.

benign prostatic hyperplasia (BPH) Nonmalignant enlargement of the prostate gland.

bicuspid valve Valve found between the left atrium and the left ventricle of the heart.

biopsy Removal of a small piece of tissue to use for diagnostic testing.

bladder Hollow, muscular organ that holds urine until the urine is released from the body.

blood pressure Force of the blood against the walls of the blood vessels.

blood urea nitrogen (BUN) Test that measures the amount of urea nitrogen in the blood.

body mechanics Use of the body based on a view of the body as a machine. A person must keep the body in good alignment and use the correct muscles when moving and lifting to prevent injury to the body.

bradykinesia Very slow movement.

bronchus Tube-like structure that extends from the trachea to the lung. There is a left and a right bronchus.

bruit Abnormal noise or sound, usually heard with a stethoscope.

buccal medications Medications held within the cheek to dissolve.

bulbourethral glands Small glands found on either side of the urethra in males.

bullae Blisters.

bursa A space near the joints; holds synovial fluid to reduce friction between tendons, bones, and ligaments.

bursitis Inflammation of the bursa.

C

cancer Uncontrolled growth of abnormal cells, which can crowd out and damage healthy tissues.

capillary The smallest type of blood vessel.

carbohydrates The major source of energy for the body.

cardiac arrest Often called "heart attack"; condition in which vital organs are deprived of blood when heart action and circulation stop or are interrupted.

cardiac conduction system System that sends electrical impulses through the heart.

cardiac dysrhythmia Irregular heart conduction cycle, rate, and rhythm.

cardiac muscle A type of involuntary muscle found only in the heart.

cardiopulmonary resuscitation (CPR) Procedure to restore spontaneous circulation in a person.

caregiver A person who helps another with activities of daily living on a regular basis.

carotene Yellow pigment that is the precursor of vitamin A.

cartilage Type of connective tissue that helps to absorb shock to the bones and allows smooth movement.

cataract A clouding of the normally clear lens of the eye.

catheter Hollow tubing that can be inserted and threaded through a vessel such as a vein.

cell The basic unit of all living organisms.

cerebellum The second largest part of the brain; concerned with coordination and movement.

cerebrum The largest part of the brain.

certificate Diploma or document given to an individual who has successfully completed a program of study.

certified medical assistant (CMA) Medical assistant who has met the criteria for certification, including passing a national certification examination of the American Association of Medical Assistants.

chancre Painless sore, often on the genitals, cervix, or anus.

chest circumference Measurement around a person's chest; routinely obtained on infants.

chief complaint (CC) The main reason or problem that made the client seek help from the health care provider.

cholecystography X-ray procedure to view the gallbladder; this procedure is currently being replaced with ultrasound.

cirrhosis Liver disorder that damages the cells of the liver.

clean-catch Method of collecting a urine sample; reduces the possibility of contamination from the area near the urinary meatus.

client The patient or person seeking help from a health care provider; also called *patient* or *health care consumer*.

clinical Medical skills and tasks regarding direct care in a health care setting.

Clinical Laboratory Improvement Amendments of 1988 (CLIA) Federal law and associated regulations that govern all testing facilities.

cognitive Intellectual ability and functioning.

colon Part of the large intestine that extends from the cecum to the rectum.

Commission on Accreditation of Allied Health Programs (CAAHEP) National organization that sets standards and accredits allied health programs such as medical assisting programs.

comorbidity Two or more separate disorders or health problems occurring at the same time.

complete blood count (CBC) A series of tests that examines all three types of blood cells.

computerized tomography (CT scan) X-ray procedure that uses a small beam of radiation to produce a cross-sectional picture.

concave Rounded or curved inward.

concussion Injury to the brain caused by trauma from outside of the head (for example, a blow to a boxer's head during a fight, or a soccer ball forcefully hitting a player's head).

conduction Transfer of heat from one object to another.

conductivity The ability to send impulses or messages.

condyloid Pertaining to a bulge or prominence that is knuckle-like.

congestive heart failure Inability of the heart to perform its work as a pump.

constipation Condition in which the feces are hard, dry, and difficult or painful to pass.

contact dermatitis Inflammation of skin caused by coming into contact with an irritant.

contamination Process of becoming dirty or infected with microorganisms.

contractibility The ability to shrink or get smaller in size.

contracture Permanent shortening of tissue that causes a deformity.

contrast medium Substance administered internally to client that helps distinguish between organs and surrounding structures during a radiological study.

convection Transfer of heat from an object to cooler air surrounding the object.

convex Rounded or curved out.

cornea Tough outer covering of the eyeball.

coronary Relating to the heart.

coronary heart disease Common term for any heart disorder.

cranial Pertaining to the skull (from which the *cranial* nerves originate)

cranial cavity Space in the head that contains the brain.

cretinism Severe hypothyroidism in children; causes mental retardation and retardation of physical development.

curette Scraping instrument with a ring or loop on one end.

Cushing's syndrome Disorder in which too much cortisol is made; a disease of the pituitary gland.

cyst A closed, defined area, like a pouch or sac, that contains liquid, dead cells, and/or waxy material.

cystitis Inflammation of the bladder.

cystocele Condition in which the bladder protrudes into the vagina.

cystography X-ray examination of the bladder.

D

dementia Steady decrease in mental ability that affects all parts of mental functioning. Dementia eventually impairs a person's ability to perform activities of daily living.

dendrite A part of the neuron that carries impulses to the cell body.

dermis True skin.

developmental level Status (usually related to age) to which the child has grown in skill and function.

diabetes insipidus Lack of antidiuretic hormone, which causes excess urination of dilute urine.

diabetes mellitus Chronic disorder affecting metabolism; associated with too little production of insulin or inability to use insulin.

diagnostic radiology The use of X-rays or radioactive substances to diagnose disorders.

diarrhea Passing of loose or liquid feces or waste material.

diastole Phase in the cardiac cycle when the heart relaxes.

diencephalon The part of the brain that contains the thalamus and hypothalamus.

digestion Process of breaking down food into smaller and simpler parts that can be used by the body.

dislocation Displacement of one or more bones at a joint.

distribution Sending out to specific sites or places.

diverticulitis Inflammation of diverticula (sacs or pouches in the intestine).

diverticulosis Formation of sacs or pouches in the intestine; does not cause any symptoms.

dorsal recumbent position Examination position in which the client lies on the back with the knees bent and feet flat on the exam table surface.

double-voided Method of collecting urine sample that involves voiding or urinating twice.

dysmenorrhea Moderate or intense pain during the menstrual blood flow.

E

ecchymosis Bruising; bleeding under the skin.

echocardiogram Graphic record of the structure and activity of the different parts of the heart.

elasticity The ability to return to original shape after being stretched or pulled.

electrocardiogram (ECG or EKG) Graphic record of the electrical impulses of the heart muscle.

electrode Consists of a wire connected to a patch that is applied to a client's skin; acts as a sensor to pick up and record electrical activity of the heart.

elimination Act of releasing or getting rid of waste products from the body.

emphysema Chronic pulmonary condition with impaired gas exchange due to damaged alveoli; often connected to smoking.

endocardium Inner layer of the heart.

endocrine glands Ductless glands that secrete hormones directly into the bloodstream.

endometriosis Tissue that looks like the endometrium but is located outside of the uterus.

endorphins Chemicals produced by the brain that help lessen pain perception.

eosinophil A type of white blood cell important in allergic reactions.

epicardium Outermost layer of the heart.

epidermis Outermost layer of the skin.

epididymis Small, tubelike organ next to the testis; holds sperm during maturation.

epiglottis Flap of tissue that prevents food and liquids from entering the larynx when swallowing.

epilepsy Disorder in which periodic misfiring of the electrical system of the brain results in a convulsion and/or partial or total loss of consciousness.

epithelial tissue Tissue that covers structures inside and on the surface of the body, thereby protecting these structures.

erythrocytes Red blood cells.

esophagus Connects the pharynx (throat) to the stomach.

estrogen Hormone produced by the ovaries; important in the menstrual cycle and responsible for secondary sex characteristics in the female.

evaporation Passing off of moisture in the form of a vapor; as the moisture becomes a gas, it cools the body.

excretion Getting rid of or moving a solid substance out of the body.

exocrine glands Glands that secrete hormones into ducts, which then open onto a body surface.

F

fallopian tubes Tubes that carry eggs from the ovaries to the uterus.

fibrinogen Plasma protein involved in blood clotting.

fibromyalgia Painful musculoskeletal condition.

fissure Crack in the skin or mucous membrane.

flatulence Excessive gas in the digestive tract.

fluoroscopy X-ray procedure done to observe movement and action inside the body.

forceps Instruments used to hold or grab tissue or blood vessels.

Fowler's position Examination position in which the client's back is supported at a 90-degree angle.

fracture To break; a break.

G

gait An individual's pattern of walking or ambulation.

gallbladder Organ that stores bile made in the liver; found under the right lobe of the liver.

gastroenteritis An inflammation of the stomach and intestine.

genetic Inherited.

genital herpes Sexually transmitted disease that is highly contagious.

genital wart Sexually transmitted condition; frequently reappears after initial treatment.

geriatrics Field of medicine related to aging and the older client.

gestational Pertains to pregnancy.

gestational diabetes Diabetes that occurs during pregnancy.

gigantism Overproduction of growth hormone during childhood.

globulin Plasma protein that protects the body from infection.

glomerular filtration Action of the kidneys that strains or filters blood.

glomerulonephritis Inflammation of the glomeruli; can harm the nephrons. This can be an acute or a chronic condition.

glomerulus The filtering unit of the kidney.

glucose Sugar; used by the body as a source of energy.

glucose tolerance test (GTT) Test to determine the metabolism of glucose in the body.

goiter Enlargement of the thyroid gland.

gonad Reproductive or sex organ (testes in the male, ovaries in the female).

gonorrhea Common sexually transmitted disease; often seen in teenagers and young adults.

Grave's disease Hyperthyroidism; condition in which the thyroid gland produces too much of the thyroid hormones.

H

hair follicle Small depression that surrounds the hair shaft; hair receives nourishment in this area.

hay fever Seasonally related form of allergic response. Sneezing, runny nose, and watery or itchy eyes are common symptoms.

head circumference Measurement around a person's head; routinely obtained on an infant.

health care team Individuals from different professions who work together to give quality health care to a client.

Health Insurance Portability and Accountability Act (HIPAA) Law passed by Congress in 1996 dealing with privacy of client information, among other matters.

hearing impairment Loss of part or all of the ability to hear.

hematocrit In blood testing, the ratio of packed red blood cells to whole blood volume.

hemoglobin Oxygen-carrying part of the blood cell.

hemophilia Genetic disorder found mostly in males; causes slow clotting of blood, which can lead to severe blood loss from even a minor cut.

hepatitis Inflammation or infection of the liver.

hernia Weakening of a muscular wall through which internal structures can protrude.

high-density lipoprotein (HDL) Also called "good" cholesterol; helps to protect against coronary artery disease.

Hodgkin's disease Malignant disorder with progressive enlargement of lymphoid tissue.

Holter monitor Similar to an electrocardiograph, but is portable, which allows recordings to be done as a client goes through daily activities.

hormone Chemical released by endocrine glands.

human immunodeficiency virus (HIV) Viral infection that weakens a person's immune system.

hydrochloric acid Secreted in the stomach; aids in the digestion of protein and kills bacteria.

hypercholesterolemia Too much cholesterol in the blood.

hyperglycemia High blood sugar levels.

hyperopia Farsightedness.

hypersensitivity disorders Overly susceptible or reactive to a substance or stimulus.

hypertension High blood pressure.

hypoglycemia Low blood sugar levels.

hypothalamus Part of the diencephalon of the brain; part of the nervous system that regulates the pituitary gland and specifically regulates body temperature.

I

immunization Process of making a person immune or resistant to a disease; usually done by injection.

immunodeficiency disorders Conditions in which the immune system does not respond, or responds insufficiently, to an invasion.

impairment Loss of the use or function of part or all of a body system; may also include an abnormality of a structure.

incision A clean, neat cut, such as that made by a scalpel.

inflammation Body's response to defend against invasion and to help heal injured tissue.

inflammatory Describes the body's response to cell or tissue injury.

influenza A respiratory infection that comes on suddenly; in frail individuals or those with chronic conditions, may be fatal. More commonly called the *flu*.

infusion pump Electronic equipment that delivers fluid at a prescribed, set rate.

insertion site Point at which a needle is put into the vein.

inspection Looking closely; a careful examination.

insulin Hormone released by the pancreas; involved in carbohydrate metabolism.

integumentary Refers to a covering, such as the skin.

interferon Protein that counteracts viruses.

interview Meeting during which one person seeks information from another in order to reach a decision (job interview, client interview).

intestinal obstruction Blockage in the intestines that interferes with movement of the contents through the intestine.

intradermal Under or within the dermis part of the skin; within the layers of the skin.

intramuscular Within the muscle layers.

intravenous Within the veins.

intravenous pyelography (IVP) X-ray examination of the kidneys, ureters, and bladder.

iodine compound A substance used in some X-ray procedures as a contrast medium; helps distinguish internal structures from each other.

irritability The ability to quickly react to something, such as a stimulus.

irritable bowel syndrome (IBS) Motility disorder of the colon that sometimes causes diarrhea and other times causes constipation.

islets of Langerhans Cells in pancreas that secrete glucagons and insulin.

isometric exercises Exercises that involve muscular contractions with sharp increase in muscle tone and very little shortening of muscle fibers.

isotonic exercises Exercises that involve muscular contractions with very little increase in muscle tone and much shortening of muscle fibers.

J

joint Point where a part of the skeleton and surrounding structures meet.

K

keratin A protein that provides a protective shield for the skin.

kidneys Organs important in waste removal, in the production of urine, and in the maintenance of homeostasis.

kyphosis Thoracic curvature of the spine; hunchback.

L

lacrimal gland Gland that makes tears; located in the eye.

large intestine Extends from the small intestine to the outside of the body at the anus.

larynx Voice box.

leadership The ability of a person to guide and direct others with influence and authority.

leads The wires that go from the electrocardiograph machine to the client.

lesion A specific difference in the appearance of the skin in a defined area.

leukemia Condition in which bone marrow makes abnormal white blood cells that the body cannot use to fight off infections.

leukocytes White blood cells.

lifestyle The typical way in which a person lives his life.

ligament Tough, strong band of tissue connecting the ends of bones.

lipids Fats.

lithotomy position Examination position in which the client is on the back with the legs bent and the feet supported in stirrups.

liver Organ found in the upper right part of the abdominal cavity; has many vital functions.

lordosis Lumbar curvature of the spine; swayback.

low-density lipoprotein (LDL) Also called "bad" cholesterol; travels through the bloodstream and then lodges in peripheral tissues.

lung cancer Cancer that affects the lungs; very frequently connected to smoking.

lymph Pale, watery fluid important in immunity and defense.

lymphocyte A type of white blood cell concerned with immunity.

M

magnetic resonance imaging (MRI) Procedure that uses a strong magnetic field and radio waves to view internal structures; does not use X-rays.

malignant melanoma Serious cancer of the melanocytes in the skin and mucous membranes.

mammary glands Glands in the breast; in females, secrete milk after childbirth.

mammogram X-ray of the breast.

manual method Method of testing in which handling of specimens and calculation of results is done by the individual laboratory worker, by hand.

Material Safety Data Sheet (MSDS) A manufacturer's document setting out directions for use and storage of a substance, identifying hazards, and specifying measures for emergency handling of the product; also, an employer's listing of potentially hazardous substances that a worker might encounter on the job.

Medicaid Joint venture between the states and the federal government to help finance health care for those who are in financial need or disabled.

medical asepsis Techniques used to decrease the number and transmission of pathogenic organisms.

medical assistant Multiskilled professional who performs both clinical and administrative tasks in a variety of health care settings.

medical clearance Statement by doctor that no known condition exists that would prevent participation in an activity such as surgery or exercise.

Medicare Federal program to help finance health care for people who are over the age of 65 or disabled.

medulla Area in the brain that controls respirations.

medulla oblongata The part of the brainstem that controls vital life processes.

melanin Pigment that gives the skin, hair, and eyes their color.

menopause The cessation of the menstrual cycle; signals the end of a female's reproductive years.

menorrhagia Excessive bleeding during the menstrual flow.

metabolism Processing of substances within the body; process of chemical changes in the body as energy is used and new material is taken in and broken down for use as fuel for the body.

metric Uses meter and kilogram as a system for measuring lengths and weights.

metrorrhagia Bleeding between menstrual flow periods.

microorganism A tiny living plant or animal that is too small to be seen with the eye unless aided by an instrument.

microscope Optical instrument that uses lenses to enlarge or magnify a specimen.

mitral valve Also called the bicuspid valve.

mobility Ability to move and change place and direction.

monitor Machine that watches and (usually) records.

monocyte A type of white blood cell; helps to kill some bacteria and viruses and neutralize toxins.

mononucleosis Increase in the number of mononuclear lymphocytes (a type of white blood cell).

multiple sclerosis Progressive disorder in which the myelin sheath of the nerves is destroyed. Frequently begins in young adulthood.

muscular dystrophy Inherited disorder characterized by progressive weakening of muscles.

myasthenia gravis Neuromuscular disorder with progressive weakening of voluntary muscles.

myocardial infarction Heart attack; complete blockage of one or more vessels to the heart.

myocardium Middle layer of the heart.

myopia Nearsightedness.

myxedema Severe form of hypothyroidism in adults; caused by lack of thyroid hormones.

N

nephron Functional or working part of the kidneys.

neurogenic Caused by the nerves.

neuroglia Nerve cells that support the neurons; the "glue" of the nervous system.

neuron Working or functional cell of the nervous system that transmits impulses.

neutropenia Decrease in the number of neutrophils, a type of white blood cell.

neutrophils Most numerous of the white blood cells.

nicotine Addictive ingredient in tobacco.

nonpathogenic Describes microorganisms that do not normally cause disease.

nonspecific immunity The body's defense against invasion by all types of foreign substances.

nonverbal sign Communication by means other than the spoken word.

nuclear medicine Branch of medicine that uses radioactive material to diagnose or treat disorders.

O

Occupational Safety and Health Administration (OSHA) Organization that regulates workplace safety and protects the health and safety of workers.

occupational therapist Rehabilitation specialist who helps clients with ADLs.

orchitis Inflammation of the testis.

organs Groups of tissue(s) that have the same function.

osseous Pertaining to bone or collagen.

osteoporosis Loss of bone mass; puts a person at risk of fractures.

otitis media Inflammation of the middle ear.

otosclerosis Condition that affects the bones in the ear and thus causes hearing loss.

ovary Female reproductive organ.

over-the-counter (OTC) medication Drugs or medicines that can be purchased without a prescription from a health care provider.

ovum Female reproductive cell.

P

pain Unpleasant bodily feeling caused by a stimulus that alerts the body to damage or a problem. May be described as sharp, dull, aching, or throbbing.

palpation Process of examining by touch, using the fingers.

pancreas Gland/organ that has both endocrine and exocrine functions.

pancreatitis Inflammation of the pancreas.

parasympathetic nervous system The part of the autonomic nervous system that controls digestion and takes over body functions during times of rest.

parathyroid One of four glands that secrete hormones to regulate levels of calcium in the blood.

Parkinson's disease Progressive neurological disorder characterized by muscle rigidity and tremors.

patch test Test to determine a person's level of allergic response to common allergens. The test involves putting a small amount of substances on the skin and covering them with a dressing. After the dressing is removed, the response on the skin is noted.

pathogen Disease-causing microorganism.

pathogenic Disease-causing.

pediatrics Medical specialty that oversees the normal growth and development of infants and children and provides care for sick infants and children.

peduncles Bands of fibers that connect parts of the brain; they look like stalks of a plant.

pelvic cavity The space in the body that contains the reproductive organs, urinary bladder, rectum, part of the large intestine, and the appendix.

pelvic inflammatory disease (PID) Infection of the pelvic organs.

penis Organ of copulation (sexual intercourse).

percussion Process of examining by tapping a surface to listen to internal sounds.

peripheral nervous system The part of the nervous system outside of the central nervous system; consists of the cranial nerves and spinal nerves.

personal protective equipment (PPE) Equipment that helps to keep workers safe from and avoid contact with hazardous materials. Examples of PPE are gloves, gowns, masks, and face shields.

phagocytosis Process by which cells surround and destroy bacteria.

pharynx Throat.

phenylketonuria (PKU) Disorder in which the amino acid phenylalanine cannot be changed to tyrosine. Untreated, PKU can lead to severe cognitive impairments. Screening is done within a few days after birth.

phlebitis Inflammation of a vein.

physical therapist Rehabilitation specialist who helps clients with use of their muscles and movement.

pineal gland Small gland in the brain that secretes melatonin.

pituitary gland Small gland in the brain that has an anterior (front) and posterior (back) area; involved in many bodily functions.

pivot Turn.

plaque A localized patch or area of skin.

plasma The liquid part of the blood.

platelet Part of the blood that is involved in blood clotting.

pleurisy Inflammation of the pleura in the thoracic (chest) cavity.

pneumonia Inflammation or infection of the lungs.

polycystic Many cysts (in the kidneys).

polycythemia Too many erythrocytes or red blood cells.

postprandial After a meal; some urine specimens are collected at a specific time after the client has eaten.

precursor Substance out of which another substance is made.

premenstrual syndrome (PMS) Symptoms that occur in some women about one week before the menstrual flow; may include bloating, breast tenderness, irritability, weight gain, and headaches.

presbyopia Condition in which the lens of the eye loses the ability of accommodation; usually occurs as a person ages.

preventive Steps taken to maintain health and avoid medical problems or disorders.

progesterone Hormone secreted by the ovaries.

prolapsed uterus Uterus that protrudes downward.

prone position Examination position in which the client lies flat with the face downward.

prostate cancer An abnormal, harmful growth of the prostate gland.

prostate gland Gland that encircles the upper end of the urethra in males, just below the bladder.

protected health information (PHI) Health information that identifies an individual.

prothrombin Plasma protein involved in the clotting process.

proximal Near the center or center point.

psoriasis A chronic condition that causes dry, elevated, silvery lesions.

pubic symphysis Also called *pelvic girdle*; place where the bones come together at the front of the pelvic region.

pulmonary Refers to the lungs.

pulmonary valve Valve found between the right ventricle and the pulmonary artery.

pulse Beating of the heart. May be felt or heard as a tapping sound in an artery near a bony prominence.

Purkinje fibers Heart fibers found in the walls of the ventricles of the heart.

pustule Small, reddened, raised or elevated vesicle containing pus.

pyelitis Inflammation of the cavities of the kidneys.

pyelonephritis Bacterial infection of the kidney; can be acute or chronic.

Q

quality control Procedures and systems to ensure that test results are reliable and accurate.

R

radiation Transfer of heat in the form of waves.

radiologist Physician who specializes in using X-rays and radioactive substances to diagnose and treat disease.

radiology Science that studies the use of X-rays and radioactive substances in diagnosis and treatment of disease.

radiolucent Lets X-rays pass through; on an X-ray film, a radiolucent structure looks black.

radiopaque Blocks X-rays; on an X-ray film, a radiopaque structure looks white.

random In urine testing, refers to a sample taken at any time of the day.

ratchets Notches on an instrument that hold the instruments closed or open at a specific degree.

reagent test strip Plastic or cardboard strips that contain specific chemicals; used to test for substances in the urine.

rectocele Condition in which the rectum protrudes into the vagina.

reference laboratory Laboratories that do complex testing; many rules and regulations govern these facilities.

refractometer Instrument used to measure the specific gravity of urine; uses a light, prism, and scale.

registered medical assistant (RMA) Medical assistant who has met the professional examination requirements set by the American Medical Technologists.

rehabilitation Process to help a client attain the highest possible level of functioning after an injury or illness.

renal threshold Level at which a substance begins to "spill over" from the kidney into the urine.

resident flora Microorganisms found in the deeper layers of the skin or the mouth; most are usually harmless, but they are not removed by routine handwashing.

respirations Taking in and letting out of air, during which oxygen and carbon dioxide are exchanged in the alveoli of the lungs. One inhalation (breathing in) and one exhalation (breathing out) is counted as one respiration.

review of systems (ROS) Organized, step-by-step review of major body systems.

rheumatic fever Autoimmune disorder in which, after an infection, the antibodies produced then attack the heart, valves, and joints.

rheumatoid arthritis Autoimmune disorder that attacks the joints.

Rinne test Test to compare bone-conduction hearing with air-conduction hearing.

roller clamp A device attached to tubing that can be opened to various degrees or completely closed to regulate the flow of fluid through the tubing.

S

salivary gland Releases saliva.

scalpel Surgical knife used to make incisions.

scoliosis Abnormal curvature of the spine; usually discovered during the early childhood years.

scrotum Saclike structure that holds the testes.

sebaceous Refers to sebum, an oily, waxy substance, secreted by certain glands.

sedative Substance that quiets, soothes, or tranquilizes.

seizures Erratic, disorganized electrical impulses discharged within the brain; sudden misfiring of the electrical rhythm of the central nervous system. Seizures occur suddenly and may have consequent muscular effects.

semen Thick, sticky fluid in which sperm cells move and are transported.

semi-Fowler's position Examination position in which the client's back is supported at a 45-degree angle.

semilunar valves Two valves found at the point where the blood leaves the ventricles.

seminal vesicles Glands that make more than half the volume of semen.

sensorineural hearing loss Hearing loss caused by nerve damage to the inner ear or auditory nerve.

serum Liquid part of the blood remaining after a clot forms.

sickle cell anemia Disorder in which red blood cells become sickle-shaped because of abnormal hemoglobin.

Sims' position A side-lying position in which the upper leg is sharply flexed.

sinus Cavity or hollow space.

skeletal muscle Voluntary muscles that connect to the skeleton and allow movement of the body.

smooth muscle A type of muscle that is involuntary; found in the internal organs.

Snellen chart A chart with letters or symbols used to measure visual acuity.

special needs General term describing clients who need either a procedure or service done somewhat differently to achieve the same results as with a client who does not have any impairment.

specific immunity The body's memory of a response to a particular foreign substance or organism.

specimen Small amount of tissue used for examination and testing; sample or part representing the whole of a tissue or substance.

speculum An instrument used to open or enlarge an area for easier viewing.

speech impairment Loss of part or all of the ability to communicate effectively with others through verbalizing.

spermatazoa (sperm) Male gamete or germ cell.

sphygmomanometer Instrument used to measure blood pressure.

spinal fusion Surgical procedure in which selected vertebrae are joined together.

spleen Vascular organ found in the upper left region of the abdominal cavity.

sprain Injury to a joint.

stethoscope Instrument used to hear sounds from inside the body; often used to listen to heart and lung sounds.

stirrups Metal supports attached to an exam table in which the client places the feet (or heels) to assume the lithotomy position; so named because the attachments look like the stirrups on a saddle.

stomach Organ found in the upper left part of the abdominal cavity; receives food, helps to break it down, and moves it to the small intestine.

strain Injury to a muscle or tendon caused by overuse.

stroke Cerebral vascular accident; sometimes called a *brain attack.*

subacute A level of care that is less intense than the acute level, but where the client is still not independent and needs skilled health care.

subcutaneous Below the skin; under the epidermal and dermal layers of the skin.

sublingual Under the tongue.

supine position Lying on the back with the face up.

surgical asepsis Sterile techniques.

suture Thread used to sew or bring together tissue in surgical procedures.

sympathetic nervous system The part of the autonomic nervous system that becomes active in "fight or flight" situations.

synovial Relating to the lubricating fluid called synovia.

syringe Cylinder-shaped instrument, usually made of plastic (sometimes glass), that holds a medication to be injected.

syringe method Method of obtaining a blood sample using a needle and a syringe; the blood from the syringe is then injected into a tube. Used most frequently on a person with small or fragile veins.

system A group of organs that work together to perform the same function.

systemic lupus erythematosus (SLE) Autoimmune disorder that can cause inflammation of one or more organs of the body.

systole Phase in the cardiac cycle when the heart contracts.

T

temperature A measurement of the hotness or coldness of the body.

tertiary Third order or stage; medical care available only in large health care centers.

testicular cancer Cancer of the testes; most commonly seen in young men.

testis Male gonad (sex organ).

testosterone Hormone made and secreted by the testes.

therapeutic radiology The use of X-rays to treat diseases.

therapeutic touch Use of the practitioner's hands and the energy from the client to promote a sense of well-being. The practitioner's hands, held a few inches off the skin, are passed over the client's body.

thermometer Instrument used to measure temperature.

thermoregulation Regulation of body temperature.

thoracic cavity The space in the body that contains the lungs, heart, trachea, esophagus, thymus gland, and large blood vessels.

thrombocytes Platelets; involved in the clotting of blood.

thrombocythemia Too many platelets in the blood.

thrombocytopenia Too few platelets in the blood.

thymus gland Gland found in the thoracic (chest) area.

thyroid Gland found in the front part of the neck; plays a major role in metabolism.

tissue A group of cells the function of which is similar.

tongue Muscle that takes part in digestion; has taste buds and is critical for speech.

tonsils Found in the oral cavity and pharynx; protect against invasion by bacteria.

topical Pertaining to the skin or mucous membranes.

tourniquet Springy material resembling a tube that is used to close off blood flow while selecting an insertion site.

trachea Also called windpipe; a tube-like structure that divides into a left and right bronchus.

transducer Piece of equipment that changes or adjusts power or a signal from one system to transfer the power or signal in a usable form to another system.

transesophageal echo (TEE) A type of echocardiogram.

transient flora Microorganisms found in and on the upper layers of skin; picked up during the course of everyday activities. These can cause disease, but can easily be removed through use of correct handwashing technique.

transient ischemic attack (TIA) Similar to a stroke, except that the symptoms resolve. A TIA may be a warning of a coming cerebral vascular accident (stroke).

tricuspid valve Valve found between the right atrium and the right ventricle; has three flaps.

triglycerides Also called *fat*; stored in adipose tissue.

tubular reabsorption Return of blood to the general circulation after filtration by the kidneys.

tubular secretion Addition of material into the urine after filtration and maximum reabsorption.

U

ultrasound Sound waves used in echocardiography.

ureter Narrow tube that carries urine from the kidneys to the bladder. There are two ureters.

urethra Tube that carries urine to the outside of the body.

urethritis Inflammation of the urethra; most common in males.

urinalysis Testing of a sample of urine; may include physical, chemical, and/or microscopic examinations.

urinary meatus Opening that allows urine to exit the body from the urethra.

urinometer Instrument used to measure specific gravity of urine; uses a float with a stem and a scale.

urticaria Hives.

uterus Hollow, muscular organ in which a fetus grows and develops.

V

vaccination Administration of a preparation of living altered or killed microorganisms for the purpose of making a person resistant to or protecting a person from a specific disease.

vacuum-tube method Method of obtaining a blood sample using a needle and color-coded vacuum tube(s).

vagina Tube that extends from the uterus to the vulva.

vas deferens Also called *ductus deferens*; carries sperm from the epididymis to the ejaculatory duct.

venipuncture Puncture of a vein for the purpose of removing blood for testing.

vesicle Elevated area of skin containing liquid.

virus Smallest of the infectious organisms.

visceral cavity The space in the body that contains abdominal organs; also called the *abdominal cavity.*

visual impairment Loss of part or all of the ability to see.

vitiligo Loss of pigment in patchy areas of the skin.

void To release urine from the body.

vulva External structure of the female genitalia.

W

Weber test Hearing test in which a vibrating tuning fork is used. The fork is held against the midline of the top of the head to determine if there is unilateral deafness.

wheal Temporary swelling of an area of skin, such as hives or an intradermal injection.

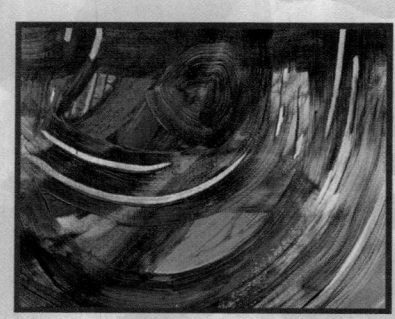

AAMA Role Delineation

Chapter	Title	Administrative Procedures	Practice Finances	Fundamental Principles
1.	The Medical Assisting Profession	X	X	X
2.	The Health Care Environment	X	X	X
3.	Infection Control	X	X	X
4.	Vital Signs	X		X
5.	Client Examination	X		X
6.	Organization of the Human Body			X
7.	Integumentary System			X
8.	Skeletal System			X
9.	Muscular System			X
10.	Nervous System and Sensory System			X
11.	Endocrine System			X
12.	Cardiovascular System			X
13.	Hematologic and Lymphatic Systems			X
14.	Immune System			X
15.	Respiratory System			X
16.	Digestive System			X
17.	Urinary System			X
18.	Male Reproductive System			X
19.	Female Reproductive System			X
20.	Integumentary System Disorders			X
21.	Skeletal System Disorders			X
22.	Muscular System Disorders			X
23.	Nervous System and Sensory System Disorders			X
24.	Endocrine System Disorders			X

Correlation Chart

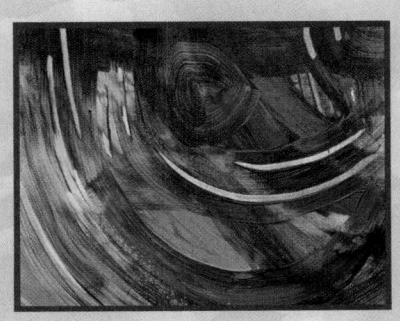

Diagnostic Orders	Patient Care	Professionalism	Communication Skills	Legal Concepts	Instruction	Operational Functions
X	X	X	X	X	X	X
X	X	X	X	X	X	X
X	X	X	X	X	X	X
X	X	X	X	X	X	
X	X	X	X	X	X	
X	X	X	X	X	X	
X	X	X	X	X	X	
X	X	X	X	X	X	
X	X	X	X	X	X	
X	X	X	X	X	X	
X	X	X	X	X	X	
	X	X	X	X	X	
	X	X	X	X	X	
	X	X	X	X	X	
	X	X	X	X	X	
X	X	X	X	X	X	
X	X	X	X	X	X	
	X	X	X	X	X	
	X	X	X	X	X	
	X	X	X	X	X	
	X	X	X	X	X	
X	X	X	X	X	X	
X	X	X	X	X	X	
X	X	X	X	X	X	

Chapter	Title	Administrative Procedures	Practice Finances	Fundamental Principles
25.	Cardiovascular System Disorders			X
26.	Hematologic and Lymphatic System Disorders			X
27.	Immune System Disorders	X		X
28.	Respiratory System Disorders			X
29.	Digestive System Disorders			X
30.	Urinary System Disorders			X
31.	Male Reproductive System Disorders			X
32.	Female Reproductive System Disorders			X
33.	The Client with Special Needs			X
34.	The Geriatric Client	X		X
35.	The Pediatric Client			X
36.	Medication and the Client Population	X		X
37.	Healthy Lifestyle in the Primary Client Population			X
38.	Minor Surgery	X		X
39.	Medical Office Emergencies and First Aid			X
40.	Physician Office Laboratory	X		X
41.	Urinalysis	X		X
42.	Hematology and Venipuncture			X
43.	Cardiac Diagnostic Laboratory			X
44.	Blood Chemistry	X		X
45.	Radiological Diagnostic Laboratory			X

Diagnostic Orders	Patient Care	Professionalism	Communication Skills	Legal Concepts	Instruction	Operational Functions
	X	X	X	X	X	
X	X	X	X	X	X	
X	X	X	X	X	X	
X	X	X	X	X	X	
X	X	X	X	X	X	
X	X	X	X	X	X	
X	X	X	X	X	X	
X	X	X	X	X	X	
X	X	X	X	X	X	
X	X	X	X	X	X	
X	X	X	X	X	X	
X	X	X	X	X	X	X
X	X	X	X	X	X	
X	X	X	X	X	X	X
X	X	X	X	X	X	X
X	X	X	X	X	X	X
X	X	X	X	X	X	X
X	X	X	X	X	X	X
X	X	X	X	X	X	X
X	X	X	X	X	X	X
X	X	X	X	X	X	X

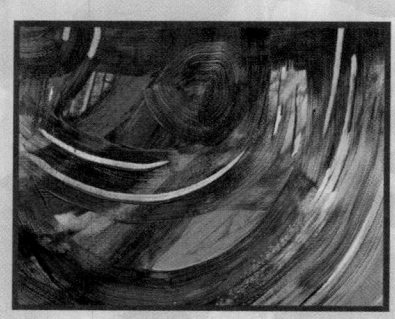

ABHES Curriculum

Chapter	Title	Orientation	Anatomy & Physiology	Medical Terminology
1.	The Medical Assisting Profession	X		X
2.	The Health Care Environment	X	X	X
3.	Infection Control		X	X
4.	Vital Signs		X	X
5.	Client Examination		X	X
6.	Organization of the Human Body		X	X
7.	Integumentary System		X	X
8.	Skeletal System		X	X
9.	Muscular System		X	X
10.	Nervous System and Sensory System		X	X
11.	Endocrine System		X	X
12.	Cardiovascular System		X	X
13.	Hematologic and Lymphatic Systems		X	X
14.	Immune System		X	X
15.	Respiratory System		X	X
16.	Digestive System		X	X
17.	Urinary System		X	X
18.	Male Reproductive System		X	X
19.	Female Reproductive System		X	X
20.	Integumentary System Disorders		X	X
21.	Skeletal System Disorders		X	X
22.	Muscular System Disorders		X	X
23.	Nervous System and Sensory System Disorders		X	X
24.	Endocrine System Disorders		X	X

Correlation Guide

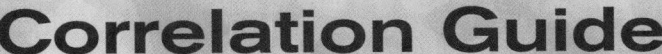
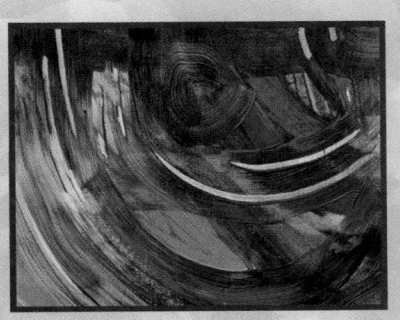

Medical Law & Ethics	Psychology of Human Relations	Pharmacology	Medical Office Business Procedures/ Management	Basic Keyboarding	Medical Office Clinical Procedures	Medical Laboratory Procedures	Career Development
X	X						X
X	X						X
X	X				X		
X	X				X		
X	X				X		
					X		
					X		
X					X		
X					X		
					X		
X					X		
					X		
					X		
					X		
X					X		
X					X		
X					X		
X					X		
X					X		
X					X		
X					X		
X					X		
X					X		
X					X		

Chapter	Title	Orientation	Anatomy & Physiology	Medical Terminology
25.	Cardiovascular System Disorders		X	X
26.	Hematologic and Lymphatic System Disorders		X	X
27.	Immune System Disorders		X	X
28.	Respiratory System Disorders		X	X
29.	Digestive System Disorders		X	X
30.	Urinary System Disorders		X	X
31.	Male Reproductive System Disorders		X	X
32.	Female Reproductive System Disorders		X	X
33.	The Client with Special Needs		X	X
34.	The Geriatric Client		X	X
35.	The Pediatric Client		X	X
36.	Medication and the Client Population		X	X
37.	Healthy Lifestyle in the Primary Client Population		X	X
38.	Minor Surgery		X	X
39.	Medical Office Emergencies and First Aid		X	X
40.	Physician Office Laboratory		X	X
41.	Urinalysis		X	X
42.	Hematology and Venipuncture		X	X
43.	Cardiac Diagnostic Laboratory		X	X
44.	Blood Chemistry		X	X
45.	Radiological Diagnostic Laboratory		X	X

Medical Law & Ethics	Psychology of Human Relations	Pharmacology	Medical Office Business Procedures/ Management	Basic Keyboarding	Medical Office Clinical Procedures	Medical Laboratory Procedures	Career Development
X					X		
X					X		
X					X		
X					X		
X					X		
X					X		
X					X		
X					X		
X	X				X		X
X	X				X		
X	X				X		
X	X	X			X		
X	X				X		
X	X				X	X	
X	X				X		
X	X				X	X	X
X	X				X	X	
X	X				X	X	
X	X				X	X	
X	X				X	X	
X	X				X	X	

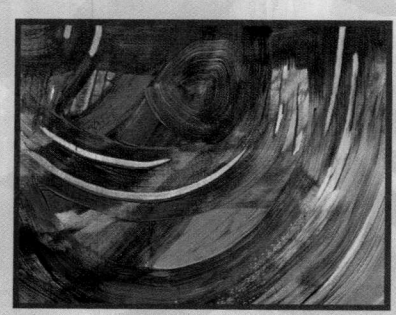

CAAHEP Curriculum

Chapter	Title	Anatomy & Physiology	Medical Terminology	Medical Law & Ethics
1.	The Medical Assisting Profession		X	X
2.	The Health Care Environment	X	X	X
3.	Infection Control	X	X	X
4.	Vital Signs	X	X	X
5.	Client Examination	X	X	X
6.	Organization of the Human Body	X	X	
7.	Integumentary System	X	X	
8.	Skeletal System	X	X	X
9.	Muscular System	X	X	X
10.	Nervous System and Sensory System	X	X	
11.	Endocrine System	X	X	X
12.	Cardiovascular System	X	X	
13.	Hematologic and Lymphatic Systems	X	X	X
14.	Immune System	X	X	
15.	Respiratory System	X	X	
16.	Digestive System	X	X	X
17.	Urinary System	X	X	
18.	Male Reproductive System	X	X	
19.	Female Reproductive System	X	X	X
20.	Integumentary System Disorders	X	X	X
21.	Skeletal System Disorders	X	X	X
22.	Muscular System Disorders	X	X	X
23.	Nervous System and Sensory System Disorders	X	X	X
24.	Endocrine System Disorders	X	X	X

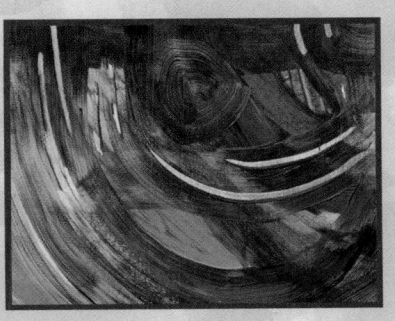

Psychology	Communication (oral and written)	Administrative Procedures	Clinical Procedures	Professional Components	Externship
X	X	X	X	X	X
X	X	X	X	X	X
X	X	X	X	X	X
X	X	X	X	X	X
X	X	X	X	X	X
X	X		X	X	
			X	X	
			X	X	
	X		X	X	
	X		X	X	
	X		X	X	
	X		X	X	
	X		X	X	
	X		X	X	
			X	X	
	X		X	X	
	X		X	X	
			X	X	
	X		X	X	
	X		X	X	
X	X		X	X	
	X		X	X	
	X		X	X	

Chapter	Title	Anatomy & Physiology	Medical Terminology	Medical Law & Ethics
25.	Cardiovascular System Disorders	X	X	X
26.	Hematologic and Lymphatic System Disorders	X	X	X
27.	Immune System Disorders	X	X	X
28.	Respiratory System Disorders	X	X	X
29.	Digestive System Disorders	X	X	X
30.	Urinary System Disorders	X	X	X
31.	Male Reproductive System Disorders	X	X	X
32.	Female Reproductive System Disorders	X	X	X
33.	The Client with Special Needs	X	X	X
34.	The Geriatric Client	X	X	X
35.	The Pediatric Client	X	X	X
36.	Medication and the Client Population	X	X	X
37.	Healthy Lifestyle in the Primary Client Population	X	X	X
38.	Minor Surgery	X	X	X
39.	Medical Office Emergencies and First Aid	X	X	X
40.	Physician Office Laboratory	X	X	X
41.	Urinalysis	X	X	X
42.	Hematology and Venipuncture	X	X	X
43.	Cardiac Diagnostic Laboratory	X	X	X
44.	Blood Chemistry	X	X	X
45.	Radiological Diagnostic Laboratory	X	X	X

Psychology	Communication (oral and written)	Administrative Procedures	Clinical Procedures	Professional Components	Externship
	X		X	X	
X	X		X	X	
X	X		X	X	
			X	X	
			X	X	
			X	X	
	X		X	X	
	X		X	X	
X	X		X	X	
X	X		X	X	
X	X		X	X	
X	X		X	X	
X	X		X	X	
X	X		X	X	
X	X	X	X	X	
X	X	X	X	X	
X	X	X	X	X	
X	X	X	X	X	
X	X	X	X	X	
X	X	X	X	X	
X	X	X	X	X	X

References

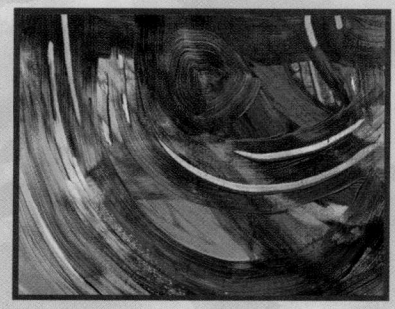

Daniels, R. (2003). *Delmar's Manual of Laboratory and Diagnostic Tests.* Clifton Park, NY: Thomson Delmar Learning.

Gersh, B. J. (Ed.). (2000). *Mayo Clinic: Heart book* (2nd ed.). New York: William Morrow.

Kier, L., Wise, B., Krebs, C. (2003). *Medical Assisting: Administrative and Clinical Competencies* (5th ed.). Clifton Park, NY: Thomson Delmar Learning.

Lindh, W. Q., Pooler, M. S., Tamparo, C. D., & Cerrato, J. U. (1998). *Delmar's Clinical Medical Assisting.* Clifton Park, NY: Thomson Delmar Learning.

Lindh, W. Q., Pooler, M. S., Tamparo, C. D., & Cerrato, J. U. (2002). *Delmar's Comprehensive Medical Assisting: Administrative and Clinical Competencies* (2nd ed.). Clifton Park, NY: Thomson Delmar Learning.

Lynch, J. M. (Ed.). *CMA Today 37* (2).

Neighbors, M. & Tannehill-Jones, R. (2000). *Human Diseases.* Clifton Park, NY: Thomson Delmar Learning.

Netter, F. H. (1997). *Atlas of Human Anatomy* (2nd ed.). East Hanover, NJ: Novartis.

Rizzo, D. C. (2001). *Delmar's Fundamentals of Anatomy & Physiology.* Clifton Park, NY: Thomson Delmar Learning.

Robb-Nicholson, C. (Ed.). (2004). *How to Release a Frozen Shoulder, Harvard Women's Health Watch 11* (8), 4-6.

Roe, Susan. (2003). *Clinical Nursing Skills and Concepts.* Clifton Park, NY: Thomson Delmar Learning.

Scott, A. S. & Fong, E. (2004). *Body Structures & Functions* (10th ed.). Clifton Park, NY: Thomson Delmar Learning.

Venes, D. (Ed.). (2001). *Taber's Cyclopedic Medical Dictionary* (19th ed.). Philadelphia, PA: F.A. Davis Company.

White, L. (2005). *Foundations of Adult Health Nursing* (2nd ed.). Clifton Park, NY: Thomson Delmar Learning.

White, L. (2005). *Foundations of Maternal and Pediatric Nursing* (2nd ed.). Clifton Park, NY: Thomson Delmar Learning.

White, L. (2005). *Foundations of Nursing* (2nd ed.). Clifton Park, NY: Thomson Delmar Learning.

American Association of Medical Assistants, http://www.aama-ntl.org/

Accrediting Bureau of Health Education Schools, http://www.abhes.org/

Occupational Safety & Health Administration, http://www.osha.gov/

Americans with Disabilities Act, http://www.usdoj.gov/crt/ada/adahom1.htm

American Academy of Allergy Asthma & Immunology, http://www.aaaai.org/

Arthritis Foundation, http://www.arthritis.org/

American Cancer Society, http://www.cancer.org/docroot/home/index.asp

National Lymphedema Network, http://www.lymphnet.org/

National Osteoporosis Foundation, http://www.nof.org/

Mayo Clinic, http://www.mayoclinic.org/

Clinical Laboratory Improvement Amendments, http://www.fda.gov/cdrh/clia/

Centers for Disease Control and Prevention, http://www.cdc.gov/

American Heart Association, http://www.americanheart.org/

American Red Cross, http://www.redcross.org/

Clinical and Laboratory Standards Institute, http://www.clsi.org/

Harvard Women's Health Watch, http://www.health.harvard.edu/women

Index

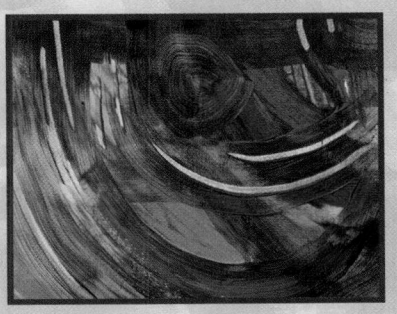